Guide to U.S.
HMOs & PPOs

2019

Thirty-first Edition

Guide to U.S. HMOs & PPOs

Detailed Profiles of U.S. Managed Healthcare
Organizations & Key Decision Makers

A SEDGWICK PRESS Book

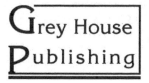

Grey House
Publishing

PRESIDENT: Richard Gottlieb
PUBLISHER: Leslie Mackenzie
EDITORIAL DIRECTOR: Laura Mars
PRODUCTION MANAGER: Kristen Hayes
EDITORIAL ASSISTANT: Olivia Parsonson
COMPOSITION: David Garoogian
MARKETING DIRECTOR: Jessica Moody

A Sedgwick Press Book
Grey House Publishing, Inc.
4919 Route 22
Amenia, NY 12501
518.789.8700   FAX 845.373.6390
www.greyhouse.com
e-mail: books@greyhouse.com

First edition published 1987
Thirty-first edition published 2019
Printed in Canada

Publisher's Cataloging-In-Publication Data
(Prepared by The Donohue Group, Inc.)

Names: Grey House Publishing, Inc., publisher.
Title: Guide to U.S. HMOs & PPOs.
Other Titles: HMOs & PPOs | Guide to U.S. HMOs and PPOs | Guide to United States health maintenance organizations & preferred provider organizations
Description: Amenia, NY : Grey House Publishing, 2018- | "Detailed profiles of U.S. managed healthcare organizations & key decision makers." | "A Sedgwick Press Book." | Includes bibliographical references and indexes.
Subjects: LCSH: Health maintenance organizations--United States--Directories. | Preferred provider organizations (Medical care)--United States--Directories. | LCGFT: Directories.
Classification: LCC RA413.5.U5 H586 | DDC 362.1042580973--dc23

ISBN: 978-1-68217-779-2 Softcover

Table of Contents

Introduction

This 31st edition of *Guide to U.S. HMOs & PPOs* profiles 857 managed care organizations in the United States. Formerly called *HMO/PPO Directory*, it lists current, comprehensive information for HMO, PPO, POS, and Vision & Dental Plans. Comprehensive coverage—from state listings to consolidations in the health insurance industry—is the cornerstone of this new edition. All entries have been reviewed and updated. This edition includes 29 brand new entries.

In addition to detailed profiles of Managed Healthcare Organizations, this edition includes:
- A 29-page report from the Census Bureau, "Health Insurance Coverage in the United States: 2017" with charts, tables and maps;
- A full page chart showing population numbers without health insurance 2013-2016 by the top 25 populous metro areas, Boston being the most insured and Houston the least insured;
- State Statistics and Rankings section with state-by-state numbers of individuals covered by type of health plans, and state ranking by number of individuals enrolled in health plans.

Praise for previous editions of *Guide to U.S. HMOs & PPOs*:

> "...of a topic that has grown exponentially more complex each year, this well-organized resource tries its best to keep it simple...The detailed user guide and five indexes enhance navigation...Written for both the consumer and the researcher, this work is a vital resource for public, academic and medical libraries."

> "...Information is clear, consistently presented, and easily located, making the guide extremely user friendly. Of particular note is the valuable...health care reform time line...A practical addition to public and medical library collections."
>
> —*Library Journal*

Arrangement

Plan profiles are arranged alphabetically by state. The first page of each state chapter is a State Summary chart of Health Insurance Coverage Status and Type of Coverage by Age. This chart includes a number of categories, from "Covered by some type of health insurance" to "Not covered at any time during the year."

Directly following the State Summary, plan listings provide crucial contact information, including key executives, often with direct phones and e-mails where available, fax numbers, web sites and hundreds of e-mail addresses. Each profile provides a detailed summary of the plan, including the following:
- Type of Plan, including Specialty and Benefits
- Type of Coverage
- Type of Payment Plan
- Subscriber Information
- Financial History
- Average Compensation Information
- Employer References
- Current Member Enrollment
- Hospital Affiliations
- Number of Primary Care and Specialty Physicians
- Federal Qualification Status
- For Profit Status
- Specialty Managed Care Partners
- Regional Business Coalitions
- Employer References
- Peer Review Information
- Accreditation Information

Additional Features

In addition to the detailed front matter, state statistics, and comprehensive plan profiles, *Guide to U.S. HMOs & PPOs* includes two Appendices and five Indexes.

- Appendix A: Glossary of Health Insurance Terms—Includes more than 150 terms such as Aggregate Indemnity, Diagnostic Related Groups, Non-participating Provider, and Waiting Period.
- Appendix B: Industry Web Sites—Contains dozens of the most valuable health care web sites and a detailed description, from Alliance of Community Health Plans to National Society of Certified Healthcare Business Consultants.
- Plan Index: Alphabetical list of insurance plans by seven plan types: HMO; PPO; HMO/PPO; Dental; Vision; Medicare; and Multiple.
- Personnel Index: Alphabetical list of all executives listed, with their affiliated organization.
- Membership Enrollment Index: List of organizations by member enrollment.
- Primary Care Physician Index: List of organizations by their number of primary care physicians.
- Referral/Specialty Care Physician Index: List of organizations by their number of referral and specialty care physicians.

To broaden its availability, the *Guide to U.S. HMOs & PPOs* is also available for subscription online at http://gold.greyhouse.com. Subscribers can search by plan details, geographic area, number of members, personnel name, title and much more. Users can print out prospect sheets or download data into their own spreadsheet or database. This database is a must for anyone in need of immediate access to contacts in the US managed care marketplace. Plus, buyers of the print directory get a free 30-day trial of the online database. Call (800) 562-2139 x118 for more information.

User Guide

Descriptive listings in the *Guide to U.S. HMOs & PPOs* are organized by state, then alphabetically by health plan. Each numbered item is described in the User Key on the following pages. Terms are defined in the Glossary.

---

1. → **U Healthcare**
2. → **3000 Riverside Road**
   Sharon, CT 06069
3. → **Toll Free: 060-364-0000**
4. → **Phone: 060-364-0001**
5. → **Fax: 060-364-0002**
6. → Info@uhealth.com
7. → www.uhealth.com
8. → Mailing Address: PO Box 729 Sharon, CT 06069-0729
9. → Subsidiary of: USA Healthcare
10. → For Profit: Yes
11. → Year Founded: 1992
12. → Physician Owned: No
13. → Owned by an IDN: No
14. → Federally Qualified: Yes 08/01/82
15. → Number of Affiliated Hospitals: 2,649
16. → Number of Primary Physicians: 4,892
17. → Number of Referral/Specialty Physicians: 6,246
18. → Current Member Enrollment: 204,000 (as of 7/1/01)
19. → State Member Enrollment: 29,000

Healthplan and Services Defined

20. → Plan Type: HMO
21. → Model Type: Staff, IPA, Group, Network
22. → Plan Specialty: ASO, Chiropractic, Dental, Disease Management, Lab, Vision, Radiology
23. → Benefits Offered: Chiropractic, Dental, Disease Management, Vision, Wellness
24. → Offers a Demand Management Patient Information Service: Yes
    DMPI Services Offered: Vision Works, Medical Imaging Institute

25. → **Type of Coverage**
    Commercial, Medicare, Supplemental Medicare, Medicaid
    Catastrophic Illness Benefit: Varies by case

26. → **Type of Payment Plans Offered**
    POS, Capitated, FFS, Combination FFS & DFFS

27. → **Geographic Areas Served**
    Connecticut, Maryland, New Jersey, Vermont, New York

Subscriber Information

28. → Average Monthly Fee Per Subscriber (Employee & Employer Contribution):
    Employee Only (Self): $8.00
    Employee & 1 Family Member: $10.00
    Employee & 2 Family Members: $15.00
    Medicare: $ 10.00
29. → Average Annual Deductible Per Subscriber:
    Employee Only (Self): $200.00

Employee & 1 Family Member: $250.00
Employee & 2 Family Members: $500.00
Medicare: $200.00
30.➤ Average Subscriber Co-Payment:
Primary Care Physician: $8.00
Non-Network Physician: $10.00
Prescription Drugs: $5.00
Hospital ER: $50.00
Home Health Care: $25.00
Home Health Care Max Days Covered/Visits: 30 days
Nursing Home: $5.00
Nursing Home Max Days/Visits Covered: 365 days

31.➤ **Network Qualifications**
Minimum Years of Practice: 10
Pre-Admission Certification: Yes

32.➤ **Peer Review Type**
Utilization Review: Yes
Second Surgical Opinion: No
Case Management: Yes

33.➤ **Accreditation Certification**
JCAHO, AAHC (formerly URAC), NCQA
Publishes and Distributes a Report Card: Yes

34.➤ **Key Personnel**
CFO...........................David Williams
Marketing.....................Clarence J. Fist
Medical Affairs..............Samantha Johnson, MD
Provider Services............Laura Falk

Average Claim Compensation
35.➤ Physician's Fee's Charged: 22%
36.➤ Hospital's Fee Charged: 34%

37.➤ **Specialty Managed Care Partners**
AMBI, Pharmaceutical Treatment, OxiTherapy

38.➤ **Enters into Contracts with Regional Business Coalitions: Yes**
New York Healthcare

39.➤ **Employer References**
Life Science Corporation

User Key

1. ➤ **Health Plan:** Formal name of health plan
2. ➤ **Address:** Physical location
3. ➤ **Toll Free:** Toll free number
4. ➤ **Phone:** Main number of organization
5. ➤ **Fax:** Fax number
6. ➤ **E-mail:** Main e-mail address of health plan, if provided
7. ➤ **Website:** Main website address of health plan, if provided
8. ➤ **Mailing Address:** If different from physical address, above.
9. ➤ **Subsidiary of:** Corporation the health plan is legally affiliated with
10. ➤ **For Profit:** Indicates if the organization was formed to make a financial profit. Non-profit organizations can make a profit, but the profits must be used to benefit the organization or purpose the corporation was created to help
11. ➤ **Year Founded:** The year the organization was recognized as a legal entity
12. ➤ **Physician Owned:** Notes if the organization is owned by a group of physicians who are recognized as a legal entity
13. ➤ **Owned by an IDN:** Notes if the organization is owned by an Integrated Delivery Network
14. ➤ **Federally Qualified:** Shows if and when the plan received federally qualified status
15. ➤ **Number of Affiliated Hospitals:** In-network hospitals contracted with the health plans
16. ➤ **Number of Primary Physicians:** In-network primary physicians contracted with the health plan
17. ➤ **Number of Referral/Specialty Physicians:** In-network referral/specialty physicians contracted with the health plan
18. ➤ **Current Member Enrollment:** The number of health plan members or subscribers using health plan benefits, and date of last enrollment count
19. ➤ **State Member Enrollment:** The number of health plan members or subscribers using health plan benefits in that state, and date of last enrollment count
20. ➤ **Plan Type:** Identifies the health plan as an HMO, PPO, Other (neither an HMO or PPO) or Multiple (both an HMO and PPO, or an HMO and TPA or POS; see Glossary for definitions of terms). Note: If a plan is both an HMO and PPO with different product information, i.e. number of hospitals or physicians, the plan is listed as two separate entries
21. ➤ **Model Type:** Describes the relationship between the health plan and its physicians
22. ➤ **Plan Specialty:** Indicates specialized services provided by the plan
23. ➤ **Benefits Offered:** Indicates specialized benefits offered in addition to standard coverage for physician services, hospitalization, diagnostic testing, and prescription drugs
24. ➤ **Offers Demand Management Patient Information Services:** Notes if Triage and other services are offered to help plan members find the most appropriate type and level of care, and what those services are
25. ➤ **Type of Coverage:** Lines of business offered
26. ➤ **Type of Payment Plans Offered:** How the insuror pays its contracted providers
27. ➤ **Geographical Areas Served:** Geographical areas the health plan services
28. ➤ **Average Monthly Fee Per Subscriber:** Monthly premium due to the carrier for each member
29. ➤ **Annual Average Deductible Per Subscriber:** The deductible each member must meet before expenses can be reimbursed
30. ➤ **Average Subscriber Co-Payment:** The co-payment each member must pay at the time services are rendered
31. ➤ **Network Qualifications:** Qualifications a physician must meet to contract with the plan
32. ➤ **Peer Review Type:** The type of on-going peer review process used by the health plan

33. ➤**Accreditation Certification:** Specific certifications the health plan achieved after rigorous review of its policies, procedures, and clinical outcomes

34. ➤**Key Personnel:** Key Executives in the most frequently contacted departments within the plans, with phone and e-mails when provided

35. ➤**Physician's Fees Charged:** The percentage of physicians' billed charges that is actually paid out by the plan

36. ➤**Hospital's Fees Charged:** The percentage of hospitals' billed charges that is actually paid out by the plan

37. ➤**Specialty Managed Care Partners:** Specialty carve-out companies that are contracted with the health plan to offer a broader array of health services to members

38. ➤**Regional Business Coalitions:** Notes if physician or business entities have formed for the sole purpose of achieving economies of scale when purchasing supplies and services, and the names of those businesses

39. ➤**Employer References:** Large employers that have contracted with the health plan and are willing to serve as references for the health plan

Health Insurance Coverage in the United States: 2017

Current Population Reports

By Edward R. Berchick, Emily Hood, and Jessica C. Barnett
Issued September 2018
P60-264

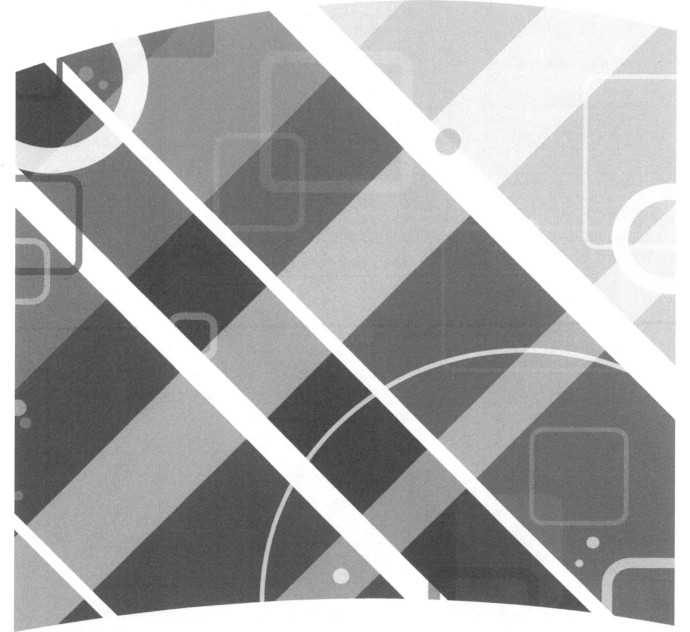

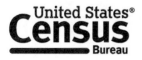

U.S. Department of Commerce
Economics and Statistics Administration
U.S. CENSUS BUREAU
census.gov

Health Insurance Coverage in the United States: 2017

Introduction

Health insurance is a means for financing a person's health care expenses. While the majority of people have private health insurance, primarily through an employer, many others obtain coverage through programs offered by the government. Other individuals do not have health insurance coverage at all (see the text box "What Is Health Insurance Coverage?").

Over time, changes in the rate of health insurance coverage and the distribution of coverage types may reflect economic trends, shifts in the demographic composition of the population, and policy changes that affect access to care. Several such policy changes occurred in 2014, when many provisions of the Patient Protection and Affordable Care Act went into effect (see the text box "Health Insurance Coverage and the Affordable Care Act").

This report presents statistics on health insurance coverage in the United States in 2017, changes in health insurance coverage rates between 2016 and 2017, as well as changes in health insurance coverage rates between 2013 and 2017.[1] The statistics in this report are based on information collected in two surveys conducted by the U.S. Census Bureau, the Current Population Survey Annual

[1] For a discussion of measuring change over time with the CPS ASEC, see Appendix B.

Social and Economic Supplement (CPS ASEC) and the American Community Survey (ACS) (see the text box "Two Measures of Health Insurance Coverage"). Throughout the report, unless otherwise noted, estimates come from the CPS ASEC.

Highlights

- In 2017, 8.8 percent of people, or 28.5 million, did not have health insurance at any point during the year. The uninsured rate and number of uninsured in 2017 were not statistically different from 2016 (8.8 percent or 28.1 million) (Figure 1 and Table 1).[2]

- The percentage of people with health insurance coverage for all or part of 2017 was 91.2 percent, not statistically different from the rate in 2016 (91.2 percent). Between 2016 and 2017, the number of people with health insurance coverage increased by 2.3 million, up to 294.6 million (Table 1).

- In 2017, private health insurance coverage continued to be more prevalent than government coverage, at 67.2 percent and 37.7 percent, respectively.[3] Of the sub-types of health insurance coverage, employer-based insurance was the most common, covering 56.0 percent of the population for some or all of the calendar year, followed by Medicaid (19.3 percent), Medicare (17.2 percent),

---

What Is Health Insurance Coverage?

Health insurance coverage in the Current Population Survey Annual Social and Economic Supplement (CPS ASEC) refers to comprehensive coverage during the calendar year.* For reporting purposes, the Census Bureau broadly classifies health insurance coverage as private insurance or government insurance. The CPS ASEC defines private health insurance as a plan provided through an employer or a union and coverage purchased directly by an individual from an insurance company or through an exchange. Government insurance coverage includes federal programs, such as Medicare, Medicaid, the Children's Health Insurance Program (CHIP), individual state health plans, TRICARE, CHAMPVA (Civilian Health and Medical Program of the Department of Veterans Affairs), as well as care provided by the Department of Veterans Affairs and the military. In the CPS ASEC, people were considered "insured" if they were covered by any type of health insurance for part or all of the previous calendar year. They were considered uninsured if, for the entire year, they were not covered by any type of health insurance. Additionally, people were considered uninsured if they only had coverage through the Indian Health Service (IHS), as IHS coverage is not considered comprehensive. For more information, see Appendix A, "Estimates of Health Insurance Coverage."

* Comprehensive health insurance covers basic healthcare needs. This definition excludes single service plans, such as accident, disability, dental, vision, or prescription medicine plans.

---

[2] For a discussion of the quality of the CPS ASEC health insurance coverage estimates, see Appendix B.
[3] Some people may have more than one coverage type during the calendar year.

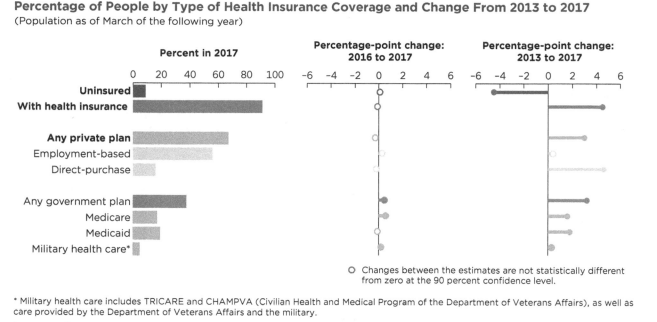

Figure 1.
Percentage of People by Type of Health Insurance Coverage and Change From 2013 to 2017
(Population as of March of the following year)

O   Changes between the estimates are not statistically different from zero at the 90 percent confidence level.

* Military health care includes TRICARE and CHAMPVA (Civilian Health and Medical Program of the Department of Veterans Affairs), as well as care provided by the Department of Veterans Affairs and the military.

Note: For information on confidentiality protection, sampling error, nonsampling error, and definitions in the Current Population Survey, see <www2.census.gov/programs-surveys/cps/techdocs/cpsmar18.pdf>.

Source: U.S. Census Bureau, Current Population Survey, 2014, 2017, and 2018 Annual Social and Economic Supplements.

direct-purchase coverage (16.0 percent), and military coverage (4.8 percent) (Table 1 and Figure 1).

- Between 2016 and 2017, the rate of Medicare coverage increased by 0.6 percentage points to cover 17.2 percent of people for part or all of 2017 (up from 16.7

percent in 2016) (Table 1 and Figure 1).[4, 5]

- The military coverage rate increased by 0.2 percentage points to 4.8 percent during this time. Coverage rates for employment-based coverage, direct-purchase coverage, and

Medicaid did not statistically change between 2016 and 2017.

- In 2017, the percentage of uninsured children under the age of 19 (5.4 percent) was not statistically different from the percentage in 2016 (Table 2).[6]

- For children under the age of 19 in poverty, the uninsured rate (7.8 percent) was higher than for children not in poverty (4.9 percent) (Figure 6).

---

[4] This increase was partly due to growth in the number of people aged 65 and over. The population 65 years and older did not have a statistically significant change in the Medicare coverage rate between 2016 and 2017. However, the percentage of the U.S. population 65 years and older increased between 2016 and 2017.

[5] Throughout this report, details may not sum to totals because of rounding.

---

[6] Throughout this report, the term "children" is used to refer to people under age 19, regardless of marital status or householder status.

- Between 2016 and 2017, the uninsured rate did not statistically change for any race or Hispanic origin group (Table 5).[7]

- In 2017, non-Hispanic Whites had the lowest uninsured rate among race and Hispanic-origin groups (6.3 percent). The uninsured rates

[7] Federal surveys give respondents the option of reporting more than one race. Therefore, two basic ways of defining a race group are possible. A group, such as Asian, may be defined as those who reported Asian and no other race (the race-alone or single-race concept) or as those who reported Asian, regardless of whether they also reported another race (the race-alone-or-in-combination concept). The body of this report (text, figures, and tables) shows data using the first approach (race alone). Use of the single-race population does not imply that it is the preferred method of presenting or analyzing data. The Census Bureau uses a variety of approaches.

In this report, the term "non-Hispanic White" refers to people who are not Hispanic and who reported White and no other race. The Census Bureau uses non-Hispanic Whites as the comparison group for other race groups and Hispanics.

Since Hispanics may be any race, data in this report for Hispanics overlap with data for race groups. Being Hispanic was reported by 15.4 percent of White householders who reported only one race, 4.8 percent of Black householders who reported only one race, and 2.2 percent of Asian householders who reported only one race.

Data users should exercise caution when interpreting aggregate results for the Hispanic population or for race groups because these populations consist of many distinct groups that differ in socioeconomic characteristics, culture, and nativity. For further information, see <www.census.gov/cps>.

for Blacks and Asians were 10.6 percent and 7.3 percent, respectively. Hispanics had the highest uninsured rate (16.1 percent) (Table 5).

- Between 2016 and 2017, the percentage of people without health insurance coverage at the time of interview decreased in three states and increased in 14 states (Table 6 and Figure 8).[8]

Estimates of Health Insurance Coverage

This report classifies health insurance coverage into three different groups: overall coverage, private coverage, and government coverage. Private coverage includes health insurance provided through an employer or union and coverage purchased directly by an individual from an insurance company or through an exchange.[9] Government coverage includes federal programs, such as Medicare, Medicaid, the

[8] Estimates are from the 2016 and 2017 American Community Survey, 1-year estimates. For more information, see the text box "Two Measures of Health Insurance Coverage."

[9] Exchanges include coverage purchased through the federal Health Insurance Marketplace, as well as other state-based marketplaces, and include both subsidized and unsubsidized plans.

Children's Health Insurance Program (CHIP), individual state health plans, TRICARE, CHAMPVA (Civilian Health and Medical Program of the Department of Veterans Affairs), as well as care provided by the Department of Veterans Affairs and the military. Individuals are considered to be uninsured if they did not have health insurance coverage at any point during the calendar year (see the text box "What Is Health Insurance Coverage?").

In 2017, most people (91.2 percent) had health insurance coverage at some point during the calendar year (Table 1 and Figure 1). More people had private health insurance (67.2 percent) than government coverage (37.7 percent).[10]

Employer-based insurance was the most common subtype of health insurance in the civilian, noninstitutionalized population (56.0 percent), followed by Medicaid (19.3 percent), Medicare (17.2 percent), direct-purchase insurance (16.0 percent), and military health care (4.8 percent) (Table 1).

[10] Some people may have more than one coverage type during the calendar year (see section on "Multiple Coverage Types").

Health Insurance Coverage and the Affordable Care Act

Since the passage of the Patient Protection and Affordable Care Act (ACA) in 2010, several of its provisions have gone into effect at different times. For example, in 2010, the Young Adult Provision enabled adults under the age of 26 to remain as dependents on their parents' health insurance plans. Many more of the main provisions went into effect on January 1, 2014, including the expansion of Medicaid eligibility and the establishment of health insurance marketplaces (e.g., healthcare.gov).

In 2014, people under the age of 65, particularly adults aged 19 to 64, may have become eligible for coverage options under the ACA. Based on family income, some people may have qualified for subsidies or tax credits to help pay for premiums associated with health insurance plans. In addition, the population with lower income may have become eligible for Medicaid coverage if they resided in one of the 31 states (or the District of Columbia) that expanded Medicaid eligibility on or before January 1, 2017. Twenty-four states and the District of Columbia expanded Medicaid eligibility by January 1, 2014. Between then and January 1, 2015, three additional states—Michigan, New Hampshire, and Pennsylvania—had expanded Medicaid eligibility. By January 1, 2016, three more states—Alaska, Indiana, and Montana—expanded Medicaid eligibility. One more state—Louisiana—expanded Medicaid eligibility by January 1, 2017.*

* For a list of the states and their Medicaid expansion status as of January 1, 2017, see Table 6: Percentage of People Without Health Insurance Coverage by State: 2013, 2016, and 2017.

Table 1.

Coverage Numbers and Rates by Type of Health Insurance: 2013, 2016, and 2017

(Numbers in thousands, margins of error in thousands or percentage points as appropriate. Population as of March of the following year. For information on confidentiality protection, sampling error, nonsampling error, and definitions, see *www.2.census.gov /programs-surveys/cps/techdocs/cpsmar18.pdf*)

Coverage type	2013				2016				2017				Change in number		Change in rate	
	Number	Margin of error[1] (±)	Rate	Margin of error[1] (±)	Number	Margin of error[1] (±)	Rate	Margin of error[1] (±)	Number	Margin of error[1] (±)	Rate	Margin of error[1] (±)	2017 less 2016	2017 less 2013	2017 less 2016	2017 less 2013
Total.................	313,401	109	X	X	320,372	96	X	X	323,156	123	X	X	X	X	X	X
Any health plan......	271,606	636	86.7	0.2	292,320	541	91.2	0.2	294,613	662	91.2	0.2	*2,293	*23,007	-0.1	*4.5
Any private plan[2,3].....	201,038	1,140	64.1	0.4	216,203	1,145	67.5	0.4	217,007	1,158	67.2	0.4	804	*15,969	-0.3	*3.0
Employment-based[2].....	174,418	1,160	55.7	0.4	178,455	1,130	55.7	0.4	181,036	1,241	56.0	0.4	*2,582	*6,618	0.3	0.4
Direct-purchase[2]........	35,755	615	11.4	0.2	51,961	874	16.2	0.3	51,821	1,008	16.0	0.3	-140	*16,066	-0.2	*4.6
Any government plan[2,4]......	108,287	1,115	34.6	0.4	119,361	1,018	37.3	0.3	121,965	1,086	37.7	0.3	*2,604	*13,678	*0.5	*3.2
Medicare[2].............	49,020	377	15.6	0.1	53,372	396	16.7	0.1	55,623	351	17.2	0.1	*2,251	*6,603	*0.6	*1.6
Medicaid[2].............	54,919	969	17.5	0.3	62,303	931	19.4	0.3	62,492	1,007	19.3	0.3	188	*7,573	-0.1	*1.8
Military health care[2,5].....	14,016	595	4.5	0.2	14,638	575	4.6	0.2	15,532	769	4.8	0.2	*893	*1,516	*0.2	*0.3
Uninsured[6]...........	41,795	614	13.3	0.2	28,052	519	8.8	0.2	28,543	634	8.8	0.2	492	*-13,252	0.1	*-4.5

X Not applicable.

* Changes between the estimates are statistically different from zero at the 90 percent confidence level.

[1] A margin of error (MOE) is a measure of an estimate's variability. The larger the MOE in relation to the size of the estimate, the less reliable the estimate. This number, when added to and subtracted from the estimate, forms the 90 percent confidence interval. MOEs shown in this table are based on standard errors calculated using replicate weights. For more information, see "Standard Errors and Their Use" at <www.2.census.gov/library/publications/2018/demo/p60-264sa.pdf>.

[2] The estimates by type of coverage are not mutually exclusive; people can be covered by more than one type of health insurance during the year.

[3] Private health insurance includes coverage provided through an employer or union, coverage purchased directly by an individual from an insurance company, or coverage through someone outside the household.

[4] Government health insurance coverage includes Medicaid, Medicare, TRICARE, CHAMPVA (Civilian Health and Medical Program of the Department of Veterans Affairs), as well as care provided by the Department of Veterans Affairs and the military.

[5] Military health care includes TRICARE and CHAMPVA (Civilian Health and Medical Program of the Department of Veterans Affairs), as well as care provided by the Department of Veterans Affairs and the military.

[6] Individuals are considered to be uninsured if they do not have health insurance coverage for the entire calendar year.

Source: U.S. Census Bureau, Current Population Survey, 2014, 2017, and 2018 Annual Social and Economic Supplements.

Two Measures of Health Insurance Coverage

This report includes two types of health insurance coverage measures: health insurance coverage during the previous calendar year and health insurance coverage at the time of the interview.

The first measure, health insurance coverage at any time during the previous calendar year, is collected with the Current Population Survey Annual Social and Economic Supplement (CPS ASEC). The CPS is the longest-running survey conducted by the U.S. Census Bureau. The key purpose of the CPS ASEC is to provide timely and detailed estimates of economic well-being, of which health insurance coverage is an important part. The Census Bureau conducts the CPS ASEC annually between February and April, and the resulting measure of health insurance coverage reflects an individual's coverage status during the previous calendar year.

The second measure, health insurance coverage at the time of the interview, is collected with the American Community Survey (ACS). The ACS is an ongoing survey that collects comprehensive information on social, economic, and housing topics. Due to its large sample size, the ACS provides estimates at many levels of geography and for smaller population groups. The Census Bureau conducts the ACS throughout the year, and the resulting measure of health coverage reflects an annual average of current health insurance coverage status.

As a result of the difference in the collection of health insurance coverage status, the resulting uninsured rates measure different concepts. The CPS ASEC uninsured rate represents the percentage of people who had no health insurance coverage at any time during the previous calendar year. The ACS uninsured rate is a measure of the percentage of people who were uninsured at the time of the interview.

As measured by the CPS ASEC, the uninsured rate was essentially unchanged between 2016 and 2017, at 8.8 percent. As measured by the ACS, the uninsured rate increased by 0.2 percentage points from 8.6 percent in 2016 to 8.7 percent in 2017 (Figure 2).

Over a longer period, as measured by the ACS, uninsured rates remained relatively stable between 2008 and 2013, but decreased sharply by 2.8 percentage points between 2013 and 2014. Uninsured rates then decreased by 2.3 percentage points between 2014 and 2015 and 0.8 percentage points between 2015 and 2016. Between 2016 and 2017, the uninsured rate increased by 0.2 percentage points.

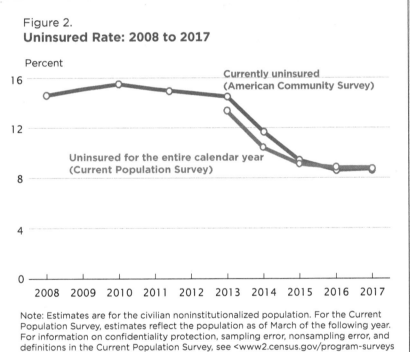

Figure 2.
Uninsured Rate: 2008 to 2017

Note: Estimates are for the civilian noninstitutionalized population. For the Current Population Survey, estimates reflect the population as of March of the following year. For information on confidentiality protection, sampling error, nonsampling error, and definitions in the Current Population Survey, see <www2.census.gov/program-surveys/cps/techdocs/cpsmar18.pdf>. For the American Community Survey, estimates reflect the population as of July of the calendar year. For information on confidentiality protection, sampling error, nonsampling error, and definitions in the American Community Survey, see <www2.census.gov/programs-surveys/acs/tech_docs/accuracy/ACS_Accuracy_of_Data_2017.pdf>.

Source: U.S. Census Bureau, Current Population Survey, 2014 to 2018 Annual Social and Economic Supplements and 2008 to 2017 American Community Survey, 1-Year Estimates.

The percentage of people covered by any type of health insurance in 2017 was not statistically different from the percentage in 2016. The percentage of people covered by private health insurance or either of the two subtypes of private health insurance (employment-based and direct-purchase) also did not statistically change between 2016 and 2017.

Between 2016 and 2017, the percentage of people with government health insurance increased by 0.5 percentage points, to 37.7 percent in 2017 (Table 1).[11] Of the three subtypes of government health insurance, both military health care and Medicare coverage rates increased between 2016 and 2017. The percentage of people covered by military health care increased by 0.2 percentage points to 4.8 percent in 2017. The rate of Medicare coverage increased by

0.6 percentage points to 17.2 percent in 2017. This increase was partly due to growth in the number of people aged 65 and over.

Multiple Coverage Types

While most people have a single type of insurance, some people may have more than one type of coverage during the calendar year. They may have multiple types of coverage at one time to supplement their primary insurance type, or they may switch coverage types over the course of the year. Of the population with health insurance coverage in 2017, 77.8 percent had one coverage type during the year and 22.2 percent had multiple coverage types over the course of the year (Figure 3).

Some types of health insurance were more likely to be held alone, while other types of health insurance coverage were more likely to be held in combination with another type of insurance at some point during the

year. Most people with employer-based health insurance coverage or Medicaid coverage did not have more than one plan type. In 2017, only 22.4 percent of people with employer-sponsored coverage and 35.0 percent with Medicaid had multiple types of coverage.

In 2017, the majority of people covered by direct-purchase, Medicare, or military health care had some other type of health insurance during the year (61.2 percent, 60.2 percent, and 62.2 percent, respectively).[12]

---

[11] All comparative statements in this report have undergone statistical testing, and unless otherwise noted, all comparisons are statistically significant at the 10 percent level.

---

[12] The percentage of people with direct-purchase coverage and another type of health insurance was not statistically different from the percentage of people with Medicare and another type of health insurance, or the percentage of people with military health care and another type of health insurance. The percentage of people with Medicare and another type of health insurance was not statistically different from the percentage of people with military health care and another type of health insurance.

Figure 3.
Percentage With One or Multiple Coverage Types: 2017
(Population as of March of the following year)

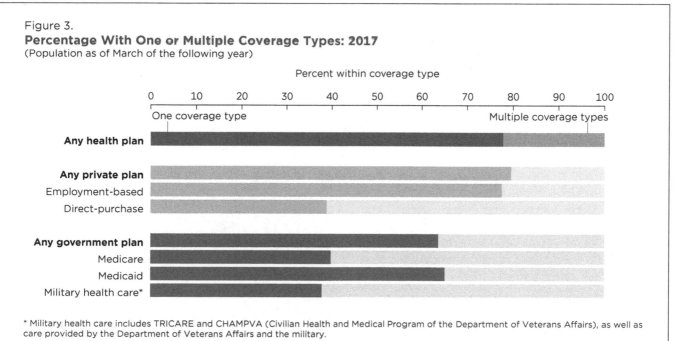

* Military health care includes TRICARE and CHAMPVA (Civilian Health and Medical Program of the Department of Veterans Affairs), as well as care provided by the Department of Veterans Affairs and the military.

Note: For information on confidentiality protection, sampling error, nonsampling error, and definitions in the Current Population Survey, see <www2.census.gov/programs-surveys/cps/techdocs/cpsmar18.pdf>.

Source: U.S. Census Bureau, Current Population Survey, 2018 Annual Social and Economic Supplement.

Table 2.

Percentage of People by Type of Health Insurance Coverage by Age: 2016 and 2017

(Numbers in thousands, margins of error in percentage points. Population as of March of the following year. For information on confidentiality protection, sampling error, nonsampling error, and definitions, see *www.2.census.gov/programs-surveys/cps/techdocs/cpsmar18.pdf*)

Characteristic	Total		Any health insurance					Private health insurance[3]					Government health insurance[4]					Uninsured[5]				
	2016 Number	2017 Number	2016 Percent	2016 Margin of error[2] (±)	2017 Percent	2017 Margin of error[2] (±)	Change (2017 less 2016)[1]*	2016 Percent	2016 Margin of error[2] (±)	2017 Percent	2017 Margin of error[2] (±)	Change (2017 less 2016)[1]*	2016 Percent	2016 Margin of error[2] (±)	2017 Percent	2017 Margin of error[2] (±)	Change (2017 less 2016)[1]*	2016 Percent	2016 Margin of error[2] (±)	2017 Percent	2017 Margin of error[2] (±)	Change (2017 less 2016)[1]*
Total	320,372	323,156	91.2	0.2	91.2	0.2	-0.1	67.5	0.4	67.2	0.4	-0.3	37.3	0.3	37.7	0.3	*0.5	8.8	0.2	8.8	0.2	0.1
Age																						
Under the age of 65 ...	271,098	272,076	89.9	0.2	89.8	0.2	-0.1	70.2	0.4	70.2	0.4	Z	27.0	0.4	27.2	0.4	0.2	10.1	0.2	10.2	0.2	0.1
Under the age of 18	74,047	73,963	94.7	0.3	94.7	0.3	Z	62.7	0.6	63.0	0.6	0.3	41.9	0.6	42.3	0.7	0.4	5.3	0.3	5.3	0.3	Z
Aged 18 to 64	197,051	198,113	88.1	0.2	87.9	0.3	-0.1	73.0	0.4	72.8	0.4	-0.1	21.4	0.3	21.6	0.4	0.2	11.9	0.2	12.1	0.3	0.1
Under the age of 19[6]	78,150	78,106	94.6	0.3	94.6	0.3	Z	62.9	0.6	63.3	0.6	0.3	41.5	0.6	41.9	0.7	0.4	5.4	0.3	5.4	0.3	Z
Aged 19 to 64	192,948	193,971	87.9	0.2	87.8	0.3	-0.1	73.1	0.4	72.9	0.4	-0.2	21.1	0.3	21.3	0.4	0.2	12.1	0.2	12.2	0.3	0.1
Aged 19 to 25[7]	29,815	29,922	86.9	0.6	86.0	0.7	*-0.9	71.3	0.8	70.2	0.9	-1.1	23.1	0.8	23.4	0.8	0.2	13.1	0.6	14.0	0.7	*0.9
Aged 26 to 34	39,736	40,152	84.3	0.6	84.4	0.6	0.1	69.7	0.7	69.9	0.8	0.2	20.4	0.6	20.3	0.7	-0.1	15.7	0.6	15.6	0.6	-0.1
Aged 35 to 44	40,046	40,659	86.9	0.5	86.7	0.5	-0.2	73.3	0.7	73.6	0.7	0.2	19.3	0.6	19.2	0.6	-0.1	13.1	0.5	13.3	0.5	0.2
Aged 45 to 64	83,351	83,237	90.6	0.3	90.7	0.3	0.1	75.2	0.5	75.1	0.5	-0.1	21.7	0.5	22.1	0.5	0.4	9.4	0.3	9.3	0.3	-0.1
Aged 65 and older	49,274	51,080	98.8	0.1	98.7	0.1	-0.1	52.8	0.8	51.1	0.8	*-1.6	93.6	0.3	93.7	0.3	0.1	1.2	0.1	1.3	0.1	0.1

* Changes between the estimates are statistically different from zero at the 90 percent confidence level.

Z Represents or rounds to zero.

[1] Details may not sum to totals because of rounding.

[2] A margin of error (MOE) is a measure of an estimate's variability. The larger the MOE in relation to the size of the estimate, the less reliable the estimate. This number, when added to and subtracted from the estimate, forms the 90 percent confidence interval. MOEs shown in this table are based on standard errors calculated using replicate weights. For more information, see "Standard Errors and Their Use" at <www.2.census.gov/library/publications/2018/demo/p60-264sa.pdf>.

[3] Private health insurance includes coverage provided through an employer or union, coverage purchased directly by an individual from an insurance company, or coverage through someone outside the household.

[4] Government health insurance coverage includes Medicaid, Medicare, TRICARE, CHAMPVA (Civilian Health and Medical Program of the Department of Veterans Affairs), as well as care provided by the Department of Veterans Affairs and the military.

[5] Individuals are considered to be uninsured if they do not have health insurance coverage for the entire calendar year.

[6] Children under the age of 19 are eligible for Medicaid/CHIP.

[7] This age is of special interest because of the Affordable Care Act's dependent coverage provision. Individuals aged 19 to 25 years may be eligible to be a dependent on a parent's health insurance plan.

Note: The estimates by type of coverage are not mutually exclusive; people can be covered by more than one type of health insurance during the year.

Source: U.S. Census Bureau, Current Population Survey, 2017 and 2018 Annual Social and Economic Supplements.

Health Insurance Coverage by Selected Characteristics

Age

Age is strongly associated with the likelihood that a person has health insurance and the type of health insurance a person has. In 2017, adults aged 65 and over and children under 19 were more likely to have had health insurance coverage (98.7 percent and 94.6 percent, respectively) compared with adults aged 19 to 64 (87.8 percent) (Table 2).

Adults aged 65 and over had the highest rate of health insurance coverage in 2017 (98.7 percent), with 93.7 percent covered by a government plan (primarily Medicare) and 51.1 percent covered by a private plan, which may have supplemented their government coverage.

Between 2016 and 2017, the rate of private coverage for adults aged 65 and over decreased by 1.6 percentage points from 52.8 percent in 2016. The rates of overall health insurance coverage and government coverage did not statistically change between 2016 and 2017 for this age group.

In 2017, children under the age of 19 were more likely to be covered by health insurance than adults aged 19 to 64 (94.6 percent and 87.8 percent, respectively). One reason for this difference could be that children from lower income families may be eligible for programs such as Medicaid or the Children's Health Insurance Program (CHIP).

In 2017, 63.3 percent of children under the age of 19 had private health insurance and 41.9 percent had government coverage. Some children were covered by both private and government coverage during the calendar year. Between 2016 and 2017, there was no statistical change in the rates of overall health insurance coverage, private coverage, or

government coverage for this age group.[13]

Working-age adults (people aged 19 to 64) had a lower rate of health insurance coverage in 2017 (87.8 percent) than both children and older adults.

Among working-age adults, the population aged 26 to 34 was the least likely to be insured, with a coverage rate of 84.4 percent. A higher percentage of adults aged 19 to 25 were insured (86.0 percent) than adults 26 to 34. For age groups between 26 and 64, the rate of health insurance coverage increased as age increased.[14]

Working-age adults were more likely than other age groups to be covered by private health insurance, with 72.9 percent of the population aged 19 to 64 having private insurance coverage in 2017. They also had a lower rate of government coverage than children under the age of 19 and adults aged 65 and over, at 21.3 percent.

Between 2016 and 2017, the percentage of adults aged 19 to 25 with any health insurance decreased by 0.9 percentage points to 86.0 percent. No other age group experienced a statistically significant change in their health insurance coverage rate during this time.

The ACS, which has a larger sample size than the CPS ASEC, provides an estimate of health insurance coverage at the time of the interview. The larger sample size offers an opportunity to look at coverage rates for

smaller groups, such as single years of age (Figure 4).[15]

Examining age across childhood and young adulthood, uninsured rates in 2017 were generally lower for children than for young adults, from 3.5 percent for infants to 17.8 percent for 26-year-olds. Two sharp differences existed between single-year ages. The percentage of 19-year-olds without coverage (13.2 percent) was 4.6 percentage points higher than the percentage for people 1 year younger. Likewise, the uninsured rate for 26-year-olds, the highest among all single years of age in 2017, was distinctly higher than for 25-year-olds (17.8 percent and 14.9 percent, respectively).

From ages 26 to 64, the uninsured rate generally declined with age. Between the ages of 64 and 65, the uninsured rate then decreased 4.9 percentage points. In 2017, 6.6 percent of 64-year-olds and 1.6 percent of 65-year-olds did not have health insurance coverage. For adults aged 65 and over, the uninsured rate varied little by age.

Between 2016 and 2017, the percentage of people without health insurance coverage at the time of interview did not statistically change for most single years of age. However, for children under the age of 19 and working-age adults between 50 and 59, the uninsured rate increased across multiple single years of age.

Between 2013 and 2017, uninsured rates fell for all single-year ages under the age of 65, with the largest declines of about 12.0 percentage points for each age between 21 and 28. An uneven downward shift in

---

[13] The Children's Health Insurance Program (CHIP) is a government program that provides health insurance to children in families with income too high to qualify for Medicaid, but who are unable to afford private health insurance.

[14] In 2017, the health insurance coverage rate for people aged 19 to 25 was not statistically different from the coverage rate for people aged 35 to 44.

[15] These estimates and estimates in the remainder of this section come from the 2013, 2016, and 2017 American Community Survey, 1-year estimates. In the ACS, health insurance coverage status corresponds to coverage at the time of the interview (see the text box "Two Measures of Health Insurance Coverage").

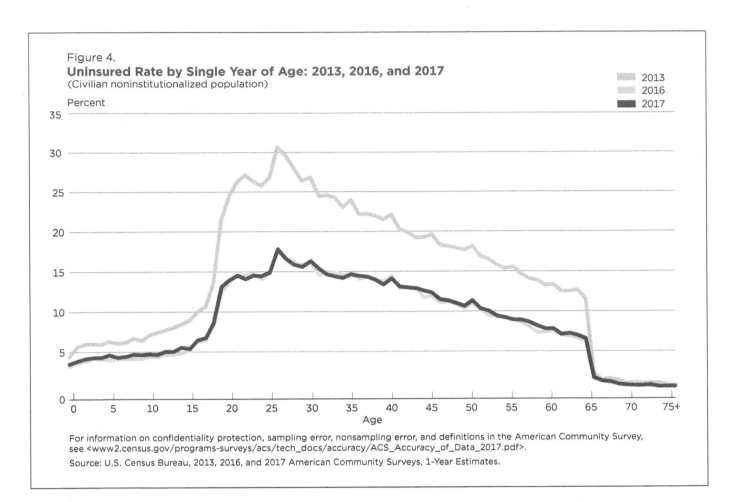

Figure 4.
Uninsured Rate by Single Year of Age: 2013, 2016, and 2017
(Civilian noninstitutionalized population)

For information on confidentiality protection, sampling error, nonsampling error, and definitions in the American Community Survey, see <www2.census.gov/programs-surveys/acs/tech_docs/accuracy/ACS_Accuracy_of_Data_2017.pdf>.

Source: U.S. Census Bureau, 2013, 2016, and 2017 American Community Surveys, 1-Year Estimates.

uninsured rates reduced some of the age-specific disparities. However, in 2017, three notable sharp differences remained between single-year ages, specifically between 18- and 19-year-olds, between 25- and 26-year-olds, and between 64- and 65-year-olds.

Marital Status

Many adults obtain health insurance coverage through their spouse. In 2017, married adults aged 19 to 64 had the highest coverage rate, at 90.9 percent (Table 3).[16] The coverage rate was lowest for people who were separated (79.7 percent). Of people who were never married, 84.0 percent were covered by health insurance. The coverage rates for people who were widowed or divorced were 86.6 percent and 86.4 percent, respectively.[17]

Between 2016 and 2017, none of the marital status groups had a statistically significant change in their rate of overall coverage.

Disability Status

Adults with a disability had a higher rate of health insurance coverage (91.2 percent) than adults with no disability (87.5 percent) in 2017 (Table 3).[18]

Adults with a disability were less likely than adults with no disability

to have private health insurance coverage and more likely to have government coverage. In 2017, 44.8 percent of adults with a disability had private coverage, compared with 75.5 percent of adults with no disability, a 30.7 percentage-point difference. At the same time, 57.8 percent of adults with a disability and 17.8 percent with no disability had government coverage, a 39.9 percentage-point difference.

Between 2016 and 2017, neither the population with a disability nor the population with no disability had statistically significant changes in their rates of overall coverage, private coverage, or government coverage.

---

[16] All estimates by marital status are for the population aged 19 to 64.

[17] In 2017, the coverage rate of people who were widowed was not statistically different from the coverage rate of people who were divorced.

[18] All estimates by disability status are for the population aged 19 to 64.

Table 3.

Percentage of People by Type of Health Insurance Coverage for Working-Age Adults Aged 19 to 64: 2016 and 2017

(Numbers in thousands, margins of error in percentage points. Population as of March of the following year. For information on confidentiality protection, sampling error, nonsampling error, and definitions, see www2.census.gov/programs-surveys/cps/techdocs/cpsmar18.pdf)

Characteristic	Number 2016	Number 2017	Any health insurance 2016 Per-cent	MOE[2] ±	2017 Per-cent	MOE[2] ±	Change (2017 less 2016)[1],*	Private health insurance[3] 2016 Per-cent	MOE[2] ±	2017 Per-cent	MOE[2] ±	Change (2017 less 2016)[1],*	Government health insurance[4] 2016 Per-cent	MOE[2] ±	2017 Per-cent	MOE[2] ±	Change (2017 less 2016)[1],*	Uninsured[5] 2016 Per-cent	MOE[2] ±	2017 Per-cent	MOE[2] ±	Change (2017 less 2016)[1],*
Total	**320,372**	**323,156**	**91.2**	**0.2**	**91.2**	**0.2**	**-0.1**	**67.5**	**0.4**	**67.2**	**0.4**	**-0.3**	**37.3**	**0.3**	**37.7**	**0.3**	***0.5**	**8.8**	**0.2**	**8.8**	**0.2**	**0.1**
Total, 19 to 64 years old	192,948	193,971	87.9	0.2	87.8	0.3	-0.1	73.1	0.4	72.9	0.4	-0.2	21.1	0.3	21.3	0.4	0.2	12.1	0.2	12.2	0.3	0.1
Marital Status																						
Married[6]	101,822	101,580	91.2	0.3	90.9	0.3	-0.3	80.1	0.5	79.7	0.4	-0.4	17.9	0.4	18.3	0.4	0.4	8.8	0.3	9.1	0.3	0.3
Widowed	3,633	3,586	86.1	1.6	86.6	1.6	0.6	58.7	2.0	57.2	2.3	-1.4	33.5	2.2	36.0	2.2	2.4	13.9	1.6	13.4	1.6	-0.6
Divorced	19,460	19,510	86.1	0.6	86.4	0.7	0.3	64.3	1.0	65.4	1.0	1.1	26.8	0.9	26.3	0.9	-0.5	13.9	0.6	13.6	0.7	-0.3
Separated	4,495	4,372	80.8	1.5	79.7	1.7	-1.1	55.9	1.9	55.4	2.0	-0.5	31.0	1.8	29.9	1.8	-1.1	19.2	1.5	20.3	1.7	1.1
Never married	63,537	64,923	84.0	0.5	84.0	0.4	Z	66.5	0.7	66.6	0.6	0.1	23.2	0.6	23.1	0.5	-0.1	16.0	0.5	16.0	0.4	Z
Disability Status[7]																						
With a disability	15,248	14,957	91.2	0.7	91.2	0.7	Z	43.5	1.2	44.8	1.2	1.3	58.6	1.1	57.8	1.2	-0.8	8.8	0.7	8.8	0.7	Z
With no disability	176,842	178,063	87.6	0.2	87.5	0.3	-0.2	75.9	0.4	75.5	0.4	-0.3	17.5	0.3	17.8	0.3	0.3	12.4	0.2	12.5	0.3	0.2
Work Experience																						
All workers	149,105	150,487	88.8	0.3	88.7	0.3	-0.2	80.1	0.3	80.2	0.3	Z	13.9	0.3	14.0	0.3	0.1	11.2	0.3	11.3	0.3	0.2
Worked full-time, year-round	107,577	109,511	90.2	0.3	90.2	0.3	Z	84.5	0.3	84.4	0.4	-0.1	10.4	0.3	10.9	0.3	*0.5	9.8	0.3	9.8	0.3	Z
Worked less than full-time, year-round	41,528	40,976	85.2	0.5	84.6	0.6	-0.6	69.0	0.6	68.9	0.7	-0.1	23.1	0.6	22.4	0.6	-0.6	14.8	0.5	15.4	0.6	0.6
Did not work at least 1 week	43,843	43,484	85.0	0.5	84.9	0.5	-0.1	49.1	0.8	47.9	0.8	*-1.1	45.6	0.7	46.5	0.9	0.9	15.0	0.5	15.1	0.5	0.1
Educational Attainment																						
Total, 26 to 64 years old	163,133	164,049	88.1	0.2	88.1	0.3	Z	73.4	0.4	73.4	0.4	Z	20.8	0.3	20.9	0.4	0.2	11.9	0.2	11.9	0.3	Z
No high school diploma	15,389	15,150	72.7	1.1	73.7	1.1	1.0	40.9	1.1	42.4	1.2	1.5	37.7	1.1	37.5	1.2	-0.3	27.3	1.1	26.3	1.1	-1.0
High school graduate (includes equivalency)	45,401	44,772	84.8	0.5	84.5	0.5	-0.4	65.0	0.7	65.4	0.7	0.4	26.3	0.6	26.3	0.6	-0.1	15.2	0.5	15.5	0.5	0.4
Some college, no degree	26,594	26,109	88.4	0.5	88.0	0.5	-0.4	71.8	0.8	70.6	0.8	*-1.2	23.8	0.7	24.7	0.8	*0.9	11.6	0.5	12.0	0.5	0.4
Associate's degree	17,739	17,659	90.7	0.6	90.5	0.7	-0.2	77.9	0.9	77.2	0.9	-0.7	19.5	0.8	19.5	0.8	0.1	9.3	0.6	9.5	0.7	0.2
Bachelor's degree	36,528	38,465	93.2	0.4	92.8	0.4	-0.4	86.8	0.5	85.5	0.5	*-1.3	11.6	0.4	12.4	0.5	*0.8	6.8	0.4	7.2	0.4	0.4
Graduate or professional degree	21,482	21,894	95.2	0.4	95.8	0.4	*0.6	90.0	0.6	90.4	0.6	0.4	9.8	0.6	10.3	0.6	0.5	4.8	0.4	4.2	0.4	*-0.6

* Changes between the estimates are statistically different from zero at the 90 percent confidence level.

Z Represents or rounds to zero.

[1] Details may not sum to totals because of rounding.

[2] A margin of error (MOE) is a measure of an estimate's variability. The larger the MOE in relation to the size of the estimate, the less reliable the estimate. This number, when added to and subtracted from the estimate, forms the 90 percent confidence interval. MOEs shown in this table are based on standard errors calculated using replicate weights. For more information, see "Standard Errors and Their Use" at <www2.census.gov/library/publications/2018/demo/p60-264sa.pdf>.

[3] Private health insurance includes coverage provided through an employer or union, coverage purchased directly by an individual from an insurance company, or coverage through someone outside the household.

[4] Government health insurance coverage includes Medicaid, Medicare, TRICARE, CHAMPVA (Civilian Health and Medical Program of the Department of Veterans Affairs), as well as care provided by the Department of Veterans Affairs and the military.

[5] Individuals are considered to be uninsured if they do not have health insurance coverage for the entire calendar year.

[6] The combined category "married" includes three individual categories: "married, civilian spouse present," "married, armed forces spouse present," and "married, spouse absent."

[7] The sum of those with and without a disability does not equal the total because disability status is not defined for individuals in the armed forces.

Note: The estimates by type of coverage are not mutually exclusive; people can be covered by more than one type of health insurance during the year.

Source: U.S. Census Bureau, Current Population Survey, 2017 and 2018 Annual Social and Economic Supplements.

Work Experience

For many adults aged 19 to 64, health insurance coverage and type of coverage is related to work status, such as working full-time, year-round; working less than full-time, year-round; or not working at all during the calendar year.[19, 20]

In 2017, 88.7 percent of all workers had health insurance coverage. Full-time, year-round workers were more likely to be covered by health insurance (90.2 percent) than the population who worked less than full-time, year-round (84.6 percent) or non-workers (84.9 percent) (Table 3).[21]

Workers were more likely than non-workers to be covered by private health insurance coverage. In 2017, 84.4 percent of full-time, year-round workers had private insurance coverage, compared with 68.9 percent of people who worked less than full-time, year-round and 47.9 percent of nonworkers.

In 2017, nonworkers were more than three times as likely to have government coverage (46.5 percent) than workers (14.0 percent). Among all workers, 10.9 percent of people who worked full-time, year-round and 22.4 percent of people who worked less than full-time, year-round had government coverage in 2017.

Between 2016 and 2017, there was no statistical difference in the health insurance coverage rates for workers or nonworkers. During this time, there were also no statistical differences in coverage rates for the population who worked full-time, year-round or

for the population who worked less than full-time, year-round.

Educational Attainment

People with higher levels of educational attainment were more likely to have health insurance coverage than people with lower levels of education. In 2017, 95.8 percent of the population aged 26 to 64 with a graduate or professional degree had health insurance coverage, compared with 92.8 percent of the population with a bachelor's degree, 88.0 percent of the population with some college (no degree), 84.5 percent of high school graduates, and 73.7 percent of the population with no high school diploma (Table 3).[22]

Between 2016 and 2017, people with a graduate or professional degree experienced a 0.6 percentage-point increase in their overall coverage rate. No other educational attainment groups saw a statistically significant change in their overall rate of coverage.

People with some college (no degree) and people with a bachelor's degree were the only educational attainment groups for which rates of private and government coverage changed between 2016 and 2017. For people with some college (no degree), the rate of private coverage decreased by 1.2 percentage points (to 70.6 percent), and the rate of government coverage increased by 0.9 percentage points (to 24.7 percent). For people with a bachelor's degree, the rate of private coverage decreased by 1.3 percentage points (to 85.5 percent), and the rate of government coverage

increased by 0.8 percentage points (to 12.4 percent).[23]

Household Income

In 2017, people in households with lower income had lower health insurance coverage rates than people in households with higher income.[24] In 2017, 86.1 percent of people in households with an annual income of less than $25,000 had health insurance coverage, compared with 92.1 percent of people in households with income of $75,000 to $99,999, and 95.7 percent of people in households with income of $125,000 or more (Table 4).[25]

People in households with lower income also had lower rates of private coverage than people with higher income, and these differences varied more for lower income groups than for higher income groups. In 2017, the private health insurance coverage rate for people in households with income of $25,000 to $49,999 (51.1 percent) was 21.0 percentage points higher than the rate for people in households with income below $25,000 (30.1 percent). At the same time, the private health insurance coverage rate for people in households with income at or above $125,000 (88.4 percent) was 4.9 percentage points higher than the rate for people in households with income of $100,000 to $124,999 (83.4 percent).

Conversely, government coverage rates decreased as income increased, and as with private coverage, rates

---

[19] In this report, a full-time, year-round worker is a person who worked 35 or more hours per week (full-time) and 50 or more weeks during the previous calendar year (year-round). For school personnel, summer vacation is counted as weeks worked if they are scheduled to return to their job in the fall.

[20] All estimates by work experience are for the population aged 19 to 64.

[21] In 2017, the health insurance coverage rate for people who worked less than full-time, year-round was not statistically different from the coverage rate for nonworkers.

[22] All estimates by educational attainment are for the population aged 26 to 64.

[23] The percentage-point difference in the private coverage rate between 2016 and 2017 for people with some college (no degree) was not statistically different from the percentage-point difference for people with a bachelor's degree. The percentage-point difference in the government coverage rate between 2016 and 2017 for people with some college, no degree was not statistically different from the percentage-point difference for people with a bachelor's degree.

[24] Income refers to the total household income, not an individual's own income.

[25] The 2016 income estimates are inflation-adjusted and presented in 2017 dollars.

differed more between lower incomes than between higher incomes. In 2017, the government coverage rate for people in households with income of less than $25,000 (68.4 percent) was 15.3 percentage points higher than the rate for people in households with income of $25,000 to $49,999 (53.0 percent). For the two highest income groups, the difference was smaller. The government coverage rate for people in households with income of $100,000 to $124,999 (24.4 percent) was 5.0 percentage points higher than the rate for people in households with income at or above $125,000 (19.4 percent).

The overall percentage of people with health insurance coverage did not statistically change between 2016 and 2017 for any income group.

Rates of private and government coverage changed for some income groups. The percentage of people with private coverage decreased for three income groups between 2016 and 2017. People in households with income of $25,000 to $49,999 had a decrease of 1.1 percentage points (from 52.3 percent in 2016). People in households with income of $50,000 to $74,999 had a decrease of 1.3 percentage points (from 68.0 percent in 2016). The private coverage rate for people in households with income of $75,000 to $99,999 decreased by 1.8 percentage points (from 79.0 percent in 2016).[26]

Between 2016 and 2017, the rate of government coverage increased by 2.3 percentage points for this same group (people in households with income of $75,000 to $99,999). The rate of government coverage also increased for people in households with income of $100,000 to $124,999 (2.0 percentage-point increase).[27] The percentage of people with government coverage did not change for any other income group.

Income-to-Poverty Ratio

People in families are classified as being in poverty if their income is less than their poverty threshold.[28] People who live alone or with nonrelatives have a poverty status that is defined based on their own income. The income-to-poverty ratio compares a family's or an unrelated individual's income with the applicable threshold.

Health insurance coverage rates are generally higher for people in higher income-to-poverty ratio groups. In 2017, people in poverty (the population living below 100 percent of poverty) had the lowest health insurance coverage rate, at 83.0 percent, while people living at or above 400 percent of poverty had the highest coverage rate, at 95.7 percent (Table 4).

Government coverage continued to be most prevalent for the population in poverty (62.8 percent) and least prevalent for the population with income-to-poverty ratios at or above

400 percent of poverty (24.2 percent) in 2017.[29]

Between 2016 and 2017, the percentage of people with any health insurance coverage did not statistically change for any income-to-poverty group.

Coverage rates for subtypes of insurance, however, changed for some groups. Two groups had offsetting changes in coverage between 2016 and 2017, with a decrease in private coverage and an increase in government coverage. For people in households with income from 200 to 299 percent of poverty, the private coverage rate decreased 1.7 percentage points and government coverage increased 2.0 percentage points. For people in households with income at or above 400 percent of poverty, the private coverage rate decreased 0.6 percentage points, while the government coverage rate increased by 1.3 percentage points.[30] During the same time, the government coverage rate decreased by 1.2 percentage points for people in households with income from 300 to 399 percent of poverty (to 30.0 percent).

In 2014, policy changes associated with the Affordable Care Act provided the option for states to expand Medicaid eligibility to people whose income-to-poverty ratio fell under a particular threshold (for more information, see the text box "Health Insurance and the Affordable Care Act"). For adults aged 19 to 64, the relationship between poverty status,

---

[26] The percentage-point difference in the private coverage rate between 2016 and 2017 for people in households with income of $25,000 to $49,999 was not statistically different from the percentage-point difference for people in households with income of $50,000 to $74,999 and with income of $75,000 to $99,999.

The percentage-point difference in the private coverage rate between 2016 and 2017 for people in households with income of $50,000 to $74,999 was not statistically different from the percentage-point difference for people in households with income of $75,000 to $99,999.

[27] The percentage-point difference in the government coverage rate between 2016 and 2017 for people in households with income of $75,000 to $99,999 was not statistically different from the percentage-point difference for people in households with income of $100,000 to $124,999.

[28] The Office of Management and Budget determined the official definition of poverty in Statistical Policy Directive 14. Appendix B of the report *Income and Poverty in the United States: 2017* provides a more detailed description of how the Census Bureau calculates poverty; see <www.census.gov/content/dam/Census/library/publications/2018/demo/p60-263.pdf>.

[29] In 2017, the government coverage rate for the population living below 100 percent of poverty was not statistically different from the coverage rate for the population living below 138 percent of poverty.

[30] The percentage-point difference between 2016 and 2017 for neither the private coverage rate nor the government coverage rate for people with income from 200 to 299 percent of poverty was statistically different from the percentage-point differences for people at or above 400 percent of poverty.

Table 4.

Percentage of People by Type of Health Insurance Coverage by Household Income and Income-to-Poverty Ratio: 2016 and 2017

(Numbers in thousands, margins of error in percentage points. Population as of March of the following year. For information on confidentiality protection, sampling error, nonsampling error, and definitions, see www.2.census.gov/programs-surveys/cps/techdocs/cpsmar18.pdf)

Characteristic	Total Number 2016	Total Number 2017	Any health insurance 2016 Percent	2016 MOE ±	2017 Percent	2017 MOE ±	Change (2017 less 2016)*	Private health insurance[3] 2016 Percent	2016 MOE ±	2017 Percent	2017 MOE ±	Change (2017 less 2016)*	Government health insurance[4] 2016 Percent	2016 MOE ±	2017 Percent	2017 MOE ±	Change (2017 less 2016)*	Uninsured[5] 2016 Percent	2016 MOE ±	2017 Percent	2017 MOE ±	Change (2017 less 2016)*
Total............	320,372	323,156	91.2	0.2	91.2	0.2	-0.1	67.5	0.4	67.2	0.4	-0.3	37.3	0.3	37.7	0.3	*0.5	8.8	0.2	8.8	0.2	0.1
Household Income[6]																						
Less than $25,000.........	47,507	46,682	86.2	0.6	86.1	0.5	-0.1	30.3	0.8	30.1	0.8	-0.2	67.9	0.8	68.4	0.7	0.5	13.8	0.6	13.9	0.5	0.1
$25,000 to $49,999.......	62,357	62,187	88.1	0.4	87.7	0.5	-0.4	52.3	0.8	51.1	0.8	*-1.1	52.5	0.7	53.0	0.8	0.6	11.9	0.4	12.3	0.5	0.4
$50,000 to $74,999.......	54,487	53,710	90.0	0.5	89.6	0.5	-0.4	68.0	0.8	66.7	0.8	*-1.3	37.4	0.8	37.3	0.8	-0.1	10.0	0.5	10.4	0.5	0.4
$75,000 to $99,999.......	43,902	44,982	92.3	0.5	92.1	0.4	-0.2	79.0	0.7	77.2	0.8	*-1.8	26.6	0.8	28.9	0.9	*2.3	7.7	0.5	7.9	0.4	0.2
$100,000 to $124,999.....	33,406	32,108	94.1	0.5	94.6	0.4	0.5	83.3	0.8	83.4	0.8	0.1	22.4	0.8	24.4	0.9	*2.0	5.9	0.5	5.4	0.4	-0.5
$125,000 or more.........	78,712	83,487	95.8	0.3	95.7	0.3	-0.1	88.5	0.5	88.4	0.4	-0.1	18.9	0.5	19.4	0.6	0.5	4.2	0.3	4.3	0.3	0.1
Income-to-Poverty Ratio																						
Below 100 percent of poverty............	40,616	39,698	83.7	0.6	83.0	0.7	-0.7	28.6	0.9	28.2	1.0	-0.4	63.6	0.8	62.8	0.9	-0.8	16.3	0.6	17.0	0.7	0.7
Below 138 percent of poverty............	61,039	61,174	84.7	0.5	84.4	0.6	-0.3	31.1	0.7	31.3	0.8	0.2	63.1	0.6	62.7	0.8	-0.5	15.3	0.5	15.6	0.6	0.3
From 100 to 199 percent of poverty....	54,629	56,004	87.4	0.5	87.2	0.6	-0.1	45.4	0.9	45.5	0.8	0.1	55.9	0.8	55.7	0.8	-0.2	12.6	0.5	12.8	0.6	0.1
From 200 to 299 percent of poverty....	51,705	51,354	89.2	0.5	89.1	0.5	-0.1	66.2	0.8	64.5	0.8	*-1.7	38.0	0.8	40.0	0.8	*2.0	10.8	0.5	10.9	0.5	0.1
From 300 to 399 percent of poverty....	42,562	41,649	92.5	0.4	92.3	0.4	-0.2	76.4	0.8	76.7	0.8	0.3	31.1	0.8	30.0	0.8	*-1.2	7.5	0.4	7.7	0.4	0.2
At or above 400 percent of poverty....	130,398	133,844	95.6	0.2	95.7	0.2	0.1	86.6	0.3	86.0	0.3	*-0.6	22.8	0.4	24.2	0.4	*1.3	4.4	0.2	4.3	0.2	-0.1

* Changes between the estimates are statistically different from zero at the 90 percent confidence level.

Z Represents or rounds to zero.

[1] Details may not sum to totals because of rounding.

[2] A margin of error (MOE) is a measure of an estimate's variability. The larger the MOE in relation to the size of the estimate, the less reliable the estimate. This number, when added to and subtracted from the estimate, forms the 90 percent confidence interval. MOEs shown in this table are based on standard errors calculated using replicate weights. For more information, see "Standard Errors and Their Use" at <www.2.census.gov/library/publications/2018/demo/p60-264sa.pdf>.

[3] Private health insurance includes coverage provided through an employer or union, coverage purchased directly by an individual from an insurance company, or coverage through someone outside the household.

[4] Government health insurance coverage includes Medicaid, Medicare, TRICARE, CHAMPVA (Civilian Health and Medical Program of the Department of Veterans Affairs), and care provided by the Department of Veterans Affairs and the military.

[5] Individuals are considered to be uninsured if they do not have health insurance coverage for the entire calendar year.

[6] The 2016 income estimates are inflation-adjusted and presented in 2017 dollars.

Note: The estimates by type of coverage are not mutually exclusive; people can be covered by more than one type of health insurance during the year.

Source: U.S. Census Bureau, Current Population Survey, 2017 and 2018 Annual Social and Economic Supplements.

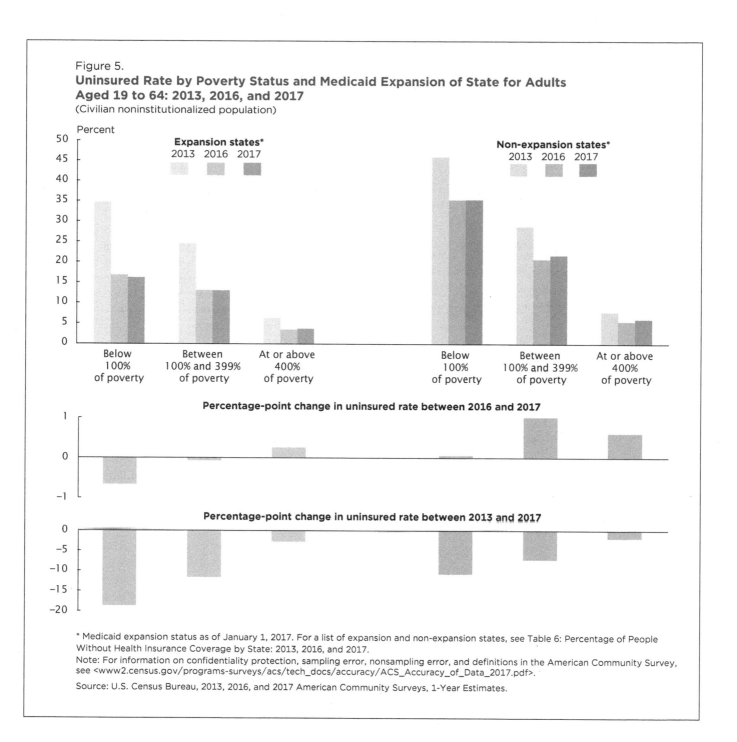

Figure 5.
Uninsured Rate by Poverty Status and Medicaid Expansion of State for Adults Aged 19 to 64: 2013, 2016, and 2017
(Civilian noninstitutionalized population)

* Medicaid expansion status as of January 1, 2017. For a list of expansion and non-expansion states, see Table 6: Percentage of People Without Health Insurance Coverage by State: 2013, 2016, and 2017.

Note: For information on confidentiality protection, sampling error, nonsampling error, and definitions in the American Community Survey, see <www2.census.gov/programs-surveys/acs/tech_docs/accuracy/ACS_Accuracy_of_Data_2017.pdf>.

Source: U.S. Census Bureau, 2013, 2016, and 2017 American Community Surveys, 1-Year Estimates.

the uninsured rate in 2017, and the change in the uninsured rate between 2016 and 2017 may be related to the state of residence and whether or not that state expanded Medicaid eligibility (Figure 5).[31, 32]

In states that expanded Medicaid eligibility on or before January 1, 2017, ("expansion states") and states that did not expand Medicaid eligibility ("non-expansion states"), the uninsured rate (based on coverage at the time of interview) decreased for adults aged 19 to 64 as the income-to-poverty ratio increased. However, in both 2016 and 2017, the uninsured rate was higher in non-expansion states than in expansion states regardless of individuals' poverty status group.

Changes in the uninsured rate between 2016 and 2017 varied by poverty status and state Medicaid expansion status. In states that expanded Medicaid eligibility, the uninsured rate decreased for persons living below 100 percent of poverty and increased for people living at or above 400 of poverty. In non-expansion states, the uninsured rate increased for both people living from 100 to 399 percent of poverty and people living at or above 400 percent of poverty.

Family Status

Many people obtain health insurance coverage through a family member's plan. The Census Bureau classifies living arrangements into three types: families, unrelated subfamilies, and unrelated individuals.[33] Families are the largest of these categories (80.7 percent of the population in 2017), followed by unrelated individuals (19.0 percent), and unrelated subfamilies (0.3 percent).

In 2017, people living in families had a higher health insurance coverage rate (91.7 percent) than unrelated individuals (88.8 percent) and people living in unrelated subfamilies (87.7 percent) (Table 5).[34] Between 2016 and 2017, there were no statistically significant changes in either the overall coverage rates or the private coverage rates for people with any of these three types of living arrangements.

During this time, the government coverage rate increased by 0.5 percentage points for people in families (to 36.9 percent). There were no statistical changes in government coverage rates for unrelated individuals and for people living in unrelated subfamilies.

Race and Hispanic Origin

In 2017, 93.7 percent of non-Hispanic Whites had health insurance coverage. This rate was higher than the coverage rate for Blacks (89.4 percent), Asians (92.7 percent), and Hispanics (83.9 percent) (Table 5).

Non-Hispanic Whites and Asians were among the most likely to have private health insurance in 2017, at 73.2 percent and 72.2 percent, respectively.[35, 36] Hispanics, who had the lowest rate of overall health insurance coverage, also had the lowest rate of private coverage, at 53.5 percent. In 2017, 56.5 percent of Blacks had private health insurance coverage.

Rates of government health coverage followed a different pattern than private health insurance coverage rates. In 2017, the government coverage rate was the highest for Blacks (44.1 percent), followed by Hispanics (39.5 percent), and non-Hispanic Whites (36.6 percent). Asians had the lowest rate of health insurance coverage through the government, at 29.6 percent in 2017.

Between 2016 and 2017, there were no statistically significant changes in overall health insurance coverage rates for any of the race and Hispanic origin groups.

Rates of private and government coverage changed for some race and Hispanic origin groups. Between 2016 and 2017, non-Hispanic Whites and Asians experienced a decrease in

---

[31] Figure 5 and estimates in the remainder of this section use data from the 2013, 2016, and 2017 American Community Survey, 1-year estimates, due to the larger sample size of the ACS compared with the CPS ASEC. The ACS measures health insurance at the time of interview. For information on how health insurance estimates differ between the ACS and CPS ASEC, see the text box "Two Measures of Health Insurance Coverage." Additionally, national statistics on income and poverty from the ACS are not identical to those from the CPS ASEC. For information on poverty estimates from the ACS and how they differ from those based on the CPS ASEC, see "Differences Between the Income and Poverty Estimates from the American Community Survey (ACS) and the Annual Social and Economic Supplement to the Current Population Survey (CPS ASEC)" at <www.census.gov/topics/income-poverty/poverty/guidance/data-sources/acs-vs-cps.html>.

[32] Thirty-one states and the District of Columbia expanded Medicaid eligibility on or before January 1, 2017. For a list of the states and their Medicaid expansion status as of January 1, 2017, see Table 6: Percentage of People Without Health Insurance Coverage by State: 2013, 2016, and 2017.

[33] Families are defined as groups of two or more related people where one of them is the householder. Family members must be related by birth, marriage, or adoption and reside together. Unrelated subfamilies are family units that reside with, but are not related to, the householder. For example, unrelated subfamilies could include a married couple with or without children, or a single parent with one or more never-married children under 18 years old living in a household. An unrelated subfamily may also include people such as partners, roommates, or resident employees and their spouses and/or children. The number of unrelated subfamily members is included in the total number of household members, but is not included in the count of family members. The remainder of the population is classified as unrelated individuals.

[34] In 2017, the health insurance coverage rate of unrelated individuals was not statistically different from the coverage rate of people living in unrelated subfamilies.

[35] The small sample size of the Asian population and the fact that the CPS does not use separate population controls for weighting the Asian sample to national totals, contributes to the large variances surrounding estimates for this group. As a result, the CPS is unable to detect statistically significant differences between some estimates for the Asian population. The ACS, based on a larger sample of the population, is a better source for estimating and identifying changes for small subgroups of the population.

[36] In 2017, the private coverage rate for non-Hispanic Whites was not statistically different from the private coverage rate for Asians.

Percentage of People by Type of Health Insurance Coverage by Selected Demographic Characteristics: 2016 and 2017

(Numbers in thousands, margins of errors in percentage points. Population as of March of the following year. For information on confidentiality protection, sampling error, nonsampling error, and definitions, see www2.census.gov/programs-surveys/cps/techdocs/cpsmar18.pdf)

Characteristic	Number 2016	Number 2017	Any health insurance 2016 Per-cent	2016 Margin of error[2] (±)	2017 Per-cent	2017 Margin of error[2] (±)	Change (2017 less 2016)[1]*	Private health insurance[3] 2016 Per-cent	2016 Margin of error[2] (±)	2017 Per-cent	2017 Margin of error[2] (±)	Change (2017 less 2016)[1]*	Government health insurance[4] 2016 Per-cent	2016 Margin of error[2] (±)	2017 Per-cent	2017 Margin of error[2] (±)	Change (2017 less 2016)[1]*	Uninsured[5] 2016 Per-cent	2016 Margin of error[2] (±)	2017 Per-cent	2017 Margin of error[2] (±)	Change (2017 less 2016)[1]*
Total	**320,372**	**323,156**	**91.2**	**0.2**	**91.2**	**0.2**	**-0.1**	**67.5**	**0.4**	**67.2**	**0.4**	**-0.3**	**37.3**	**0.3**	**37.7**	**0.3**	**0.3**	**8.8**	**0.2**	**8.8**	**0.2**	**0.1**
Family Status																						
In families	259,863	260,709	91.8	0.2	91.7	0.2	-0.1	68.7	0.4	68.3	0.4	-0.3	36.4	0.4	36.9	0.4	0.5	8.2	0.2	8.3	0.2	0.1
Householder	82,854	83,103	91.6	0.3	91.2	0.3	*-0.4	71.2	0.4	70.0	0.4	*-1.1	36.3	0.4	37.0	0.4	0.7	8.4	0.3	8.8	0.3	*0.4
Related children under the age of 18	72,674	72,532	94.8	0.3	94.7	0.3	Z	63.0	0.6	63.4	0.6	0.4	41.5	0.7	41.8	0.7	0.3	5.2	0.3	5.3	0.3	Z
Related children under the age of 6	23,531	23,574	94.2	0.4	94.0	0.5	-0.2	58.9	1.0	59.2	1.0	0.3	45.1	1.0	44.9	1.0	-0.1	5.8	0.4	6.0	0.5	0.2
In unrelated subfamilies	1,208	1,054	86.5	2.9	87.7	2.8	1.2	48.5	5.3	52.5	5.5	4.1	48.6	4.9	45.4	5.2	-3.2	13.5	2.9	12.3	2.8	-1.2
Unrelated individuals	59,301	61,393	88.7	0.3	88.8	0.4	0.1	62.8	0.6	62.5	0.7	-0.3	40.6	0.5	41.2	0.6	0.6	11.3	0.3	11.2	0.4	-0.1
Residence[6]																						
Inside metropolitan statistical areas	276,682	280,048	91.3	0.2	91.2	0.2	-0.1	68.5	0.4	68.0	0.4	*-0.5	35.9	0.4	36.6	0.4	*0.6	8.7	0.2	8.8	0.2	0.1
Inside principal cities	103,365	104,068	90.2	0.3	89.6	0.4	*-0.6	64.0	0.6	63.1	0.6	-0.8	37.9	0.7	38.2	0.6	0.3	9.8	0.3	10.4	0.4	*0.6
Outside principal cities	173,317	175,980	92.0	0.3	92.2	0.2	0.2	71.2	0.5	70.8	0.5	-0.4	34.8	0.4	35.6	0.5	*0.8	8.0	0.3	7.8	0.3	-0.2
Outside metropolitan statistical areas[7]	43,689	43,108	90.6	0.6	90.8	0.5	0.2	61.1	1.1	61.9	1.1	0.8	45.6	1.1	45.5	1.1	-0.1	9.4	0.6	9.2	0.5	-0.2
Race[8] and Hispanic Origin																						
White	246,310	247,695	91.6	0.2	91.5	0.2	-0.1	69.4	0.4	69.0	0.4	-0.4	36.6	0.3	37.1	0.4	*0.5	8.4	0.2	8.5	0.2	0.1
White, not Hispanic	195,453	195,530	93.7	0.2	93.7	0.2	Z	73.9	0.4	73.2	0.4	*-0.7	35.9	0.4	36.6	0.4	0.7	6.3	0.2	6.3	0.2	Z
Black	42,040	42,564	89.5	0.5	89.4	0.5	-0.1	56.5	1.0	56.5	0.9	Z	43.7	0.9	44.1	0.9	0.4	10.5	0.5	10.6	0.5	0.1
Asian	18,897	19,484	92.4	0.7	92.7	0.7	0.4	74.2	1.2	72.2	1.4	-2.0	27.1	1.2	29.6	1.2	*2.5	7.6	0.7	7.3	0.7	-0.4
Hispanic (any race)	57,670	59,227	84.0	0.5	83.9	0.6	Z	52.4	0.8	53.5	0.9	*1.1	40.1	0.7	39.5	0.7	-0.6	16.0	0.5	16.1	0.6	Z
Nativity																						
Native born	276,518	277,748	92.7	0.2	92.5	0.2	-0.2	68.7	0.4	68.2	0.4	-0.5	38.1	0.3	38.7	0.4	*0.5	7.3	0.2	7.5	0.2	*0.2
Foreign born	43,854	45,408	82.0	0.6	83.2	0.6	*1.2	59.9	0.7	60.6	0.8	0.7	31.7	0.7	32.0	0.7	0.3	18.0	0.6	16.8	0.6	*-1.2
Naturalized citizen	20,409	21,854	91.5	0.6	91.1	0.5	-0.4	67.3	1.0	65.6	1.0	*-1.6	37.2	1.0	37.5	1.0	0.3	8.5	0.6	8.9	0.5	0.4
Not a citizen	23,445	23,554	73.8	1.0	75.9	1.0	*2.1	53.5	1.1	55.9	1.0	*2.4	27.0	1.0	27.0	0.9	Z	26.2	1.0	24.1	1.0	*-2.1

* Changes between the estimates are statistically different from zero at the 90 percent confidence level.

Z Represents or rounds to zero.

[1] Details may not sum to totals because of rounding.

[2] A margin of error (MOE) is a measure of an estimate's variability. The larger the MOE in relation to the size of the estimate, the less reliable the estimate. This number, when added to and subtracted from the estimate, forms the 90 percent confidence interval. MOEs shown in this table are based on standard errors calculated using replicate weights. For more information, see "Standard Errors and Their Use" at <www2.census.gov/library/publications/2018/demo/p60-264sa.pdf>.

[3] Private health insurance includes coverage provided through an employer or union, coverage purchased directly by an individual from an insurance company, or coverage through someone outside the household.

[4] Government health insurance coverage includes Medicaid, Medicare, TRICARE, CHAMPVA (Civilian Health and Medical Program of the Department of Veterans Affairs) and care provided by the Department of Veterans Affairs and the military.

[5] Individuals are considered to be uninsured if they do not have health insurance coverage for the entire calendar year.

[6] The 2016 estimates presented for residence may not match the previously published estimates due to a correction in the assignment of principal city status for a small number of households. For the definition of metropolitan statistical areas and principal cites, see <www.census.gov/programs-surveys/metro-micro/about/glossary.html>.

[7] The "Outside metropolitan statistical areas" category includes both micropolitan statistical areas and territory outside of metropolitan and micropolitan statistical areas. For more information, see "About Metropolitan and Micropolitan Statistical Areas" at <www.census.gov/population/metro/about>.

[8] Federal surveys now give respondents the option of reporting more than one race. Therefore, two basic ways of defining a race group are possible. A group such as Asian may be defined as those who reported Asian and no other race (the race-alone or single-race concept) or as those who reported Asian regardless of whether they also reported another race (the race-alone-or-in-combination concept). This table shows data using the first approach (race alone). The use of the single-race population does not imply that it is the preferred method of presenting or analyzing data. The Census Bureau uses a variety of approaches. Information on people who reported more than one race, such as White and American Indian and Alaska Native or Asian and Black or African American, is available from the 2010 Census through American FactFinder. About 2.9 percent of people reported more than one race in the 2010 Census. Data for American Indians and Alaska Natives, Native Hawaiians and Other Pacific Islanders, and those reporting two or more races are not shown separately.

Note: The estimates by type of coverage are not mutually exclusive; people can be covered by more than one type of health insurance during the year.

Source: U.S. Census Bureau, Current Population Survey, 2017 and 2018 Annual Social and Economic Supplements.

their private coverage rate (0.7 and 2.0 percentage points, respectively).[37] The private coverage rate for Hispanics increased by 1.1 percentage points. There was no statistical change in the private coverage rate for Blacks.

The percentage of non-Hispanic Whites and Asians with government coverage increased between 2016 and 2017 (0.7 and 2.5 percentage points, respectively). There was no statistically significant change in the government coverage rate for Blacks and Hispanics.

Nativity

In 2017, the overall health insurance coverage rate for the native-born population (92.5 percent) was larger than that of naturalized citizens (91.1 percent) and noncitizens (75.9 percent) (Table 5).

Between 2016 and 2017, the percentage of the native-born population with health insurance coverage decreased by 0.2 percentage points to 92.5 percent. The percentage of

---

[37] The percentage-point difference in the private coverage rate between 2016 and 2017 for non-Hispanic Whites was not statistically different from the percentage-point difference for Asians.

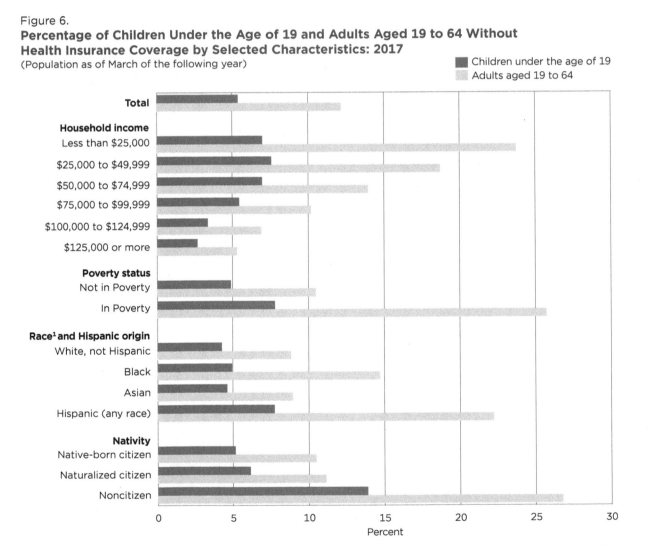

Figure 6.
Percentage of Children Under the Age of 19 and Adults Aged 19 to 64 Without Health Insurance Coverage by Selected Characteristics: 2017
(Population as of March of the following year)

Legend:
- Children under the age of 19
- Adults aged 19 to 64

[1] Federal surveys give respondents the option of reporting more than one race. This figure shows data using the race-alone concept. For example, Asian refers to people who reported Asian and no other race.

For information on confidentiality protection, sampling error, nonsampling error, and definitions in the Current Population Survey, see <www2.census.gov/programs-surveys/cps/techdocs/cpsmar18.pdf>.

Source: U.S. Census Bureau, Current Population Survey, 2018 Annual Social and Economic Supplement.

the foreign born with health insurance increased by 1.2 percentage points to 83.2 percent. Among the foreign-born population, the health insurance coverage rate for noncitizens increased by 2.1 percentage points to 75.9 percent. For this group, the rate of private coverage increased by 2.4 percentage points, and the rate of government coverage did not statistically change.[38]

Children and Adults Without Health Insurance Coverage

In 2017, 5.4 percent of children under the age of 19 and 12.2 percent of adults aged 19 to 64 did not have health insurance coverage. For all selected characteristics, the percentage of adults without health insurance coverage was significantly higher than for children (under 19 years of age) (Figure 6). Additionally, differences in the uninsured rates between demographic and socioeconomic groups were generally larger among adults than among children.[39]

For example, the difference in the uninsured rate by poverty status was larger among adults than among children. In 2017, 7.8 percent of children in poverty were uninsured, compared with 4.9 percent of children not in poverty, a 2.9 percentage-point difference. The uninsured rates for adults in poverty and not in poverty were 25.7

percent and 10.5 percent, respectively, a 15.2 percentage-point difference.

In 2017, non-Hispanic White children had an uninsured rate of 4.3 percent. Asian children had an uninsured rate of 4.6 percent, and Black children had an uninsured rate of 4.9 percent.[40] Hispanic children had the highest uninsured rate, at 7.7 percent. For all race and Hispanic origin groups, the uninsured rate for adults was significantly larger than the uninsured rate for children.

The uninsured rate for noncitizen children in 2017 was 13.9 percent, compared with 5.2 percent for native-born citizen children, an 8.7 percentage-point difference. For adults in 2017, 26.8 percent of noncitizen adults and 10.5 percent of native-born adults were uninsured, a 16.3 percentage-point difference.

State Estimates of Health Insurance Coverage

During 2017, the state with the lowest percentage of people without health insurance at the time of interview was Massachusetts (2.8 percent), while the state with the highest percentage was Texas (17.3 percent) (Table 6 and Figure 7).[41] Twenty-five states and the District of Columbia had an uninsured rate of 8.0 percent or less, among which six states (Hawaii, Iowa, Massachusetts, Minnesota, Rhode Island, and Vermont) and the District of Columbia had an uninsured rate of 5.0 percent or less. Two states, Oklahoma and Texas, had an uninsured rate of 14.0 percent or more.[42]

Between 2016 and 2017, the percentage of people without health insurance coverage decreased in three states and increased in 14 states (Table 6 and Figure 8).[43] Decreases ranged from 0.2 percentage points to 1.9 percentage points, and increases ranged from 0.3 percentage points to 1.0 percentage point. Thirty-three states and the District of Columbia did not have a statistically significant change in their uninsured rate.

As part of the Patient Protection and Affordable Care Act, 31 states and the District of Columbia expanded Medicaid eligibility on or before January 1, 2017, in (see the text box "Health Insurance Coverage and the Affordable Care Act").

In general, the uninsured rate in states that expanded Medicaid eligibility prior to January 1, 2017, was lower than in states that did not expand eligibility (Figure 7). In states that expanded Medicaid eligibility ("expansion states"), the uninsured rate in 2017 was 6.5 percent, compared with 12.2 percent in states that did not expand Medicaid eligibility ("non-expansion states"). Many Medicaid expansion states had uninsured rates lower than the national average, while many non-expansion states had uninsured rates above the national average (Figure 8).

The uninsured rates by state ranged from 2.8 percent to 13.7 percent in expansion states, and from 5.4 percent to 17.3 percent in non-expansion states.

Between 2016 and 2017, the uninsured rate did not statistically change in expansion states and increased by 0.4 percentage points in non-expansion states.

---

[38] The percentage-point difference in the private coverage rate between 2016 and 2017 for noncitizens was not statistically different from the percentage-point difference in the overall coverage rate for this group.

[39] In 2017, the percentage-point difference in the uninsured rate between children in households with income between $100,000 and $124,999 and children in households with income at or above $125,000 was not statistically different from the percentage-point difference between adults in households with income between $100,000 and $124,999 and adults in households with income at or above $125,000. In 2017, the percentage-point difference in the uninsured rate between native-born children and naturalized children was not statistically different from the percentage-point difference between native-born adults and naturalized adults. In 2017, the percentage-point difference in the uninsured rate between non-Hispanic White children and Asian children was not statistically different from the percentage-point difference between non-Hispanic White adults and Asian adults.

[40] In 2017, the uninsured rate for non-Hispanic White children was not statistically different from the uninsured rate for Black children or Asian children. In 2017, the uninsured rate for Black children was not statistically different from the uninsured rate for Asian children.

[41] The estimates in this section come from the 2013, 2016, and 2017 American Community Survey 1-year estimates, which measures insurance coverage at the time of interview. The ACS, which has a much larger sample size than the CPS, is also a useful source for estimating and identifying changes in the uninsured population at the state level.

[42] Consistent with Figure 7, classification into these categories is based on unrounded uninsured rates.

[43] For additional information on coverage types by state, see <www.census.gov/topics/2018/demo/health-insurance/p60-264.html>.

Table 6.

Percentage of People Without Health Insurance Coverage by State: 2013, 2016, and 2017

(Civilian noninstitutionalized population. For information on confidentiality protection, sampling error, nonsampling error, and definitions, see www2.census.gov/programs-surveys/acs/tech_docs/accuracy/ACS_Accuracy_of_Data_2017.pdf)

State	Medicaid expansion state? Yes (Y) or No (N)[1]	2013 uninsured		2016 uninsured		2017 uninsured		Difference in uninsured			
								2017 less 2016		2017 less 2013	
		Percent	Margin of error[2] (±)	Percent	Margin of error[2] (±)	Percent	Margin of error[2] (±)	Percent	Margin of error[2] (±)	Percent	Margin of error[2] (±)
United States	X	14.5	0.1	8.6	0.1	8.7	0.1	*0.2	0.1	*-5.8	0.1
Alabama	N	13.6	0.4	9.1	0.3	9.4	0.3	0.3	0.5	*-4.2	0.5
Alaska	+Y	18.5	1.0	14.0	0.9	13.7	0.8	-0.4	1.2	*-4.8	1.3
Arizona	Y	17.1	0.4	10.0	0.3	10.1	0.3	0.1	0.4	*-7.1	0.5
Arkansas	Y	16.0	0.5	7.9	0.4	7.9	0.3	Z	0.5	*-8.1	0.6
California................	Y	17.2	0.2	7.3	0.1	7.2	0.1	*-0.2	0.1	*-10.0	0.2
Colorado	Y	14.1	0.3	7.5	0.3	7.5	0.2	Z	0.4	*-6.6	0.4
Connecticut	Y	9.4	0.4	4.9	0.3	5.5	0.3	*0.6	0.5	*-3.9	0.5
Delaware................	Y	9.1	0.7	5.7	0.5	5.4	0.6	-0.3	0.7	*-3.7	0.9
District of Columbia	Y	6.7	0.6	3.9	0.6	3.8	0.6	-0.1	0.9	*-2.8	0.8
Florida...................	N	20.0	0.2	12.5	0.2	12.9	0.2	*0.4	0.3	*-7.1	0.3
Georgia	N	18.8	0.3	12.9	0.3	13.4	0.3	*0.5	0.4	*-5.4	0.4
Hawaii	Y	6.7	0.4	3.5	0.4	3.8	0.4	0.3	0.5	*-2.9	0.5
Idaho	N	16.2	0.8	10.1	0.5	10.1	0.5	Z	0.7	*-6.0	0.9
Illinois...................	Y	12.7	0.2	6.5	0.2	6.8	0.2	*0.3	0.2	*-5.9	0.3
Indiana..................	+Y	14.0	0.3	8.1	0.3	8.2	0.3	0.1	0.4	*-5.8	0.4
Iowa....................	Y	8.1	0.3	4.3	0.2	4.7	0.3	*0.4	0.4	*-3.4	0.4
Kansas	N	12.3	0.4	8.7	0.3	8.7	0.4	Z	0.5	*-3.5	0.6
Kentucky	Y	14.3	0.3	5.1	0.2	5.4	0.3	0.3	0.4	*-8.9	0.4
Louisiana................	#Y	16.6	0.4	10.3	0.4	8.4	0.3	*-1.9	0.5	*-8.3	0.5
Maine...................	N	11.2	0.5	8.0	0.5	8.1	0.5	0.1	0.7	*-3.1	0.7
Maryland.................	Y	10.2	0.3	6.1	0.3	6.1	0.2	Z	0.4	*-4.0	0.4
Massachusetts.............	Y	3.7	0.2	2.5	0.2	2.8	0.1	*0.3	0.2	*-0.9	0.2
Michigan	^Y	11.0	0.2	5.4	0.1	5.2	0.2	-0.2	0.2	*-5.8	0.2
Minnesota................	Y	8.2	0.3	4.1	0.2	4.4	0.2	*0.3	0.3	*-3.8	0.3
Mississippi................	N	17.1	0.5	11.8	0.4	12.0	0.5	0.2	0.7	*-5.0	0.7
Missouri.................	N	13.0	0.3	8.9	0.2	9.1	0.3	0.2	0.4	*-3.9	0.4
Montana	+Y	16.5	0.8	8.1	0.5	8.5	0.5	0.3	0.8	*-8.0	0.9
Nebraska.................	N	11.3	0.5	8.6	0.5	8.3	0.4	-0.3	0.6	*-3.0	0.6
Nevada	Y	20.7	0.6	11.4	0.5	11.2	0.4	-0.1	0.6	*-9.4	0.8
New Hampshire............	^Y	10.7	0.5	5.9	0.4	5.8	0.4	-0.1	0.6	*-4.9	0.7
New Jersey...............	Y	13.2	0.2	8.0	0.2	7.7	0.2	-0.2	0.3	*-5.5	0.3
New Mexico	Y	18.6	0.6	9.2	0.5	9.1	0.6	-0.1	0.8	*-9.5	0.9
New York.................	Y	10.7	0.2	6.1	0.1	5.7	0.1	*-0.4	0.2	*-5.0	0.2
North Carolina.............	N	15.6	0.3	10.4	0.2	10.7	0.2	0.3	0.3	*-5.0	0.4
North Dakota..............	Y	10.4	0.8	7.0	0.6	7.5	0.6	0.5	0.9	*-2.8	1.0
Ohio....................	Y	11.0	0.2	5.6	0.2	6.0	0.2	*0.3	0.2	*-5.1	0.3
Oklahoma................	N	17.7	0.3	13.8	0.3	14.2	0.3	0.4	0.4	*-3.5	0.5
Oregon	Y	14.7	0.4	6.2	0.2	6.8	0.3	*0.6	0.4	*-7.8	0.5
Pennsylvania..............	^Y	9.7	0.2	5.6	0.2	5.5	0.2	-0.1	0.2	*-4.2	0.2
Rhode Island	Y	11.6	0.7	4.3	0.5	4.6	0.4	0.3	0.6	*-7.0	0.8
South Carolina.............	N	15.8	0.4	10.0	0.3	11.0	0.3	*1.0	0.4	*-4.8	0.5
South Dakota..............	N	11.3	0.7	8.7	0.5	9.1	0.6	0.3	0.8	*-2.2	0.9
Tennessee................	N	13.9	0.3	9.0	0.2	9.5	0.3	*0.5	0.4	*-4.4	0.4
Texas	N	22.1	0.2	16.6	0.2	17.3	0.2	*0.7	0.3	*-4.8	0.3
Utah....................	N	14.0	0.5	8.8	0.4	9.2	0.4	0.4	0.6	*-4.8	0.6
Vermont	Y	7.2	0.6	3.7	0.4	4.6	0.4	*0.8	0.6	*-2.7	0.8
Virginia	N	12.3	0.3	8.7	0.3	8.8	0.3	0.1	0.4	*-3.5	0.4
Washington	Y	14.0	0.3	6.0	0.2	6.1	0.2	0.2	0.3	*-7.9	0.4
West Virginia	Y	14.0	0.5	5.3	0.3	6.1	0.4	*0.8	0.5	*-7.9	0.7
Wisconsin................	N	9.1	0.2	5.3	0.2	5.4	0.2	0.1	0.3	*-3.7	0.3
Wyoming	N	13.4	0.9	11.5	1.0	12.3	1.2	0.7	1.6	*-1.2	1.5

* Statistically different from zero at the 90 percent confidence level.

\+ Expanded Medicaid eligibility after January 1, 2015, and on or before January 1, 2016.

X Not applicable.

^ Expanded Medicaid eligibility after January 1, 2014, and on or before January 1, 2015.

\# Expanded Medicaid eligibility after January 1, 2016, and on or before January 1, 2017.

Z Represents or rounds to zero.

[1] Medicaid expansion status as of January 1, 2017. For more information, see <www.medicaid.gov/state-overviews/index.html>.

[2] Data are based on a sample and are subject to sampling variability. A margin of error is a measure of an estimate's variability. The larger the margin of error is in relation to the size of the estimate, the less reliable the estimate. This number, when added to and subtracted from the estimate, forms the 90 percent confidence interval.

Note: Differences are calculated with unrounded numbers, which may produce different results from using the rounded values in the table.

Source: U.S. Census Bureau, 2013, 2016, and 2017 American Community Survey 1-Year Estimates.

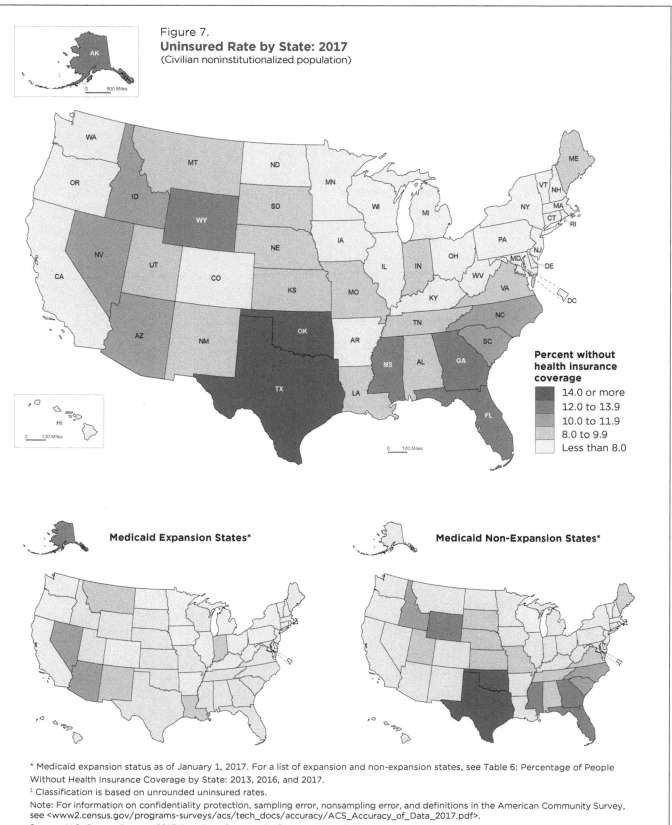

Figure 7.
Uninsured Rate by State: 2017
(Civilian noninstitutionalized population)

Percent without health insurance coverage

- 14.0 or more
- 12.0 to 13.9
- 10.0 to 11.9
- 8.0 to 9.9
- Less than 8.0

Medicaid Expansion States*

Medicaid Non-Expansion States*

* Medicaid expansion status as of January 1, 2017. For a list of expansion and non-expansion states, see Table 6: Percentage of People Without Health Insurance Coverage by State: 2013, 2016, and 2017.

[1] Classification is based on unrounded uninsured rates.

Note: For information on confidentiality protection, sampling error, nonsampling error, and definitions in the American Community Survey, see <www2.census.gov/programs-surveys/acs/tech_docs/accuracy/ACS_Accuracy_of_Data_2017.pdf>.

Source: U.S. Census Bureau, 2017 American Community Survey, 1-Year Estimates.

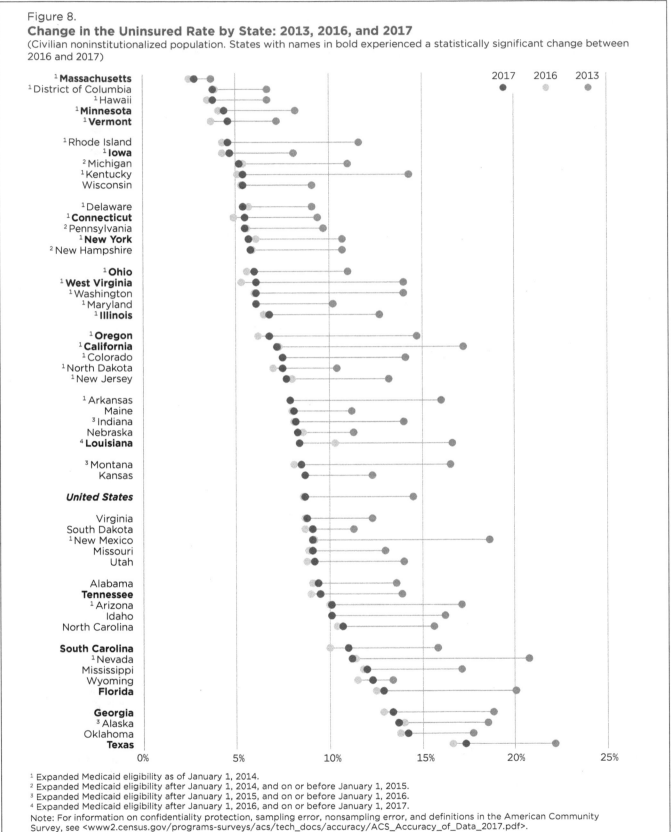

Figure 8.

Change in the Uninsured Rate by State: 2013, 2016, and 2017

(Civilian noninstitutionalized population. States with names in bold experienced a statistically significant change between 2016 and 2017)

[1] Expanded Medicaid eligibility as of January 1, 2014.
[2] Expanded Medicaid eligibility after January 1, 2014, and on or before January 1, 2015.
[3] Expanded Medicaid eligibility after January 1, 2015, and on or before January 1, 2016.
[4] Expanded Medicaid eligibility after January 1, 2016, and on or before January 1, 2017.

Note: For information on confidentiality protection, sampling error, nonsampling error, and definitions in the American Community Survey, see <www2.census.gov/programs-surveys/acs/tech_docs/accuracy/ACS_Accuracy_of_Data_2017.pdf>.

Source: U.S. Census Bureau, 2013, 2016, and 2017 American Community Surveys, 1-Year Estimates.

More Information About Health Insurance Coverage

Additional Data and Contacts

Detailed tables, historical tables, press releases, and briefings are available on the Census Bureau's Health Insurance Web site. The Web site can be accessed at <www.census.gov /topics/health/health-insurance .html>.

Microdata are available for download on the Census Bureau's Web site. Disclosure protection techniques have been applied to CPS microdata to protect respondent confidentiality.

State and Local Estimates of Health Insurance Coverage

The Census Bureau publishes annual estimates of health insurance coverage by state and other smaller geographic units based on data collected in the ACS. Single-year estimates are available for geographic units with populations of 65,000 or more. Five-year estimates are available for all geographic units, including census tracts and block groups.

The Census Bureau's Small Area Health Insurance Estimates (SAHIE) program also produces single-year estimates of health insurance for states and all counties. These estimates are based on models using data from a variety of sources, including current surveys, administrative records, and intercensal population estimates. In general, SAHIE estimates have lower variances than ACS estimates but are released later because they incorporate these additional data into their models.

Small Area Health Insurance Estimates are available at <www.census.gov /programs-surveys/sahie.html>. The most recent estimates are for 2016.

Comments

The Census Bureau welcomes the comments and advice of data and report users. If you have suggestions or comments on the health insurance coverage report, please write to:

Sharon Stern
Assistant Division Chief, Employment
   Characteristics
Social, Economic, and Housing
   Statistics Division
U.S. Census Bureau
Washington, DC 20233-8500

or e-mail
<sharon.m.stern@census.gov>.

Sources of Estimates

The majority of the estimates in this report are from the 2014, 2017, and 2018 Current Population Survey Annual Social and Economic Supplements (CPS ASEC) and were collected in the 50 states and the District of Columbia. These data do not represent residents of Puerto Rico and the U.S. Island Areas.[44] These data are based on a sample of about 92,000 addresses. The estimates in this report are controlled to independent national population estimates by age, sex, race, and Hispanic origin for March of the year in which the data are collected. Beginning with 2010, estimates are based on 2010 Census population counts and are updated annually taking into account births, deaths, emigration, and immigration.

The CPS is a household survey primarily used to collect employment data. The sample universe for the basic CPS consists of the resident civilian noninstitutionalized population

of the United States. People in institutions, such as prisons, long-term care hospitals, and nursing homes are not eligible to be interviewed in the CPS. Students living in dormitories are included in the estimates only if information about them is reported in an interview at their parents' home. Since the CPS is a household survey, people who are homeless and not living in shelters are not included in the sample. The sample universe for the CPS ASEC is slightly larger than that of the basic CPS since it includes military personnel who live in a household with at least one other civilian adult, regardless of whether they live off post or on post. All other armed forces are excluded. For further documentation about the CPS ASEC, see <www2.census.gov/programs -surveys/cps/techdocs/cpsmar18 .pdf>.

Additional estimates in this report are from the American Community Survey (ACS). The ACS is an ongoing, nationwide survey designed to provide demographic, social, economic, and housing data at different levels of geography. While the ACS includes Puerto Rico and the group quarters population, the ACS data in this report focus on the civilian noninstitutionalized population of the United States (excluding Puerto Rico and some people living in group quarters). It has an annual sample size of about 3.5 million addresses. For information on the ACS sample design and other topics, visit <www.census.gov/programs-surveys /acs/>.

Statistical Accuracy

The estimates in this report (which may be shown in text, figures, and tables) are based on responses from a sample of the population. Sampling

---

[44] The U.S. Island Areas include American Samoa, Guam, the Commonwealth of the Northern Mariana Islands, and the Virgin Islands of the United States.

error is the uncertainty between an estimate based on a sample and the corresponding value that would be obtained if the estimate were based on the entire population (as from a census). All comparative statements in this report have undergone statistical testing, and comparisons are significant at the 90 percent level unless otherwise noted. Data are subject to error arising from a variety of sources. Measures of sampling error are provided in the form of margins of error, or confidence intervals, for all estimates included in this report. In addition to sampling error, nonsampling error may be introduced during any of the operations used to collect and process survey data, such as editing, reviewing, or keying data from questionnaires. In this report, the variances

of estimates were calculated using the Fay and Train (1995) Successive Difference Replication (SDR) method.

Most of the data from the 2018 CPS ASEC were collected in March (with some data collected in February and April). Each year, the CPS ASEC sample ranges between 92,000 and 100,000 addresses. In 2018, the CPS ASEC sample had 92,000 addresses, as 5,000 randomly selected addresses were removed from the March sample. The 5,000 addresses were given the pre-2013 health insurance questions in order to fulfill budgetary requirements for the 2018 fiscal year.[45, 46] Adjustments

[45] Public Law 113-235, 2017.
[46] The series of questions asking about health insurance coverage in calendar year 2012 and earlier.

to the weights were made to account for the reduction in sample. Further information about the source and accuracy of the CPS ASEC estimates is available at <www2.census.gov /library/publications/2018/demo /p60-264sa.pdf>.

The remaining data presented in this report are based on the ACS sample collected from January 2017 through December 2017. For more information on sampling and estimation methods, confidentiality protection, and sampling and nonsampling errors, please see the 2017 ACS Accuracy of the Data document located at <www2.census.gov /programs-surveys/acs/tech_docs /accuracy/ACS_Accuracy_of_Data _2017.pdf>.

Table A-1.
Number of People by Type of Health Insurance Coverage by Age: 2016 and 2017

(Numbers in thousands, margins of error in thousands. Population as of March of the following year. For information on confidentiality protection, sampling error, nonsampling error, and definitions, see *www2.census.gov/programs-surveys/cps/techdocs/cpsmar18.pdf*)

Characteristic	Total 2016 Number	Total 2017 Number	Any health insurance 2016 Number	2017 Number	2017 Margin of error[2] (±)	Change (2017 less 2016)[1,*]	Private health insurance 2016 Number	2016 Margin of error[2] (±)	2017 Number	2017 Margin of error[2] (±)	Change (2017 less 2016)[1,*]	Government health insurance[4] 2016 Number	2016 Margin of error[2] (±)	2017 Number	2017 Margin of error[2] (±)	Change (2017 less 2016)[1,*]	Uninsured[5] 2016 Number	2016 Margin of error[2] (±)	2017 Number	2017 Margin of error[2] (±)	Change (2017 less 2016)[*]
Total............	320,372	323,156	292,320	294,613	541	*2,293	216,203	1,145	217,007	1,158	804	119,361	1,018	121,965	1,086	*2,604	28,052	519	28,543	634	492
Age																					
Under age 65..........	271,098	272,076	243,645	244,211	582	566	190,198	1,051	190,882	1,064	684	73,220	991	74,082	1,042	862	27,453	508	27,865	612	412
Under age 18.........	74,047	73,963	70,123	70,033	246	-90	46,393	438	46,570	488	177	31,020	481	31,277	482	258	3,924	192	3,930	238	6
Aged 18 to 64........	197,051	198,113	173,521	174,178	535	657	143,805	772	144,312	760	507	42,200	689	42,804	729	604	23,530	438	23,935	498	405
Under age 19[6].......	78,150	78,106	73,948	73,884	240	-63	49,185	452	49,419	504	235	32,439	501	32,748	509	309	4,203	205	4,221	252	19
Aged 19 to 64........	192,948	193,971	169,697	170,327	525	630	141,013	750	141,463	749	449	40,781	662	41,334	717	553	23,251	435	23,644	489	393
Aged 19 to 25[7].......	29,815	29,922	25,917	25,727	274	-190	21,247	290	21,002	304	-244	6,898	263	6,994	260	96	3,898	179	4,195	204	*297
Aged 26 to 34........	39,736	40,152	33,499	33,875	267	*376	27,692	313	28,047	329	355	8,097	258	8,154	295	57	6,237	224	6,277	229	40
Aged 35 to 44........	40,046	40,659	34,794	35,253	197	*459	29,373	270	29,912	272	*540	7,728	228	7,825	240	97	5,252	192	5,407	199	154
Aged 45 to 64........	83,351	83,237	75,487	75,472	342	-15	62,702	449	62,501	469	-201	18,058	408	18,361	421	303	7,863	257	7,765	282	-98
Aged 65 and older.....	49,274	51,080	48,675	50,402	225	*1,726	26,005	378	26,125	441	120	46,140	259	47,883	232	*1,743	598	69	678	71	80

* Changes between the estimates are statistically different from zero at the 90 percent confidence level.
[1] Details may not sum to totals because of rounding.
[2] A margin of error (MOE) is a measure of an estimate's variability. The larger the MOE in relation to the size of the estimate, the less reliable the estimate. This number, when added to and subtracted from the estimate, forms the 90 percent confidence interval. MOEs shown in this table are based on standard errors calculated using replicate weights. For more information, see "Standard Errors and Their Use" at <www2.census.gov/library/publications/2018/demo/p60-264sa.pdf>.
[3] Private health insurance includes coverage provided through an employer or union, coverage purchased directly by an individual from an insurance company, or coverage through someone outside the household.
[4] Government health insurance coverage includes Medicaid, Medicare, TRICARE, CHAMPVA (Civilian Health and Medical Program of the Department of Veterans Affairs), and care provided by the Department of Veterans Affairs and the military.
[5] Individuals are considered to be uninsured if they do not have health insurance coverage for the entire calendar year.
[6] Children under the age of 19 are eligible for Medicaid/CHIP.
[7] This age is of special interest because of the Affordable Care Act's dependent coverage provision. Individuals aged 19 to 25 may be eligible to be a dependent on a parent's health insurance plan. This age group are not mutually exclusive; people can be covered by more than one type of health insurance during the year.
Note: The estimates by type of coverage are not mutually exclusive; people can be covered by more than one type of health insurance during the year.
Source: U.S. Census Bureau, Current Population Survey, 2017 and 2018 Annual Social and Economic Supplements.

Table A-2.

Number of People by Type of Health Insurance Coverage for Working-Age Adults Aged 19 to 64: 2016 and 2017

(Numbers in thousands, margins of error in thousands. Population as of March of the following year. For information on confidentiality protection, sampling error, nonsampling error, and definitions, see www2.census.gov/programs-surveys/cps/techdocs/cpsmar18.pdf)

Characteristic	Total 2016 Number	Total 2017 Number	Any health insurance 2016 Number	2016 Margin of error² (±)	2017 Number	2017 Margin of error² (±)	Change (2017 less 2016)*	Private health insurance³ 2016 Number	2016 Margin² (±)	2017 Number	2017 Margin² (±)	Change (2017 less 2016)*	Government health insurance⁴ 2016 Number	2016 Margin² (±)	2017 Number	2017 Margin² (±)	Change (2017 less 2016)*	Uninsured⁵ 2016 Number	2016 Margin² (±)	2017 Number	2017 Margin² (±)	Change (2017 less 2016)*
Total	320,372	323,156	292,320	541	294,613	662	*2,293	216,203	1,145	217,007	1,158	804	119,361	1,018	121,965	1,086	*2,604	28,052	519	28,543	634	492
Total, 19 to 64 years old	192,948	193,971	169,697	525	170,327	561	630	141,013	750	141,463	749	449	40,781	662	41,334	717	553	23,251	435	23,644	489	393
Marital Status																						
Married⁶	101,822	101,580	92,821	670	92,318	805	-503	81,594	666	80,988	773	-606	18,230	447	18,597	476	367	9,001	333	9,262	314	261
Widowed	3,633	3,586	3,127	158	3,107	162	-20	2,131	117	2,053	134	-79	1,218	101	1,290	99	71	506	61	479	62	-27
Divorced	19,460	19,510	16,753	363	16,858	380	105	12,503	317	12,753	338	250	5,223	212	5,136	203	-86	2,707	132	2,652	146	-55
Separated	4,495	4,372	3,632	169	3,486	161	-146	2,512	144	2,423	139	-89	1,394	96	1,309	90	-85	863	73	886	84	23
Never married	63,537	64,923	53,364	547	54,558	570	*1,195	42,272	552	43,246	517	*973	14,716	392	15,002	388	286	10,174	320	10,365	304	191
Disability Status⁷																						
With a disability	15,248	14,957	13,899	358	13,641	350	-258	6,633	231	6,702	240	70	8,933	287	8,639	300	-294	1,349	109	1,317	100	-32
With no disability	176,842	178,063	154,940	572	155,735	585	*796	134,162	765	134,502	751	340	30,989	558	31,744	572	*755	21,902	417	22,327	466	425
Work Experience																						
All workers	149,105	150,487	132,422	587	133,419	738	*996	119,497	661	120,622	767	*1,125	20,797	474	21,115	500	318	16,682	385	17,068	379	386
Worked full-time, year-round	107,577	109,511	97,049	652	98,770	713	*1,722	90,853	669	92,394	721	*1,540	11,224	313	11,927	367	*703	10,528	292	10,741	286	213
Worked less than full-time, year-round	41,528	40,976	35,374	514	34,648	511	*-725	28,643	441	28,228	468	-416	9,573	286	9,189	283	*-385	6,154	225	6,327	244	173
Did not work at east 1 week	43,843	43,484	37,275	507	36,908	547	-367	21,517	413	20,841	419	-676	19,984	395	20,218	484	235	6,568	247	6,576	256	8
Educational Attainment																						
Total, 26 to 64 years old	163,133	164,049	143,780	473	144,599	534	*819	119,766	685	120,460	691	694	33,883	547	34,340	594	457	19,353	386	19,449	446	96
No high school diploma	15,389	15,150	11,184	300	11,161	297	-23	6,293	218	6,425	228	132	5,806	218	5,677	217	-129	4,205	189	3,989	197	-216
High school graduate (includes equivalency)	45,401	44,772	38,511	605	37,814	579	*-697	29,512	541	29,273	510	-239	11,961	328	11,756	328	-205	6,890	232	6,958	261	67
Some college, no degree	26,594	26,109	23,512	407	22,977	381	*-536	19,102	383	18,445	343	*-656	6,324	227	6,439	221	115	3,082	147	3,133	155	51
Associate's degree	17,739	17,659	16,096	354	15,987	348	-110	13,820	323	13,627	328	-193	3,454	171	3,449	153	-5	1,642	110	1,673	127	30
Bachelor's degree	36,528	38,465	34,032	503	35,690	577	*1,658	31,698	498	32,889	576	*1,191	4,239	172	4,765	204	*525	2,496	133	2,775	160	*279
Graduate or professional degree	21,482	21,894	20,444	437	20,971	431	*527	19,342	432	19,801	419	459	2,098	122	2,254	130	156	1,038	86	922	82	*-116

* Changes between the estimates are statistically different from zero at the 90 percent confidence level.
¹ Details may not sum to totals because of rounding.
² A margin of error (MOE) is a measure of an estimate's variability. The larger the MOE in relation to the size of the estimate, the less reliable the estimate. This number, when added to and subtracted from the estimate, forms the 90 percent confidence interval. MOEs shown in this table are based on standard errors calculated using replicate weights. For more information, see "Standard Errors and Their Use" at <www2.census.gov/library/publications/2018/demo/p60-264sa.pdf>.
³ Private health insurance includes coverage provided through an employer or union, coverage purchased directly by an individual from an insurance company, or coverage through someone outside the household.
⁴ Government health insurance coverage includes Medicaid, Medicare, CHAMPVA (Civilian Health and Medical Program of the Department of Veterans Affairs), and care provided by the Department of Veterans Affairs and the military.
⁵ Individuals are considered to be uninsured if they do not have health insurance coverage for the entire calendar year.
⁶ The combined category "married" includes three individual categories: "married, civilian spouse present," "married, armed forces spouse present," and "married, spouse absent."
⁷ The sum of those with and without a disability does not equal the total because disability status is not defined for individuals in the armed forces.
Note: The estimates by type of coverage are not mutually exclusive; people can be covered by more than one type of health insurance during the year.
Source: U.S. Census Bureau, Current Population Survey, 2017 and 2018 Annual Social and Economic Supplements.

Table A-3.

Number of People by Type of Health Insurance Coverage by Household Income and Income-to-Poverty Ratio: 2016 and 2017

(Numbers in thousands, margins of error in thousands. Population as of March of the following year. For information on confidentiality protection, sampling error, nonsampling error, and definitions, see www2.census.gov/programs-surveys/cps/techdocs/cpsmar18.pdf)

Characteristic	Total		Any health insurance					Private health insurance[3]					Government health insurance[4]					Uninsured[5]				
	2016	2017	2016		2017		Change	2016		2017		Change	2016		2017		Change	2016		2017		Change
	Number	Number	Number	Margin of error[2] (±)	Number	Margin of error[2] (±)	(2017 less 2016)[1,*]	Number	Margin of error[2] (±)	Number	Margin of error[2] (±)	(2017 less 2016)[1,*]	Number	Margin of error[2] (±)	Number	Margin of error[2] (±)	(2017 less 2016)[1,*]	Number	Margin of error[2] (±)	Number	Margin of error[2] (±)	(2017 less 2016)[1,*]
Total	320,372	323,156	292,320	541	294,613	662	*2,293	216,203	1,145	217,007	1,158	804	119,361	1,018	124,965	1,086	*2,604	28,052	519	28,543	634	492
Household income[6]																						
Less than $25,000	47,507	46,682	40,958	779	40,199	797	-758	14,398	461	14,071	460	-327	32,259	668	31,920	664	-339	6,550	288	6,482	304	-67
$25,000 to $49,999	62,357	62,187	54,940	967	54,569	981	-371	32,584	685	31,800	706	-784	32,708	744	32,986	756	278	7,417	294	7,618	350	201
$50,000 to $74,999	54,487	53,710	49,036	901	48,141	860	-895	37,049	783	35,844	732	*-1,205	20,369	531	20,031	524	-338	5,452	266	5,570	298	118
$75,000 to $99,999	43,902	44,982	40,533	797	41,436	864	903	34,696	729	34,733	805	38	11,697	389	13,014	483	*1,318	3,369	216	3,546	206	177
$100,000 to $124,999	33,406	32,108	31,425	730	30,367	769	*-1,057	27,822	656	26,787	703	*-1,035	7,483	342	7,831	351	348	1,982	171	1,741	147	*-241
$125,000 or more	78,712	83,487	75,429	1,034	79,900	1,251	*4,472	69,654	1,050	73,771	1,204	*4,117	14,845	458	16,182	523	*1,337	3,283	223	3,587	229	304
Income-to-Poverty Ratio																						
Below 100 percent of poverty	40,616	39,698	34,004	683	32,950	806	*-1,053	11,620	420	11,185	490	-434	25,826	585	24,934	647	*-892	6,612	261	6,748	311	135
Below 138 percent of poverty	61,039	61,174	51,681	820	51,632	927	-49	19,001	537	19,159	577	158	38,522	692	38,329	798	-193	9,357	316	9,542	392	185
From 100 to 199 percent of poverty	54,629	56,004	47,735	876	48,862	906	1,127	24,786	671	25,492	632	706	30,518	651	31,192	667	674	6,894	309	7,142	348	248
From 200 to 299 percent of poverty	51,705	51,354	46,131	825	45,756	850	-375	34,216	742	33,119	692	*-1,097	19,631	478	20,519	559	*887	5,574	258	5,598	262	23
From 300 to 399 percent of poverty	42,562	41,649	39,359	753	38,432	860	-927	32,525	640	31,940	790	-585	13,258	448	12,478	420	*-780	3,204	192	3,218	189	14
At or above 400 percent of poverty	130,398	133,844	124,665	1,256	128,044	1,343	*3,378	112,884	1,217	115,059	1,301	*2,175	29,793	575	32,376	629	*2,583	5,733	272	5,801	262	68

* Changes between the estimates are statistically different from zero at the 90 percent confidence level.

[1] Details may not sum to totals because of rounding.

[2] A margin of error (MOE) is a measure of an estimate's variability. The larger the MOE in relation to the size of the estimate, the less reliable the estimate. This number, when added to and subtracted from the estimate, forms the 90 percent confidence interval. MOEs shown in this table are based on standard errors calculated using replicate weights. For more information, see "Standard Errors and Their Use" at <www2.census.gov/library/publications/2018/demo/p60-264sa.pdf>.

[3] Private health insurance includes coverage provided through an employer or union, coverage purchased directly by an individual from an insurance company, or coverage through someone outside the household.

[4] Government health insurance coverage includes Medicaid, Medicare, TRICARE, CHAMPVA (Civilian Health and Medical Program of the Department of Veterans Affairs), and care provided by the Department of Veterans Affairs and the military.

[5] Individuals are considered to be uninsured if they do not have health insurance coverage for the entire calendar year.

[6] The 2016 income estimates are inflation-adjusted and presented in 2017 dollars.

Note: The estimates by type of coverage are not mutually exclusive; people can be covered by more than one type of health insurance during the year.

Source: U.S. Census Bureau, Current Population Survey, 2017 and 2018 Annual Social and Economic Supplements.

Table A-4.

Number of People by Type of Health Insurance Coverage by Selected Demographic Characteristics: 2016 and 2017

(Numbers in thousands, margins of errors in thousands. Population as of March of the following year. For information on confidentiality protection, sampling error, nonsampling error, and definitions, see www.census.gov/programs-surveys/cps/techdocs/cpsmar18.pdf)

Characteristic	Total 2016 Number	Total 2017 Number	Any health insurance 2016 Number	2016 MOE (±)	2017 Number	2017 MOE (±)	Change (2017 less 2016)*	Private health insurance[3] 2016 Number	2016 MOE (±)	2017 Number	2017 MOE (±)	Change (2017 less 2016)*	Government health insurance[4] 2016 Number	2016 MOE (±)	2017 Number	2017 MOE (±)	Change (2017 less 2016)*	Uninsured[5] 2016 Number	2016 MOE (±)	2017 Number	2017 MOE (±)	Change (2017 less 2016)*
Total	320,372	323,156	292,320	541	294,613	662	*2,293	216,203	1,145	217,007	1,158	804	119,361	1,018	121,965	1,086	*2,604	28,052	519	28,543	634	492
Family Status																						
In families	259,863	260,709	238,655	883	239,167	1,016	512	178,401	1,203	178,086	1,216	-315	94,707	936	96,220	1,084	*1,513	21,208	504	21,542	581	334
Householder	82,854	83,103	75,899	437	75,756	466	-143	58,954	458	58,182	458	*-773	30,074	335	30,712	435	*638	6,956	217	7,347	220	*391
Related children under age 18	72,674	72,532	68,867	261	68,701	289	-166	45,793	440	45,988	487	195	30,180	481	30,327	473	148	3,807	194	3,831	234	24
Related children under age 6	23,531	23,574	22,175	128	22,165	136	-10	13,848	224	13,950	236	101	10,603	238	10,594	235	-9	1,355	105	1,408	110	53
In unrelated subfamilies	1,208	1,054	1,045	135	924	117	-120	585	102	553	84	-32	587	89	479	83	-108	163	37	129	30	-34
Unrelated individuals	59,301	61,393	52,621	729	54,521	779	*1,901	37,217	645	38,368	645	*1,151	24,067	437	25,266	492	*1,199	6,680	227	6,872	278	192
Residence[6]																						
Inside metropolitan statistical areas	276,682	280,048	252,748	2,587	255,475	2,663	*2,727	189,505	2,011	190,316	2,218	811	99,424	1,584	102,358	1,570	*2,934	23,935	582	24,573	654	638
Inside principal cities	103,365	104,068	93,278	1,882	93,280	1,843	2	66,111	1,329	65,713	1,497	-398	39,170	1,108	39,721	1,033	551	10,088	405	10,788	463	*700
Outside principal cities	173,317	175,980	159,470	2,442	162,195	2,437	*2,725	123,393	1,906	124,603	2,021	1,209	60,254	1,265	62,637	1,268	*2,383	13,847	491	13,785	459	-62
Outside metropolitan statistical areas[7]	43,689	43,108	39,572	2,525	39,138	2,524	-434	26,699	1,723	26,691	1,747	-8	19,936	1,395	19,607	1,404	-329	4,117	371	3,970	343	-147
Race[8] and Hispanic Origin																						
White	246,310	247,695	225,497	491	226,621	552	*1,124	170,839	949	170,913	965	74	90,220	847	91,952	929	*1,732	20,813	455	21,075	526	262
White, not Hispanic	195,453	195,530	183,139	422	183,168	437	29	144,398	839	143,181	793	*-1,216	70,136	701	71,550	804	*1,415	12,314	360	12,362	395	48
Black	42,040	42,564	37,612	227	38,052	211	*439	23,739	415	24,041	401	302	18,377	378	18,792	376	415	4,428	223	4,512	204	84
Asian	18,897	19,484	17,455	208	18,071	237	*616	14,013	260	14,068	305	55	5,124	237	5,761	253	*637	1,442	134	1,413	133	-29
Hispanic (any race)	57,670	59,227	48,433	319	49,719	360	*1,286	30,192	453	31,672	562	*1,480	23,125	419	23,414	426	289	9,237	316	9,508	356	271
Nativity																						
Native born	276,518	277,748	256,338	767	256,827	849	488	189,946	1,126	189,503	1,104	-443	105,440	982	107,421	1,068	*1,981	20,180	438	20,921	513	*742
Foreign born	43,854	45,408	35,982	538	37,786	664	*1,804	26,258	469	27,504	577	*1,247	13,921	389	14,544	396	*623	7,872	312	7,622	316	-250
Naturalized citizen	20,409	21,854	18,684	405	19,918	468	*1,235	13,726	346	14,342	414	*616	7,591	259	8,191	280	*601	1,726	125	1,936	116	*210
Not a citizen	23,445	23,554	17,298	380	17,868	450	*570	12,532	346	13,162	359	*630	6,330	262	6,353	266	22	6,147	269	5,687	263	*-460

* Changes between the estimates are statistically different from zero at the 90 percent confidence level.

[1] Details may not sum to totals because of rounding.

[2] A margin of error (MOE) is a measure of an estimate's variability. The larger the MOE in relation to the size of the estimate, the less reliable the estimate. This number, when added to and subtracted from the estimate, forms the 90 percent confidence interval. MOEs shown in this table are based on standard errors calculated using replicate weights. For more information, see "Standard Errors and Their Use" at <www2.census.gov/library/publications/2018/demo/p60-264sa.pdf>.

[3] Private health insurance includes coverage provided through an employer or union, coverage purchased directly by an individual from an insurance company, or coverage through someone outside the household.

[4] Government health insurance coverage includes Medicaid, Medicare, TRICARE, CHAMPVA (Civilian Health and Medical Program of the Department of Veterans Affairs), and care provided by the Department of Veterans Affairs and the military.

[5] Individuals are considered to be uninsured if they do not have health insurance coverage for the entire calendar year.

[6] The 2016 estimates presented for residence may not match the previously published estimates due to a correction in the assignment of principal city status for a small number of households. For the definition of metropolitan statistical areas and principal cities, see <www.census.gov/programs-surveys/metro-micro/about/glossary.html>.

[7] The "Outside metropolitan statistical areas" category includes both micropolitan statistical areas and territory outside of metropolitan and micropolitan statistical areas. For more information, see "About Metropolitan and Micropolitan Statistical Areas" at <www.census.gov/population/metro/about>.

[8] Federal surveys now give respondents the option of reporting more than one race. Therefore, two basic ways of defining a race group are possible. A group such as Asian may be defined as those who reported Asian and no other race (the race-alone or single-race concept) or as those who reported Asian regardless of whether they also reported another race (the race-alone-or-in-combination concept). This table shows data using the first approach (race alone). The use of the single-race population does not imply that it is the preferred method of presenting or analyzing data. The Census Bureau uses a variety of approaches. Information on people who reported more than one race, such as White and American Indian and Alaska Native or Asian and Black or African American, is available from the 2010 Census through American FactFinder. About 2.9 percent of people reported more than one race in the 2010 Census. Data for American Indians and Alaska Natives, Native Hawaiians and Other Pacific Islanders, and those reporting two or more races are not shown separately.

Note: The estimates by type of coverage are not mutually exclusive; people can be covered by more than one type of health insurance during the year.

Source: U.S. Census Bureau, Current Population Survey, 2017 and 2018 Annual Social and Economic Supplements.

Table A-5.
Number of People Without Health Insurance Coverage by State: 2013, 2016, and 2017

(Numbers in thousands. Civilian noninstitutionalized population. For information on confidentiality protection, sampling error, nonsampling error, and definitions, see www2.census.gov/programs-surveys/acs/tech_docs/accuracy/ACS_Accuracy_of_Data_2017.pdf)

| State | Medicaid expansion state? Yes (Y) or No (N)[1] | 2013 uninsured | | 2016 uninsured | | 2017 uninsured | | Difference in uninsured | | | |
| | | | | | | | | 2017 less 2016 | | 2017 less 2013 | |
		Number	Margin of error[2] (±)	Number	Margin of error[2] (±)	Number	Margin of error[2] (±)	Number	Margin of error[2] (±)	Number	Margin of error[2] (±)
United States.		45,181	200	27,304	162	28,019	188	*715	248	*-17,161	275
Alabama	N	645	17	435	14	449	16	14	22	*-197	23
Alaska	+Y	132	7	101	6	98	6	-3	9	*-34	9
Arizona	Y	1,118	24	681	21	695	20	14	29	*-423	32
Arkansas.	Y	465	14	232	12	232	10	27	16	*-233	17
California.	Y	6,500	57	2,844	41	2,797	34	-47	53	*-3,704	67
Colorado.	Y	729	18	410	14	414	13	4	19	*-315	22
Connecticut	Y	333	14	172	11	194	12	*22	16	*-139	19
Delaware.	Y	83	6	53	5	51	5	-2	7	*-32	8
District of Columbia	Y	42	4	26	4	26	4	Z	6	*-16	6
Florida	N	3,853	43	2,544	47	2,676	43	*132	64	*-1,177	61
Georgia	N	1,846	30	1,310	30	1,375	29	*66	42	*-471	42
Hawaii	Y	91	6	49	5	53	5	4	7	*-38	7
Idaho	N	257	12	168	8	172	9	4	12	*-85	15
Illinois.	Y	1,618	27	817	20	859	23	*43	31	*-759	35
Indiana.	+Y	903	19	530	17	536	18	6	25	*-367	26
Iowa	Y	248	9	132	8	146	8	*14	11	*-102	12
Kansas	N	348	12	249	9	249	11	Z	14	*-99	16
Kentucky	Y	616	14	223	10	235	12	12	16	*-381	19
Louisiana.	#Y	751	17	470	17	383	13	*-87	22	*-369	21
Maine	N	147	7	106	7	107	6	1	9	*-40	10
Maryland	Y	593	17	363	16	366	15	2	22	*-228	23
Massachusetts	Y	247	10	171	10	190	10	*19	14	*-57	14
Michigan	^Y	1,072	19	527	14	510	15	-17	20	*-562	24
Minnesota	Y	440	14	225	10	243	11	*18	15	*-197	18
Mississippi.	N	500	16	346	12	352	15	6	19	*-148	22
Missouri.	N	773	18	532	14	548	17	16	22	*-225	25
Montana	+Y	165	8	83	6	88	6	4	8	*-77	10
Nebraska.	N	209	9	161	9	157	7	-4	12	*-52	12
Nevada	Y	570	17	330	13	333	13	2	19	*-237	21
New Hampshire.	^Y	140	7	78	6	77	5	-1	8	*-63	9
New Jersey.	Y	1,160	22	705	19	688	17	-17	26	*-472	28
New Mexico	Y	382	13	188	10	187	12	-1	16	*-195	18
New York.	Y	2,070	30	1,183	26	1,113	27	*-70	38	*-957	41
North Carolina	N	1,509	26	1,038	21	1,076	24	*38	32	*-433	36
North Dakota	Y	73	6	52	5	56	5	3	7	*-18	7
Ohio	Y	1,258	21	644	18	686	22	*42	28	*-572	31
Oklahoma	N	666	13	530	13	545	12	16	17	*-120	17
Oregon	Y	571	15	253	10	281	12	*28	16	*-290	19
Pennsylvania	^Y	1,222	22	708	21	692	21	-16	30	*-530	31
Rhode Island	Y	120	7	45	5	48	4	3	7	*-72	8
South Carolina	N	739	18	486	14	542	17	*56	22	*-197	25
South Dakota	N	93	5	74	4	77	5	3	7	*-16	7
Tennessee.	N	887	20	592	16	629	19	*37	25	*-258	27
Texas	N	5,748	55	4,545	55	4,817	48	*272	73	*-931	73
Utah	N	402	13	265	12	282	12	17	17	*-120	18
Vermont	Y	45	4	23	2	28	3	*5	4	*-17	5
Virginia	N	991	22	715	21	729	21	14	30	*-261	31
Washington	Y	960	22	428	15	446	15	18	21	*-514	26
West Virginia	Y	255	10	96	6	109	7	*13	9	*-146	12
Wisconsin	N	518	14	300	10	309	11	9	15	*-208	17
Wyoming	N	77	5	67	6	70	7	3	9	-7	8

* Statistically different from zero at the 90 percent confidence level.
^ Expanded Medicaid eligibility after January 1, 2014, and on or before January 1, 2015.
+ Expanded Medicaid eligibility after January 1, 2015, and on or before January 1, 2016.
# Expanded Medicaid eligibility after January 1, 2016, and on or before January 1, 2017.
Z Represents or rounds to zero.
[1] Medicaid expansion status as of January 1, 2017. For more information, see <www.medicaid.gov/state-overviews/index.html>.
[2] Data are based on a sample and are subject to sampling variability. A margin of error is a measure of an estimate's variability. The larger the margin of error is in relation to the size of the estimate, the less reliable the estimate. This number, when added to and subtracted from the estimate, forms the 90 percent confidence interval.
Note: Differences are calculated with unrounded numbers, which may produce different results from using the rounded values in the table.
Source: U.S. Census Bureau, 2013, 2016, and 2017 American Community Survey 1-Year Estimates.

Population Without Health Insurance Coverage
The 25 Most Populous Metro Areas

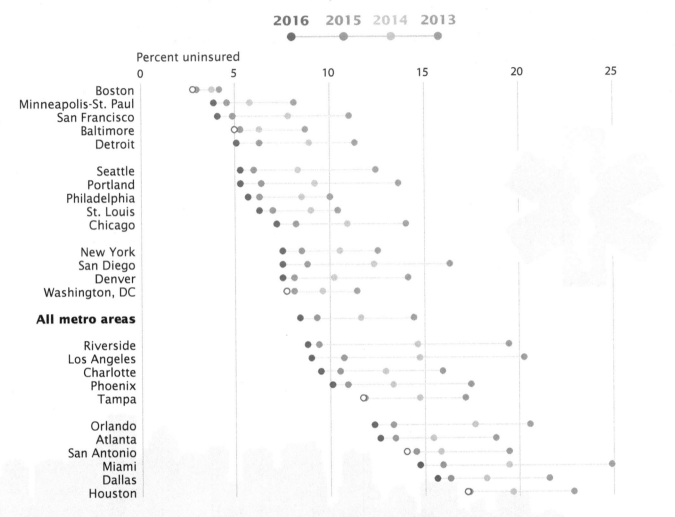

2016   2015   2014   2013

State Statistics & Rankings

Covered by Some Type of Health Insurance

All Persons		Under 18 Years		Under 65 Years	
State	**Percent**	**State**	**Percent**	**State**	**Percent**
Massachusetts	97.2 (0.1)	District of Columbia	98.8 (0.7)	Massachusetts	96.7 (0.2)
District of Columbia	96.2 (0.6)	Massachusetts	98.5 (0.2)	District of Columbia	95.8 (0.7)
Hawaii	96.2 (0.4)	Vermont	98.4 (0.6)	Hawaii	95.4 (0.4)
Minnesota	95.6 (0.2)	Rhode Island	97.9 (0.6)	Minnesota	94.9 (0.2)
Rhode Island	95.4 (0.4)	Hawaii	97.8 (0.5)	Iowa	94.5 (0.3)
Vermont	95.4 (0.4)	New Hampshire	97.7 (0.5)	Rhode Island	94.5 (0.5)
Iowa	95.3 (0.3)	Washington	97.4 (0.3)	Vermont	94.5 (0.5)
Michigan	94.8 (0.2)	West Virginia	97.4 (0.5)	Michigan	93.9 (0.2)
Delaware	94.6 (0.6)	New York	97.3 (0.2)	Kentucky	93.7 (0.3)
Kentucky	94.6 (0.3)	Illinois	97.1 (0.2)	Connecticut	93.6 (0.4)
Wisconsin	94.6 (0.2)	Michigan	97.0 (0.2)	Delaware	93.6 (0.7)
Connecticut	94.5 (0.3)	Alabama	96.9 (0.4)	Wisconsin	93.6 (0.2)
Pennsylvania	94.5 (0.2)	California	96.9 (0.1)	New York	93.4 (0.2)
New York	94.3 (0.1)	Connecticut	96.9 (0.5)	Pennsylvania	93.4 (0.2)
New Hampshire	94.2 (0.4)	Iowa	96.9 (0.4)	New Hampshire	93.1 (0.5)
Ohio	94.0 (0.2)	Louisiana	96.9 (0.4)	Maryland	93.0 (0.3)
Maryland	93.9 (0.2)	Minnesota	96.6 (0.3)	Ohio	93.0 (0.2)
Washington	93.9 (0.2)	Delaware	96.5 (1.0)	Washington	92.9 (0.2)
West Virginia	93.9 (0.4)	Oregon	96.4 (0.5)	West Virginia	92.5 (0.5)
Illinois	93.2 (0.2)	New Jersey	96.3 (0.3)	Illinois	92.2 (0.2)
Oregon	93.2 (0.3)	Kentucky	96.2 (0.6)	California	91.9 (0.1)
California	92.8 (0.1)	Maryland	96.2 (0.4)	Oregon	91.8 (0.4)
Colorado	92.5 (0.2)	Wisconsin	96.1 (0.3)	Colorado	91.4 (0.3)
North Dakota	92.5 (0.6)	Colorado	95.7 (0.4)	North Dakota	91.2 (0.8)
New Jersey	92.3 (0.2)	Arkansas	95.6 (0.6)	New Jersey	91.0 (0.2)
Arkansas	92.1 (0.3)	Pennsylvania	95.6 (0.3)	Arkansas	90.7 (0.4)
Maine	91.9 (0.5)	Tennessee	95.6 (0.5)	Indiana	90.5 (0.3)
Indiana	91.8 (0.3)	Ohio	95.5 (0.4)	Nebraska	90.4 (0.5)
Nebraska	91.7 (0.4)	Idaho	95.4 (0.7)	Louisiana	90.3 (0.3)
Louisiana	91.6 (0.3)	Mississippi	95.2 (0.7)	Maine	90.0 (0.6)
Montana	91.5 (0.5)	North Carolina	95.2 (0.3)	Utah	89.9 (0.4)
Kansas	91.3 (0.4)	Maine	95.1 (0.7)	Kansas	89.8 (0.4)
United States	91.3 (0.1)	United States	95.0 (0.1)	Montana	89.8 (0.7)
Virginia	91.2 (0.3)	Missouri	94.9 (0.4)	United States	89.8 (0.1)
Missouri	90.9 (0.3)	Nebraska	94.9 (0.7)	Virginia	89.8 (0.3)
New Mexico	90.9 (0.6)	New Mexico	94.9 (0.7)	New Mexico	89.3 (0.7)
South Dakota	90.9 (0.6)	South Carolina	94.9 (0.5)	South Dakota	89.3 (0.7)
Utah	90.8 (0.4)	Virginia	94.9 (0.4)	Missouri	89.2 (0.3)
Alabama	90.6 (0.3)	Kansas	94.8 (0.6)	Alabama	88.9 (0.4)
Tennessee	90.5 (0.3)	Montana	94.2 (1.0)	Tennessee	88.8 (0.3)
Arizona	89.9 (0.3)	South Dakota	93.8 (1.0)	Idaho	88.1 (0.6)
Idaho	89.9 (0.5)	Indiana	93.7 (0.5)	Arizona	88.0 (0.3)
North Carolina	89.3 (0.2)	Florida	92.7 (0.3)	North Carolina	87.4 (0.3)
South Carolina	89.0 (0.3)	Utah	92.7 (0.6)	Nevada	87.0 (0.5)
Nevada	88.8 (0.4)	Georgia	92.5 (0.4)	South Carolina	86.8 (0.4)
Mississippi	88.0 (0.5)	North Dakota	92.5 (1.4)	Mississippi	85.8 (0.6)
Wyoming	87.7 (1.2)	Arizona	92.3 (0.5)	Wyoming	85.5 (1.4)
Florida	87.1 (0.2)	Nevada	92.0 (0.8)	Alaska	84.7 (0.9)
Georgia	86.6 (0.3)	Oklahoma	91.9 (0.5)	Georgia	84.6 (0.3)
Alaska	86.3 (0.8)	Wyoming	90.5 (2.0)	Florida	84.1 (0.3)
Oklahoma	85.8 (0.3)	Alaska	90.4 (1.7)	Oklahoma	83.4 (0.3)
Texas	82.7 (0.2)	Texas	89.3 (0.3)	Texas	80.6 (0.2)

Note: Numbers in thousands; Figures cover civilian noninstitutionalized population in 2017; N/A indicates that data was not available; Z represents or rounds to zero; Margin of error appears in parenthesis and is calculated using replicate weights.
Source: U.S. Census Bureau, American Community Survey, Table HIC-4_ACS. Health Insurance Coverage Status and Type of Coverage by State—All People: 2008 to 2017, Table HIC-5_ACS. Health Insurance Coverage Status and Type of Coverage by State—Children Under 18: 2008 to 2017, Table HIC-6_ACS. Health Insurance Coverage Status and Type of Coverage by State—Persons Under 65: 2008 to 2017

Covered by Private Health Insurance

All Persons		Under 18 Years		Under 65 Years	
State	Percent	State	Percent	State	Percent
North Dakota	79.8 *(1.2)*	Utah	76.7 *(1.1)*	North Dakota	80.9 *(1.4)*
Utah	78.4 *(0.6)*	North Dakota	75.0 *(2.7)*	Utah	80.5 *(0.6)*
Hawaii	77.0 *(0.9)*	Minnesota	70.9 *(0.7)*	Hawaii	78.3 *(1.0)*
New Hampshire	76.7 *(0.8)*	Virginia	70.7 *(0.8)*	New Hampshire	78.1 *(0.9)*
Virginia	76.2 *(0.4)*	New Hampshire	70.2 *(1.8)*	Nebraska	77.9 *(0.8)*
Minnesota	76.0 *(0.3)*	Wyoming	70.1 *(3.0)*	Virginia	77.5 *(0.4)*
Nebraska	75.9 *(0.8)*	Wisconsin	69.9 *(0.9)*	Iowa	77.4 *(0.6)*
Iowa	75.8 *(0.5)*	Massachusetts	69.7 *(0.8)*	Wisconsin	77.4 *(0.5)*
Wisconsin	75.2 *(0.4)*	Hawaii	69.6 *(1.9)*	Minnesota	77.0 *(0.4)*
Kansas	74.5 *(0.6)*	Nebraska	69.6 *(1.5)*	Kansas	75.9 *(0.6)*
Maryland	74.3 *(0.5)*	Iowa	69.4 *(1.2)*	Massachusetts	75.2 *(0.5)*
Massachusetts	73.8 *(0.4)*	New Jersey	67.6 *(0.7)*	Delaware	75.1 *(1.4)*
Delaware	73.6 *(1.3)*	Maine	67.3 *(1.8)*	South Dakota	75.1 *(1.1)*
South Dakota	73.2 *(1.0)*	Kansas	66.9 *(1.2)*	Maryland	74.9 *(0.5)*
Pennsylvania	72.5 *(0.3)*	Delaware	66.6 *(2.6)*	New Jersey	74.1 *(0.4)*
Wyoming	72.5 *(1.7)*	Maryland	66.6 *(1.0)*	Pennsylvania	73.6 *(0.3)*
New Jersey	72.0 *(0.3)*	Connecticut	66.4 *(1.2)*	Wyoming	73.6 *(1.9)*
Connecticut	71.4 *(0.6)*	South Dakota	66.2 *(1.9)*	Connecticut	73.3 *(0.7)*
Michigan	71.4 *(0.3)*	Pennsylvania	64.8 *(0.6)*	Missouri	72.8 *(0.5)*
Washington	70.8 *(0.5)*	Rhode Island	64.4 *(2.3)*	Maine	72.7 *(1.1)*
Indiana	70.7 *(0.5)*	Missouri	64.1 *(1.1)*	Washington	72.0 *(0.5)*
Missouri	70.6 *(0.5)*	Colorado	63.5 *(1.0)*	Colorado	71.9 *(0.5)*
Maine	70.5 *(0.9)*	Michigan	63.4 *(0.6)*	Indiana	71.9 *(0.5)*
District of Columbia	70.1 *(1.2)*	Indiana	63.2 *(1.0)*	Rhode Island	71.6 *(1.3)*
Colorado	70.0 *(0.4)*	Ohio	62.8 *(0.8)*	Illinois	71.4 *(0.4)*
Illinois	69.9 *(0.4)*	Washington	62.8 *(1.0)*	Michigan	71.2 *(0.4)*
Idaho	69.8 *(0.8)*	Illinois	62.5 *(0.7)*	Idaho	71.0 *(0.9)*
Rhode Island	69.6 *(1.2)*	Idaho	62.0 *(1.8)*	District of Columbia	70.7 *(1.3)*
Ohio	69.1 *(0.4)*	New York	61.7 *(0.6)*	Ohio	70.5 *(0.4)*
United States	67.6 *(0.1)*	Oregon	60.6 *(1.3)*	United States	69.1 *(0.1)*
Oregon	67.5 *(0.5)*	Nevada	60.4 *(1.3)*	New York	68.6 *(0.4)*
Montana	67.2 *(1.2)*	United States	60.0 *(0.2)*	Oregon	68.5 *(0.6)*
North Carolina	67.0 *(0.4)*	Tennessee	58.0 *(1.0)*	Montana	68.3 *(1.4)*
Alabama	66.9 *(0.6)*	Arizona	57.0 *(1.0)*	North Carolina	68.1 *(0.5)*
New York	66.9 *(0.3)*	California	56.9 *(0.4)*	Tennessee	67.7 *(0.6)*
Vermont	66.5 *(1.3)*	Montana	56.7 *(2.6)*	Alabama	67.6 *(0.7)*
Tennessee	66.3 *(0.5)*	Georgia	56.6 *(0.9)*	Georgia	67.5 *(0.5)*
Georgia	66.1 *(0.5)*	Alaska	56.4 *(2.4)*	Nevada	67.4 *(0.8)*
South Carolina	65.4 *(0.5)*	Kentucky	56.4 *(1.3)*	Vermont	67.1 *(1.5)*
Nevada	64.9 *(0.7)*	North Carolina	56.3 *(0.8)*	South Carolina	66.3 *(0.6)*
Kentucky	64.5 *(0.7)*	District of Columbia	55.2 *(2.8)*	California	65.7 *(0.2)*
Oklahoma	64.0 *(0.5)*	South Carolina	55.1 *(1.1)*	Kentucky	65.1 *(0.7)*
California	63.6 *(0.2)*	Alabama	55.0 *(1.1)*	Florida	64.9 *(0.3)*
Alaska	63.2 *(1.3)*	Vermont	54.1 *(2.4)*	Arizona	64.5 *(0.6)*
Arizona	63.0 *(0.5)*	West Virginia	53.5 *(1.6)*	Oklahoma	64.2 *(0.5)*
Texas	62.2 *(0.3)*	Texas	52.7 *(0.5)*	Alaska	63.4 *(1.3)*
Florida	62.1 *(0.3)*	Oklahoma	52.6 *(1.1)*	Texas	63.4 *(0.3)*
West Virginia	62.0 *(0.9)*	Florida	52.5 *(0.6)*	Arkansas	61.9 *(0.9)*
Arkansas	61.3 *(0.8)*	Louisiana	49.2 *(1.2)*	West Virginia	61.6 *(1.0)*
Louisiana	60.3 *(0.7)*	Mississippi	48.0 *(1.4)*	Mississippi	61.4 *(1.0)*
Mississippi	60.3 *(0.8)*	Arkansas	47.2 *(1.5)*	Louisiana	61.3 *(0.7)*
New Mexico	54.4 *(1.1)*	New Mexico	44.3 *(1.7)*	New Mexico	54.7 *(1.2)*

Note: Numbers in thousands; Figures cover civilian noninstitutionalized population in 2017; N/A indicates that data was not available; Z represents or rounds to zero; Margin of error appears in parenthesis and is calculated using replicate weights.

Source: U.S. Census Bureau, American Community Survey, Table HIC-4_ACS. Health Insurance Coverage Status and Type of Coverage by State—All People: 2008 to 2017, Table HIC-5_ACS. Health Insurance Coverage Status and Type of Coverage by State—Children Under 18: 2008 to 2017, Table HIC-6_ACS. Health Insurance Coverage Status and Type of Coverage by State—Persons Under 65: 2008 to 2017

Covered by Private Health Insurance: Employer-based

All Persons		Under 18 Years		Under 65 Years	
State	Percent	State	Percent	State	Percent
Utah	64.8 (0.7)	Utah	66.6 (1.3)	New Hampshire	69.3 (0.9)
New Hampshire	63.8 (0.8)	Wisconsin	64.8 (0.8)	Wisconsin	69.2 (0.5)
Maryland	63.5 (0.5)	Minnesota	64.7 (0.7)	Minnesota	69.1 (0.4)
Hawaii	63.3 (1.0)	North Dakota	63.7 (2.7)	Utah	68.5 (0.8)
Massachusetts	62.8 (0.4)	New Hampshire	63.6 (1.9)	Iowa	67.8 (0.7)
Minnesota	62.6 (0.3)	Massachusetts	63.3 (0.9)	North Dakota	67.4 (1.4)
Wisconsin	62.4 (0.4)	Iowa	61.6 (1.1)	Massachusetts	66.9 (0.5)
Delaware	62.3 (1.4)	New Jersey	61.1 (0.7)	Delaware	66.6 (1.5)
New Jersey	62.0 (0.4)	Nebraska	60.6 (1.6)	New Jersey	66.2 (0.4)
North Dakota	61.5 (1.2)	Wyoming	60.5 (3.1)	Hawaii	66.0 (1.2)
Iowa	60.8 (0.6)	Delaware	59.7 (2.7)	Nebraska	66.0 (0.9)
Michigan	60.7 (0.4)	Connecticut	59.6 (1.3)	Maryland	65.8 (0.6)
Connecticut	60.1 (0.6)	Maryland	59.2 (1.1)	Pennsylvania	64.9 (0.3)
Nebraska	59.7 (0.7)	Maine	58.9 (1.8)	Connecticut	64.6 (0.6)
Virginia	59.6 (0.4)	Pennsylvania	58.5 (0.6)	Kansas	64.6 (0.7)
Pennsylvania	59.3 (0.3)	Michigan	58.1 (0.6)	Indiana	64.1 (0.6)
Indiana	59.0 (0.5)	Indiana	57.5 (1.0)	Michigan	63.4 (0.4)
Ohio	58.9 (0.4)	Ohio	57.3 (0.7)	Ohio	63.4 (0.4)
Illinois	58.7 (0.4)	Illinois	57.1 (0.7)	Virginia	63.4 (0.5)
Kansas	58.6 (0.6)	Virginia	57.0 (0.8)	Illinois	63.2 (0.5)
District of Columbia	58.2 (1.5)	Kansas	56.9 (1.2)	Missouri	62.5 (0.6)
Wyoming	57.2 (1.6)	Rhode Island	56.6 (2.3)	Wyoming	62.5 (1.8)
Washington	57.1 (0.5)	Missouri	55.7 (1.2)	South Dakota	62.0 (1.3)
Missouri	56.9 (0.5)	Hawaii	55.2 (1.9)	Rhode Island	61.9 (1.3)
Rhode Island	56.9 (1.2)	South Dakota	55.0 (2.1)	Washington	61.7 (0.5)
New York	55.9 (0.3)	Washington	53.9 (0.9)	Maine	61.5 (1.1)
South Dakota	55.6 (1.1)	Nevada	53.2 (1.5)	Colorado	59.5 (0.5)
Colorado	55.4 (0.5)	Oregon	53.0 (1.2)	District of Columbia	59.3 (1.6)
Maine	55.2 (0.9)	Colorado	52.5 (1.1)	United States	59.1 (0.1)
United States	55.0 (0.1)	United States	52.0 (0.2)	New York	59.0 (0.3)
Nevada	53.9 (0.7)	Idaho	51.8 (2.0)	Nevada	58.7 (0.8)
Georgia	53.7 (0.4)	New York	51.7 (0.5)	Oregon	58.3 (0.7)
Kentucky	53.3 (0.6)	Tennessee	50.4 (1.1)	Idaho	57.9 (1.2)
Alabama	53.2 (0.6)	Kentucky	49.9 (1.2)	Tennessee	57.9 (0.6)
Oregon	53.0 (0.6)	Arizona	49.2 (1.0)	Vermont	57.7 (1.5)
Tennessee	53.0 (0.5)	Vermont	49.1 (2.3)	Alabama	57.0 (0.7)
Vermont	53.0 (1.3)	West Virginia	49.1 (1.6)	Georgia	56.9 (0.5)
Idaho	52.8 (1.1)	California	48.8 (0.4)	Kentucky	56.9 (0.6)
West Virginia	52.4 (0.9)	Georgia	48.5 (0.9)	North Carolina	55.8 (0.5)
California	52.0 (0.2)	Alabama	47.3 (1.2)	South Carolina	55.5 (0.6)
North Carolina	51.8 (0.4)	South Carolina	47.0 (1.1)	West Virginia	55.5 (1.0)
Texas	51.5 (0.3)	North Carolina	46.0 (0.8)	California	55.4 (0.2)
Alaska	51.4 (1.4)	Texas	45.7 (0.5)	Arizona	55.2 (0.6)
South Carolina	51.3 (0.6)	Montana	44.7 (2.4)	Texas	54.4 (0.3)
Oklahoma	50.6 (0.5)	Oklahoma	44.4 (1.0)	Oklahoma	54.2 (0.5)
Arizona	50.1 (0.5)	Alaska	43.5 (2.4)	Montana	54.0 (1.4)
Louisiana	49.1 (0.6)	Louisiana	42.7 (1.2)	Louisiana	52.2 (0.7)
Montana	48.5 (1.2)	District of Columbia	42.4 (3.3)	Alaska	52.0 (1.5)
Arkansas	46.7 (0.7)	Florida	41.3 (0.6)	Arkansas	51.4 (0.8)
Mississippi	46.7 (0.8)	Arkansas	40.3 (1.4)	Mississippi	51.1 (0.9)
Florida	45.0 (0.3)	Mississippi	39.6 (1.2)	Florida	50.2 (0.4)
New Mexico	43.2 (1.1)	New Mexico	37.1 (1.7)	New Mexico	45.7 (1.2)

Note: Numbers in thousands; Figures cover civilian noninstitutionalized population in 2017; N/A indicates that data was not available; Z represents or rounds to zero; Margin of error appears in parenthesis and is calculated using replicate weights.
Source: U.S. Census Bureau, American Community Survey, Table HIC-4_ACS. Health Insurance Coverage Status and Type of Coverage by State—All People: 2008 to 2017, Table HIC-5_ACS. Health Insurance Coverage Status and Type of Coverage by State—Children Under 18: 2008 to 2017, Table HIC-6_ACS. Health Insurance Coverage Status and Type of Coverage by State—Persons Under 65: 2008 to 2017

Covered by Private Health Insurance: Direct Purchase

All Persons		Under 18 Years		Under 65 Years	
State	Percent	State	Percent	State	Percent
North Dakota	19.0 (0.6)	District of Columbia	11.9 (2.5)	Florida	14.4 (0.2)
Montana	18.7 (0.8)	New York	10.9 (0.4)	District of Columbia	14.2 (1.1)
South Dakota	17.8 (0.8)	Montana	10.3 (1.5)	Montana	13.9 (0.9)
Florida	17.1 (0.2)	Utah	10.2 (0.8)	North Dakota	13.7 (0.7)
Idaho	17.0 (0.7)	North Dakota	10.1 (1.4)	Idaho	12.8 (0.7)
Nebraska	17.0 (0.5)	Florida	9.8 (0.4)	South Dakota	12.8 (0.9)
Iowa	16.9 (0.4)	South Dakota	9.2 (1.1)	Utah	12.8 (0.5)
Kansas	16.7 (0.4)	Idaho	9.0 (1.1)	Nebraska	12.4 (0.5)
Maine	15.9 (0.6)	Nebraska	8.5 (0.8)	Virginia	11.5 (0.3)
Oregon	15.6 (0.3)	Virginia	8.4 (0.4)	Kansas	11.4 (0.4)
Wyoming	15.6 (0.9)	Wyoming	8.4 (1.5)	Maine	11.4 (0.6)
District of Columbia	15.4 (1.1)	Colorado	8.3 (0.6)	Colorado	11.3 (0.4)
Minnesota	15.3 (0.2)	Kansas	8.1 (0.6)	North Carolina	11.3 (0.3)
Pennsylvania	15.2 (0.2)	California	7.9 (0.2)	New York	11.1 (0.2)
North Carolina	15.1 (0.3)	Missouri	7.9 (0.5)	Wyoming	11.0 (0.9)
Vermont	14.9 (0.9)	Iowa	7.8 (0.5)	California	10.9 (0.1)
Virginia	14.9 (0.3)	Maine	7.7 (1.0)	Oregon	10.9 (0.3)
Arkansas	14.6 (0.4)	Rhode Island	7.6 (1.4)	Iowa	10.8 (0.4)
Utah	14.6 (0.5)	Arizona	7.5 (0.5)	Rhode Island	10.7 (0.9)
Wisconsin	14.5 (0.3)	North Carolina	7.5 (0.4)	Alabama	10.6 (0.4)
Missouri	14.4 (0.3)	Oregon	7.5 (0.6)	Missouri	10.6 (0.3)
New Hampshire	14.4 (0.6)	United States	7.3 (0.1)	Arkansas	10.4 (0.4)
Rhode Island	14.4 (0.9)	Mississippi	7.1 (0.7)	United States	10.3 (0.1)
Alabama	14.0 (0.3)	Massachusetts	7.0 (0.4)	Vermont	10.2 (0.9)
Colorado	13.9 (0.3)	Washington	7.0 (0.5)	Georgia	10.1 (0.3)
South Carolina	13.8 (0.3)	Connecticut	6.9 (0.6)	South Carolina	10.1 (0.3)
Tennessee	13.5 (0.3)	New Jersey	6.9 (0.4)	Connecticut	9.9 (0.3)
United States	13.5 (0.1)	Oklahoma	6.7 (0.5)	Mississippi	9.9 (0.4)
Washington	13.5 (0.3)	Pennsylvania	6.7 (0.3)	Pennsylvania	9.8 (0.2)
Indiana	13.4 (0.3)	Alabama	6.6 (0.6)	Massachusetts	9.7 (0.3)
Oklahoma	13.4 (0.3)	Minnesota	6.6 (0.4)	Oklahoma	9.7 (0.3)
Arizona	13.3 (0.3)	Georgia	6.5 (0.4)	Tennessee	9.7 (0.3)
Connecticut	13.3 (0.3)	Hawaii	6.5 (0.9)	Washington	9.7 (0.3)
Massachusetts	13.3 (0.3)	Nevada	6.5 (0.7)	Louisiana	9.5 (0.4)
Mississippi	13.3 (0.4)	Maryland	6.4 (0.4)	Arizona	9.4 (0.3)
New York	13.2 (0.2)	Tennessee	6.4 (0.4)	Illinois	9.4 (0.2)
Illinois	13.1 (0.2)	Texas	6.3 (0.3)	New Hampshire	9.4 (0.7)
Michigan	13.1 (0.2)	New Hampshire	6.1 (0.9)	Wisconsin	9.4 (0.3)
California	12.6 (0.1)	Indiana	6.0 (0.4)	Hawaii	9.3 (0.6)
Delaware	12.5 (0.7)	South Carolina	6.0 (0.5)	Maryland	9.2 (0.3)
Georgia	12.4 (0.3)	Illinois	5.9 (0.3)	Minnesota	9.2 (0.3)
Hawaii	12.2 (0.6)	Arkansas	5.8 (0.6)	Texas	9.1 (0.2)
Ohio	12.1 (0.2)	Delaware	5.8 (1.1)	New Jersey	9.0 (0.3)
Kentucky	12.0 (0.3)	Louisiana	5.8 (0.6)	Indiana	8.9 (0.3)
Louisiana	12.0 (0.4)	Michigan	5.8 (0.3)	Michigan	8.9 (0.2)
Maryland	12.0 (0.3)	New Mexico	5.5 (0.8)	Nevada	8.5 (0.5)
New Jersey	11.9 (0.3)	Ohio	5.5 (0.3)	Delaware	8.4 (0.8)
Texas	11.1 (0.2)	Wisconsin	5.5 (0.4)	New Mexico	8.2 (0.5)
Nevada	10.9 (0.4)	Kentucky	5.4 (0.5)	Kentucky	8.0 (0.3)
New Mexico	10.8 (0.5)	Vermont	5.3 (1.1)	Ohio	8.0 (0.2)
West Virginia	10.4 (0.4)	Alaska	5.2 (1.3)	Alaska	6.7 (0.9)
Alaska	7.6 (0.7)	West Virginia	3.9 (0.6)	West Virginia	6.4 (0.4)

Note: Numbers in thousands; Figures cover civilian noninstitutionalized population in 2017; N/A indicates that data was not available; Z represents or rounds to zero; Margin of error appears in parenthesis and is calculated using replicate weights.

Source: U.S. Census Bureau, American Community Survey, Table HIC-4_ACS. Health Insurance Coverage Status and Type of Coverage by State—All People: 2008 to 2017, Table HIC-5_ACS. Health Insurance Coverage Status and Type of Coverage by State—Children Under 18: 2008 to 2017, Table HIC-6_ACS. Health Insurance Coverage Status and Type of Coverage by State—Persons Under 65: 2008 to 2017

Covered by Private Health Insurance: TRICARE

All Persons		Under 18 Years		Under 65 Years	
State	Percent	State	Percent	State	Percent
Alaska	9.8 *(0.9)*	Hawaii	13.5 *(1.1)*	Alaska	9.5 *(1.0)*
Hawaii	9.0 *(0.5)*	Alaska	12.4 *(1.7)*	Hawaii	8.9 *(0.6)*
Virginia	8.0 *(0.2)*	Virginia	8.5 *(0.5)*	Virginia	7.1 *(0.2)*
South Carolina	4.8 *(0.2)*	North Carolina	4.9 *(0.3)*	North Carolina	3.8 *(0.2)*
Alabama	4.5 *(0.2)*	Colorado	4.5 *(0.5)*	Colorado	3.6 *(0.2)*
North Carolina	4.4 *(0.2)*	Kansas	4.4 *(0.5)*	South Carolina	3.6 *(0.2)*
Colorado	4.3 *(0.2)*	Washington	4.3 *(0.3)*	Washington	3.6 *(0.2)*
Mississippi	4.3 *(0.3)*	South Dakota	4.1 *(0.9)*	Kansas	3.5 *(0.3)*
New Mexico	4.3 *(0.3)*	South Carolina	3.9 *(0.5)*	Georgia	3.4 *(0.2)*
Washington	4.3 *(0.2)*	Georgia	3.8 *(0.3)*	Mississippi	3.3 *(0.3)*
Georgia	4.1 *(0.2)*	North Dakota	3.7 *(0.9)*	New Mexico	3.3 *(0.3)*
Kansas	3.9 *(0.2)*	Delaware	3.5 *(0.9)*	North Dakota	3.3 *(0.5)*
North Dakota	3.9 *(0.5)*	Oklahoma	3.5 *(0.4)*	South Dakota	3.3 *(0.5)*
Oklahoma	3.9 *(0.2)*	Maryland	3.4 *(0.4)*	Alabama	3.2 *(0.2)*
South Dakota	3.9 *(0.6)*	Nebraska	3.4 *(0.6)*	Oklahoma	3.1 *(0.2)*
Arkansas	3.7 *(0.3)*	New Mexico	3.4 *(0.6)*	Delaware	2.9 *(0.5)*
Delaware	3.7 *(0.4)*	Wyoming	3.3 *(1.1)*	Maryland	2.9 *(0.2)*
Florida	3.6 *(0.1)*	Mississippi	3.2 *(0.5)*	Wyoming	2.9 *(0.6)*
Wyoming	3.6 *(0.6)*	Montana	3.1 *(0.8)*	Nebraska	2.8 *(0.3)*
Idaho	3.5 *(0.4)*	Alabama	3.0 *(0.4)*	Florida	2.7 *(0.1)*
Maryland	3.5 *(0.2)*	District of Columbia	3.0 *(1.3)*	Montana	2.7 *(0.5)*
Montana	3.4 *(0.4)*	Florida	2.9 *(0.2)*	Tennessee	2.7 *(0.2)*
Tennessee	3.4 *(0.2)*	Maine	2.9 *(0.7)*	Arkansas	2.5 *(0.3)*
Maine	3.3 *(0.3)*	Tennessee	2.7 *(0.3)*	Idaho	2.5 *(0.4)*
Nebraska	3.3 *(0.3)*	Rhode Island	2.6 *(0.9)*	Maine	2.5 *(0.3)*
Nevada	3.3 *(0.2)*	Nevada	2.5 *(0.5)*	Arizona	2.4 *(0.2)*
Arizona	3.2 *(0.1)*	Arkansas	2.4 *(0.5)*	Nevada	2.4 *(0.2)*
Texas	3.0 *(0.1)*	Idaho	2.4 *(0.7)*	Texas	2.3 *(0.1)*
Kentucky	2.8 *(0.2)*	Kentucky	2.4 *(0.3)*	Kentucky	2.2 *(0.2)*
Louisiana	2.7 *(0.2)*	Texas	2.4 *(0.1)*	Louisiana	2.1 *(0.2)*
United States	2.7 *(Z)*	United States	2.4 *(Z)*	United States	2.1 *(Z)*
Missouri	2.6 *(0.2)*	Arizona	2.2 *(0.2)*	Missouri	2.0 *(0.2)*
Vermont	2.5 *(0.4)*	Louisiana	2.1 *(0.3)*	District of Columbia	1.9 *(0.5)*
District of Columbia	2.3 *(0.5)*	Missouri	2.1 *(0.3)*	Vermont	1.8 *(0.4)*
Utah	2.3 *(0.2)*	California	1.6 *(0.1)*	Utah	1.6 *(0.2)*
New Hampshire	2.2 *(0.3)*	Iowa	1.6 *(0.4)*	Rhode Island	1.5 *(0.3)*
Rhode Island	2.2 *(0.3)*	West Virginia	1.6 *(0.5)*	California	1.4 *(Z)*
West Virginia	2.1 *(0.2)*	Utah	1.5 *(0.3)*	West Virginia	1.4 *(0.2)*
Oregon	2.0 *(0.2)*	Vermont	1.5 *(0.7)*	Iowa	1.3 *(0.2)*
California	1.7 *(Z)*	Connecticut	1.4 *(0.3)*	Ohio	1.3 *(0.1)*
Iowa	1.7 *(0.2)*	Ohio	1.4 *(0.2)*	New Hampshire	1.2 *(0.2)*
Ohio	1.7 *(0.1)*	New Hampshire	1.3 *(0.4)*	Oregon	1.2 *(0.2)*
Indiana	1.5 *(0.1)*	Oregon	1.3 *(0.3)*	Indiana	1.1 *(0.1)*
Pennsylvania	1.5 *(0.1)*	Indiana	1.2 *(0.2)*	Connecticut	1.0 *(0.1)*
Minnesota	1.4 *(0.1)*	Massachusetts	1.1 *(0.2)*	Minnesota	1.0 *(0.1)*
Wisconsin	1.4 *(0.1)*	Minnesota	1.0 *(0.2)*	Pennsylvania	1.0 *(0.1)*
Connecticut	1.3 *(0.1)*	New Jersey	1.0 *(0.2)*	Wisconsin	1.0 *(0.1)*
Michigan	1.3 *(0.1)*	Michigan	0.9 *(0.1)*	Illinois	0.9 *(0.1)*
Massachusetts	1.2 *(0.1)*	Pennsylvania	0.9 *(0.1)*	Massachusetts	0.9 *(0.1)*
Illinois	1.1 *(0.1)*	Wisconsin	0.9 *(0.1)*	Michigan	0.9 *(0.1)*
New Jersey	1.0 *(0.1)*	Illinois	0.8 *(0.1)*	New Jersey	0.7 *(0.1)*
New York	0.8 *(Z)*	New York	0.8 *(0.1)*	New York	0.7 *(Z)*

Note: Numbers in thousands; Figures cover civilian noninstitutionalized population in 2017; N/A indicates that data was not available; Z represents or rounds to zero; Margin of error appears in parenthesis and is calculated using replicate weights.
Source: U.S. Census Bureau, American Community Survey, Table HIC-4_ACS. Health Insurance Coverage Status and Type of Coverage by State—All People: 2008 to 2017, Table HIC-5_ACS. Health Insurance Coverage Status and Type of Coverage by State—Children Under 18: 2008 to 2017, Table HIC-6_ACS. Health Insurance Coverage Status and Type of Coverage by State—Persons Under 65: 2008 to 2017

Covered by Public Health Insurance

All Persons		Under 18 Years		Under 65 Years	
State	**Percent**	**State**	**Percent**	**State**	**Percent**
New Mexico	49.2 (0.9)	New Mexico	55.8 (1.7)	New Mexico	39.7 (1.0)
West Virginia	47.6 (0.8)	Arkansas	52.9 (1.4)	West Virginia	35.7 (1.0)
Arkansas	44.4 (0.7)	Louisiana	52.2 (1.2)	Arkansas	34.0 (0.8)
Vermont	44.2 (1.1)	Mississippi	51.2 (1.3)	Louisiana	33.4 (0.6)
Kentucky	43.2 (0.5)	Vermont	50.7 (2.3)	Kentucky	33.1 (0.7)
Louisiana	42.6 (0.5)	West Virginia	49.1 (1.8)	Vermont	32.2 (1.4)
Oregon	39.7 (0.5)	District of Columbia	48.3 (2.8)	California	29.4 (0.2)
New York	39.6 (0.2)	Alabama	45.8 (1.0)	New York	29.3 (0.3)
Mississippi	39.3 (0.6)	Oklahoma	44.4 (0.9)	Mississippi	28.6 (0.7)
Arizona	39.2 (0.4)	Kentucky	44.0 (1.3)	District of Columbia	28.4 (1.2)
Michigan	38.6 (0.3)	California	43.8 (0.4)	Oregon	27.9 (0.6)
Montana	38.6 (1.1)	Florida	43.5 (0.6)	Arizona	27.2 (0.5)
California	38.4 (0.2)	South Carolina	43.2 (1.1)	Alaska	27.0 (1.2)
Rhode Island	38.0 (1.1)	Tennessee	42.1 (1.0)	Michigan	27.0 (0.3)
Alabama	37.8 (0.4)	North Carolina	42.0 (0.8)	Rhode Island	26.9 (1.3)
Ohio	37.6 (0.3)	New York	41.7 (0.5)	Alabama	26.1 (0.5)
Florida	37.3 (0.2)	Montana	41.3 (2.7)	Ohio	26.1 (0.4)
South Carolina	37.2 (0.4)	Oregon	40.6 (1.2)	Massachusetts	25.8 (0.5)
Pennsylvania	36.8 (0.2)	Alaska	39.5 (2.5)	Montana	25.7 (1.3)
Tennessee	36.8 (0.4)	Arizona	39.2 (0.9)	Tennessee	25.5 (0.5)
Massachusetts	36.7 (0.4)	Georgia	39.1 (0.9)	Washington	25.2 (0.4)
Delaware	36.5 (1.2)	Washington	39.1 (1.0)	South Carolina	24.7 (0.4)
Maine	36.2 (0.7)	Texas	39.0 (0.5)	United States	24.4 (0.1)
District of Columbia	36.1 (1.1)	United States	39.0 (0.2)	Pennsylvania	24.2 (0.3)
Washington	35.8 (0.4)	Idaho	38.6 (1.9)	Illinois	23.5 (0.3)
United States	35.5 (0.1)	Michigan	38.4 (0.6)	Connecticut	23.4 (0.7)
Connecticut	35.2 (0.6)	Rhode Island	38.1 (2.3)	Oklahoma	23.4 (0.4)
Hawaii	35.2 (0.7)	Illinois	37.8 (0.8)	Colorado	23.3 (0.5)
Alaska	34.7 (1.1)	Ohio	37.1 (0.8)	Delaware	23.3 (1.4)
North Carolina	34.7 (0.3)	Pennsylvania	36.6 (0.6)	Nevada	23.1 (0.7)
Oklahoma	34.6 (0.4)	Colorado	35.9 (1.2)	North Carolina	22.9 (0.4)
Illinois	34.2 (0.3)	Delaware	35.4 (2.6)	Florida	22.6 (0.3)
Nevada	34.2 (0.6)	Nevada	35.3 (1.5)	Indiana	22.2 (0.5)
Iowa	33.9 (0.5)	Connecticut	34.6 (1.3)	Idaho	22.0 (0.9)
Idaho	33.5 (0.8)	Massachusetts	34.6 (0.9)	Hawaii	21.9 (0.9)
Indiana	33.5 (0.4)	Indiana	34.5 (0.9)	Iowa	21.6 (0.5)
Colorado	33.2 (0.4)	Missouri	34.1 (1.1)	Minnesota	21.6 (0.4)
Minnesota	33.0 (0.3)	Iowa	33.9 (1.2)	Maryland	21.5 (0.5)
Wisconsin	32.7 (0.4)	Hawaii	33.5 (1.8)	Maine	21.3 (0.8)
Missouri	32.4 (0.3)	Maryland	32.7 (1.1)	Georgia	20.6 (0.4)
Maryland	32.2 (0.4)	South Dakota	32.7 (2.0)	Wisconsin	20.2 (0.4)
New Hampshire	31.8 (0.7)	New Jersey	31.9 (0.8)	Missouri	19.9 (0.4)
New Jersey	31.4 (0.3)	Kansas	31.7 (1.1)	Texas	19.9 (0.2)
South Carolina	30.9 (0.8)	Maine	31.6 (1.8)	New Jersey	19.8 (0.3)
Georgia	30.7 (0.3)	Wisconsin	31.5 (0.9)	New Hampshire	18.4 (0.8)
Kansas	29.6 (0.4)	New Hampshire	30.9 (2.0)	South Dakota	18.3 (1.0)
Texas	28.9 (0.2)	Minnesota	30.2 (0.7)	Kansas	17.6 (0.4)
Wyoming	28.3 (1.1)	Nebraska	28.6 (1.6)	Virginia	15.9 (0.3)
Nebraska	27.8 (0.6)	Virginia	27.4 (0.7)	Nebraska	15.6 (0.7)
Virginia	27.8 (0.3)	Wyoming	23.7 (2.6)	Wyoming	15.5 (1.2)
North Dakota	25.8 (1.0)	North Dakota	21.8 (2.5)	North Dakota	13.9 (1.1)
Utah	21.4 (0.5)	Utah	19.4 (1.0)	Utah	12.5 (0.5)

Note: Numbers in thousands; Figures cover civilian noninstitutionalized population in 2017; N/A indicates that data was not available; Z represents or rounds to zero; Margin of error appears in parenthesis and is calculated using replicate weights.
Source: U.S. Census Bureau, American Community Survey, Table HIC-4_ACS. Health Insurance Coverage Status and Type of Coverage by State—All People: 2008 to 2017, Table HIC-5_ACS. Health Insurance Coverage Status and Type of Coverage by State—Children Under 18: 2008 to 2017, Table HIC-6_ACS. Health Insurance Coverage Status and Type of Coverage by State—Persons Under 65: 2008 to 2017

Covered by Public Health Insurance: Medicaid

All Persons		Under 18 Years		Under 65 Years	
State	Percent	State	Percent	State	Percent
New Mexico	33.2 (0.8)	New Mexico	55.5 (1.7)	New Mexico	36.4 (1.0)
Louisiana	28.5 (0.5)	Arkansas	52.3 (1.4)	West Virginia	31.6 (0.9)
West Virginia	27.9 (0.8)	Louisiana	51.9 (1.2)	Louisiana	30.6 (0.6)
Arkansas	27.3 (0.7)	Mississippi	50.7 (1.3)	Arkansas	29.8 (0.8)
District of Columbia	27.0 (1.1)	Vermont	50.5 (2.3)	Vermont	29.8 (1.3)
Kentucky	27.0 (0.6)	West Virginia	49.0 (1.8)	Kentucky	29.4 (0.6)
Vermont	26.8 (1.1)	District of Columbia	47.9 (2.8)	New York	27.6 (0.3)
California	26.6 (0.2)	Alabama	45.3 (1.0)	California	27.5 (0.2)
New York	26.3 (0.3)	Kentucky	43.5 (1.3)	District of Columbia	26.9 (1.2)
Mississippi	24.4 (0.6)	Oklahoma	43.2 (0.9)	Mississippi	25.3 (0.7)
Rhode Island	23.2 (1.1)	California	43.1 (0.4)	Oregon	25.2 (0.6)
Massachusetts	23.1 (0.4)	Florida	43.0 (0.6)	Rhode Island	24.8 (1.3)
Oregon	23.0 (0.5)	South Carolina	42.7 (1.1)	Arizona	24.7 (0.5)
Alaska	22.7 (1.2)	North Carolina	41.7 (0.9)	Michigan	24.6 (0.3)
Arizona	22.5 (0.4)	New York	41.5 (0.5)	Massachusetts	24.4 (0.5)
Michigan	22.5 (0.3)	Tennessee	41.2 (0.9)	Alaska	23.7 (1.3)
Ohio	21.0 (0.3)	Montana	41.0 (2.7)	Ohio	23.3 (0.4)
Washington	21.0 (0.4)	Oregon	40.4 (1.1)	Montana	22.8 (1.3)
Tennessee	20.6 (0.4)	Alaska	39.4 (2.5)	Washington	22.6 (0.4)
United States	20.6 (0.1)	Arizona	39.0 (0.9)	Tennessee	21.9 (0.5)
Alabama	20.5 (0.4)	Washington	38.8 (1.0)	United States	21.9 (0.1)
Connecticut	20.5 (0.6)	Texas	38.7 (0.5)	Alabama	21.8 (0.5)
Montana	20.4 (1.1)	United States	38.6 (0.2)	Connecticut	21.6 (0.7)
Illinois	20.0 (0.3)	Georgia	38.3 (1.0)	Illinois	21.5 (0.4)
Pennsylvania	19.7 (0.2)	Idaho	38.3 (1.9)	Pennsylvania	21.4 (0.3)
Colorado	19.5 (0.5)	Michigan	38.3 (0.6)	Colorado	20.9 (0.5)
South Carolina	19.4 (0.4)	Rhode Island	38.0 (2.3)	South Carolina	20.9 (0.5)
Nevada	18.9 (0.6)	Illinois	37.5 (0.8)	Delaware	20.6 (1.3)
Florida	18.6 (0.2)	Ohio	36.8 (0.8)	Nevada	20.3 (0.7)
Delaware	18.5 (1.1)	Pennsylvania	36.2 (0.6)	Iowa	19.8 (0.5)
North Carolina	18.5 (0.3)	Colorado	35.4 (1.2)	Florida	19.7 (0.2)
Iowa	18.1 (0.5)	Delaware	35.1 (2.6)	North Carolina	19.7 (0.4)
Oklahoma	18.1 (0.3)	Nevada	34.9 (1.5)	Hawaii	19.5 (0.9)
Idaho	18.0 (0.7)	Connecticut	34.4 (1.3)	Indiana	19.5 (0.4)
Indiana	18.0 (0.4)	Massachusetts	34.4 (0.9)	Minnesota	19.5 (0.3)
Hawaii	17.9 (0.7)	Indiana	34.2 (0.9)	Oklahoma	19.4 (0.4)
Maryland	17.9 (0.4)	Iowa	33.7 (1.2)	Idaho	19.2 (0.9)
Minnesota	17.9 (0.3)	Missouri	33.5 (1.0)	Maryland	19.1 (0.5)
Maine	17.8 (0.7)	Hawaii	33.1 (1.8)	Maine	18.3 (0.8)
Georgia	17.4 (0.3)	South Dakota	32.5 (2.0)	New Jersey	18.0 (0.3)
New Jersey	17.2 (0.3)	Maryland	32.0 (1.1)	Wisconsin	18.0 (0.4)
Texas	17.1 (0.2)	New Jersey	31.6 (0.8)	Georgia	17.7 (0.3)
Wisconsin	17.1 (0.4)	Kansas	31.2 (1.1)	Texas	17.6 (0.2)
Missouri	15.0 (0.3)	Wisconsin	31.1 (0.9)	Missouri	16.3 (0.4)
South Dakota	14.5 (0.7)	Maine	30.9 (1.8)	South Dakota	15.4 (0.9)
Kansas	14.1 (0.4)	New Hampshire	30.6 (2.0)	New Hampshire	15.3 (0.8)
New Hampshire	13.8 (0.7)	Minnesota	30.1 (0.7)	Kansas	14.8 (0.4)
Nebraska	13.0 (0.6)	Nebraska	28.3 (1.6)	Nebraska	13.5 (0.7)
Wyoming	12.2 (1.0)	Virginia	26.4 (0.7)	Wyoming	12.8 (1.2)
Virginia	11.8 (0.3)	Wyoming	23.5 (2.6)	Virginia	12.3 (0.3)
North Dakota	11.2 (0.9)	North Dakota	21.4 (2.5)	North Dakota	11.6 (1.1)
Utah	10.8 (0.4)	Utah	19.2 (1.0)	Utah	11.0 (0.5)

Note: Numbers in thousands; Figures cover civilian noninstitutionalized population in 2017; N/A indicates that data was not available; Z represents or rounds to zero; Margin of error appears in parenthesis and is calculated using replicate weights.
Source: U.S. Census Bureau, American Community Survey, Table HIC-4_ACS. Health Insurance Coverage Status and Type of Coverage by State—All People: 2008 to 2017, Table HIC-5_ACS. Health Insurance Coverage Status and Type of Coverage by State—Children Under 18: 2008 to 2017, Table HIC-6_ACS. Health Insurance Coverage Status and Type of Coverage by State—Persons Under 65: 2008 to 2017

Covered by Public Health Insurance: Medicare

All Persons		Under 18 Years		Under 65 Years	
State	Percent	State	Percent	State	Percent
West Virginia	23.0 (0.3)	Oklahoma	1.6 (0.3)	Arkansas	5.4 (0.3)
Maine	22.7 (0.3)	Arkansas	1.4 (0.5)	West Virginia	5.3 (0.3)
Florida	21.7 (0.1)	District of Columbia	1.4 (1.1)	Alabama	5.2 (0.2)
Vermont	21.1 (0.4)	Vermont	1.2 (0.8)	Kentucky	5.0 (0.2)
Arkansas	20.4 (0.3)	California	1.1 (0.1)	Mississippi	4.9 (0.3)
Alabama	20.3 (0.2)	Delaware	1.1 (0.7)	Maine	4.6 (0.3)
Delaware	20.1 (0.5)	Kentucky	1.1 (0.2)	Missouri	4.0 (0.2)
South Carolina	20.0 (0.2)	Georgia	1.0 (0.2)	South Carolina	4.0 (0.2)
Pennsylvania	19.9 (0.1)	Tennessee	1.0 (0.2)	Vermont	4.0 (0.4)
Montana	19.6 (0.3)	Maine	0.9 (0.5)	Oklahoma	3.9 (0.2)
Kentucky	19.5 (0.2)	Maryland	0.9 (0.3)	Tennessee	3.9 (0.2)
New Mexico	19.3 (0.3)	Virginia	0.9 (0.2)	Louisiana	3.8 (0.2)
Mississippi	19.2 (0.3)	Colorado	0.8 (0.2)	New Mexico	3.8 (0.3)
New Hampshire	19.2 (0.3)	Missouri	0.8 (0.2)	Pennsylvania	3.7 (0.1)
Missouri	19.1 (0.1)	Rhode Island	0.8 (0.4)	Michigan	3.6 (0.1)
Michigan	19.0 (0.1)	Florida	0.7 (0.1)	North Carolina	3.4 (0.1)
Oregon	18.9 (0.2)	Idaho	0.7 (0.2)	Delaware	3.3 (0.5)
Arizona	18.7 (0.1)	Kansas	0.7 (0.2)	Indiana	3.3 (0.2)
Hawaii	18.6 (0.2)	Pennsylvania	0.7 (0.1)	New Hampshire	3.3 (0.3)
Tennessee	18.6 (0.1)	United States	0.7 (Z)	Ohio	3.3 (0.1)
Ohio	18.5 (0.1)	Wisconsin	0.7 (0.1)	Florida	3.2 (0.1)
North Carolina	18.2 (0.1)	Alabama	0.6 (0.1)	Georgia	3.1 (0.1)
Rhode Island	18.1 (0.4)	Louisiana	0.6 (0.1)	Rhode Island	3.1 (0.3)
Wisconsin	18.1 (0.1)	Nevada	0.6 (0.2)	Idaho	3.0 (0.3)
Oklahoma	18.0 (0.2)	New York	0.6 (0.1)	United States	3.0 (Z)
Connecticut	17.8 (0.2)	Ohio	0.6 (0.1)	District of Columbia	2.9 (0.5)
Iowa	17.8 (0.2)	South Carolina	0.6 (0.2)	Kansas	2.8 (0.2)
South Dakota	17.6 (0.3)	Indiana	0.5 (0.2)	New York	2.8 (0.1)
Idaho	17.4 (0.3)	Mississippi	0.5 (0.2)	Oregon	2.8 (0.2)
Indiana	17.4 (0.1)	New Hampshire	0.5 (0.2)	Virginia	2.8 (0.1)
Louisiana	17.4 (0.2)	New Jersey	0.5 (0.1)	Wisconsin	2.8 (0.1)
United States	17.3 (Z)	New Mexico	0.5 (0.2)	Arizona	2.6 (0.1)
Wyoming	17.3 (0.4)	Texas	0.5 (0.1)	Connecticut	2.6 (0.2)
New York	17.2 (0.1)	Washington	0.5 (0.1)	Montana	2.6 (0.3)
Kansas	16.9 (0.2)	Connecticut	0.4 (0.2)	Washington	2.6 (0.1)
Massachusetts	16.9 (0.1)	Hawaii	0.4 (0.2)	Wyoming	2.6 (0.4)
New Jersey	16.8 (0.1)	Illinois	0.4 (0.1)	Iowa	2.5 (0.2)
Nevada	16.7 (0.2)	Massachusetts	0.4 (0.1)	Maryland	2.5 (0.2)
Virginia	16.6 (0.1)	Michigan	0.4 (0.1)	Nevada	2.5 (0.2)
Washington	16.6 (0.1)	Montana	0.4 (0.2)	New Jersey	2.5 (0.1)
Minnesota	16.5 (0.1)	North Dakota	0.4 (0.2)	South Dakota	2.5 (0.3)
Nebraska	16.3 (0.2)	Oregon	0.4 (0.1)	Illinois	2.4 (0.1)
Illinois	16.2 (0.1)	South Dakota	0.4 (0.2)	Massachusetts	2.4 (0.1)
Maryland	16.0 (0.2)	Arizona	0.3 (0.1)	California	2.3 (0.1)
Georgia	15.5 (0.1)	Iowa	0.3 (0.1)	Minnesota	2.3 (0.1)
North Dakota	15.4 (0.3)	Minnesota	0.3 (0.1)	Texas	2.3 (0.1)
California	15.1 (0.1)	Nebraska	0.3 (0.2)	Colorado	2.2 (0.1)
Colorado	15.1 (0.1)	North Carolina	0.3 (0.1)	Nebraska	2.2 (0.2)
District of Columbia	13.6 (0.4)	Wyoming	0.3 (0.3)	North Dakota	1.8 (0.2)
Texas	13.4 (0.1)	Utah	0.2 (0.1)	Alaska	1.7 (0.3)
Alaska	12.1 (0.3)	West Virginia	0.2 (0.1)	Hawaii	1.7 (0.2)
Utah	11.6 (0.1)	Alaska	0.1 (0.1)	Utah	1.5 (0.1)

Note: Numbers in thousands; Figures cover civilian noninstitutionalized population in 2017; N/A indicates that data was not available; Z represents or rounds to zero; Margin of error appears in parenthesis and is calculated using replicate weights.

Source: U.S. Census Bureau, American Community Survey, Table HIC-4_ACS. Health Insurance Coverage Status and Type of Coverage by State—All People: 2008 to 2017, Table HIC-5_ACS. Health Insurance Coverage Status and Type of Coverage by State—Children Under 18: 2008 to 2017, Table HIC-6_ACS. Health Insurance Coverage Status and Type of Coverage by State—Persons Under 65: 2008 to 2017

Covered by Public Health Insurance: VA Care

All Persons		Under 18 Years		Under 65 Years	
State	Percent	State	Percent	State	Percent
Alaska	4.4 *(0.4)*	Mississippi	0.4 *(0.2)*	Alaska	3.1 *(0.4)*
Montana	4.2 *(0.3)*	Virginia	0.4 *(0.1)*	Montana	2.1 *(0.2)*
South Dakota	3.9 *(0.3)*	Idaho	0.3 *(0.2)*	Virginia	2.0 *(0.1)*
Arkansas	3.6 *(0.2)*	Montana	0.3 *(0.2)*	Arkansas	1.9 *(0.2)*
Maine	3.6 *(0.2)*	Nevada	0.3 *(0.2)*	Oklahoma	1.9 *(0.1)*
Wyoming	3.4 *(0.3)*	Tennessee	0.3 *(0.1)*	South Dakota	1.9 *(0.3)*
New Mexico	3.3 *(0.2)*	Alabama	0.2 *(0.1)*	Alabama	1.8 *(0.1)*
West Virginia	3.3 *(0.2)*	Delaware	0.2 *(0.2)*	Maine	1.8 *(0.2)*
Idaho	3.2 *(0.2)*	Hawaii	0.2 *(0.1)*	New Mexico	1.8 *(0.2)*
Oklahoma	3.2 *(0.1)*	Kansas	0.2 *(0.1)*	South Carolina	1.8 *(0.1)*
South Carolina	3.2 *(0.1)*	Kentucky	0.2 *(0.1)*	Wyoming	1.8 *(0.3)*
Alabama	3.0 *(0.1)*	Maine	0.2 *(0.1)*	Idaho	1.7 *(0.2)*
Florida	3.0 *(0.1)*	Missouri	0.2 *(0.1)*	North Carolina	1.7 *(0.1)*
Kentucky	3.0 *(0.1)*	North Carolina	0.2 *(0.1)*	Tennessee	1.7 *(0.1)*
Oregon	3.0 *(0.1)*	Oklahoma	0.2 *(0.1)*	Florida	1.6 *(0.1)*
Arizona	2.9 *(0.1)*	Texas	0.2 *(Z)*	Hawaii	1.6 *(0.2)*
Nevada	2.9 *(0.2)*	Alaska	0.1 *(0.1)*	Mississippi	1.6 *(0.2)*
Virginia	2.9 *(0.1)*	Arizona	0.1 *(0.1)*	Nevada	1.6 *(0.2)*
Mississippi	2.8 *(0.2)*	Arkansas	0.1 *(0.1)*	Oregon	1.6 *(0.1)*
Missouri	2.8 *(0.1)*	California	0.1 *(Z)*	Washington	1.6 *(0.1)*
North Carolina	2.8 *(0.1)*	Colorado	0.1 *(0.1)*	West Virginia	1.6 *(0.2)*
Hawaii	2.7 *(0.2)*	District of Columbia	0.1 *(0.1)*	Arizona	1.5 *(0.1)*
Kansas	2.7 *(0.1)*	Florida	0.1 *(Z)*	Colorado	1.5 *(0.1)*
Nebraska	2.7 *(0.2)*	Georgia	0.1 *(0.1)*	Georgia	1.5 *(0.1)*
North Dakota	2.7 *(0.3)*	Illinois	0.1 *(Z)*	Kansas	1.5 *(0.1)*
Tennessee	2.7 *(0.1)*	Indiana	0.1 *(Z)*	Kentucky	1.5 *(0.1)*
Vermont	2.7 *(0.3)*	Iowa	0.1 *(0.1)*	Missouri	1.4 *(0.1)*
Minnesota	2.6 *(0.1)*	Louisiana	0.1 *(0.1)*	North Dakota	1.4 *(0.2)*
Washington	2.6 *(0.1)*	Maryland	0.1 *(Z)*	Louisiana	1.3 *(0.1)*
Colorado	2.5 *(0.1)*	Michigan	0.1 *(Z)*	Nebraska	1.3 *(0.1)*
New Hampshire	2.5 *(0.2)*	Minnesota	0.1 *(Z)*	Texas	1.3 *(Z)*
Georgia	2.4 *(0.1)*	Nebraska	0.1 *(0.1)*	Delaware	1.2 *(0.3)*
Iowa	2.4 *(0.1)*	New Hampshire	0.1 *(0.1)*	Indiana	1.2 *(0.1)*
Wisconsin	2.4 *(0.1)*	New Mexico	0.1 *(0.1)*	Maryland	1.2 *(0.1)*
Delaware	2.3 *(0.3)*	New York	0.1 *(Z)*	New Hampshire	1.2 *(0.2)*
Indiana	2.3 *(0.1)*	North Dakota	0.1 *(0.1)*	Ohio	1.2 *(0.1)*
Ohio	2.3 *(0.1)*	Ohio	0.1 *(0.1)*	United States	1.2 *(Z)*
United States	2.3 *(Z)*	Oregon	0.1 *(0.1)*	Vermont	1.2 *(0.2)*
Louisiana	2.2 *(0.2)*	Pennsylvania	0.1 *(Z)*	Minnesota	1.1 *(0.1)*
Pennsylvania	2.1 *(0.1)*	South Carolina	0.1 *(0.1)*	Wisconsin	1.1 *(0.1)*
Rhode Island	2.1 *(0.2)*	United States	0.1 *(Z)*	Iowa	1.0 *(0.1)*
Texas	2.1 *(Z)*	Utah	0.1 *(0.1)*	Michigan	1.0 *(Z)*
Maryland	2.0 *(0.1)*	Vermont	0.1 *(0.2)*	District of Columbia	0.9 *(0.2)*
Michigan	2.0 *(0.1)*	Washington	0.1 *(0.1)*	Pennsylvania	0.9 *(Z)*
Illinois	1.7 *(Z)*	West Virginia	0.1 *(0.1)*	Rhode Island	0.9 *(0.2)*
Massachusetts	1.6 *(0.1)*	Wisconsin	0.1 *(Z)*	California	0.8 *(Z)*
Utah	1.6 *(0.1)*	Wyoming	0.1 *(0.1)*	Illinois	0.8 *(Z)*
California	1.5 *(Z)*	Connecticut	Z *(Z)*	Massachusetts	0.7 *(0.1)*
Connecticut	1.5 *(0.1)*	Massachusetts	Z *(Z)*	Utah	0.7 *(0.1)*
District of Columbia	1.4 *(0.2)*	New Jersey	Z *(Z)*	Connecticut	0.6 *(0.1)*
New York	1.3 *(Z)*	Rhode Island	Z *(Z)*	New York	0.6 *(Z)*
New Jersey	1.1 *(0.1)*	South Dakota	Z *(Z)*	New Jersey	0.4 *(Z)*

Note: Numbers in thousands; Figures cover civilian noninstitutionalized population in 2017; N/A indicates that data was not available; Z represents or rounds to zero; Margin of error appears in parenthesis and is calculated using replicate weights.
Source: U.S. Census Bureau, American Community Survey, Table HIC-4_ACS. Health Insurance Coverage Status and Type of Coverage by State—All People: 2008 to 2017, Table HIC-5_ACS. Health Insurance Coverage Status and Type of Coverage by State—Children Under 18: 2008 to 2017, Table HIC-6_ACS. Health Insurance Coverage Status and Type of Coverage by State—Persons Under 65: 2008 to 2017

Not Covered by Health Insurance at any Time During the Year

All Persons		Under 18 Years		Under 65 Years	
State	Percent	State	Percent	State	Percent
Texas	17.3 *(0.2)*	Texas	10.7 *(0.3)*	Texas	19.4 *(0.2)*
Oklahoma	14.2 *(0.3)*	Alaska	9.6 *(1.7)*	Oklahoma	16.6 *(0.3)*
Alaska	13.7 *(0.8)*	Wyoming	9.5 *(2.0)*	Florida	15.9 *(0.3)*
Georgia	13.4 *(0.3)*	Oklahoma	8.1 *(0.5)*	Georgia	15.4 *(0.3)*
Florida	12.9 *(0.2)*	Nevada	8.0 *(0.8)*	Alaska	15.3 *(0.9)*
Wyoming	12.3 *(1.2)*	Arizona	7.7 *(0.5)*	Wyoming	14.5 *(1.4)*
Mississippi	12.0 *(0.5)*	Georgia	7.5 *(0.4)*	Mississippi	14.2 *(0.6)*
Nevada	11.2 *(0.4)*	North Dakota	7.5 *(1.4)*	South Carolina	13.2 *(0.4)*
South Carolina	11.0 *(0.3)*	Florida	7.3 *(0.3)*	Nevada	13.0 *(0.5)*
North Carolina	10.7 *(0.2)*	Utah	7.3 *(0.6)*	North Carolina	12.6 *(0.3)*
Arizona	10.1 *(0.3)*	Indiana	6.3 *(0.5)*	Arizona	12.0 *(0.3)*
Idaho	10.1 *(0.5)*	South Dakota	6.2 *(1.0)*	Idaho	11.9 *(0.6)*
Tennessee	9.5 *(0.3)*	Montana	5.8 *(1.0)*	Tennessee	11.2 *(0.3)*
Alabama	9.4 *(0.3)*	Kansas	5.2 *(0.6)*	Alabama	11.1 *(0.4)*
Utah	9.2 *(0.4)*	Missouri	5.1 *(0.4)*	Missouri	10.8 *(0.3)*
Missouri	9.1 *(0.3)*	Nebraska	5.1 *(0.7)*	New Mexico	10.7 *(0.7)*
New Mexico	9.1 *(0.6)*	New Mexico	5.1 *(0.7)*	South Dakota	10.7 *(0.7)*
South Dakota	9.1 *(0.6)*	South Carolina	5.1 *(0.5)*	Kansas	10.2 *(0.4)*
Virginia	8.8 *(0.3)*	Virginia	5.1 *(0.4)*	Montana	10.2 *(0.7)*
Kansas	8.7 *(0.4)*	United States	5.0 *(0.1)*	United States	10.2 *(0.1)*
United States	8.7 *(0.1)*	Maine	4.9 *(0.7)*	Virginia	10.2 *(0.3)*
Montana	8.5 *(0.5)*	Mississippi	4.8 *(0.7)*	Utah	10.1 *(0.4)*
Louisiana	8.4 *(0.3)*	North Carolina	4.8 *(0.3)*	Maine	10.0 *(0.6)*
Nebraska	8.3 *(0.4)*	Idaho	4.6 *(0.7)*	Louisiana	9.7 *(0.3)*
Indiana	8.2 *(0.3)*	Ohio	4.5 *(0.4)*	Nebraska	9.6 *(0.5)*
Maine	8.1 *(0.5)*	Arkansas	4.4 *(0.6)*	Indiana	9.5 *(0.3)*
Arkansas	7.9 *(0.3)*	Pennsylvania	4.4 *(0.3)*	Arkansas	9.3 *(0.4)*
New Jersey	7.7 *(0.2)*	Tennessee	4.4 *(0.5)*	New Jersey	9.0 *(0.2)*
Colorado	7.5 *(0.2)*	Colorado	4.3 *(0.4)*	North Dakota	8.8 *(0.8)*
North Dakota	7.5 *(0.6)*	Wisconsin	3.9 *(0.3)*	Colorado	8.6 *(0.3)*
California	7.2 *(0.1)*	Kentucky	3.8 *(0.6)*	Oregon	8.2 *(0.4)*
Illinois	6.8 *(0.2)*	Maryland	3.8 *(0.4)*	California	8.1 *(0.1)*
Oregon	6.8 *(0.3)*	New Jersey	3.7 *(0.3)*	Illinois	7.8 *(0.2)*
Maryland	6.1 *(0.2)*	Oregon	3.6 *(0.5)*	West Virginia	7.5 *(0.5)*
Washington	6.1 *(0.2)*	Delaware	3.5 *(1.0)*	Washington	7.1 *(0.2)*
West Virginia	6.1 *(0.4)*	Minnesota	3.4 *(0.3)*	Maryland	7.0 *(0.3)*
Ohio	6.0 *(0.2)*	Alabama	3.1 *(0.4)*	Ohio	7.0 *(0.2)*
New Hampshire	5.8 *(0.4)*	California	3.1 *(0.1)*	New Hampshire	6.9 *(0.5)*
New York	5.7 *(0.1)*	Connecticut	3.1 *(0.5)*	New York	6.6 *(0.2)*
Connecticut	5.5 *(0.3)*	Iowa	3.1 *(0.4)*	Pennsylvania	6.6 *(0.2)*
Pennsylvania	5.5 *(0.2)*	Louisiana	3.1 *(0.4)*	Connecticut	6.4 *(0.4)*
Delaware	5.4 *(0.6)*	Michigan	3.0 *(0.2)*	Delaware	6.4 *(0.7)*
Kentucky	5.4 *(0.3)*	Illinois	2.9 *(0.2)*	Wisconsin	6.4 *(0.2)*
Wisconsin	5.4 *(0.2)*	New York	2.7 *(0.2)*	Kentucky	6.3 *(0.3)*
Michigan	5.2 *(0.2)*	Washington	2.6 *(0.3)*	Michigan	6.1 *(0.2)*
Iowa	4.7 *(0.3)*	West Virginia	2.6 *(0.5)*	Iowa	5.5 *(0.3)*
Rhode Island	4.6 *(0.4)*	New Hampshire	2.3 *(0.5)*	Rhode Island	5.5 *(0.5)*
Vermont	4.6 *(0.4)*	Hawaii	2.2 *(0.5)*	Vermont	5.5 *(0.5)*
Minnesota	4.4 *(0.2)*	Rhode Island	2.1 *(0.6)*	Minnesota	5.1 *(0.2)*
District of Columbia	3.8 *(0.6)*	Vermont	1.6 *(0.6)*	Hawaii	4.6 *(0.4)*
Hawaii	3.8 *(0.4)*	Massachusetts	1.5 *(0.2)*	District of Columbia	4.2 *(0.7)*
Massachusetts	2.8 *(0.1)*	District of Columbia	1.2 *(0.7)*	Massachusetts	3.3 *(0.2)*

Note: Numbers in thousands; Figures cover civilian noninstitutionalized population in 2017; N/A indicates that data was not available; Z represents or rounds to zero; Margin of error appears in parenthesis and is calculated using replicate weights.

Source: U.S. Census Bureau, American Community Survey, Table HIC-4_ACS. Health Insurance Coverage Status and Type of Coverage by State—All People: 2008 to 2017, Table HIC-5_ACS. Health Insurance Coverage Status and Type of Coverage by State—Children Under 18: 2008 to 2017, Table HIC-6_ACS. Health Insurance Coverage Status and Type of Coverage by State—Persons Under 65: 2008 to 2017

Managed Care Organizations Ranked by Total Enrollment

State	Total Enrollment	Organization	Plan Type
Alabama	30,000,000	Trinity Health of Alabama	Other
Alabama	502,000	Behavioral Health Systems	PPO
Alabama	90,000	VIVA Health	HMO
Alabama	66,000	North Alabama Managed Care Inc	PPO
Alabama	45,000	Health Choice of Alabama	PPO
Alaska	800,000	Moda Health Alaska	Multiple
Arizona	7,800,000	United Concordia of Arizona	Dental
Arizona	3,500,000	Avesis: Arizona	Multiple
Arizona	1,500,000	Blue Cross & Blue Shield of Arizona	HMO/PPO
Arizona	325,000	Mercy Care Plan/Mercy Care Advantage	Multiple
Arizona	175,000	Arizona Foundation for Medical Care	Multiple
Arizona	130,000	Employers Dental Services	Dental
Arizona	115,000	Health Choice Arizona	HMO
Arizona	50,000	Care1st Health Plan Arizona	HMO
Arkansas	2,000,000	Delta Dental of Arkansas	Dental
Arkansas	500,000	HealthSCOPE Benefits	Other
California	118,000,000	Kaiser Permanente Northern California	HMO/PPO
California	30,000,000	Trinity Health of California	Other
California	25,900,000	American Specialty Health	HMO
California	11,800,000	Kaiser Permanente	HMO/PPO
California	11,800,000	Kaiser Permanente Southern California	Multiple
California	7,800,000	United Concordia of California	Dental
California	7,300,000	Managed Health Network, Inc.	Other
California	6,600,000	Dental Benefit Providers: California	Dental
California	6,100,000	Health Net, Inc.	HMO
California	4,000,000	eHealthInsurance Services, Inc.	Multiple
California	3,000,000	Liberty Dental Plan of California	Dental
California	2,900,000	Health Net Federal Services	Multiple
California	2,000,000	First Health	PPO
California	2,000,000	L.A. Care Health Plan	HMO
California	560,000	Partnership HealthPlan of California	Other
California	413,795	CalOptima	HMO
California	390,000	Dental Alternatives Insurance Services	Dental
California	338,000	Pacific Health Alliance	PPO
California	320,000	Care1st Health Plan Blue Shield of California Promise	HMO
California	315,440	Western Dental Services	Dental
California	250,000	Lakeside Community Healthcare Network	HMO
California	250,000	Santa Clara Family Health Foundations Inc	HMO
California	210,000	Central California Alliance for Health	HMO
California	175,000	CenCal Health	HMO
California	150,000	Landmark Healthplan of California	HMO/PPO
California	146,000	Community Health Group	HMO
California	140,000	Alameda Alliance for Health	HMO
California	140,000	Contra Costa Health Services	HMO
California	128,272	SCAN Health Plan	HMO
California	125,000	Premier Access Insurance/Access Dental	PPO
California	123,880	Access Dental Services	Dental
California	120,000	Sant, Community Physicians	HMO/PPO
California	109,000	Health Plan of San Joaquin	HMO
California	97,000	Kern Family Health Care	HMO

State	Total Enrollment	Organization	Plan Type
California	92,000	Western Health Advantage	HMO
California	90,000	BEST Life and Health Insurance Co.	PPO
California	90,000	Dental Health Services of California	Dental
California	87,740	Health Plan of San Mateo	HMO
California	55,000	San Francisco Health Plan	HMO
California	49,000	Sharp Health Plan	HMO
California	17,000	Primecare Dental Plan	Dental
California	14,600	Inter Valley Health Plan	Medicare
California	13,582	Chinese Community Health Plan	HMO
California	12,000	Medica HealthCare Plans, Inc	Medicare
California	1,000	On Lok Lifeways	HMO
Colorado	11,800,000	Kaiser Permanente Northern Colorado	HMO
Colorado	11,800,000	Kaiser Permanente Southern Colorado	HMO/PPO
Colorado	326,000	Colorado Health Partnerships	HMO
Colorado	236,962	Rocky Mountain Health Plans	HMO/PPO
Colorado	60,000	Boulder Valley Individual Practice Association	PPO
Colorado	15,000	Denver Health Medical Plan	HMO
Colorado	5,000	Friday Health Plans	HMO
Connecticut	46,700,000	Aetna Inc.	Multiple
Connecticut	30,000,000	Trinity Health of Connecticut	Other
Delaware	30,000,000	Trinity Health of Delaware	Other
District of Columbia	90,000	Quality Plan Administrators	HMO/PPO
Florida	30,000,000	Trinity Health of Florida	Other
Florida	7,800,000	United Concordia of Florida	Dental
Florida	5,000,000	Coventry Health Care of Florida	HMO/PPO
Florida	3,700,000	WellCare Health Plans	Medicare
Florida	2,000,000	Liberty Dental Plan of Florida	Dental
Florida	340,000	AvMed	Medicare
Florida	340,000	AvMed Ft. Lauderdale	Medicare
Florida	340,000	AvMed Gainesville	HMO
Florida	340,000	AvMed Orlando	HMO
Florida	125,000	Capital Health Plan	HMO
Florida	111,000	CarePlus Health Plans	Medicare
Florida	108,000	Neighborhood Health Partnership	HMO
Florida	45,000	Preferred Care Partners	Multiple
Florida	27,000	Leon Medical Centers Health Plan	HMO
Georgia	30,000,000	Trinity Health of Georgia	Other
Georgia	7,800,000	United Concordia of Georgia	Dental
Georgia	5,000,000	Coventry Health Care of Georgia	HMO/PPO
Georgia	68,000	Secure Health PPO Newtork	PPO
Georgia	15,000	Alliant Health Plans	HMO/PPO
Hawaii	70,000	AlohaCare	HMO
Idaho	30,000,000	Trinity Health of Idaho	Other
Idaho	2,400,000	Regence BlueShield of Idaho	Multiple
Idaho	563,000	Blue Cross of Idaho Health Service, Inc.	HMO/PPO
Illinois	105,000,000	BlueCross BlueShield Association	Medicare
Illinois	30,000,000	Trinity Health of Illinois	Other

State	Total Enrollment	Organization	Plan Type
Illinois	15,000,000	Health Care Service Corporation	HMO/PPO
Illinois	8,100,000	Blue Cross & Blue Shield of Illinois	HMO/PPO
Illinois	6,200,000	Dental Network of America	Dental
Illinois	2,000,000	Liberty Dental Plan of Illinois	Dental
Illinois	1,500,000	OSF Healthcare	HMO
Illinois	1,100,000	CoreSource	PPO
Illinois	750,000	Meridian Health Plan of Illinois	Medicare
Illinois	475,000	Trustmark Companies	PPO
Illinois	316,000	Preferred Network Access	PPO
Illinois	255,494	Health Alliance Medicare	Medicare
Indiana	30,000,000	Trinity Health of Indiana	Other
Indiana	1,000,000	CareSource Indiana	Medicare
Indiana	900,000	Anthem Blue Cross & Blue Shield of Indiana	HMO/PPO
Iowa	50,000	Sanford Health Plan	HMO
Iowa	45,000	Medical Associates	HMO
Kansas	5,000,000	PCC Preferred Chiropractic Care	PPO
Kansas	400,000	Preferred Mental Health Management	Multiple
Kansas	152,000	ProviDRs Care Network	PPO
Kansas	134,000	Advance Insurance Company of Kansas	Multiple
Kansas	95,000	Health Partners of Kansas	PPO
Kentucky	1,000,000	CareSource Kentucky	Medicare
Kentucky	170,000	Passport Health Plan	HMO
Kentucky	136,472	Baptist Health Plan	HMO/PPO
Louisiana	1,300,000	Blue Cross and Blue Shield of Louisiana	HMO/PPO
Louisiana	50,000	Peoples Health	HMO
Louisiana	50,000	Vantage Health Plan	HMO
Louisiana	14,000	Vantage Medicare Advantage	Medicare
Maine	70,000	Martin's Point HealthCare	Multiple
Maryland	30,000,000	Trinity Health of Maryland	Other
Maryland	17,000,000	Spectera Eyecare Networks	Multiple
Maryland	7,800,000	United Concordia of Maryland	Dental
Maryland	6,600,000	Dental Benefit Providers	Dental
Maryland	3,500,000	Avesis: Maryland	PPO
Maryland	3,200,000	CareFirst BlueCross BlueShield	HMO/PPO
Maryland	614,350	Kaiser Permanente Mid-Atlantic	Multiple
Maryland	205,000	American Postal Workers Union (APWU) Health Plan	PPO
Maryland	185,000	Priority Partners Health Plans	HMO
Maryland	10,000	Denta-Chek of Maryland	Dental
Massachusetts	30,000,000	Trinity Health of Massachusetts	Other
Massachusetts	14,000,000	Dentaquest	Dental
Massachusetts	3,500,000	Avesis: Massachusetts	PPO
Massachusetts	3,000,000	Blue Cross & Blue Shield of Massachusetts	HMO
Massachusetts	737,411	Tufts Health Plan	Multiple
Massachusetts	430,000	Neighborhood Health Plan	HMO
Massachusetts	250,000	Araz Group	PPO
Massachusetts	240,890	Medical Center Healthnet Plan	HMO
Massachusetts	200,000	Health New England	HMO/PPO

State	Total Enrollment	Organization	Plan Type
Michigan	30,000,000	Trinity Health	Other
Michigan	30,000,000	Trinity Health of Michigan	Other
Michigan	14,100,000	Delta Dental of Michigan	Dental
Michigan	7,800,000	United Concordia of Michigan	Dental
Michigan	5,800,000	Blue Cross Blue Shield of Michigan	Multiple
Michigan	4,500,000	DenteMax	Dental
Michigan	2,500,000	Cofinity	PPO
Michigan	807,000	Blue Care Network of Michigan	HMO
Michigan	750,000	Meridian Health Plan	HMO
Michigan	650,000	HAP-Health Alliance Plan: Flint	HMO/PPO
Michigan	650,000	Health Alliance Plan	HMO/PPO
Michigan	596,220	Priority Health	HMO
Michigan	390,000	SVS Vision	Vision
Michigan	383,000	Health Alliance Medicare	Medicare
Michigan	187,000	Paramount Care of Michigan	HMO/PPO
Michigan	130,000	Golden Dental Plans	Dental
Michigan	90,000	Total Health Care	HMO
Michigan	68,942	Physicians Health Plan of Mid-Michigan	HMO/PPO
Michigan	47,000	Upper Peninsula Health Plan	HMO
Michigan	17,000	ConnectCare	PPO
Michigan	14,000	HAP-Health Alliance Plan: Senior Medicare Plan	Medicare
Minnesota	70,000,000	UnitedHealth Group	Medicare
Minnesota	3,500,000	Avesis: Minnesota	PPO
Minnesota	2,700,000	Blue Cross & Blue Shield of Minnesota	HMO
Minnesota	1,700,000	Medica	HMO
Minnesota	147,000	UCare	Multiple
Minnesota	10,500	Hennepin Health	HMO
Mississippi	155,070	Health Link PPO	PPO
Missouri	11,000,000	Centene Corporation	HMO/PPO
Missouri	3,000,000	Liberty Dental Plan of Missouri	Dental
Missouri	1,700,000	Dental Health Alliance	Dental
Missouri	942,000	American Health Care Alliance	PPO
Missouri	60,000	Essence Healthcare	Medicare
Missouri	49,976	Children's Mercy Pediatric Care Network	HMO
Missouri	5,000	Cox Healthplans	HMO/PPO
Montana	250,000	Blue Cross & Blue Shield of Montana	HMO
Montana	80,000	First Choice Health	PPO
Nebraska	5,000,000	Coventry Health Care of Nebraska	HMO/PPO
Nebraska	717,000	Blue Cross & Blue Shield of Nebraska	PPO
Nebraska	615,000	Midlands Choice	PPO
Nebraska	54,418	Mutual of Omaha Health Plans	HMO/PPO
Nevada	2,000,000	Liberty Dental Plan of Nevada	Dental
Nevada	418,000	Health Plan of Nevada	HMO
Nevada	150,000	Nevada Preferred Healthcare Providers	PPO
Nevada	32,000	Hometown Health Plan	Multiple
New Jersey	30,000,000	Trinity Health of New Jersey	Other
New Jersey	3,000,000	Liberty Dental Plan of New Jersey	Dental
New Jersey	975,000	CHN PPO	PPO
New Jersey	750,000	QualCare	Multiple

State	Total Enrollment	Organization	Plan Type
New Jersey	727,000	Horizon NJ Health	PPO
New Jersey	265,000	AmeriHealth New Jersey	HMO/PPO
New Jersey	150,000	Atlanticare Health Plans	HMO/PPO
New Mexico	7,800,000	United Concordia of New Mexico	Dental
New Mexico	400,000	Presbyterian Health Plan	HMO
New Mexico	367,000	Blue Cross & Blue Shield of New Mexico	HMO/PPO
New York	55,000,000	Davis Vision	Vision
New York	30,000,000	Trinity Health of New York	Other
New York	7,800,000	United Concordia of New York	Dental
New York	3,500,000	Healthplex	Dental
New York	2,000,000	Liberty Dental Plan of New York	Dental
New York	2,000,000	Universal American Medicare Plans	Medicare
New York	1,500,000	Excellus BlueCross BlueShield	HMO
New York	1,500,000	Univera Healthcare	HMO
New York	1,326,000	MagnaCare	PPO
New York	700,000	MVP Health Care	Multiple
New York	625,000	Fidelis Care	Multiple
New York	555,405	BlueCross BlueShield of Western New York	HMO/PPO
New York	400,000	CDPHP Medicare Plan	Medicare
New York	365,000	Independent Health	HMO/PPO
New York	350,000	CDPHP: Capital District Physicians' Health Plan	HMO/PPO
New York	332,128	MetroPlus Health Plan	Medicare
New York	210,000	Nova Healthcare Administrators	Multiple
New York	205,677	Guardian Life Insurance Company of America	HMO/PPO
New York	193,498	BlueShield of Northeastern New York	HMO/PPO
New York	154,162	Aetna Health of New York	HMO/PPO
New York	134,837	Affinity Health Plan	HMO
New York	53,000	GHI Medicare Plan	Medicare
New York	52,000	Island Group Administration, Inc.	PPO
New York	19,000	Quality Health Plans of New York	Medicare
New York	16,000	Elderplan	Medicare
North Carolina	7,800,000	United Concordia of North Carolina	Dental
North Carolina	5,000,000	Coventry Health Care of the Carolinas	HMO/PPO
North Carolina	3,890,000	Blue Cross Blue Shield of North Carolina	HMO/PPO
North Carolina	670,000	MedCost	PPO
North Carolina	40,000	Crescent Health Solutions	PPO
North Carolina	13,000	FirstCarolinaCare	HMO
North Dakota	1,600,000	Medica: North Dakota	HMO
North Dakota	1,000	Heart of America Health Plan	HMO
Ohio	43,000,000	EyeMed Vision Care	Vision
Ohio	30,000,000	Trinity Health of Ohio	Other
Ohio	1,000,000	CareSource Ohio	Medicare
Ohio	500,000	Aultcare Corporation	HMO/PPO
Ohio	380,000	The Health Plan of the Ohio Valley/Mountaineer Region	HMO/PPO
Ohio	370,000	Ohio Health Choice	PPO
Ohio	300,000	The Dental Care Plus Group	Multiple
Ohio	187,000	Paramount Elite Medicare Plan	Medicare
Ohio	187,000	Paramount Health Care	HMO/PPO
Ohio	144,000	Medical Mutual Services	PPO
Ohio	100,000	OhioHealth Group	PPO
Ohio	55,000	MediGold	Medicare

State	Total Enrollment	Organization	Plan Type
Ohio	52,000	Ohio State University Health Plan Inc.	Multiple
Ohio	26,000	SummaCare Medicare Advantage Plan	Medicare
Ohio	20,000	Prime Time Health Medicare Plan	Medicare
Oklahoma	1,000,000	Delta Dental of Oklahoma	Dental
Oklahoma	600,000	Blue Cross & Blue Shield of Oklahoma	HMO/PPO
Oklahoma	500,000	CommunityCare	Multiple
Oregon	7,800,000	United Concordia of Oregon	Dental
Oregon	2,400,000	Regence BlueCross BlueShield of Oregon	Multiple
Oregon	275,000	PacificSource Health Plans	HMO/PPO
Oregon	275,000	PacificSource Health Plans	Multiple
Oregon	250,000	CareOregon Health Plan	Medicare
Oregon	125,000	Managed HealthCare Northwest	PPO
Oregon	54,000	AllCare Health	Medicare
Pennsylvania	30,000,000	Trinity Health of Pennsylvania	Other
Pennsylvania	22,000,000	Value Behavioral Health of Pennsylvania	PPO
Pennsylvania	9,500,000	Independence Blue Cross	HMO/PPO
Pennsylvania	7,800,000	United Concordia Dental	Dental
Pennsylvania	7,800,000	United Concordia of Pennsylvania	Dental
Pennsylvania	5,300,000	Highmark Blue Shield	PPO
Pennsylvania	540,000	Geisinger Health Plan	HMO/PPO
Pennsylvania	265,000	AmeriHealth Pennsylvania	HMO/PPO
Pennsylvania	263,200	Health Partners Plans	Medicare
Pennsylvania	174,309	Valley Preferred	Multiple
Pennsylvania	101,000	UPMC Health Plan	Multiple
Pennsylvania	33,000	South Central Preferred Health Network	PPO
Pennsylvania	2,375	Vale-U-Health	PPO
Puerto Rico	300,000	Medical Card System (MCS)	Multiple
Puerto Rico	180,000	First Medical Health Plan	Multiple
Puerto Rico	126,000	MMM Holdings	Multiple
Puerto Rico	53,000	PMC Medicare Choice	Medicare
Rhode Island	70,000,000	CVS CareMark	Other
Rhode Island	1,018,589	Tufts Health Plan: Rhode Island	Multiple
Rhode Island	600,000	Blue Cross & Blue Shield of Rhode Island	HMO
Rhode Island	190,000	Neighborhood Health Plan of Rhode Island	HMO
South Carolina	950,000	Blue Cross & Blue Shield of South Carolina	HMO/PPO
South Carolina	330,000	Select Health of South Carolina	HMO
South Carolina	205,000	BlueChoice Health Plan of South Carolina	Multiple
South Carolina	30,000	InStil Health	Medicare
South Dakota	60,000,000	Delta Dental of South Dakota	Dental
South Dakota	1,800,000	Wellmark Blue Cross & Blue Shield of South Dakota	Multiple
South Dakota	118,600	DakotaCare	HMO
South Dakota	87,000	First Choice of the Midwest	PPO
South Dakota	63,000	Avera Health Plans	HMO
Tennessee	3,000,000	Blue Cross & Blue Shield of Tennessee	Multiple
Tennessee	518,000	Health Choice LLC	PPO
Tennessee	423,244	Baptist Health Services Group	Other
Tennessee	345,000	Cigna-HealthSpring	Medicare
Tennessee	200,000	Initial Group	PPO

State	Total Enrollment	Organization	Plan Type
Texas	7,800,000	United Concordia of Texas	Dental
Texas	5,427,579	USA Managed Care Organization	PPO
Texas	5,000,000	American National Insurance Company	PPO
Texas	3,500,000	Avesis: Texas	PPO
Texas	3,500,000	Galaxy Health Network	PPO
Texas	3,000,000	Liberty Dental Plan of Texas	Dental
Texas	2,000,000	MHNet Behavioral Health	Multiple
Texas	1,000,000	HealthSmart	PPO
Texas	200,000	Scott & White Health Plan	Multiple
Texas	120,000	Horizon Health Corporation	PPO
Texas	110,000	Community First Health Plans	HMO/PPO
Texas	80,000	Alliance Regional Health Network	PPO
Texas	44,000	Sterling Insurance	Medicare
Texas	42,000	TexanPlus Medicare Advantage HMO	Multiple
Texas	22,000	Valley Baptist Health Plan	HMO
Texas	15,000	Seton Healthcare Family	HMO
Texas	1,000	UTMB HealthCare Systems	HMO
Utah	2,400,000	Regence BlueCross BlueShield of Utah	Multiple
Utah	750,000	Intermountain Healthcare	HMO
Utah	177,854	Public Employees Health Program	PPO
Utah	150,000	Opticare of Utah	Vision
Utah	148,000	Altius Health Plans	Multiple
Utah	86,000	University Health Plans	HMO/PPO
Utah	6,000	Emi Health	HMO/PPO
Vermont	180,000	Blue Cross & Blue Shield of Vermont	PPO
Virginia	68,000,000	Delta Dental of Virginia	Dental
Virginia	24,000,000	Dominion Dental Services	Dental
Virginia	7,800,000	United Concordia of Virginia	Dental
Virginia	3,400,000	CareFirst Blue Cross & Blue Shield of Virginia	HMO/PPO
Virginia	2,800,000	Anthem Blue Cross & Blue Shield of Virginia	HMO
Virginia	430,000	Optima Health Plan	HMO/PPO
Virginia	88,366	MedCost Virginia	PPO
Virginia	30,000	Piedmont Community Health Plan	Multiple
Washington	7,800,000	United Concordia of Washington	Dental
Washington	1,900,000	LifeWise	PPO
Washington	300,000	Community Health Plan of Washington	Multiple
Washington	90,000	Dental Health Services of Washington	Dental
Washington	71,000	Asuris Northwest Health	Multiple
Washington	17,000	Soundpath Health	Medicare
West Virginia	5,300,000	Highmark BCBS West Virginia	PPO
West Virginia	1,000,000	CareSource West Virginia	Medicare
West Virginia	80,000	UniCare West Virginia	Multiple
Wisconsin	247,881	Dean Health Plan	Multiple
Wisconsin	200,000	Care Plus Dental Plans	Dental
Wisconsin	187,000	Security Health Plan of Wisconsin	Multiple
Wisconsin	175,000	Wisconsin Physician's Service	Multiple
Wisconsin	150,000	ChiroCare of Wisconsin	PPO
Wisconsin	130,000	Managed Health Services	HMO
Wisconsin	119,712	Prevea Health Network	PPO

State	Total Enrollment	Organization	Plan Type
Wisconsin	118,000	Network Health Plan of Wisconsin	HMO
Wisconsin	112,000	Physicians Plus Insurance Corporation	HMO/PPO
Wisconsin	90,000	Gundersen Lutheran Health Plan	HMO
Wisconsin	90,000	Unity Health Insurance	Multiple
Wisconsin	80,000	Group Health Cooperative of South Central Wisconsin	HMO
Wisconsin	75,000	Group Health Cooperative of Eau Claire	HMO
Wisconsin	34,000	Health Tradition	HMO
Wisconsin	5,000	Trilogy Health Insurance	PPO
Wyoming	100,000	Blue Cross & Blue Shield of Wyoming	HMO

Managed Care Organizations Ranked by State Enrollment

State	State Enrollment	Organization	Plan Type
Alabama	3,000,000	Blue Cross and Blue Shield of Alabama	HMO/PPO
Alabama	90,000	VIVA Health	HMO
Alabama	45,000	Health Choice of Alabama	PPO
Arizona	1,500,000	Blue Cross & Blue Shield of Arizona	HMO/PPO
Arizona	892,000	Delta Dental of Arizona	Dental
Arizona	325,000	Mercy Care Plan/Mercy Care Advantage	Multiple
Arizona	130,000	Employers Dental Services	Dental
California	8,521,345	Kaiser Permanente	HMO/PPO
California	4,390,019	Kaiser Permanente Southern California	Multiple
California	4,131,326	Kaiser Permanente Northern California	HMO/PPO
California	3,000,000	Blue Shield of California	HMO/PPO
California	585,000	First Health	PPO
California	402,000	CalOptima	HMO
California	250,000	Lakeside Community Healthcare Network	HMO
California	250,000	Santa Clara Family Health Foundations Inc	HMO
California	197,000	Pacific Health Alliance	PPO
California	190,000	Central California Alliance for Health	HMO
California	146,000	Community Health Group	HMO
California	110,000	Alameda Alliance for Health	HMO
California	109,000	Health Plan of San Joaquin	HMO
California	92,000	Western Health Advantage	HMO
California	90,074	Kern Family Health Care	HMO
California	87,740	Health Plan of San Mateo	HMO
California	55,000	San Francisco Health Plan	HMO
California	49,000	Sharp Health Plan	HMO
California	12,283	SCAN Health Plan	HMO
California	6,336	Chinese Community Health Plan	HMO
California	942	On Lok Lifeways	HMO
Colorado	1,000,000	Delta Dental of Colorado	Dental
Colorado	675,279	Kaiser Permanente Northern Colorado	HMO
Colorado	675,279	Kaiser Permanente Southern Colorado	HMO/PPO
Colorado	236,962	Rocky Mountain Health Plans	HMO/PPO
Florida	375,000	Coventry Health Care of Florida	HMO/PPO
Florida	340,000	AvMed	Medicare
Florida	340,000	AvMed Ft. Lauderdale	Medicare
Florida	340,000	AvMed Gainesville	HMO
Florida	340,000	AvMed Orlando	HMO
Florida	141,178	Neighborhood Health Partnership	HMO
Florida	125,000	Capital Health Plan	HMO
Florida	111,000	CarePlus Health Plans	Medicare
Georgia	269,962	Kaiser Permanente Georgia	HMO
Georgia	200,000	Coventry Health Care of Georgia	HMO/PPO
Georgia	68,000	Secure Health PPO Newtork	PPO
Georgia	15,000	Alliant Health Plans	HMO/PPO
Hawaii	700,000	Hawaii Medical Service Association	HMO/PPO
Hawaii	242,978	Kaiser Permanente Hawaii	HMO
Idaho	700,000	Trinity Health of Idaho	Other

State	State Enrollment	Organization	Plan Type
Idaho	563,000	Blue Cross of Idaho Health Service, Inc.	HMO/PPO
Idaho	160,000	Regence BlueShield of Idaho	Multiple
Illinois	15,000,000	Health Care Service Corporation	HMO/PPO
Illinois	8,100,000	Blue Cross & Blue Shield of Illinois	HMO/PPO
Illinois	2,000,000	Delta Dental of Illinois	Dental
Illinois	316,000	Preferred Network Access	PPO
Illinois	240,000	Meridian Health Plan of Illinois	Medicare
Kansas	880,000	Blue Cross and Blue Shield of Kansas	HMO
Kansas	95,000	Health Partners of Kansas	PPO
Kentucky	170,000	Passport Health Plan	HMO
Kentucky	65,428	Baptist Health Plan	HMO/PPO
Louisiana	1,300,000	Blue Cross and Blue Shield of Louisiana	HMO/PPO
Louisiana	50,000	Vantage Health Plan	HMO
Louisiana	4,707	Peoples Health	HMO
Maryland	205,000	American Postal Workers Union (APWU) Health Plan	PPO
Maryland	185,000	Priority Partners Health Plans	HMO
Massachusetts	3,000,000	Blue Cross & Blue Shield of Massachusetts	HMO
Massachusetts	430,000	Neighborhood Health Plan	HMO
Massachusetts	240,890	Medical Center Healthnet Plan	HMO
Massachusetts	200,000	Health New England	HMO/PPO
Massachusetts	160,000	Araz Group	PPO
Michigan	4,500,000	Blue Cross Blue Shield of Michigan	Multiple
Michigan	650,000	HAP-Health Alliance Plan: Flint	HMO/PPO
Michigan	650,000	Health Alliance Plan	HMO/PPO
Michigan	235,000	UnitedHealthcare Great Lakes Health Plan	HMO
Michigan	90,000	Total Health Care	HMO
Michigan	68,942	Physicians Health Plan of Mid-Michigan	HMO/PPO
Michigan	47,000	Upper Peninsula Health Plan	HMO
Michigan	36,000	ConnectCare	PPO
Michigan	20,000	Dencap Dental Plans	Dental
Michigan	14,000	HAP-Health Alliance Plan: Senior Medicare Plan	Medicare
Minnesota	2,700,000	Blue Cross & Blue Shield of Minnesota	HMO
Minnesota	245,000	Americas PPO	PPO
Missouri	1,700,000	Delta Dental of Missouri	Dental
Missouri	860,000	American Health Care Alliance	PPO
Missouri	49,976	Children's Mercy Pediatric Care Network	HMO
Missouri	26,000	Med-Pay	Other
Missouri	1,964	Cox Healthplans	HMO/PPO
Montana	250,000	Blue Cross & Blue Shield of Montana	HMO
Montana	56,000	First Choice Health	PPO
Nebraska	717,000	Blue Cross & Blue Shield of Nebraska	PPO
Nebraska	28,978	Mutual of Omaha Health Plans	HMO/PPO
Nevada	150,000	Nevada Preferred Healthcare Providers	PPO
Nevada	25,576	Health Plan of Nevada	HMO

State	State Enrollment	Organization	Plan Type
Nevada	10,000	Hometown Health Plan	Multiple
New Jersey	3,800,000	Horizon Blue Cross Blue Shield of New Jersey	HMO/PPO
New Jersey	750,000	QualCare	Multiple
New Jersey	467,000	Horizon NJ Health	PPO
New Jersey	150,000	Atlanticare Health Plans	HMO/PPO
New Mexico	400,000	Presbyterian Health Plan	HMO
New Mexico	390,000	Delta Dental of New Mexico	Dental
New Mexico	367,000	Blue Cross & Blue Shield of New Mexico	HMO/PPO
New York	1,500,000	Univera Healthcare	HMO
New York	928,200	MagnaCare	PPO
New York	625,000	Fidelis Care	Multiple
New York	365,000	Independent Health	HMO/PPO
New York	350,000	CDPHP: Capital District Physicians' Health Plan	HMO/PPO
New York	332,128	MetroPlus Health Plan	Medicare
New York	197,194	BlueCross BlueShield of Western New York	HMO/PPO
New York	154,162	Aetna Health of New York	HMO/PPO
New York	134,837	Affinity Health Plan	HMO
New York	72,563	BlueShield of Northeastern New York	HMO/PPO
New York	15,000	Elderplan	Medicare
North Carolina	670,000	MedCost	PPO
North Carolina	187,000	Coventry Health Care of the Carolinas	HMO/PPO
North Carolina	40,000	Crescent Health Solutions	PPO
North Carolina	13,000	FirstCarolinaCare	HMO
North Dakota	2,049	Heart of America Health Plan	HMO
Ohio	380,000	The Health Plan of the Ohio Valley/Mountaineer Region	HMO/PPO
Ohio	370,000	Ohio Health Choice	PPO
Ohio	100,000	OhioHealth Group	PPO
Ohio	73,724	SummaCare Medicare Advantage Plan	Medicare
Ohio	55,000	MediGold	Medicare
Ohio	52,000	Ohio State University Health Plan Inc.	Multiple
Ohio	20,000	Prime Time Health Medicare Plan	Medicare
Ohio	5,151	Aultcare Corporation	HMO/PPO
Oklahoma	600,000	Blue Cross & Blue Shield of Oklahoma	HMO/PPO
Oregon	730,000	Regence BlueCross BlueShield of Oregon	Multiple
Oregon	523,967	Kaiser Permanente Northwest	HMO
Oregon	250,000	CareOregon Health Plan	Medicare
Oregon	54,000	AllCare Health	Medicare
Pennsylvania	2,500,000	Independence Blue Cross	HMO/PPO
Pennsylvania	300,000	Gateway Health	HMO
Pennsylvania	209,211	UPMC Health Plan	Multiple
Pennsylvania	174,209	Valley Preferred	Multiple
Pennsylvania	33,000	South Central Preferred Health Network	PPO
Puerto Rico	180,000	First Medical Health Plan	Multiple
Rhode Island	190,000	Neighborhood Health Plan of Rhode Island	HMO

State	State Enrollment	Organization	Plan Type
South Carolina	950,000	Blue Cross & Blue Shield of South Carolina	HMO/PPO
South Carolina	330,000	Select Health of South Carolina	HMO
South Carolina	205,000	BlueChoice Health Plan of South Carolina	Multiple
South Dakota	340,000	Delta Dental of South Dakota	Dental
South Dakota	300,000	Wellmark Blue Cross & Blue Shield of South Dakota	Multiple
South Dakota	63,000	Avera Health Plans	HMO
South Dakota	25,000	First Choice of the Midwest	PPO
South Dakota	24,310	DakotaCare	HMO
Tennessee	3,000,000	Blue Cross & Blue Shield of Tennessee	Multiple
Tennessee	1,500,000	Delta Dental of Tennessee	Dental
Tennessee	518,000	Health Choice LLC	PPO
Tennessee	106,364	Initial Group	PPO
Tennessee	17,844	Cigna-HealthSpring	Medicare
Texas	4,700,000	Blue Cross & Blue Shield of Texas	HMO/PPO
Texas	3,200,000	Galaxy Health Network	PPO
Texas	1,118,582	USA Managed Care Organization	PPO
Texas	200,000	Scott & White Health Plan	Multiple
Texas	110,000	Community First Health Plans	HMO/PPO
Texas	79,500	Alliance Regional Health Network	PPO
Texas	44,000	Sterling Insurance	Medicare
Texas	12,004	Valley Baptist Health Plan	HMO
Texas	1,500	Dental Source: Dental Health Care Plans	Dental
Utah	330,000	Regence BlueCross BlueShield of Utah	Multiple
Utah	177,854	Public Employees Health Program	PPO
Utah	150,000	Opticare of Utah	Vision
Utah	84,000	Altius Health Plans	Multiple
Utah	65,000	Emi Health	HMO/PPO
Utah	50,000	University Health Plans	HMO/PPO
Vermont	54,023	Blue Cross & Blue Shield of Vermont	PPO
Virginia	2,800,000	Anthem Blue Cross & Blue Shield of Virginia	HMO
Virginia	2,000,000	Delta Dental of Virginia	Dental
Virginia	490,000	Dominion Dental Services	Dental
Virginia	430,000	Optima Health Plan	HMO/PPO
Virginia	88,366	MedCost Virginia	PPO
Virginia	30,000	Piedmont Community Health Plan	Multiple
Washington	300,000	Community Health Plan of Washington	Multiple
Washington	17,000	Soundpath Health	Medicare
West Virginia	500,000	Highmark BCBS West Virginia	PPO
Wisconsin	223,000	Wisconsin Physician's Service	Multiple
Wisconsin	187,000	Security Health Plan of Wisconsin	Multiple
Wisconsin	164,700	Managed Health Services	HMO
Wisconsin	112,000	Physicians Plus Insurance Corporation	HMO/PPO
Wisconsin	90,000	Gundersen Lutheran Health Plan	HMO
Wisconsin	75,000	Unity Health Insurance	Multiple
Wisconsin	67,812	Network Health Plan of Wisconsin	HMO
Wisconsin	40,000	Health Tradition	HMO
Wisconsin	15,706	Prevea Health Network	PPO

State	State Enrollment	Organization	Plan Type
Wyoming	100,000	Blue Cross & Blue Shield of Wyoming	HMO

HMO/PPO Profiles

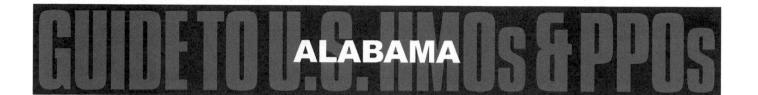
Health Insurance Coverage Status and Type of Coverage by Age

Category	All Persons		Under 18 years		Under 65 years	
	Number	%	Number	%	Number	%
Total population	4,794	-	1,169	-	4,011	-
Covered by some type of health insurance	4,345 *(16)*	90.6 *(0.3)*	1,133 *(6)*	96.9 *(0.4)*	3,565 *(17)*	88.9 *(0.4)*
Covered by private health insurance	3,205 *(27)*	66.9 *(0.6)*	643 *(12)*	55.0 *(1.1)*	2,710 *(26)*	67.6 *(0.7)*
Employer-based	2,552 *(28)*	53.2 *(0.6)*	553 *(14)*	47.3 *(1.2)*	2,286 *(27)*	57.0 *(0.7)*
Direct purchase	671 *(16)*	14.0 *(0.3)*	77 *(7)*	6.6 *(0.6)*	424 *(15)*	10.6 *(0.4)*
TRICARE	215 *(10)*	4.5 *(0.2)*	36 *(5)*	3.0 *(0.4)*	130 *(9)*	3.2 *(0.2)*
Covered by public health insurance	1,812 *(21)*	37.8 *(0.4)*	536 *(12)*	45.8 *(1.0)*	1,047 *(21)*	26.1 *(0.5)*
Medicaid	983 *(20)*	20.5 *(0.4)*	530 *(12)*	45.3 *(1.0)*	875 *(19)*	21.8 *(0.5)*
Medicare	972 *(8)*	20.3 *(0.2)*	7 *(2)*	0.6 *(0.1)*	208 *(8)*	5.2 *(0.2)*
VA Care	142 *(6)*	3.0 *(0.1)*	3 *(1)*	0.2 *(0.1)*	71 *(4)*	1.8 *(0.1)*
Not covered at any time during the year	449 *(16)*	9.4 *(0.3)*	36 *(4)*	3.1 *(0.4)*	446 *(16)*	11.1 *(0.4)*

Note: Numbers in thousands; Figures cover civilian noninstitutionalized population in 2017; N/A indicates that data was not available; Z represents or rounds to zero; Margin of error appears in parenthesis and is calculated using replicate weights.
Source: U.S. Census Bureau, American Community Survey, Table HIC-4_ACS. Health Insurance Coverage Status and Type of Coverage by State—All People: 2008 to 2017, Table HIC-5_ACS. Health Insurance Coverage Status and Type of Coverage by State—Children Under 18: 2008 to 2017, Table HIC-6_ACS. Health Insurance Coverage Status and Type of Coverage by State—Persons Under 65: 2008 to 2017

Alabama

1 Aetna Health of Alabama

151 Farmington Avenue
Hartford, CT 06156
Toll-Free: 800-872-3862
Phone: 860-273-0123
www.aetna.com
Subsidiary of: Aetna Inc.
For Profit Organization: Yes

Healthplan and Services Defined
PLAN TYPE: PPO
Model Type: Network
Plan Specialty: Behavioral Health, Lab, PBM, Radiology
Benefits Offered: Behavioral Health, Dental, Disease
  Management, Long-Term Care, Physical Therapy,
  Podiatry, Prescription, Psychiatric, Vision, Wellness, Life,
  LTD, STD

Type of Coverage
Commercial, Supplemental Medicare, Student health

Type of Payment Plans Offered
POS, FFS

Geographic Areas Served
Statewide

Key Personnel
Sales Executive . . . . Cathleen Coyne
Market Pres., GA/LA/AL/MS. . . . . Frank Ulibarri

2 Ascension At Home

St Vincent's Home Health & Hospice
1400 Urban Center Drive, Suite 240
Birmingham, AL 35242
Phone: 205-313-2800
ascensionathome.com
Subsidiary of: Ascension
Non-Profit Organization: Yes

Healthplan and Services Defined
PLAN TYPE: Other
Plan Specialty: Disease Management
Benefits Offered: Dental, Disease Management, Home Care,
  Wellness, Ambulance & Transportation; Nursing Service;
  Short-and-long-term care management planning; Hospice

Geographic Areas Served
Texas, Alabama, Indiana, Kansas, Michigan, Mississippi,
Oklahoma, Wisconsin

Key Personnel
President. . . . . Kirk Allen
Dir., Home Health Service . . . . Darcy Burthay

3 Behavioral Health Systems

2 Metroplex Drive
Suite 500
Birmingham, AL 35209
Toll-Free: 800-245-1150
www.behavioralhealthsystems.com

Secondary Address: John Hancock Center, 875 N Michigan
  Avenue, Suite 3137, Chicago, IL 60611
For Profit Organization: Yes
Year Founded: 1989
Total Enrollment: 502,000

Healthplan and Services Defined
PLAN TYPE: PPO
Plan Specialty: Behavioral Health
Benefits Offered: Behavioral Health, Psychiatric, Wellness,
  Worker's Compensation, EAP, Drug Testing

Geographic Areas Served
Nationwide

Network Qualifications
Minimum Years of Practice: 5
Pre-Admission Certification: Yes

Peer Review Type
Utilization Review: Yes
Case Management: Yes

Publishes and Distributes Report Card: Yes

Accreditation Certification
AAAHC, TJC, URAC, CARF
Utilization Review, Pre-Admission Certification, Quality
  Assurance Program

Key Personnel
Founder, Chairman & CEO . . . . Deborah L. Stephens
President, Safety First . . . . Danny Cooner
Executive Vice President . . . . Kyle Strange
Chief Financial Officer . . . . Mark Gordon
Medical Director . . . . William M. Patterson, MD
Chief Information Officer . . . . Richard Convington
Vice President, Business . . . . Judi Braswell
Public & Corp. Relations . . . . Shannon Flanagan
  205-443-5483

Specialty Managed Care Partners
State of Alabama, Drummond Co, MTD Products
Enters into Contracts with Regional Business Coalitions: Yes
Employers Coalition on Healthcare Options (ECHO),
  Louisiana Business Group on Health (LBGH), Louisiana
  Health Care Alliance (LHCA)

4 Blue Cross and Blue Shield of Alabama

450 Riverchase Parkway East
Birmingham, AL 35244
Toll-Free: 888-267-2955
www.bcbsal.org
Year Founded: 1936
State Enrollment: 3,000,000

Healthplan and Services Defined
PLAN TYPE: HMO/PPO
Model Type: IPA
Plan Specialty: Behavioral Health, Dental, Lab
Benefits Offered: Behavioral Health, Dental, Physical
  Therapy, Prescription, Wellness

Type of Coverage
Commercial, Individual, Medicare, Supplemental Medicare

Geographic Areas Served
Statewide

Accreditation Certification
URAC

Key Personnel
President & CEO.......................... Tim Vines

5   Bright Health Alabama

219 N 2nd Street
Suite 310
Minneapolis, MN 55401
Phone: 844-426-4086
brighthealthplan.com
Year Founded: 2016
Number of Primary Care Physicians: 1,500

Healthplan and Services Defined
PLAN TYPE: HMO
Benefits Offered: Wellness

Key Personnel
Chief Executive Officer .... Bob Sheehy
Chief Medical Officer .... Tom Valdivia
President.............................. Kyle Rolfing

6   Health Choice of Alabama

2800 University Boulevard
Suite 304
Birmingham, AL 35233
Toll-Free: 866-508-4800
Phone: 205-939-7030
Fax: 205-930-2349
www.healthchoiceofalabama.com
Subsidiary of: St. Vincent's Hospital
Non-Profit Organization: Yes
Year Founded: 1984
Number of Affiliated Hospitals: 90
Number of Primary Care Physicians: 4,600
Total Enrollment: 45,000
State Enrollment: 45,000

Healthplan and Services Defined
PLAN TYPE: PPO
Model Type: Group, Network
Plan Specialty: Chiropractic
Benefits Offered: Chiropractic

Type of Coverage
Commercial

Type of Payment Plans Offered
POS, DFFS, FFS

Geographic Areas Served
Statewide

Specialty Managed Care Partners
Aetna, Superien, MNHO

7   Humana Health Insurance of Alabama

8213 Highway 72 W
Suite C
Madison, AL 35758
Toll-Free: 800-942-0605
Phone: 256-755-3282
Fax: 256-430-3468
www.humana.com
Secondary Address: 2204 Lakeshore Drive, Suite 100,
  Birmingham, AL 35209, 205-879-7374
Subsidiary of: Humana
For Profit Organization: Yes

Healthplan and Services Defined
PLAN TYPE: HMO/PPO
Model Type: Network
Plan Specialty: Dental, Vision
Benefits Offered: Dental, Vision, Life, LTD, STD

Type of Coverage
Commercial, Medicare, Medicaid

Geographic Areas Served
Statewide

Accreditation Certification
URAC, NCQA, CORE

Key Personnel
Market VP, GA/AL................... John Dammann

8   North Alabama Managed Care Inc

699-A Gallatin Street
Suite A1
Huntsville, AL 35801
Toll-Free: 800-636-2624
Phone: 256-532-2755
Fax: 256-532-2756
mamie.sheldrick@namci.com
www.namci.com
Non-Profit Organization: Yes
Year Founded: 1991
Number of Affiliated Hospitals: 100
Number of Primary Care Physicians: 13,000
Total Enrollment: 66,000

Healthplan and Services Defined
PLAN TYPE: PPO
Model Type: Network
Plan Specialty: Group Health
Benefits Offered: Behavioral Health, Chiropractic, Physical
  Therapy, Podiatry, Psychiatric, Vision, PPO Network;
  Radiology; Durable Medical Equipment; Chemical
  Dependency Recovery Facilities; Kidney Dialysis Centers

Type of Coverage
Commercial, Individual

Type of Payment Plans Offered
Combination FFS & DFFS

Geographic Areas Served
North Alabama: Colbert, Cullman, Franklin, Jackson,
  Lauderdale, Lawrence, Limestone, Madison, Marshall,
  Morgan and Winston

Subscriber Information
Average Subscriber Co-Payment:
Primary Care Physician: Varies by plan
Nursing Home: Varies

Network Qualifications
Pre-Admission Certification: Yes

Key Personnel
Executive Director . . . . Sherree Clark
sherree.clark@namci.com
Operations Manager . . . . Brenda Willoughby
brenda.willoughby@namci.com
Services Coordinator . . . . Judy Marks
judy.marks@namci.com

Specialty Managed Care Partners
Enters into Contracts with Regional Business Coalitions: Yes
ECHO

Employer References
Huntsville HospitalSunshine Homes

---

9   Trinity Health of Alabama

Mercy LIFE
2900 Springhill Avenue
Mobile, AL 36607
Phone: 251-287-8420
www.trinity-health.org
Secondary Address: 20555 Victor Parkway, Livonia, MI
48152-7018, 734-343-1000
Subsidiary of: Trinity Health
Non-Profit Organization: Yes
Year Founded: 2013
Number of Affiliated Hospitals: 93
Total Enrollment: 30,000,000

Healthplan and Services Defined
  PLAN TYPE: Other
Benefits Offered: Disease Management, Home Care,
Long-Term Care, Physical Therapy, Psychiatric, Hospice
programs, PACE (Program of All Inclusive Care for the
Elderly), occupational therapy

Geographic Areas Served
Gulf Coast region

Key Personnel
Executive Director . . . . Diane Brown
251-287-8420
dianeb@mercymedical.com
Sales/Marketing Manager . . . . Gemma Campbell
251-287-8427
gemmac@mercymedical.com

---

10   UnitedHealthcare of Alabama

Birmingham, AL 35242
Toll-Free: 888-545-5205
www.uhc.com
Subsidiary of: UnitedHealth Group
For Profit Organization: Yes
Year Founded: 1991

Healthplan and Services Defined
  PLAN TYPE: HMO/PPO
Model Type: Network
Plan Specialty: Behavioral Health, Dental, Disease
Management, PBM, Vision
Benefits Offered: Behavioral Health, Dental, Disease
Management, Long-Term Care, Prescription, Vision,
Wellness, AD&D, Life, LTD, STD

Type of Coverage
Commercial, Individual, Medicare, Supplemental Medicare,
Medicaid, Family, Military, Veterans, Group,

Geographic Areas Served
Statewide

Accreditation Certification
NCQA

Key Personnel
Executive Director . . . . Michael Jones
Senior Analyst . . . . Lisa Powell

---

11   VIVA Health

417 20th Street N
Suite 100
Birmingham, AL 35203
Toll-Free: 800-294-7780
Phone: 205-558-7474
www.vivahealth.com
Secondary Address: Viva Medicare Member Services,
Birmingham, AL , 800-633-1542
Year Founded: 1995
Number of Affiliated Hospitals: 70
Total Enrollment: 90,000
State Enrollment: 90,000

Healthplan and Services Defined
  PLAN TYPE: HMO
Other Type: Medicare
Plan Specialty: Medicare
Benefits Offered: Prescription, Medicare

Type of Coverage
Medicare, Supplemental Medicare

Geographic Areas Served
Statewide

Key Personnel
CEO/President . . . . Brad Rollow
Chief Operating Officer . . . . Cardwell Feagin
VP of Provider Services . . . . Terry Knight
Provider Network Dev. . . . . Megan Schrimsher

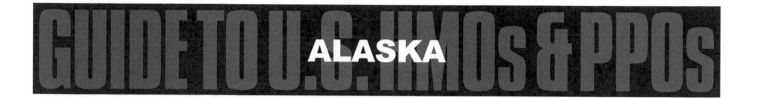

Health Insurance Coverage Status and Type of Coverage by Age

Category	All Persons		Under 18 years		Under 65 years	
	Number	%	Number	%	Number	%
Total population	716	-	194	-	635	-
Covered by some type of health insurance	618 (6)	86.3 (0.8)	176 (3)	90.4 (1.7)	538 (6)	84.7 (0.9)
Covered by private health insurance	453 (9)	63.2 (1.3)	110 (5)	56.4 (2.4)	402 (8)	63.4 (1.3)
Employer-based	368 (10)	51.4 (1.4)	85 (5)	43.5 (2.4)	330 (9)	52.0 (1.5)
Direct purchase	55 (5)	7.6 (0.7)	10 (3)	5.2 (1.3)	42 (6)	6.7 (0.9)
TRICARE	70 (6)	9.8 (0.9)	24 (3)	12.4 (1.7)	61 (6)	9.5 (1.0)
Covered by public health insurance	248 (8)	34.7 (1.1)	77 (5)	39.5 (2.5)	172 (8)	27.0 (1.2)
Medicaid	163 (9)	22.7 (1.2)	76 (5)	39.4 (2.5)	150 (8)	23.7 (1.3)
Medicare	87 (2)	12.1 (0.3)	Z (Z)	0.1 (0.1)	11 (2)	1.7 (0.3)
VA Care	31 (3)	4.4 (0.4)	Z (Z)	0.1 (0.1)	19 (3)	3.1 (0.4)
Not covered at any time during the year	98 (6)	13.7 (0.8)	19 (3)	9.6 (1.7)	97 (6)	15.3 (0.9)

Note: Numbers in thousands; Figures cover civilian noninstitutionalized population in 2017; N/A indicates that data was not available; Z represents or rounds to zero; Margin of error appears in parenthesis and is calculated using replicate weights.
Source: U.S. Census Bureau, American Community Survey, Table HIC-4_ACS. Health Insurance Coverage Status and Type of Coverage by State—All People: 2008 to 2017, Table HIC-5_ACS. Health Insurance Coverage Status and Type of Coverage by State—Children Under 18: 2008 to 2017, Table HIC-6_ACS. Health Insurance Coverage Status and Type of Coverage by State—Persons Under 65: 2008 to 2017

Alaska

12 Aetna Health of Alaska

151 Farmington Avenue
Hartford, CT 06156
Toll-Free: 800-872-3862
Phone: 860-273-0123
www.aetna.com
Subsidiary of: Aetna Inc.
For Profit Organization: Yes

Healthplan and Services Defined
PLAN TYPE: PPO
Other Type: POS
Model Type: Network
Plan Specialty: Behavioral Health, EPO, Lab, PBM,
   Radiology
Benefits Offered: Behavioral Health, Dental, Disease
   Management, Long-Term Care, Physical Therapy,
   Podiatry, Prescription, Psychiatric, Vision, Wellness, Life,
   LTD, STD

Type of Coverage
Commercial, Supplemental Medicare, Student health

Type of Payment Plans Offered
POS, FFS

Geographic Areas Served
Statewide

Subscriber Information
Average Monthly Fee Per Subscriber
   (Employee + Employer Contribution):
      Employee Only (Self): Varies
      Employee & 2 Family Members: Varies
Average Annual Deductible Per Subscriber:
      Employee Only (Self): Varies
      Employee & 2 Family Members: Varies
Average Subscriber Co-Payment:
      Primary Care Physician: Varies
      Prescription Drugs: Varies

Key Personnel
Network Market Head. . . . . John J. Wagner

13 Humana Health Insurance of Alaska

1498 SE Tech Center Place
Suite 300
Vancouver, WA 98683
Toll-Free: 800-781-4203
Phone: 360-253-7523
Fax: 360-253-7524
www.humana.com
For Profit Organization: Yes
Year Founded: 1961
Federally Qualified: Yes

Healthplan and Services Defined
PLAN TYPE: HMO/PPO
Model Type: IPA

Benefits Offered: Behavioral Health, Chiropractic, Dental,
   Prescription, Psychiatric, Transplant, Vision, Worker's
   Compensation

Type of Coverage
Commercial, Individual

Geographic Areas Served
Statewide

Accreditation Certification
TJC, URAC, NCQA, CORE

Key Personnel
Market Manager . . . . Catherine Field

14 Moda Health Alaska

510 L Street
Suite 270
Anchorage, AK 99501-6303
Toll-Free: 877-605-3229
www.modahealth.com
Mailing Address: P.O. Box 40384, Portland, OR 97240-0384
Year Founded: 1955
Total Enrollment: 800,000

Healthplan and Services Defined
PLAN TYPE: Multiple
Other Type: PPO, POS, Dental
Plan Specialty: Dental
Benefits Offered: Chiropractic, Dental, Disease Management,
   Home Care, Inpatient SNF, Physical Therapy, Podiatry,
   Prescription, Psychiatric, Vision, Wellness

Type of Coverage
Commercial, Individual, Medicare

Subscriber Information
Average Monthly Fee Per Subscriber
   (Employee + Employer Contribution):
      Employee Only (Self): Varies
      Medicare: Varies
Average Annual Deductible Per Subscriber:
      Employee Only (Self): Varies
      Medicare: Varies
Average Subscriber Co-Payment:
      Primary Care Physician: Varies
      Non-Network Physician: Varies
      Prescription Drugs: Varies
      Hospital ER: Varies
      Home Health Care: Varies
      Home Health Care Max. Days/Visits Covered: Varies
      Nursing Home: Varies
      Nursing Home Max. Days/Visits Covered: Varies

Accreditation Certification
URAC

Key Personnel
Chief Executive Officer . . . . Robert Gootee
President . . . . William Johnson
Executive Vice President . . . . Steve Wynee
Senior Vice President . . . . Robin Richardson
Senior Vice President. . . . . Tracie Murphy
Senior Vice President . . . . Dave Evans

Senior Vice President . . . . Kraig Anderson
Senior Vice President . . . . Jay Lamb
Strategic Communications . . . . Jonathan Nicholas
    503-219-3673
    jonathan.nicholas@modahealth.com

Key Personnel
  President, West Region . . . . David Hansen

---

15   Premera Blue Cross Blue Shield of Alaska

3800 Centerpoint Drive
Suite 940
Anchorage, AK 99503
Toll-Free: 800-508-4722
www.premera.com/ak/visitor
Secondary Address: P.O. 91060, Seattle, WA 98111-9160
Subsidiary of: Premera
For Profit Organization: Yes
Year Founded: 1952
Number of Primary Care Physicians: 3,300

Healthplan and Services Defined
  PLAN TYPE: PPO
  Other Type: EPO
  Model Type: Network
  Plan Specialty: Dental, Vision
  Benefits Offered: Behavioral Health, Dental, Home Care,
    Inpatient SNF, Long-Term Care, Prescription, Vision, Life,
    LTD, STD

Type of Coverage
  Commercial, Individual, Medicare, Supplemental Medicare

Geographic Areas Served
  Alaska and Washington, excluding Clark County

Accreditation Certification
  AAAHC, URAC, TJC

Key Personnel
  President & CEO . . . . Jim Grazko
  VP, Sales and Service . . . . Lynn Rust Henderson

---

16   UnitedHealthcare of Alaska

5995 Plaza Drive
Cypress, CA 90630
Phone: 657-214-3662
www.uhc.com
Subsidiary of: UnitedHealth Group
For Profit Organization: Yes

Healthplan and Services Defined
  PLAN TYPE: HMO/PPO
  Model Type: Network
  Plan Specialty: Behavioral Health, Dental, Disease
    Management, PBM, Vision
  Benefits Offered: Behavioral Health, Dental, Disease
    Management, Long-Term Care, Prescription, Vision,
    Wellness, Life, LTD, STD

Type of Coverage
  Commercial, Individual, Medicare, Supplemental Medicare,
    Medicaid, Family, Group

Geographic Areas Served
  Statewide. Alaska is covered by the California branch

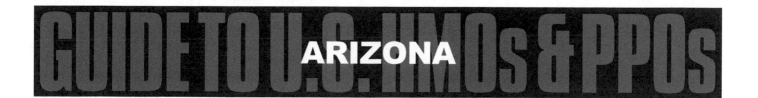
Health Insurance Coverage Status and Type of Coverage by Age

Category	All Persons		Under 18 years		Under 65 years	
	Number	%	Number	%	Number	%
Total population	6,908	-	1,729	-	5,719	-
Covered by some type of health insurance	6,213 *(21)*	89.9 *(0.3)*	1,596 *(10)*	92.3 *(0.5)*	5,034 *(20)*	88.0 *(0.3)*
Covered by private health insurance	4,352 *(34)*	63.0 *(0.5)*	985 *(18)*	57.0 *(1.0)*	3,689 *(33)*	64.5 *(0.6)*
Employer-based	3,460 *(36)*	50.1 *(0.5)*	851 *(18)*	49.2 *(1.0)*	3,158 *(34)*	55.2 *(0.6)*
Direct purchase	917 *(22)*	13.3 *(0.3)*	130 *(8)*	7.5 *(0.5)*	539 *(19)*	9.4 *(0.3)*
TRICARE	224 *(10)*	3.2 *(0.1)*	39 *(4)*	2.2 *(0.2)*	135 *(9)*	2.4 *(0.2)*
Covered by public health insurance	2,705 *(29)*	39.2 *(0.4)*	678 *(15)*	39.2 *(0.9)*	1,557 *(29)*	27.2 *(0.5)*
Medicaid	1,554 *(29)*	22.5 *(0.4)*	675 *(15)*	39.0 *(0.9)*	1,411 *(29)*	24.7 *(0.5)*
Medicare	1,292 *(8)*	18.7 *(0.1)*	5 *(1)*	0.3 *(0.1)*	146 *(8)*	2.6 *(0.1)*
VA Care	198 *(6)*	2.9 *(0.1)*	2 *(1)*	0.1 *(0.1)*	87 *(5)*	1.5 *(0.1)*
Not covered at any time during the year	695 *(20)*	10.1 *(0.3)*	133 *(9)*	7.7 *(0.5)*	685 *(20)*	12.0 *(0.3)*

Note: Numbers in thousands; Figures cover civilian noninstitutionalized population in 2017; N/A indicates that data was not available; Z represents or rounds to zero; Margin of error appears in parenthesis and is calculated using replicate weights.
Source: U.S. Census Bureau, American Community Survey, Table HIC-4_ACS. Health Insurance Coverage Status and Type of Coverage by State—All People: 2008 to 2017, Table HIC-5_ACS. Health Insurance Coverage Status and Type of Coverage by State—Children Under 18: 2008 to 2017, Table HIC-6_ACS. Health Insurance Coverage Status and Type of Coverage by State—Persons Under 65: 2008 to 2017

Arizona

17   Aetna Health of Arizona

151 Farmington Avenue
Hartford, CT 06156
Toll-Free: 866-217-1953
azbenefitoptionsplans@aetna.com
www.aetnastateaz.com
Subsidiary of: Aetna Inc.
For Profit Organization: Yes
Year Founded: 1988

Healthplan and Services Defined
PLAN TYPE: HMO
Other Type: POS
Model Type: Network
Plan Specialty: Behavioral Health, Dental, Lab, PBM, Vision, Radiology
Benefits Offered: Behavioral Health, Dental, Disease Management, Long-Term Care, Physical Therapy, Podiatry, Prescription, Psychiatric, Vision, Wellness, Life, LTD, STD

Type of Coverage
Commercial, Supplemental Medicare, Catastrophic

Type of Payment Plans Offered
POS, Capitated, Combination FFS & DFFS

Geographic Areas Served
Statewide

Network Qualifications
Minimum Years of Practice: 2
Pre-Admission Certification: Yes

Peer Review Type
Utilization Review: Yes

Publishes and Distributes Report Card: Yes

Accreditation Certification
NCQA

Specialty Managed Care Partners
Behavioral Health, Prescription, Dental, Vision

18   AHCCS/Medicaid

1 East Washington Street
Suite 1700
Phoenix, AZ 85004
Toll-Free: 888-724-4018
www.uhc.com
Subsidiary of: UnitedHealth Group
For Profit Organization: Yes

Healthplan and Services Defined
PLAN TYPE: Other
Other Type: Medicaid
Model Type: Network
Benefits Offered: Dental, Disease Management, Prescription, Vision, Wellness

Type of Coverage
Medicaid

Geographic Areas Served
Available in Apache, Cochise, Coconino, Graham, Greenlee, La Paz, Maricopa, Mohave, Navajo, Pima, Santa Cruz, Yavapai, Yuma

Key Personnel
VP, Business Development . . . . Roger Brown
CEO, Community Plan . . . . Joe Gaudio
Medical Director . . . . Leslie Paulus

19   Arizona Foundation for Medical Care

2700 N Central Avenue
Suite 810
Phoenix, AZ 85004-1162
Toll-Free: 800-624-4277
Phone: 602-252-4042
info@azfmc.com
www.azfmc.com
Non-Profit Organization: Yes
Year Founded: 1969
Number of Affiliated Hospitals: 77
Number of Primary Care Physicians: 4,516
Total Enrollment: 175,000

Healthplan and Services Defined
PLAN TYPE: Multiple
Other Type: HMO, PPO, POS, EPO
Model Type: Group, Network
Plan Specialty: Chiropractic, Disease Management, EPO, Worker's Compensation, PPO, POS, Medical Management, Case Management, Utilization Management, Wellness Services, 24/7 Nurse Line
Benefits Offered: Disease Management, Wellness, Maternity Management
Offers Demand Management Patient Information Service: Yes
DMPI Services Offered: 24-Hour Nurse Care Line

Type of Coverage
Commercial, Individual, Indemnity

Type of Payment Plans Offered
POS

Geographic Areas Served
Statewide

Network Qualifications
Pre-Admission Certification: Yes

Peer Review Type
Utilization Review: Yes
Case Management: Yes

Accreditation Certification
TJC, URAC, NCQA

Key Personnel
Administration Director . . . . Kerry Kovaleski
Executive Vice President . . . . Tracey Mitchell

Specialty Managed Care Partners
American Health Holding

20　Avesis: Arizona

10400 N 25th Avenue
Suite 200
Phoenix, AZ 85012
Toll-Free: 800-522-0258
www.avesis.com
Secondary Address: Executive Offic, 10324 S Dilfield Road,
　Owings Mills, MD 21117, 800-643-1132
Subsidiary of: Guardian Life Insurance Company
Year Founded: 1978
Number of Primary Care Physicians: 25,000
Total Enrollment: 3,500,000

Healthplan and Services Defined
　PLAN TYPE: Multiple
　Model Type: Network
　Plan Specialty: Dental, Vision, Hearing, Medicare/Medicaid
　Benefits Offered: Dental, Vision

Type of Coverage
　Commercial, Medicare, Supplemental Medicare, Medicaid

Type of Payment Plans Offered
　POS, Capitated, Combination FFS & DFFS

Geographic Areas Served
　Statewide

Publishes and Distributes Report Card: Yes

Accreditation Certification
　AAAHC
　TJC Accreditation

Key Personnel
　Chief Executive Officer . . . . Chris Swanker
　Finance Director. . . . . Amy Jackson
　Business Development. . . . . Alan Cohn
　Chief Information Officer . . . . Laura Gill

21　Blue Cross & Blue Shield of Arizona

2444 West Las Palmaritas Drive
Phoenix, AZ 85021
Phone: 602-864-4100
www.azblue.com
Secondary Address: Flagstaff Customer Service Officer, 1500
　E Cedar Avenue, Suite 56, Flagstaff, AZ 86004
Non-Profit Organization: Yes
Year Founded: 1939
Number of Affiliated Hospitals: 65
Number of Primary Care Physicians: 1,611
Total Enrollment: 1,500,000
State Enrollment: 1,500,000

Healthplan and Services Defined
　PLAN TYPE: HMO/PPO
　Model Type: Network
　Benefits Offered: Behavioral Health, Chiropractic, Dental,
　　Prescription, Wellness, STD

Type of Coverage
　Commercial, Individual, Indemnity, Supplemental Medicare

Geographic Areas Served
　Statewide

Accreditation Certification
　URAC
　TJC Accreditation, Medicare Approved, Utilization Review,
　　Pre-Admission Certification, State Licensure, Quality
　　Assurance Program

Key Personnel
　Chief Executive Officer . . . . Pam Kehaly
　Chief Strategy Officer. . . . . Beth Ginzinger
　Chief Medical Officer. . . . . Woodrow A. Mayers, Jr.
　Chief Growth Officer . . . . Paige Rothermel
　Chief HR Officer . . . . Greg Wells
　Chief Legal Officer. . . . . Deanna Salazar
　VP & Interim CFO . . . . Bill Arthur
　Media Contact . . . . Jeremy Adler
　　310-360-5782
　　jeremy.adler@dpnww.com

22　Care1st Health Plan Arizona

2355 E Camelback Road
Suite 300
Phoenix, AZ 85016
Toll-Free: 866-560-4042
Phone: 602-778-1800
Fax: 602-778-1863
www.care1staz.com/az
Subsidiary of: Care1st Health Plan
For Profit Organization: Yes
Year Founded: 1994
Total Enrollment: 50,000

Healthplan and Services Defined
　PLAN TYPE: HMO
　Benefits Offered: Disease Management, Wellness

Type of Coverage
　Medicare

Geographic Areas Served
　Maricopa County and Pima County

Accreditation Certification
　NCQA

Key Personnel
　State President. . . . . Scott Cummings
　Director, Operations . . . . Brent Ratterree
　VP, Field Finance . . . . Deena Sigel
　Senior Medical Director . . . . Satya Sarma
　Dir., Sales & Marketing. . . . . Anna Maria Maldonado
　Dir., Quality Improvement. . . . . Nancy DeRosa
　Value Based Partnerships . . . . Kathy Thurman
　Dir., Customer Services. . . . . Mike Ferguson
　Dir., Network Management. . . . . Jessica Sedita-Igneri

23　CareCentrix: Arizona

7740 N 16th Street
Suite 100
Phoenix, AZ 85020
Toll-Free: 800-808-1902
carecentrix.com
Year Founded: 1996
Number of Primary Care Physicians: 8,000

Healthplan and Services Defined
  PLAN TYPE: HMO
  Benefits Offered: Home Care, Physical Therapy, Durable
    Medical Equipment; Occupational & Respiratory Therapy;
    Orthotics; Prosthetics

Key Personnel
  Dir., Network Management . . . . David L. Chartrand

24 Cigna HealthCare of Arizona

509 W Clark Street
Mesa, AZ 85201
Toll-Free: 800-244-6224
Phone: 678-210-6310
www.cigna.com
For Profit Organization: Yes

Healthplan and Services Defined
  PLAN TYPE: HMO/PPO
  Other Type: POS
  Model Type: IPA, Network
  Benefits Offered: Behavioral Health, Chiropractic,
    Complementary Medicine, Disease Management, Home
    Care, Inpatient SNF, Long-Term Care, Physical Therapy,
    Podiatry, Prescription, Psychiatric, Transplant, Vision,
    Wellness

Type of Coverage
  Commercial, Individual, Medicare

Type of Payment Plans Offered
  POS

Accreditation Certification
  NCQA

Key Personnel
  Market President. . . . . Kim Shepard

25 Cigna Medical Group

25500 N Norterra Drive
Phoenix, AZ 85085
Phone: 481-987-6917
CMGservice@cigna.com
www.cigna.com/cmgaz
Subsidiary of: Cigna Corporation
For Profit Organization: Yes

Healthplan and Services Defined
  PLAN TYPE: HMO
  Model Type: Staff
  Plan Specialty: Primary care, pediatrics
  Benefits Offered: Podiatry, Prescription, Vision, After-Hours
    Nurseline, General Surgery, Hearing, Ophthalmology,
    Outpatient Surgery,

Key Personnel
  Chief Financial Officer . . . . Keith Swan

26 Delta Dental of Arizona

5656 West Talavi Boulevard
Glendale, AZ 85306
Toll-Free: 800-352-6132
Phone: 602-938-3131
www.deltadentalaz.com
Mailing Address: P.O. Box 43000, Phoenix, AZ 85080-3000
Non-Profit Organization: Yes
Year Founded: 1972
State Enrollment: 892,000

Healthplan and Services Defined
  PLAN TYPE: Dental
  Other Type: Vision
  Model Type: Network
  Plan Specialty: Dental, Vision
  Benefits Offered: Dental, Vision

Type of Coverage
  Commercial, Individual, Indemnity

Type of Payment Plans Offered
  FFS

Geographic Areas Served
  Statewide

Accreditation Certification
  NCQA

Key Personnel
  President & CEO . . . . Allan Allford
  VP, Financial Officer . . . . Mark Anderson
  VP, Business Development . . . . Brad Clothier
  VP of Operations. . . . . Craig Livesay
  VP of Marketing & Comm. . . . . Scott Pederson

27 Employers Dental Services

3430 E Sunrise
Suite 160
Tuscon, AZ 85718
Toll-Free: 800-722-9772
Phone: 520-696-4343
edscs@exchange.principal.com
www.employersdental.com
Subsidiary of: Principal Financial Group
Year Founded: 1974
Owned by an Integrated Delivery Network (IDN): Yes
Number of Primary Care Physicians: 1,340
Total Enrollment: 130,000
State Enrollment: 130,000

Healthplan and Services Defined
  PLAN TYPE: Dental
  Model Type: Group, Individual
  Plan Specialty: Dental, Vision
  Benefits Offered: Dental, Prescription, Vision, Prepaid

Type of Coverage
  DHMO, Orthodontic

Geographic Areas Served
  Arizona Statewide

Peer Review Type
  Utilization Review: Yes

Case Management: Yes

Accreditation Certification
Utilization Review, Quality Assurance Program

Key Personnel
Chairman, President & CEO . . . . Daniel J. Houston

Specialty Managed Care Partners
Enters into Contracts with Regional Business Coalitions: Yes

---

28   Health Choice Arizona

410 N 44th Street
Suite 920
Phoenix, AZ 85008
Toll-Free: 800-322-8670
Phone: 480-968-6866
comments@healthchoiceaz.com
www.healthchoiceaz.com
Subsidiary of: IASIS Healthcare
For Profit Organization: Yes
Year Founded: 1990
Number of Affiliated Hospitals: 4
Number of Primary Care Physicians: 132
Total Enrollment: 115,000

Healthplan and Services Defined
PLAN TYPE: HMO
Model Type: IPA
Plan Specialty: Services to AHCCCS members
Benefits Offered: Behavioral Health, Dental, Disease
Management, Prescription, Wellness, Care Coordination,
Maternal Child Health

Type of Coverage
Medicaid, Managed Medicaid

Geographic Areas Served
Apache, Coconino, Gila, Maricopa, Mohave, Navajo, Pima,
Pinal counties

Network Qualifications
Pre-Admission Certification: Yes

Peer Review Type
Utilization Review: Yes
Second Surgical Opinion: Yes
Case Management: Yes

Accreditation Certification
URAC
Utilization Review

Key Personnel
Chief Operating Officer. . . . . Troy Smith
VP, Operations . . . . Diana Alvarez

---

29   Humana Health Insurance of Arizona

2231 E Camelback Road
Suite 400
Phoenix, AZ 85016
Toll-Free: 800-889-0301
Phone: 602-760-1700
www.humana.com

Secondary Address: 5210 E Williams Circle, Suite 200,
Tucson, AZ 85711, 520-571-6548
For Profit Organization: Yes
Year Founded: 1984

Healthplan and Services Defined
PLAN TYPE: HMO/PPO
Model Type: IPA
Benefits Offered: Dental, Disease Management, Prescription,
Transplant, Vision, Wellness, Life, LTD, STD

Type of Coverage
Commercial, Individual, Medicare, Medicaid

Type of Payment Plans Offered
POS, Combination FFS & DFFS

Geographic Areas Served
Apache, Cochise, Coconino, Gila, Graham, Greenlee, La Paz,
Maricipa, Mohave, Navajo, Pima, Pinal, Santa Cruz, Yavapai,
Yuma counties

Peer Review Type
Utilization Review: Yes
Second Surgical Opinion: Yes
Case Management: Yes

Publishes and Distributes Report Card: Yes

Accreditation Certification
URAC, NCQA, CORE
TJC Accreditation

Key Personnel
Regional Vice President. . . . . Charles Ritz

Specialty Managed Care Partners
Enters into Contracts with Regional Business Coalitions: Yes

---

30   Magellan Health

4800 N Schottsdale Road
Suite 4400
Scottsdale, AZ 85251
MagellanHealthComInquiries@magellanhealth.com
www.magellanhealth.com
For Profit Organization: Yes

Healthplan and Services Defined
PLAN TYPE: Other
Plan Specialty: ASO, Behavioral Health, Diagnostic imaging
& specialty pharma services
Benefits Offered: Behavioral Health, Long-Term Care,
Prescription

Type of Coverage
Medicare, Medicaid

Key Personnel
Chairman & CEO . . . . Barry M. Smith
Chief Financial Officer . . . . Jonathan N. Rubin
General Counsel . . . . Daniel N. Gregoire
Human Resources. . . . . Caskie Lewis-Clapper
Chief Medical Officer . . . . Karen Amstutz
Chief Information Officer . . . . Srini Koushik

31   Magellan Rx Management

101 Billerica Avenue
Building 4
North Billeria, MA 01862
Toll-Free: 978-856-2345
Fax: 978-856-2335
info@magellandx.com
www.magellanrx.com
Subsidiary of: Magellan Health
For Profit Organization: Yes

Healthplan and Services Defined
   PLAN TYPE: Other
   Other Type: PBM
   Plan Specialty: PBM

Key Personnel
   President & CEO . . . . Amy Winslow
   Chief Operating Officer . . . . Hossein Maleknia
   Director of Sales . . . . Jennifer Zonderman
   Director of Finance . . . . Janine LeBlanc

32   Mercy Care Plan/Mercy Care Advantage

4350 East Cotton Center Boulevard
Building D
Phoenix, AZ 85040
Toll-Free: 800-624-3879
Phone: 602-263-3000
www.mercycareplan.com
Subsidiary of: Southwest Catholic Health Network
Non-Profit Organization: Yes
Year Founded: 1985
Total Enrollment: 325,000
State Enrollment: 325,000

Healthplan and Services Defined
   PLAN TYPE: Multiple
   Other Type: HMO, Medicare
   Model Type: Group
   Benefits Offered: Disease Management, Long-Term Care,
      Prescription, Wellness

Type of Coverage
   Medicare, Medicaid

Geographic Areas Served
   Cochise, Gila, Graham, Greenlee, La Paz, Maricopa, Pima,
   Pinal, Santa Cruz, Yavapai, Yuma counties

Key Personnel
   Deputy CEO . . . . Lorry Bottrill
   VP, Health Operations . . . . John Monte
   Chief Medical Officer . . . . Charlton Wilson

33   NIA Magellan

4800 N Scottsdale Road
Suite 4400
Scottsdale, AZ 85251
Toll-Free: 877-NIA-9762
www.niahealthcare.com
Subsidiary of: Magellan Health
For Profit Organization: Yes

Year Founded: 1995

Healthplan and Services Defined
   PLAN TYPE: Other
   Plan Specialty: Radiology, Radiology benefits management

Key Personnel
   Chief Medical Officer . . . . Michael J. Pentecost
   SVP, Sales . . . . Edie Jardine
   VP, Finance . . . . William F. Henderson
   VP, Client Services . . . . Annalisa Cooper

34   Outlook Benefit Solutions

1550 E McKellips Road
Suite 112
Mesa, AZ 85203
Toll-Free: 800-342-7188
Phone: 480-461-9001
Fax: 480-461-9021
customerservice@outlookvision.com
www.outlookvision.com
Year Founded: 1990
Federally Qualified: Yes

Healthplan and Services Defined
   PLAN TYPE: Vision
   Plan Specialty: Vision
   Benefits Offered: Prescription, Vision, Hearing

Type of Coverage
   Commercial, Individual

Geographic Areas Served
   Available nationwide, except for AK, CT, MT, RI, VT and
   WA

35   Phoenix Health Plan

7878 North 16th Street
Suite 105
Phoenix, AZ 85020
Toll-Free: 800-747-7997
Phone: 602-824-3700
www.phoenixhealthplan.com
Non-Profit Organization: Yes
Year Founded: 1983
Number of Affiliated Hospitals: 28
Number of Primary Care Physicians: 3,780

Healthplan and Services Defined
   PLAN TYPE: HMO
   Model Type: IPA
   Benefits Offered: Behavioral Health, Dental, Disease
      Management, Prescription, Wellness, Nurse Advice Line;
      Transportation

Type of Coverage
   Medicaid

Type of Payment Plans Offered
   POS, Combination FFS & DFFS

Geographic Areas Served
   Maricopa County

Publishes and Distributes Report Card: Yes

Accreditation Certification
NCQA
TJC Accreditation, Medicare Approved, Utilization Review, Pre-Admission Certification, State Licensure, Quality Assurance Program

Specialty Managed Care Partners
Enters into Contracts with Regional Business Coalitions: Yes

36 Pivot Health

29308 N 108th Place
Scottdales, AZ 85262
Toll-Free: 866-566-2707
pivothealth.com
Year Founded: 2015

Healthplan and Services Defined
PLAN TYPE: Other
Other Type: Supplemental

Type of Coverage
Short-term; Supplemental; Zero Dedu

Geographic Areas Served
Alabama, Arizona, Arkansas, the District of Columbia, Florida, Georgia, Illinois, Indiana, Iowa, Kentucky, Michigan, Mississippi, Nebraska, Ohio, Oklahoma, Pennsylvania, Tennessee, Texas, Virginia, West Virginia, and Wisconsin

Key Personnel
Chief Executive Officer . . . . Jeff Smedsrud
VP of Sales & Marketing . . . . Kyle Dietz

37 Preferred Therapy Providers

23460 North 19th Avenue
Suite 250
Phoenix, AZ 85027
Toll-Free: 800-664-5240
Phone: 623-869-9101
www.preferredtherapy.com
For Profit Organization: Yes
Year Founded: 1992
Physician Owned Organization: No
Federally Qualified: No
Number of Referral/Specialty Physicians: 3,000

Healthplan and Services Defined
PLAN TYPE: HMO/PPO
Model Type: Network
Plan Specialty: Physical, Occupational, Speech Therapies
Benefits Offered: Physical Therapy, Ocupational Therapy, Speech Therapy
Offers Demand Management Patient Information Service: No

Type of Coverage
Commercial

Geographic Areas Served
35 states

Network Qualifications
Pre-Admission Certification: No

Publishes and Distributes Report Card: No

Accreditation Certification
NCQA, AAPPO

Key Personnel
President . . . . Steven Allred

Specialty Managed Care Partners
Enters into Contracts with Regional Business Coalitions: No

38 Premier Access Insurance/Access Dental

P.O. Box 659010
Sacramento, CA 95865-9010
Toll-Free: 888-634-6074
Phone: 916-920-2500
Fax: 916-563-9000
info@premierlife.com
www.premierppo.com
Subsidiary of: Guardian Life Insurance Co.
For Profit Organization: Yes
Year Founded: 1989
Number of Primary Care Physicians: 1,000

Healthplan and Services Defined
PLAN TYPE: PPO
Other Type: Dental
Plan Specialty: Dental
Benefits Offered: Dental

Key Personnel
President & CEO . . . . Deanna M. Mulligan

39 SilverScript

P.O. Box 52067
Phoenix, AZ 85072-2067
Toll-Free: 866-362-6212
silverscript.com
Subsidiary of: CVS Health
Year Founded: 2006

Healthplan and Services Defined
PLAN TYPE: Medicare
Plan Specialty: Medicare Part D
Benefits Offered: Prescription

Type of Coverage
Medicare

Geographic Areas Served
SilverScript Choice: Nationwide and the District of Columbia; SilverScript Plus: Nationwide and the District of Columbia, except Alaska

Key Personnel
President & CEO . . . . Larry J. Merlo

40   ## Total Dental Administrators

2111 E Highland Avenue
Suite 250
Phoenix, AZ 85016-4735
Toll-Free: 888-422-1995
Phone: 602-266-1995
Fax: 602-266-1948
www.tdadental.com
Secondary Address: 6985 Union Park Center, Suite 675,
Cottonwood Heights, UT 84047, 800-880-3536
Subsidiary of: Companion Life Insurance Co.

Healthplan and Services Defined
  PLAN TYPE: Dental
  Plan Specialty: PPO, Prepaid
  Benefits Offered: Dental

Type of Coverage
  Indemnity

Key Personnel
  President/CEO . . . . Jeremy Spencer
  Provider Relations Mgr. . . . . Meg Pipkin
  Director of Operations . . . . Jeff Wilkinson
  Digital Marketing Manager . . . . Brent Singleton
  Director of Information. . . . . Chris Parrott

41   ## United Concordia of Arizona

2198 E Camelback Road
Suite 260
Phoenix, AZ 85016
Phone: 602-667-2200
www.unitedconcordia.com
For Profit Organization: Yes
Year Founded: 1971
Number of Primary Care Physicians: 97,300
Total Enrollment: 7,800,000

Healthplan and Services Defined
  PLAN TYPE: Dental
  Model Type: Network
  Plan Specialty: Dental
  Benefits Offered: Dental

Type of Coverage
  Commercial, Individual, Military personnel & families

Geographic Areas Served
  Nationwide

Accreditation Certification
  URAC

42   ## UnitedHealthcare of Arizona

1 East Washington Street
Suite 1700
Phoenix, AZ 85004
Toll-Free: 888-724-4018
www.uhc.com
Subsidiary of: UnitedHealth Group
For Profit Organization: Yes

Healthplan and Services Defined
  PLAN TYPE: HMO/PPO

Model Type: Network
Plan Specialty: Behavioral Health, Dental, Vision
Benefits Offered: Behavioral Health, Dental, Disease
  Management, Prescription, Vision, Wellness, AD&D, Life

Type of Coverage
  Commercial, Individual, Medicare, Supplemental Medicare,
  Medicaid

Geographic Areas Served
  Statewide

Key Personnel
  VP, Business Development . . . . Roger Brown
  CEO, Community Plan . . . . Joe Gaudio
  Medical Director . . . . Leslie Paulus

43   ## University Care Advantage

2701 E Elvira Road
Tuscon, AZ 85756
Toll-Free: 877-874-3930
universitycareadvantage.com
Subsidiary of: University of Arizona Health Plans

Healthplan and Services Defined
  PLAN TYPE: HMO
  Benefits Offered: Chiropractic, Dental, Podiatry, Prescription,
  Vision

Geographic Areas Served
  Cochise, Gila, Graham, Greenlee, La Paz, Pima, Pinal, Santa
  Cruz, Yavapai, Yuma counties

Key Personnel
  Chief Executive Officer . . . . Kathleen Oestreich

44   ## University Family Care Health Plan

2701 E Elvira Road
Tucson, AZ 85756
Toll-Free: 800-582-8686
Phone: 520-874-5290
www.ufcaz.com
Subsidiary of: University Physicians Health Plans
Non-Profit Organization: Yes

Healthplan and Services Defined
  PLAN TYPE: HMO

Type of Coverage
  Individual

Geographic Areas Served
  Cochise, Gila, Graham, Greenlee, La Paz, Pima, Pinal, Santa
  Cruz, Yavapai, and Yuma counties

Key Personnel
  CEO . . . . Kathleen Oestreich

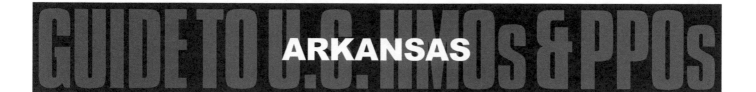
Health Insurance Coverage Status and Type of Coverage by Age

Category	All Persons		Under 18 years		Under 65 years	
	Number	%	Number	%	Number	%
Total population	2,949	-	752	-	2,469	-
Covered by some type of health insurance	2,718 (10)	92.1 (0.3)	718 (5)	95.6 (0.6)	2,238 (10)	90.7 (0.4)
Covered by private health insurance	1,807 (23)	61.3 (0.8)	355 (11)	47.2 (1.5)	1,528 (21)	61.9 (0.9)
Employer-based	1,377 (20)	46.7 (0.7)	303 (10)	40.3 (1.4)	1,270 (19)	51.4 (0.8)
Direct purchase	431 (12)	14.6 (0.4)	43 (4)	5.8 (0.6)	258 (11)	10.4 (0.4)
TRICARE	108 (7)	3.7 (0.3)	18 (3)	2.4 (0.5)	61 (6)	2.5 (0.3)
Covered by public health insurance	1,309 (21)	44.4 (0.7)	398 (11)	52.9 (1.4)	839 (20)	34.0 (0.8)
Medicaid	806 (21)	27.3 (0.7)	393 (11)	52.3 (1.4)	736 (20)	29.8 (0.8)
Medicare	602 (8)	20.4 (0.3)	10 (3)	1.4 (0.5)	133 (7)	5.4 (0.3)
VA Care	105 (5)	3.6 (0.2)	1 (Z)	0.1 (0.1)	47 (4)	1.9 (0.2)
Not covered at any time during the year	232 (10)	7.9 (0.3)	33 (4)	4.4 (0.6)	231 (10)	9.3 (0.4)

Note: Numbers in thousands; Figures cover civilian noninstitutionalized population in 2017; N/A indicates that data was not available; Z represents or rounds to zero; Margin of error appears in parenthesis and is calculated using replicate weights.
Source: U.S. Census Bureau, American Community Survey, Table HIC-4_ACS. Health Insurance Coverage Status and Type of Coverage by State—All People: 2008 to 2017, Table HIC-5_ACS. Health Insurance Coverage Status and Type of Coverage by State—Children Under 18: 2008 to 2017, Table HIC-6_ACS. Health Insurance Coverage Status and Type of Coverage by State—Persons Under 65: 2008 to 2017

Arkansas

45 Arkansas Blue Cross Blue Shield

P.O. Box 2181
Little Rock, AR 72203-2181
Toll-Free: 800-238-8379
www.arkansasbluecross.com
Non-Profit Organization: Yes
Year Founded: 1948

Healthplan and Services Defined
  PLAN TYPE: Multiple
  Other Type: HMO, Medicare
  Model Type: Network
  Plan Specialty: Dental, Vision
  Benefits Offered: Chiropractic, Dental, Home Care, Inpatient
    SNF, Physical Therapy, Podiatry, Prescription, Vision,
    Worker's Compensation, Life, Mental Health, Substance
    Abuse, Emergency, Short-Term, Federal Employees

Type of Coverage
  Commercial, Individual, Medicare, Supplemental Medicare
  Catastrophic Illness Benefit: Varies per case

Geographic Areas Served
  Statewide

Subscriber Information
  Average Subscriber Co-Payment:
    Home Health Care: Varies
    Nursing Home: Varies

Accreditation Certification
  TJC, URAC, NCQA

Key Personnel
  President/CEO. . . . . Curtis Barnett
  EVP/Chief Admin Officer . . . . David Bridges
  EVP/CFO/Treasurer . . . . Gray Dillard
  VP, Claims Administration . . . . Marcus James
  SVP/Chief Legal Officer . . . . Tim Gauger
  SVP, Provider Services . . . . Alicia Berkemeyer
  VP/Chief Medical Officer . . . . Connie Meeks, MD
  VP/Chief Actuary. . . . . Sam Vorderstrasse
  VP, Info Technology . . . . Melvin Hardy

46 Delta Dental of Arkansas

1513 Country Club Road
Sherwood, AR 72120
Toll-Free: 800-462-5410
Phone: 501-835-3400
www.deltadentalar.com
Mailing Address: P.O. Box 15965, Little Rock, AR 72231
Non-Profit Organization: Yes
Year Founded: 1982
Total Enrollment: 2,000,000

Healthplan and Services Defined
  PLAN TYPE: Dental
  Other Type: Vision
  Model Type: Network
  Plan Specialty: Dental, Vision
  Benefits Offered: Dental, Vision

Type of Coverage
  Commercial, Individual, Group

Type of Payment Plans Offered
  DFFS

Geographic Areas Served
  Statewide

Publishes and Distributes Report Card: Yes

Key Personnel
  President & CEO . . . . Ed Choate

47 Frazier Insurance Agency

808 Reservoir Road
Suite B
Little Rock, AR 72227
Phone: 501-225-1818
Fax: 501-223-8682
frazieragency.com

Healthplan and Services Defined
  PLAN TYPE: HMO/PPO
  Benefits Offered: Wellness, AD&D, Life

Type of Coverage
  Medicare

Geographic Areas Served
  Statewide

48 HealthSCOPE Benefits

27 Corporate Hill Drive
Little Rock, AR 72205
Toll-Free: 800-972-3025
www.healthscopebenefits.com
For Profit Organization: Yes
Year Founded: 1985
Total Enrollment: 500,000

Healthplan and Services Defined
  PLAN TYPE: Other
  Plan Specialty: Healthcare management services

Type of Coverage
  Catastrophic Illness Benefit: Maximum $1M

Type of Payment Plans Offered
  POS, DFFS, FFS, Combination FFS & DFFS

Geographic Areas Served
  Nationwide

Network Qualifications
  Minimum Years of Practice: 3
  Pre-Admission Certification: Yes

Peer Review Type
  Utilization Review: Yes
  Second Surgical Opinion: Yes
  Case Management: Yes

Accreditation Certification
  TJC, URAC
  Utilization Review, State Licensure

Key Personnel
Chief Executive Officer. . . . . Joe Edwards
President . . . . Mary Catherine Person
VP, Business Development . . . . Tom Bartlett
VP, Quality/Assurance . . . . Cathleen Armstrong
SVP, Solutions & Legal . . . . Brett Edwards
VP of Sales . . . . Pepper Schafer
Chief Information Officer . . . . Tim Beasley

Specialty Managed Care Partners
American Health Holdings, PHCS, Advance PCS, Caremark, CCN
Enters into Contracts with Regional Business Coalitions: Yes
Alaska Business Coalition

Employer References
American Greetings, Alcoa, MedCath, Whirlpool

---

49   Humana Health Insurance of Arkansas

5206 Village Parkway
Suite 4
Rogers, AR 72758
Toll-Free: 800-434-4207
Phone: 479-418-7140
Fax: 479-273-2516
www.humana.com
Subsidiary of: Humana
For Profit Organization: Yes

Healthplan and Services Defined
PLAN TYPE: HMO/PPO
Model Type: Network
Plan Specialty: Dental, Vision
Benefits Offered: Dental, Prescription, Vision, Life, LTD, STD

Type of Coverage
Commercial, Medicare

Geographic Areas Served
Statewide

Accreditation Certification
URAC, NCQA, CORE

Key Personnel
Regional President. Jeremy Gaskill

---

50   Mercy Clinic Arkansas

207 Carter Street
Berryville, AR 72616
Phone: 870-423-6661
mercy.net
Subsidiary of: IBM Watson Health
Non-Profit Organization: Yes
Year Founded: 1986
Number of Affiliated Hospitals: 44
Number of Primary Care Physicians: 700
Number of Referral/Specialty Physicians: 2,000

Healthplan and Services Defined
PLAN TYPE: HMO
Benefits Offered: Behavioral Health, Disease Management, Home Care, Inpatient SNF, Physical Therapy, Podiatry,

Vision, Wellness, Non-Surgical Weight Loss; Urgent Care; Dermatology; Rehabilitation; Breast Cancer; Orthopedics; Ostoclerosis; Pediatrics

Geographic Areas Served
Arkansas, Kansas, Missouri, and Oklahoma

Key Personnel
President, Arkansas . . . . Stephen Goss, MD

---

51   NovaSys Health

10801 Executive Center Drive
Little Rock, AR 72221
Toll-Free: 800-294-3557
Phone: 501-219-4444
novasyshealth.com
Year Founded: 1996
Number of Affiliated Hospitals: 67
Number of Primary Care Physicians: 4,000

Healthplan and Services Defined
PLAN TYPE: PPO
Model Type: Network
Plan Specialty: Integrated provider network & administrative services

Geographic Areas Served
Statewide

Key Personnel
Chief Executive Officer . . . . John P. Ryan

---

52   UnitedHealthcare of Arkansas

Little Rock, AR 72201
Toll-Free: 888-545-5205
www.uhc.com
Subsidiary of: UnitedHealth Group
For Profit Organization: Yes

Healthplan and Services Defined
PLAN TYPE: HMO/PPO
Model Type: Network
Plan Specialty: Behavioral Health, Dental, Disease Management, PBM, Vision
Benefits Offered: Behavioral Health, Dental, Disease Management, Long-Term Care, Prescription, Vision, Wellness, Life, LTD, STD

Type of Coverage
Commercial, Individual, Medicare, Supplemental Medicare, Medicaid, Family

Type of Payment Plans Offered
POS, FFS

Geographic Areas Served
Statewide

Network Qualifications
Pre-Admission Certification: Yes

Peer Review Type
Utilization Review: Yes

Publishes and Distributes Report Card: Yes

Accreditation Certification

URAC, NCQA

TJC Accreditation, Medicare Approved, Utilization Review, Pre-Admission Certification, State Licensure, Quality Assurance Program

Key Personnel

CFO, Tennessee/Arkansas . . . . Eric H. Johnson

Specialty Managed Care Partners

Enters into Contracts with Regional Business Coalitions: Yes

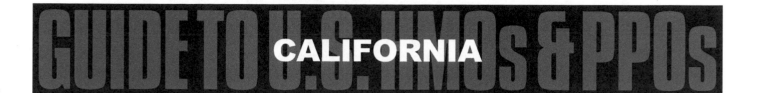

Health Insurance Coverage Status and Type of Coverage by Age

Category	All Persons		Under 18 years		Under 65 years	
	Number	%	Number	%	Number	%
Total population	39,047	-	9,567	-	33,637	-
Covered by some type of health insurance	36,250 *(35)*	92.8 *(0.1)*	9,267 *(16)*	96.9 *(0.1)*	30,898 *(35)*	91.9 *(0.1)*
Covered by private health insurance	24,824 *(74)*	63.6 *(0.2)*	5,448 *(35)*	56.9 *(0.4)*	22,107 *(71)*	65.7 *(0.2)*
Employer-based	20,288 *(83)*	52.0 *(0.2)*	4,673 *(35)*	48.8 *(0.4)*	18,646 *(79)*	55.4 *(0.2)*
Direct purchase	4,913 *(50)*	12.6 *(0.1)*	760 *(18)*	7.9 *(0.2)*	3,675 *(43)*	10.9 *(0.1)*
TRICARE	679 *(16)*	1.7 *(Z)*	156 *(9)*	1.6 *(0.1)*	457 *(16)*	1.4 *(Z)*
Covered by public health insurance	14,992 *(71)*	38.4 *(0.2)*	4,195 *(36)*	43.8 *(0.4)*	9,881 *(70)*	29.4 *(0.2)*
Medicaid	10,383 *(73)*	26.6 *(0.2)*	4,125 *(38)*	43.1 *(0.4)*	9,256 *(72)*	27.5 *(0.2)*
Medicare	5,887 *(26)*	15.1 *(0.1)*	107 *(9)*	1.1 *(0.1)*	784 *(23)*	2.3 *(0.1)*
VA Care	601 *(13)*	1.5 *(Z)*	7 *(2)*	0.1 *(Z)*	283 *(9)*	0.8 *(Z)*
Not covered at any time during the year	2,797 *(34)*	7.2 *(0.1)*	301 *(12)*	3.1 *(0.1)*	2,739 *(34)*	8.1 *(0.1)*

Note: Numbers in thousands; Figures cover civilian noninstitutionalized population in 2017; N/A indicates that data was not available; Z represents or rounds to zero; Margin of error appears in parenthesis and is calculated using replicate weights.
Source: U.S. Census Bureau, American Community Survey, Table HIC-4_ACS. Health Insurance Coverage Status and Type of Coverage by State—All People: 2008 to 2017, Table HIC-5_ACS. Health Insurance Coverage Status and Type of Coverage by State—Children Under 18: 2008 to 2017, Table HIC-6_ACS. Health Insurance Coverage Status and Type of Coverage by State—Persons Under 65: 2008 to 2017

California

53   Access Dental Services

P.O. Box 659005
Sacramento, CA 95865-9005
Toll-Free: 866-682-9904
Fax: 916-646-9000
info@accessdental.com
www.accessdental.com
For Profit Organization: Yes
Year Founded: 1989
Number of Primary Care Physicians: 2,000
Total Enrollment: 123,880

Healthplan and Services Defined
   PLAN TYPE: Dental
   Model Type: Staff
   Plan Specialty: Dental
   Benefits Offered: Dental

Type of Coverage
   Commercial, Individual, Medicare, Supplemental Medicare,
   Medicaid

Geographic Areas Served
   Statewide

Key Personnel
   Chief Executive Officer. . . . . George Neal
   Chief Clinical Officer . . . . Cherag Sarkari
   VP, Operations. . . . . Payam Pardis

54   Aetna Health of California

10260 Meanley Drive
San Diego, CA 92131
Toll-Free: 855-772-9076
Fax: 844-453-1150
www.aetnabetterhealth.com/california
Subsidiary of: Aetna Inc.
For Profit Organization: Yes

Healthplan and Services Defined
   PLAN TYPE: HMO/PPO
   Other Type: POS
   Model Type: Network
   Plan Specialty: Behavioral Health, EPO, Lab, PBM,
      Radiology
   Benefits Offered: Behavioral Health, Dental, Disease
      Management, Long-Term Care, Physical Therapy,
      Podiatry, Prescription, Psychiatric, Vision, Wellness, Life,
      LTD, STD

Type of Coverage
   Commercial, Supplemental Medicare, Catastrophic, Student
   health

Geographic Areas Served
   Statewide

55   Alameda Alliance for Health

1240 South Loop Road
Alameda, CA 94502
Toll-Free: 877-932-2738
Phone: 510-747-4500
www.alamedaalliance.org
Non-Profit Organization: Yes
Year Founded: 1996
Federally Qualified: Yes
Number of Affiliated Hospitals: 15
Number of Primary Care Physicians: 4,000
Total Enrollment: 140,000
State Enrollment: 110,000

Healthplan and Services Defined
   PLAN TYPE: HMO
   Model Type: Network
   Plan Specialty: Dental
   Benefits Offered: Dental, Prescription, Vision, Medi-Cal,
      Healthy Families, Alliance Group Care

Type of Coverage
   Individual, Government Sponsored Programs

Type of Payment Plans Offered
   POS

Geographic Areas Served
   Alameda County

Peer Review Type
   Second Surgical Opinion: Yes

Accreditation Certification
   NCQA
   State Licensure

Key Personnel
   Chief Executive Officer. . . . . Scott E. Coffin
   Chief Operations Officer. . . . . Matthew Woodruff
   Chief Financial Officer . . . . Gil Riojas
   Chief Medical Officer. . . . . Steve O'Brien, MD
   Chief Analytics Officer. . . . . Tiffany Cheang

56   Alameda Medi-Cal Plan

1240 South Loop Road
Alameda, CA 94502
Toll-Free: 800-698-1118
Phone: 510-777-2300
www.alamedaalliance.org
Subsidiary of: Alameda Alliance for Health
Non-Profit Organization: Yes
Federally Qualified: Yes
Number of Affiliated Hospitals: 15
Number of Primary Care Physicians: 4,000

Healthplan and Services Defined
   PLAN TYPE: Other
   Plan Specialty: Serving families and children, people with
      disabilities, and seniors
   Benefits Offered: Dental, Inpatient SNF, Vision, Wellness

Geographic Areas Served
   Alameda County

Key Personnel
Chief Executive Officer . . . . Scott Coffin
Chief Operations Officer . . . . Matthew Woodruff
Chief Financial Officer . . . . Gil Riojas
General Counsel . . . . Matthew Levin
Chief Information Officer . . . . Aman Bahsin

57 Alignment Health Plan
1100 W Town and Country Road
Suite 1600
Orange, CA 92868
Toll-Free: 866-634-2247
Phone: 323-728-7232
Fax: 323-728-8494
www.alignmenthealthplan.com

Healthplan and Services Defined
PLAN TYPE: Medicare

Type of Coverage
Medicare, Supplemental Medicare

Geographic Areas Served
Los Angeles, Northern Orange County, San Bernardino, Riverside, Stanislaus, San Joaquin and Santa Clara

Key Personnel
President & CEO . . . . John Kao

58 Allied Pacific IPA
1668 S. Garfield Avenue
2nd Floor
Alhambra, CA 91801
Toll-Free: 877-282-8272
Phone: 626-282-0288
CustomerService.Dept@nmm.cc
www.alliedipa.com
Secondary Address: 568 W. Garvey Avenue, Monterey Park, CA 91754, 888-888-7424
Year Founded: 1992
Physician Owned Organization: Yes
Number of Primary Care Physicians: 800

Healthplan and Services Defined
PLAN TYPE: HMO
Other Type: IPA
Model Type: IPA
Benefits Offered: Disease Management, Wellness

Type of Coverage
Commercial, Individual

59 American Specialty Health
10221 Wateridge Circle
San Diego, CA 92121
Toll-Free: 800-848-3555
Phone: 619-578-2000
www.ashcompanies.com
For Profit Organization: Yes
Year Founded: 1987
Total Enrollment: 25,900,000

Healthplan and Services Defined
PLAN TYPE: HMO
Model Type: Network
Plan Specialty: Chiropractic
Benefits Offered: Chiropractic, Complementary Medicine, Acupuncture

Type of Coverage
Commercial, Supplemental Medicare

Type of Payment Plans Offered
POS, Capitated

Geographic Areas Served
Nationwide - ASH Network, California - ASH Plans

Network Qualifications
Pre-Admission Certification: Yes

Peer Review Type
Utilization Review: Yes
Case Management: Yes

Accreditation Certification
URAC, NCQA, HITRUST

Key Personnel
Vice President . . . . Rik Lee

Specialty Managed Care Partners
Enters into Contracts with Regional Business Coalitions: Yes

60 Anthem Blue Cross of California
2000 Corporate Center Drive
Newbury Park, CA 91320
Toll-Free: 866-791-5538
Phone: 805-713-3007
www.anthem.com
Subsidiary of: Anthem, Inc.
For Profit Organization: Yes

Healthplan and Services Defined
PLAN TYPE: HMO/PPO
Model Type: Network
Plan Specialty: Behavioral Health, Dental, Disease Management, Lab, PBM, Vision, Radiology
Benefits Offered: Behavioral Health, Dental, Disease Management, Inpatient SNF, Physical Therapy, Prescription, Psychiatric, Transplant, Vision, Wellness, Life

Type of Coverage
Commercial, Individual, Medicare, Supplemental Medicare, Minimum coverage

Geographic Areas Served
Santa Clara, San Joaquin, Stanislaus, Merced, and Tulare

Accreditation Certification
URAC

Key Personnel
President/CEO . . . . Paul Markovich

61   BEST Life and Health Insurance Co.

17701 Mitchell N
Irvine, CA 92614-6028
Toll-Free: 800-433-0088
Fax: 208-893-5040
cs@bestlife.com
www.bestlife.com
Mailing Address: P.O. Box 890, Meridian, ID 83680-0890
For Profit Organization: Yes
Year Founded: 1970
Number of Affiliated Hospitals: 5,005
Number of Primary Care Physicians: 772,292
Total Enrollment: 90,000

Healthplan and Services Defined
  PLAN TYPE: PPO
  Model Type: PPO/Indemnity
  Benefits Offered: Dental, Disease Management, Vision,
    Wellness, Life, STD

Type of Coverage
  Commercial

Geographic Areas Served
  AK, AL, AR, AZ, CA, CO, DC, FL, GA, HI, ID, IL, IN, KS,
  KY, LA, MD, MI, MS, MO, MT, NC, ND, NE, NM, NV, OH,
  OK, OR, PA, SC, SD, TN, TX, UT, VA, WA, WY

Network Qualifications
  Pre-Admission Certification: Yes

Peer Review Type
  Case Management: Yes

Accreditation Certification
  URAC, NCQA
  Quality Assurance Program

Key Personnel
  President.............................. Paul Peatross

62   Blue Shield of California

50 Beale Street
San Francisco, CA 94105-1808
Toll-Free: 800-393-6130
Phone: 415-229-5000
www.blueshieldca.com
Mailing Address: P.O. Box 272540, Chico, CA 95927-2540
Non-Profit Organization: Yes
Year Founded: 1939
State Enrollment: 3,000,000

Healthplan and Services Defined
  PLAN TYPE: HMO/PPO
  Plan Specialty: Dental, Vision
  Benefits Offered: Behavioral Health, Chiropractic, Dental,
    Home Care, Inpatient SNF, Podiatry, Prescription, Vision,
    Life, Benefits vary depending on the plan

Type of Coverage
  Commercial, Individual, Medicare, Supplemental Medicare,
    Medicaid

Geographic Areas Served
  Statewide

Accreditation Certification
  NCQA

Key Personnel
  President/CEO .... Paul Markovich
  SVP/CFO.......................... Michael Murray
  SVP/General Counsel .... Seth Jacobs, Esq
  SVP/Chief Actuary......................... Amy Yao
  SVP/Chief Info Officer............... Michael Mathias

63   Brand New Day HMO

5455 Garden Grove Boulevard
Suite 500
Westminster, CA 92683
Toll-Free: 866-255-4795
Fax: 657-400-1208
bndhmo.com
For Profit Organization: Yes
Year Founded: 1985

Healthplan and Services Defined
  PLAN TYPE: HMO
  Plan Specialty: Behavioral Health
  Benefits Offered: Behavioral Health, Dental, Disease
    Management, Prescription, Psychiatric, Vision, Wellness

Type of Coverage
  Individual, Medicare, Medicaid

Geographic Areas Served
  Statewide

Key Personnel
  CEO.................................... Jeff Davis

64   Bright Now! Dental

3358 South Bristol Street
Santa Ana, CA 92704
Toll-Free: 844-400-7645
Phone: 714-361-2141
www.brightnow.com
Secondary Address: 1601 W 17th Street, Suite G, Santa Ana,
  CA 92706, 714-567-9255
Subsidiary of: Smile Brands Inc.
Year Founded: 1998
Number of Primary Care Physicians: 300
Number of Referral/Specialty Physicians: 416

Healthplan and Services Defined
  PLAN TYPE: Dental
  Model Type: Staff, Network
  Plan Specialty: Dental
  Benefits Offered: Dental

Type of Payment Plans Offered
  Capitated

Geographic Areas Served
  AZ, CA, CO, FL, IN, MD, OH, OR, PA, TN, TX, UT, VA,
  WA

Subscriber Information
  Average Monthly Fee Per Subscriber
    (Employee + Employer Contribution):
      Employee Only (Self): $40.00

Employee & 1 Family Member: $75.00
Employee & 2 Family Members: $110.00

Network Qualifications
Pre-Admission Certification: Yes

Key Personnel
President/CEO . . . . Steven Bilt
CFO . . . . Brad Schmidt
CIO . . . . George Suda

Specialty Managed Care Partners
Enters into Contracts with Regional Business Coalitions: No

---

65   California Dental Network

23291 Mill Creek Drive
Suite 100
Laguna Hills, CA 92653
Toll-Free: 877-433-6825
Fax: 949-830-1655
www.caldental.net

Healthplan and Services Defined
PLAN TYPE: Dental
Plan Specialty: Dental
Benefits Offered: Dental

Type of Coverage
Individual

Geographic Areas Served
Statewide

Key Personnel
CEO . . . . Brian Watts
President, DentaQuest . . . . Steve Pollock

---

66   California Foundation for Medical Care

3993 Jurupa Avenue
Riverside, CA 92506
Toll-Free: 800-334-7341
Fax: 951-686-1692
www.cfmcnet.org
For Profit Organization: Yes
Number of Affiliated Hospitals: 250
Number of Primary Care Physicians: 30,000
Number of Referral/Specialty Physicians: 5,000

Healthplan and Services Defined
PLAN TYPE: PPO
Plan Specialty: Behavioral Health, EPO, Lab, Worker's
Compensation, UR, Chemical Dependency Centers.
Surgical Centers
Benefits Offered: Worker's Compensation

Geographic Areas Served
Statewide

Key Personnel
President . . . . Debi Hardwick
831-754-3800
dhardwick@costalmgmt.com
Vice President . . . . Carolyn Temple
661-616-4814
ctemple@kernfmc.com

Chief Executive Officer . . . . Dolores L. Green
951-686-9049
dgreen@rcmanet.com
Administration Director . . . . Ester M. Sanchez
800-334-7341
esanchez@rfasi.com

---

67   CalOptima

505 City Parkway West
Orange, CA 92868
Toll-Free: 888-587-8088
Phone: 714-246-8500
www.caloptima.org
For Profit Organization: Yes
Year Founded: 1993
Owned by an Integrated Delivery Network (IDN): Yes
Number of Primary Care Physicians: 3,500
Total Enrollment: 413,795
State Enrollment: 402,000

Healthplan and Services Defined
PLAN TYPE: HMO
Model Type: Group
Plan Specialty: ASO, Behavioral Health, Chiropractic, Dental,
Disease Management, EPO, Lab, MSO, PBM, Vision,
Radiology, Worker's Compensation
Benefits Offered: Behavioral Health, Chiropractic, Dental,
Disease Management, Home Care, Prescription, Vision,
Wellness

Type of Coverage
Individual, Supplemental Medicare, Medicaid, Medi-Cal

Geographic Areas Served
Orange County

Key Personnel
Chief Executive Officer . . . . Michael Schrader
Chief Counsel . . . . Gary Crockett
Chief Information Officer . . . . Len Rosignoli
Chief Financial Officer . . . . Greg Hamblin
Chief Operating Officer . . . . Ladan Khamseh
Chief Medical Officer . . . . Richard Helmer, MD

---

68   Care1st Cal MediConnect Plan

601 Potrero Grande Drive
Montery Park, CA 91755
Toll-Free: 855-905-3825
Fax: 323-889-2100
care1st.com
Subsidiary of: Care1st Health Plan

Healthplan and Services Defined
PLAN TYPE: Other
Plan Specialty: Combines Medicare and Medi-Cal benefits
into a single plan.
Benefits Offered: Behavioral Health, Long-Term Care,
Prescription

Type of Coverage
Medicare

Geographic Areas Served
Los Angeles and San Diego counties

Key Personnel
Associate Vice President . . . . Maria Lackner

69   Care1st Health Plan Blue Shield of California Promise

601 Potrero Grande Drive
Monterey Park, CA 91755
Toll-Free: 800-544-0088
Phone: 323-889-6638
Fax: 323-889-6255
www.care1st.com
Secondary Address: 3131 Camino del Rio North, Suite 1300, San Diego, CA 92108, 619-528-4800
Subsidiary of: Blue Shield California
For Profit Organization: Yes
Year Founded: 1994
Total Enrollment: 320,000

Healthplan and Services Defined
PLAN TYPE: HMO
Benefits Offered: Dental, Disease Management, Wellness, Medi-Cal Health, Medi-Cal Dental, Healthy Families

Type of Coverage
Commercial, Medicare, Supplemental Medicare, Medicaid

Geographic Areas Served
Los Angeles, Orange, San Bernardino, Riverside and San Diego counties

Accreditation Certification
NCQA

Key Personnel
President/CEO . . . . Greg Buchert, MD
Chief Financial Officer . . . . Barry Staton
VP/Chief Medical Officer. . . . . Tanya Dansky, MD
Chief Legal Officer . . . . Kristen Cerf
Chief Operating Officer . . . . Amanda Flaum
Chief Compliance Officer. . . . . Michael Osorio

70   Care1st Medicare Advantage Plan

601 Potrero Grande Drive
Monterey Park, CA 91755
Toll-Free: 800-544-0088
Fax: 323-889-2101
www.care1st.com
Year Founded: 1994

Healthplan and Services Defined
PLAN TYPE: Medicare
Benefits Offered: Disease Management, Wellness

Type of Coverage
Medicare, Supplemental Medicare

Geographic Areas Served
California, Texas

Accreditation Certification
NCQA

71   CareMore Health Plan

12900 Park Plaza Drive
Suite 150, MS-6150
Cerritos, CA 90703
Toll-Free: 800-499-2793
Fax: 562-741-4406
www.caremore.com

Healthplan and Services Defined
PLAN TYPE: Medicare
Plan Specialty: Seniors healthcare
Benefits Offered: Home Care

Type of Coverage
Medicare

Geographic Areas Served
Arizona, California, Iowa, Nevada, Ohio, Tennessee, Virginia

Key Personnel
President & CEO . . . . Sachin H. Jain
Chief Operations Officer. . . . . Karen Sugano
Chief Financial Officer . . . . Michael Plumb
Chief Medical Officer . . . . Zubin Eapen
Chief Quality Officer. . . . . David Ramirez

72   CenCal Health

4050 Calle Real
Santa Barbara, CA 93110
Toll-Free: 800-421-2560
Phone: 805-685-9525
info@cencalhealth.org
www.cencalhealth.org
Secondary Address: 1288 Morro Street, Suite 100, San Luis Obispo, CA 93401
Non-Profit Organization: Yes
Year Founded: 1983
Number of Primary Care Physicians: 260
Number of Referral/Specialty Physicians: 1,300
Total Enrollment: 175,000

Healthplan and Services Defined
PLAN TYPE: HMO
Benefits Offered: Complementary Medicine, Disease Management, Prescription, Wellness

Type of Coverage
Individual, Medicare, Medicaid, Medi-Cal, Healthy Families

Geographic Areas Served
Santa Barbara and San Luis Obispo counties

Key Personnel
Chief Executive Officer . . . . Bob Freeman
Chief Operating Officer . . . . Paul Jaconette
Chief Financial Officer. . . . . David Ambrose
Chief Information Officer . . . . Barrie Parker
Human Resources . . . . Karyn Fish
Chief Medical Officer. . . . . Takashi Michael Wada, MD
Director of Pharmacy. . . . . Jeff Januska

73 Central California Alliance for Health

1600 Green Hills Road
Suite 101
Scotts Valley, CA 95066-4981
Toll-Free: 800-700-3874
Phone: 831-430-5500
www.ccah-alliance.org
Secondary Address: 950 East Blanco Road, Suite 101, Salinas, CA 93901-3400, 831-755-6000
Non-Profit Organization: Yes
Year Founded: 1996
Physician Owned Organization: No
Federally Qualified: No
Number of Primary Care Physicians: 1,590
Total Enrollment: 210,000
State Enrollment: 190,000

Healthplan and Services Defined
  PLAN TYPE: HMO
  Model Type: County Org Health System
  Benefits Offered: Chiropractic, Long-Term Care, Vision, Medi-Cal, Healthy Families, Healthy Kids, Alliance Care Access for Infants and Mothers, Alliance Care IHSS
  Offers Demand Management Patient Information Service: No

Geographic Areas Served
  Santa Cruz, Monterey and Merced counties

Network Qualifications
  Pre-Admission Certification: No

Publishes and Distributes Report Card: No

Key Personnel
  Chief Executive Officer . . . . Stephanie Sonnenshine
  Chief Financial Officer . . . . Lisa Ba
  Chief Medical Officer . . . . Dale Bishop, MD
  Administrative Officer . . . . Scott Fortner
  Chief Information Officer . . . . Dory Hicks
  Chief Operating Officer . . . . Marina Owen
  Health Services Officer . . . . Suzanne Skerness
  Pharmacy Director . . . . Michael Blatt
  Utilization Management . . . . Mary Brusuelas, RN
  Government Relations . . . . Danita Carlson
  Accounting Director . . . . Joy Cubbin
  Medical Director . . . . Ghislaine Guez, MD
  Human Resources Director . . . . Lisa Hauck
  Chief Compliance Officer . . . . Jenifer Mandella
  Communications Director . . . . Eric McKeeby

Specialty Managed Care Partners
  Enters into Contracts with Regional Business Coalitions: No

74 Central Health Medicare Plan

1540 Bridgegate Drive
Diamond Bar, CA 91765
Toll-Free: 866-314-2427
mbrsvcs@centralhealthplan.com
www.centralhealthplan.com
Year Founded: 2004

Healthplan and Services Defined
  PLAN TYPE: Medicare
  Other Type: HMO

Benefits Offered: Chiropractic, Dental, Home Care, Inpatient SNF, Physical Therapy, Podiatry, Vision, Wellness, Diagnostics/Labs/Imaging; Rehabilitation; Medical Equipment

Type of Coverage
  Medicare, Supplemental Medicare

Geographic Areas Served
  Los Angeles, Orange, San Bernardino and Ventura counties

Key Personnel
  Chief Executive Officer . . . . Lee Suyenaga

75 Chinese Community Health Plan

445 Grant Avenue
Suite 700
San Francisco, CA 94108
Toll-Free: 888-775-7888
Phone: 415-955-8800
Fax: 415-955-8818
www.cchphealthplan.com
Secondary Address: 845 Jackson Street, San Francisco, CA 94133, 415-834-2118
For Profit Organization: Yes
Year Founded: 1986
Owned by an Integrated Delivery Network (IDN): Yes
Number of Affiliated Hospitals: 10
Number of Primary Care Physicians: 1,700
Number of Referral/Specialty Physicians: 144
Total Enrollment: 13,582
State Enrollment: 6,336

Healthplan and Services Defined
  PLAN TYPE: HMO
  Model Type: IPA
  Benefits Offered: Prescription, Vision, Wellness, Acupuncture Services, Worldwide Emergency

Type of Coverage
  Medicare

Geographic Areas Served
  San Francisco, Northern San Mateo

Subscriber Information
  Average Monthly Fee Per Subscriber
    (Employee + Employer Contribution):
      Employee Only (Self): $218.00
      Employee & 1 Family Member: $419.00
      Employee & 2 Family Members: $384.53
  Average Subscriber Co-Payment:
      Primary Care Physician: $10.00
      Non-Network Physician: Not covered
      Prescription Drugs: $6.00
      Hospital ER: $25.00
      Home Health Care Max. Days/Visits Covered: None except mental
      Nursing Home Max. Days/Visits Covered: 10 days

Network Qualifications
  Pre-Admission Certification: Yes

Peer Review Type
  Utilization Review: Yes

Second Surgical Opinion: Yes
Case Management: Yes

Accreditation Certification
TJC Accreditation, Medicare Approved, Utilization Review,
Pre-Admission Certification, State Licensure, Quality
Assurance Program

Key Personnel
Sales Manager . . . . Yolanda Lee
415-955-8000
Yolanda.Lee@CCHPHealthPlan.com
President/CEO . . . . Brenda Yee, RN

Specialty Managed Care Partners
Enters into Contracts with Regional Business Coalitions: No

---

76   ChiroSource, Inc.
PO Box 130
Clayton, CA 94517
Toll-Free: 800-680-9997
Fax: 925-844-3124
info@chirosource.com
www.chpc.com
For Profit Organization: Yes
Year Founded: 1997

Healthplan and Services Defined
PLAN TYPE: Multiple
Model Type: Network
Plan Specialty: Chiropractic, Physical Medicine,
Accupuncture, Massage
Benefits Offered: Worker's Compensation, Health-Group &
Individual, Medicare Advantage, IME Networks

Type of Coverage
PPO, EPO, POS, MPN, HCN, IME

Type of Payment Plans Offered
FFS

Geographic Areas Served
National

Network Qualifications
Pre-Admission Certification: Yes

Peer Review Type
Utilization Review: Yes

Publishes and Distributes Report Card: No

Specialty Managed Care Partners
Enters into Contracts with Regional Business Coalitions: Yes

---

77   Cigna HealthCare of California
900 Cottage Grove Road
Bloomfield, CT 06002
Toll-Free: 800-244-6224
www.cigna.com
For Profit Organization: Yes

Healthplan and Services Defined
PLAN TYPE: Multiple
Other Type: POS
Plan Specialty: Behavioral Health, Dental, Substance Abuse
Centers

Benefits Offered: Behavioral Health, Dental, Life

Type of Coverage
Commercial, Individual

Key Personnel
President/General Manager . . . . Peter Welch

---

78   Coastal TPA, Inc.
928 East Blanco Road
Suite 235
Salinas, CA 93901
Toll-Free: 800-564-7475
Phone: 831-754-3800
Fax: 831-754-3830
info@coastalmgmt.com
www.coastalmgmt.com
For Profit Organization: Yes
Year Founded: 1961

Healthplan and Services Defined
PLAN TYPE: PPO
Plan Specialty: Third party claims administration and
proprietary regional PPO.
Benefits Offered: Dental, Disease Management, Prescription,
Vision, PPO Network

Type of Coverage
Commercial
Catastrophic Illness Benefit: Unlimited

Type of Payment Plans Offered
FFS

Geographic Areas Served
Monterey, Santa Cruz, San Benito, San Luis Obispo and Santa
Clara counties

Peer Review Type
Utilization Review: No
Second Surgical Opinion: Yes
Case Management: No

Accreditation Certification
NCQA

Average Claim Compensation
Physician's Fees Charged: 70%
Hospital's Fees Charged: 85%

---

79   Community Health Group
2420 Fenton Street
Chula Vista, CA 91914
Toll-Free: 800-224-7766
Phone: 619-422-0422
info@chgsd.com
www.chgsd.com
Non-Profit Organization: Yes
Year Founded: 1982
Number of Affiliated Hospitals: 28
Number of Primary Care Physicians: 488
Number of Referral/Specialty Physicians: 1,820
Total Enrollment: 146,000
State Enrollment: 146,000

Healthplan and Services Defined
   PLAN TYPE: HMO
   Model Type: Network
   Plan Specialty: Behavioral Health, Disease Management,
      Lab, Vision, Radiology, UR
   Benefits Offered: Behavioral Health, Disease Management,
      Home Care, Inpatient SNF, Physical Therapy, Podiatry,
      Prescription, Psychiatric, Transplant, Wellness
   Offers Demand Management Patient Information Service:
      Yes

Type of Coverage
   Medi-Cal, CommuniCare Advantage
   Catastrophic Illness Benefit: None

Type of Payment Plans Offered
   Capitated, FFS

Geographic Areas Served
   San Diego county

Network Qualifications
   Pre-Admission Certification: Yes

Peer Review Type
   Utilization Review: Yes
   Second Surgical Opinion: Yes
   Case Management: Yes

Publishes and Distributes Report Card: Yes

Accreditation Certification
   NCQA
   Utilization Review, Pre-Admission Certification, State
      Licensure, Quality Assurance Program

Key Personnel
   Chief Executive Officer . . . . Norma Diaz

Specialty Managed Care Partners
   Enters into Contracts with Regional Business Coalitions: No

---

80 CONCERN: Employee Assistance Program
1503 Grant Road
Suite 120
Mountain View, CA 94040
Toll-Free: 800-344-4222
info@concern-eap.com
www.concern-eap.com
Non-Profit Organization: Yes

Healthplan and Services Defined
   PLAN TYPE: Other
   Other Type: EAP
   Benefits Offered: Behavioral Health, Psychiatric, Wellness

Type of Coverage
   Commercial, EAP

Geographic Areas Served
   Silicon Valley

Key Personnel
   Chief Executive Officer . . . . Cecile Currier

---

81 Contra Costa Health Services
50 Douglas Drive
Suite 310
Martinez, CA 94553
Toll-Free: 800-232-4636
cchealth.org
Non-Profit Organization: Yes
Year Founded: 1973
Federally Qualified: Yes
Number of Affiliated Hospitals: 1
Total Enrollment: 140,000

Healthplan and Services Defined
   PLAN TYPE: HMO
   Model Type: Staff, Network
   Benefits Offered: Behavioral Health, Disease Management,
      Wellness, 24-hour psychiatric emergency services

Geographic Areas Served
   Contra Costa County

Peer Review Type
   Utilization Review: Yes
   Second Surgical Opinion: Yes
   Case Management: Yes

Publishes and Distributes Report Card: Yes

Accreditation Certification
   URAC Accreditation
   TJC Accreditation, Medicare Approved, Utilization Review,
      State Licensure, Quality Assurance Program

Key Personnel
   Director . . . . Anna Roth, RN, MS
      925-957-5403
   Health Officer . . . . Chris Farnitano
   COO/CFO . . . . Patrick Godley
      925-957-5405
   Communications Officer . . . . Victoria Balladeres
      925-313-6268

Specialty Managed Care Partners
   Enters into Contracts with Regional Business Coalitions: Yes

---

82 Coventry Health Care of California
2200 W Orangewood Avenue
Suite 120
Orange, CA 92868
Phone: 714-450-4463
www.coventryhealthcare.com
Subsidiary of: Aetna Inc.
For Profit Organization: Yes

Healthplan and Services Defined
   PLAN TYPE: HMO/PPO
   Model Type: Network
   Plan Specialty: Behavioral Health, Dental, Worker's
      Compensation
   Benefits Offered: Behavioral Health, Dental, Prescription,
      Wellness, Worker's Compensation

Type of Coverage
   Commercial, Individual, Medicare, Medicaid

Plan Specialty: Dental
Benefits Offered: Dental
Offers Demand Management Patient Information Service: Yes

Network Qualifications
Pre-Admission Certification: Yes

Peer Review Type
Utilization Review: Yes
Second Surgical Opinion: Yes
Case Management: Yes

Publishes and Distributes Report Card: Yes

Accreditation Certification
NCQA

Specialty Managed Care Partners
Enters into Contracts with Regional Business Coalitions: Yes

Key Personnel
Director, HR. . . . . Norman Sedgwick

83   Delta Dental of California
P.O. Box 997330
Sacramento, CA 95899-7330
Toll-Free: 800-765-6003
www.deltadentalins.com
Secondary Address: DeltaCare USA Customer Service, P.O.
Box 1803, Alpharetta, GA 30023, 800-422-4234
Non-Profit Organization: Yes
Year Founded: 1955

Healthplan and Services Defined
PLAN TYPE: Dental
Other Type: Dental PPO
Model Type: Network
Plan Specialty: Dental
Benefits Offered: Dental

Type of Coverage
Commercial, Individual

Type of Payment Plans Offered
DFFS, Capitated, FFS

Geographic Areas Served
Statewide

Network Qualifications
Pre-Admission Certification: No

Peer Review Type
Utilization Review: Yes
Second Surgical Opinion: Yes
Case Management: Yes

Publishes and Distributes Report Card: Yes

Key Personnel
President & CEO . . . . Anthony S. Barth
Chief Financial Officer . . . . Michael Castro
Chief Operating Officer . . . . Nilesh Patel
Chief Information Officer . . . . Kirsten Garen
Chief Legal Officer . . . . Michael Hankinson

Specialty Managed Care Partners
PMI Dental Health Plan
Enters into Contracts with Regional Business Coalitions: Yes

84   Dental Alternatives Insurance Services
Toll-Free: 800-445-8119
Fax: 714-429-1261
info@gotodais.com
www.gotodais.com
Subsidiary of: SafeGuard Health Plans, Inc.
For Profit Organization: Yes
Year Founded: 1977
Total Enrollment: 390,000

Healthplan and Services Defined
PLAN TYPE: Dental
Model Type: IPA

85   Dental Benefit Providers: California
425 Market Street
Suite 12
San Francisco, CA 94105
Phone: 415-778-3800
www.dbp.com
Subsidiary of: UnitedHealth Group
For Profit Organization: Yes
Year Founded: 1984
Number of Primary Care Physicians: 125,000
Total Enrollment: 6,600,000

Healthplan and Services Defined
PLAN TYPE: Dental
Model Type: IPA
Plan Specialty: ASO, Dental, EPO, DHMO, PPO, CSO,
Preventive, Claims Repricing and Network Access
Benefits Offered: Dental

Type of Coverage
Indemnity, Medicare, Medicaid

Type of Payment Plans Offered
POS, DFFS, Capitated, FFS

Geographic Areas Served
48 states including District of Columbia, Puerto Rico and
Virgin Islands

Accreditation Certification
NCQA

86   Dental Health Services of California
3833 Atlantic Avenue
Long Beach, CA 90807
Toll-Free: 800-637-6453
Phone: 562-595-6000
Fax: 562-424-0150
www.dentalhealthservices.com
For Profit Organization: Yes
Year Founded: 1974
Physician Owned Organization: Yes
Federally Qualified: Yes
Number of Primary Care Physicians: 1,000
Number of Referral/Specialty Physicians: 400

Total Enrollment: 90,000

Healthplan and Services Defined
  PLAN TYPE: Dental
  Model Type: Network
  Plan Specialty: Dental
  Benefits Offered: Dental

Type of Coverage
  Commercial, Individual
  Catastrophic Illness Benefit: None

Type of Payment Plans Offered
  DFFS

Geographic Areas Served
  California, Washington, and Oregon

Subscriber Information
  Average Monthly Fee Per Subscriber
    (Employee + Employer Contribution):
      Employee Only (Self): Varies
      Employee & 1 Family Member: Varies
      Employee & 2 Family Members: Varies

Network Qualifications
  Pre-Admission Certification: Yes

Peer Review Type
  Second Surgical Opinion: Yes
  Case Management: Yes

Publishes and Distributes Report Card: Yes

Accreditation Certification
  Dhm
  TJC Accreditation, Utilization Review, State Licensure,
    Quality Assurance Program

Key Personnel
  Founder . . . . Godfrey Pernell

Specialty Managed Care Partners
  United Association, 7up
  Enters into Contracts with Regional Business Coalitions: No

---

87   **Dentistat**
1688 Dell Avenue
Suite 210
Campbell, CA 95008
Toll-Free: 800-336-8250
Phone: 408-376-0336
Fax: 408-376-0736
info@dentistat.com
www.dentistat.com
For Profit Organization: Yes
Year Founded: 1968
Number of Primary Care Physicians: 80,000

Healthplan and Services Defined
  PLAN TYPE: Dental
  Model Type: Network
  Plan Specialty: Dental
  Benefits Offered: Dental

Type of Payment Plans Offered
  DFFS, Capitated, FFS, Combination FFS & DFFS

Geographic Areas Served
  Nationwide

Accreditation Certification
  NCQA
  Utilization Review, Quality Assurance Program

Key Personnel
  President . . . . Bret Guenther
  Chief Information Officer . . . . Sondra Zambino

Specialty Managed Care Partners
  Enters into Contracts with Regional Business Coalitions: Yes

---

88   **eHealthInsurance Services, Inc.**
440 E Middlefield Road
Mountain View, CA 94043
Toll-Free: 877-456-7180
headquarters@ehealth.com
www.ehealthinsurance.com
Subsidiary of: eHealth, Inc.
Year Founded: 1997
Total Enrollment: 4,000,000

Healthplan and Services Defined
  PLAN TYPE: Multiple
  Plan Specialty: Dental, Vision
  Benefits Offered: Behavioral Health, Chiropractic, Dental,
    Disease Management, Home Care, Inpatient SNF, Podiatry,
    Prescription, Vision, Wellness, Life, STD, Benefits vary
    according to plan

Type of Coverage
  Commercial, Individual, Medicare, Supplemental Medicare

Geographic Areas Served
  Nationwide, including the District of Columbia

Key Personnel
  Chief Executive Officer . . . . Scott N. Flanders
  Chief Operating Officer . . . . Dave Francis
  Chief Financial Officer . . . . Derek Yung
  Chief Technology Officer . . . . Ian Kalin
  Chief Marketing Officer . . . . Tim Hannan
  SVP, Human Resources . . . . Rena Lane
  SVP, Sales & Operations . . . . Dave Nicklaus
  SVP/General Counsel . . . . Scott Giesler

---

89   **First Health**
Toll-Free: 800-226-5116
www.firsthealth.com
Subsidiary of: Aetna, Inc.
For Profit Organization: Yes
Year Founded: 1984
Number of Affiliated Hospitals: 134
Number of Primary Care Physicians: 1,923
Number of Referral/Specialty Physicians: 5,744
Total Enrollment: 2,000,000
State Enrollment: 585,000

Healthplan and Services Defined
  PLAN TYPE: PPO
  Model Type: Network
  Benefits Offered: Disease Management, Wellness

Type of Payment Plans Offered
DFFS

Geographic Areas Served
State of Oklahoma and contiguous border cities of Missouri, Arkansas, Kansas and Texas

Key Personnel
Executive Director . . . . Paul Lavin
VP, Business Development . . . . Kara Dornig
VP, Account Management . . . . Susan Korth
Wholesale Operations . . . . Ron Gibb

Average Claim Compensation
Physician's Fees Charged: 72%
Hospital's Fees Charged: 62%

---

90 Foundation f. Medical Care f. Kern & Santa Barbara Counties

5701 Truxtun Avenue
Suite 100
Bakersfield, CA 93309
Phone: 661-327-7581
Fax: 661-327-5129
www.kernfmc.com
Number of Affiliated Hospitals: 400
Number of Primary Care Physicians: 30,000
Number of Referral/Specialty Physicians: 7,000

Healthplan and Services Defined
PLAN TYPE: PPO
Model Type: IPA, Group, Network
Benefits Offered: Dental, Disease Management, Prescription, Wellness
Offers Demand Management Patient Information Service: Yes

Type of Payment Plans Offered
POS, DFFS, FFS, Combination FFS & DFFS

Geographic Areas Served
Kern and Santa Barbara counties

Network Qualifications
Pre-Admission Certification: Yes

Peer Review Type
Utilization Review: Yes
Second Surgical Opinion: Yes
Case Management: Yes

Accreditation Certification
TJC Accreditation, Medicare Approved, Utilization Review, Pre-Admission Certification, State Licensure

Key Personnel
Chief Executive Officer. . . . . Carolyn J Temple
ctemple@kernfmc.com
Chief Operating Officer. . . . . Deborah Hankins
dhankinskernfmc.com
Executive Assistant. . . . . Lisa Garzelli
lgarzelli@kernfmc.com
Manager, Customer Service . . . . Annette Charlton
acharlton@kernfmc.com
Provider Relations . . . . Kelly Swartz
kswartz@kernfmc.com

Exec Admin Supervisor . . . . Lisa Garzelli
lgarzelli@kernfmc.com

Specialty Managed Care Partners
Enters into Contracts with Regional Business Coalitions: No

---

91 GEMCare Health Plan

4550 California Avenue
Suite 500
Bakersfield, CA 93309
Phone: 661-716-7100
Fax: 661-716-9200
gemcare.com
Year Founded: 1992
Number of Primary Care Physicians: 120

Healthplan and Services Defined
PLAN TYPE: Medicare
Model Type: IPA

Type of Coverage
Medicare, Supplemental Medicare

Geographic Areas Served
Kern County, including Bakersfield and the outlying communities of Arvin, Delano, Lake Isabella, Shafter, Taft, Tehachapi and Wasco

Key Personnel
President & CEO . . . . Michael R Myers
Chief Operating Officer . . . . Tonya Rhoades
Chief Financial Officer . . . . Jeff Mihal
Chief Medical Officer . . . . Stephan Bass, MD

---

92 Golden West Dental & Vision

5171 Verdugo Way
Camarillo, CA 93012
Toll-Free: 800-219-9216
www.goldenwestdental.com
Subsidiary of: Anthem
For Profit Organization: Yes
Year Founded: 1974

Healthplan and Services Defined
PLAN TYPE: Multiple
Plan Specialty: Dental, Vision
Benefits Offered: Dental, Vision
Offers Demand Management Patient Information Service: Yes

Type of Payment Plans Offered
Capitated, Combination FFS & DFFS

Geographic Areas Served
Statewide

Peer Review Type
Second Surgical Opinion: Yes

Publishes and Distributes Report Card: Yes

Key Personnel
CFO . . . . Steve Sheehan
CIO. . . . . Shenoy Manju
Marketing . . . . Chris McConathy
Dental Director . . . . Karen Feldman

Average Claim Compensation
Physician's Fees Charged: 80%

Specialty Managed Care Partners
Enters into Contracts with Regional Business Coalitions: Yes

93 Health Net Dental

340 Commerce
Suite 100
Irvine, CA 92602
Toll-Free: 800-977-7307
www.hndental.com
For Profit Organization: Yes

Healthplan and Services Defined
PLAN TYPE: Dental
Model Type: Network
Plan Specialty: Dental
Benefits Offered: Dental

Type of Coverage
Individual, Dental coverage for Healthy Familie

Geographic Areas Served
Los Angeles and Sacramento County

94 Health Net Federal Services

2025 Aerojet Road
Mail Code CA-169-01-27
Rancho Cordova, CA 95742
Toll-Free: 800-440-3114
www.hnfs.com
Subsidiary of: Health Net
For Profit Organization: Yes
Total Enrollment: 2,900,000

Healthplan and Services Defined
PLAN TYPE: Multiple
Model Type: Network
Plan Specialty: Behavioral Health
Benefits Offered: Behavioral Health, Anger management;
    DUI program; alcohol & drug assessments

Type of Coverage
Commercial, Individual, Medicare, Supplemental Medicare

Geographic Areas Served
Alaska, Arizona, California, Colorado, Hawaii, Idaho, Iowa
(except the Rock Island Arsenal area), Kansas, Minnesota,
Missouri, (except the St. Louis area), Montana, Nebraska,
Nevada, New Mexico, North Dakota, Oregon, South Dakota,
Texas (areas of Western Texas only), Utah, Washington, and
Wyoming

Key Personnel
President. . . . . Billy Maynard
Media Contact . . . . Molly Tuttle
    molly.m.tuttle@healthnet.com

95 Health Net Insurance

P.O. Box 10420
Van Nuys, CA 91410-0420
Toll-Free: 877-527-8409
www.healthnet.com
Subsidiary of: Centene Corporation
For Profit Organization: Yes

Healthplan and Services Defined
PLAN TYPE: Multiple
Model Type: Network
Plan Specialty: Behavioral Health

Type of Coverage
Commercial, Individual, Medicare, Supplemental Medicare,
    Medi-Cal

Geographic Areas Served
Arizona, California, Oregon, Washington

96 Health Net, Inc.

21650 Oxnard Street
Woodland Hills, CA 91367
Toll-Free: 877-878-7983
www.healthnet.com
Subsidiary of: Centene Corporation
For Profit Organization: Yes
Year Founded: 1977
Total Enrollment: 6,100,000

Healthplan and Services Defined
PLAN TYPE: HMO
Model Type: IPA, Group
Plan Specialty: Behavioral Health, PBM, Substance abuse and
    employee assistance programs.
Benefits Offered: Behavioral Health, Chiropractic, Dental,
    Disease Management, Prescription, Vision, Wellness,
    Benefits vary according to plan
Offers Demand Management Patient Information Service: Yes

Type of Coverage
Commercial, Individual, Medicare, Supplemental Medicare,
    Health Net Medi-Cal
Catastrophic Illness Benefit: Covered

Type of Payment Plans Offered
POS, DFFS, FFS

Geographic Areas Served
Nationwide, including the District of Columbia

Peer Review Type
Utilization Review: Yes
Second Surgical Opinion: Yes
Case Management: Yes

Publishes and Distributes Report Card: Yes

Accreditation Certification
NCQA
TJC Accreditation, Medicare Approved, Utilization Review,
    Pre-Admission Certification, State Licensure, Quality
    Assurance Program

Key Personnel
President/CEO . . . . Jay Gellert

Chief Financial Officer . . . . Joseph C. Capezza
Chief Operating Officer . . . . James Woys
Contact, Federal Services . . . . Molly Tuttle
molly.tuttle@healthnet.com

Specialty Managed Care Partners
Enters into Contracts with Regional Business Coalitions: Yes

---

97 Health Plan of San Joaquin

7751 South Manthey Road
French Camp, CA 95231-9802
Toll-Free: 888-936-7526
Phone: 209-942-6340
Fax: 209-942-6305
www.hpsj.com
Secondary Address: 1025 J. Street, Modesto, CA 95354
Non-Profit Organization: Yes
Year Founded: 1996
Number of Primary Care Physicians: 180
Number of Referral/Specialty Physicians: 1,400
Total Enrollment: 109,000
State Enrollment: 109,000

Healthplan and Services Defined
PLAN TYPE: HMO
Benefits Offered: Behavioral Health, Dental, Inpatient SNF, Podiatry, Prescription, Vision, Wellness
Offers Demand Management Patient Information Service: Yes
DMPI Services Offered: 24 Hour Nurse Advice Hotline

Type of Coverage
Commercial, Medicaid, Medi-Cal

Geographic Areas Served
San Joaquin and Stanislaus counties

Key Personnel
CEO. . . . . Amy Shin
CFO . . . . Michelle Tetreault
Medical Director . . . . Dorcas C. Yao, MD
VP, External Affairs. David Hurst

---

98 Health Plan of San Mateo

801 Gateway Boulevard
Suite 100
South San Francisco, CA 94080
Toll-Free: 800-735-2929
Phone: 650-616-0050
Fax: 650-616-0060
info@hpsm.org
www.hpsm.org
Non-Profit Organization: Yes
Year Founded: 1987
Number of Affiliated Hospitals: 12
Number of Primary Care Physicians: 197
Total Enrollment: 87,740
State Enrollment: 87,740

Healthplan and Services Defined
PLAN TYPE: HMO
Model Type: IPA

Benefits Offered: Dental, Disease Management, Long-Term Care, Prescription, Vision, Wellness

Type of Coverage
Medi-Cal, Healthy Families, Healthy

Type of Payment Plans Offered
Capitated, FFS

Geographic Areas Served
San Mateo county

Key Personnel
CEO. . . . . Maya Altman
CFO . . . . Michael Smigielski
CIO . . . . Eben Yong
CCO . . . . Ian Johansson
Chief Strategy Officer . . . . Khoa Nguyen
Chief HR Officer . . . . Vicki Simpson

---

99 Health Services Los Angeles County

313 N Figueroa Street
Los Angeles, CA 90012
dhs.lacounty.gov/wps/portal/dhs
Subsidiary of: Los Angeles County Department of Health Services
Non-Profit Organization: Yes
Federally Qualified: Yes
Number of Affiliated Hospitals: 4

Healthplan and Services Defined
PLAN TYPE: Other
Model Type: municipal health system
Plan Specialty: Juvenile Justice System, children in Foster Care
Benefits Offered: Disease Management, Prescription, Wellness, AIDS Drug Assistance Program; Pediatrics

Type of Coverage
Catastrophic Illness Benefit: Unlimited

Geographic Areas Served
Los Angeles County

Subscriber Information
Average Monthly Fee Per Subscriber
(Employee + Employer Contribution):
Employee Only (Self): $143.05
Employee & 1 Family Member: $286.15
Employee & 2 Family Members: $332.01
Average Subscriber Co-Payment:
Primary Care Physician: $5.00
Prescription Drugs: $4.00
Home Health Care Max. Days/Visits Covered: Unlimited
Nursing Home Max. Days/Visits Covered: 60 days

Network Qualifications
Pre-Admission Certification: Yes

Peer Review Type
Utilization Review: Yes
Second Surgical Opinion: Yes
Case Management: Yes

Accreditation Certification
TJC Accreditation, Medicare Approved, Utilization Review, State Licensure, Quality Assurance Program

Key Personnel
Director . . . . Mitchell Katz, MD
Chief Financial Officer . . . . Allan Wecker
Chief Operations Officer . . . . Christina Ghaly, MD
Chief Information Officer . . . . Kevin Lynch
Chief Medical Officer . . . . Hal F. Yee Jr., MD

100 Humana Health Insurance of California

1 Park Plaza
Suite 470
Irvine, CA 92614
Phone: 949-623-1447
www.humana.com
Secondary Address: 516 W Shaw Avenue, Suite 200, Fresno, CA 93704, 559-221-2522
Subsidiary of: Humana
For Profit Organization: Yes

Healthplan and Services Defined
 PLAN TYPE: HMO/PPO
 Model Type: Network
 Plan Specialty: Dental, Vision
 Benefits Offered: Dental, Prescription, Vision, Life, LTD, STD, Benefits vary according to plan

Type of Coverage
 Commercial, Medicare

Geographic Areas Served
 Statewide

Accreditation Certification
 URAC, NCQA, CORE

Key Personnel
 Market Director . . . . Yuliya Parra

101 Inter Valley Health Plan

300 S Park Avenue
P.O. Box 6002
Pomona, CA 91769-6002
Toll-Free: 800-251-8191
info@ivhp.com
www.ivhp.com
Non-Profit Organization: Yes
Year Founded: 1979
Owned by an Integrated Delivery Network (IDN): No
Federally Qualified: Yes
Number of Affiliated Hospitals: 24
Number of Primary Care Physicians: 1,161
Number of Referral/Specialty Physicians: 4,791
Total Enrollment: 14,600

Healthplan and Services Defined
 PLAN TYPE: Medicare
 Model Type: Network
 Benefits Offered: Behavioral Health, Dental, Home Care, Inpatient SNF, Physical Therapy, Prescription, Psychiatric, Transplant, Wellness

Type of Coverage
 Medicare
 Catastrophic Illness Benefit: Unlimited

Type of Payment Plans Offered
 Capitated

Geographic Areas Served
 Southern California counties including Los Angeles, Riverside, San Bernardino, and Orange

Network Qualifications
 Pre-Admission Certification: No

Peer Review Type
 Utilization Review: Yes
 Second Surgical Opinion: Yes
 Case Management: Yes

Accreditation Certification
 URAC, PBGH, CCHRI
 TJC Accreditation, Medicare Approved, Utilization Review, State Licensure, Quality Assurance Program

Key Personnel
 President/CEO . . . . Ronald H. Bolding
 VP, Finance/CFO . . . . Paul Biberkraut
 VP, Health Plan Operation . . . . Susan Tenorio
 VP, Medical Services/CMO . . . . Kenneth E. Smith, MD

Average Claim Compensation
 Physician's Fees Charged: 75%
 Hospital's Fees Charged: 55%

Specialty Managed Care Partners
 Vision Service Plan

102 Kaiser Permanente

1 Kaiser Plaza
Oakland, CA 94612
Phone: 510-271-5910
www.kaiserpermanente.org
Non-Profit Organization: Yes
Year Founded: 1945
Number of Affiliated Hospitals: 39
Number of Primary Care Physicians: 17,791
Total Enrollment: 11,800,000
State Enrollment: 8,521,345

Healthplan and Services Defined
 PLAN TYPE: HMO/PPO
 Model Type: Group
 Benefits Offered: Dental, Disease Management, Home Care, Inpatient SNF, Long-Term Care, Physical Therapy, Podiatry, Prescription, Psychiatric, Transplant, Vision, Wellness, Benefits vary according to plan
 Offers Demand Management Patient Information Service: Yes

Type of Coverage
 Commercial, Individual, Medicare, Supplemental Medicare, Medicaid
 Catastrophic Illness Benefit: Covered

Type of Payment Plans Offered
 POS

Geographic Areas Served
 California, Colorado, Georgia, Hawaii, Maryland, Oregon, Virginia, Washington and the District of Columbia

Network Qualifications
Pre-Admission Certification: Yes

Peer Review Type
Utilization Review: Yes
Second Surgical Opinion: Yes
Case Management: Yes

Publishes and Distributes Report Card: Yes

Accreditation Certification
NCQA
TJC Accreditation, Medicare Approved, Utilization Review, Pre-Admission Certification, State Licensure, Quality Assurance Program

Key Personnel
Chairman/CEO........................ Bernard Tyson
EVP/CIO .... Richard Daniels
EVP/CFO .... Kathy Lancaster
SVP, Government Relations......... Anthony A. Barrueta
SVP/Commuications Officer............. Kathryn Beiser
SVP/CCM .... Vanessa M. Benavides
SVP/Chief HR Officer .... Chuck Columbus
SVP/General Counsel .... Mark S. Zemelman
EVP/CMO.................... Patrick Courneya, MD

Specialty Managed Care Partners
Enters into Contracts with Regional Business Coalitions: No

---

103 Kaiser Permanente Northern California
1950 Franklin Street
Oakland, CA 94612
Phone: 510-987-1000
thrive.kaiserpermanente.org/care-near-northern-california
Subsidiary of: Kaiser Permanente
Non-Profit Organization: Yes
Year Founded: 1945
Number of Affiliated Hospitals: 21
Number of Primary Care Physicians: 8,500
Total Enrollment: 118,000,000
State Enrollment: 4,131,326

Healthplan and Services Defined
PLAN TYPE: HMO/PPO
Model Type: Group, Network
Benefits Offered: Disease Management, Home Care, Inpatient SNF, Long-Term Care, Physical Therapy, Podiatry, Prescription, Psychiatric, Transplant, Vision, Wellness

Type of Coverage
Commercial, Individual, Medicare, Medicaid

Type of Payment Plans Offered
POS, Combination FFS & DFFS

Geographic Areas Served
Alameda, Amador, Contra Costa, El Dorado, Fresno, Kings, Madera, Marin, Mariposa, Napa, Placer, Sacramento, San Francisco, San Joaquin, San Mateo, Santa Clara, Solano, Sonoma, Stanislaus, Sutter, Tulcare, Yolo & Yuba counties

Subscriber Information
Average Monthly Fee Per Subscriber
(Employee + Employer Contribution):

Employee Only (Self): Varies by plan

Network Qualifications
Pre-Admission Certification: Yes

Publishes and Distributes Report Card: Yes

Accreditation Certification
TJC Accreditation, Medicare Approved, Utilization Review, Pre-Admission Certification, State Licensure, Quality Assurance Program

Key Personnel
President, No.California .... Janet Liang
Executive Medic. Director .... Edward M. Ellison, MD
Media Contact..................... Jessie Mangaliman
510-301-5414

Specialty Managed Care Partners
Enters into Contracts with Regional Business Coalitions: Yes

---

104 Kaiser Permanente Southern California
9455 Clairemont Mesa Boulevard
San Diego, CA 92123
thrive.kaiserpermanente.org/care-near-you/southern-califor
ni
Subsidiary of: Kaiser Permanente
Non-Profit Organization: Yes
Year Founded: 1945
Number of Affiliated Hospitals: 15
Number of Primary Care Physicians: 7,274
Total Enrollment: 11,800,000
State Enrollment: 4,390,019

Healthplan and Services Defined
PLAN TYPE: Multiple
Model Type: Network
Benefits Offered: Disease Management, Home Care, Inpatient SNF, Long-Term Care, Physical Therapy, Podiatry, Prescription, Psychiatric, Transplant, Vision, Wellness

Type of Coverage
Commercial, Individual, Medicare, Medicaid

Geographic Areas Served
Antelope Valley, Baldwin Park, Downey, Kern County, Los Angeles, Orange County, Panorama City, Riverside County, San Bernadino County, San Diego, South Bay, Ventura County, West Los Angeles, Woodland Hills

Key Personnel
President, South. Cali .... Julie Miller-Phipps
Media Contact...................... Lowell Goodman
626-405-3004

---

105 Kern Family Health Care
5701 Truxtun Avenue
Suite 201
Bakersfield, CA 93309
Toll-Free: 800-391-2000
Phone: 661-664-5000
louiei@khs-net.com
www.kernfamilyhealthcare.com
Secondary Address: 9700 Stockdale Highway, Bakersfield, CA 93311, 661-632-1590

Subsidiary of: Kern Health Systems
Non-Profit Organization: Yes
Number of Affiliated Hospitals: 10
Number of Primary Care Physicians: 213
Number of Referral/Specialty Physicians: 400
Total Enrollment: 97,000
State Enrollment: 90,074

Healthplan and Services Defined
  PLAN TYPE: HMO
  Model Type: Network
  Benefits Offered: Dental, Disease Management, Prescription,
    Vision, Wellness
  Offers Demand Management Patient Information Service:
    Yes
  DMPI Services Offered: 24 Hour Nurse Advice Hotline

Type of Coverage
  Individual, Medicaid, Medi-Cal

Key Personnel
  Chief Executive Officer . . . . Doug Hayward
  Chief Financial Officer . . . . Robert Landis
  Chief Operations Officer . . . . Alan Avery
  Chief Medical Officer . . . . Dr. Martha E. Tasinga
  Chief Information Officer . . . . Richard Pruitt
  Manager, Marketing . . . . Louis Iturriria
    661-664-5120
    louiei@khs-net.com

106   L.A. Care Health Plan
1055 W 7th Street
10th Floor
Los Angeles, CA 90017
Toll-Free: 888-452-2273
www.lacare.org
Non-Profit Organization: Yes
Year Founded: 1997
Total Enrollment: 2,000,000

Healthplan and Services Defined
  PLAN TYPE: HMO
  Benefits Offered: Behavioral Health, Dental, Home Care,
    Inpatient SNF, Physical Therapy, Prescription, Transplant,
    Vision, Wellness, Asthma Care; Cancer Clinical Trials;
    Diabetic Care; Diagnostic/Labs/Imaging Services; Durable
    Medical Equipment; Hospice

Type of Coverage
  Individual, Medicare, Medicaid

Key Personnel
  Chief Executive Officer . . . . John Baackes
  Chief Operating Officer . . . . Dino Kasdagly
  Chief Financial Officer . . . . Marie Montgomery
  Chief Medical Officer . . . . Richard Seidman
  General Counsel . . . . Augustavia Haydel
  Chief Compliance Officer . . . . Tom Mapp
  Chief Information Officer . . . . Tom Schwaninger

107   L.A. Care Health Plan
1055 W 7th Street
10th Floor
Los Angeles, CA 90017
Toll-Free: 888-452-2273
www.lacare.org
Non-Profit Organization: Yes
Year Founded: 1997
Number of Affiliated Hospitals: 83
Number of Primary Care Physicians: 3,555
Number of Referral/Specialty Physicians: 6,286
Total Enrollment: 857,252
State Enrollment: 836,724

Healthplan and Services Defined
  PLAN TYPE: HMO
  Model Type: Staff
  Benefits Offered: Dental, Home Care, Podiatry, Prescription,
    Vision, Comprehensive Health Coverage, Medical

Type of Coverage
  Medicaid, Medi-Cal, L.A. Care Covered, Cal Me

Geographic Areas Served
  Los Angeles County

Key Personnel
  CEO . . . . John Baackes
  COO . . . . Dino Kasdagly
  CFO . . . . Marie Montgomery
  CCO . . . . Tom Mapp
  General Counsel . . . . Augustavia J. Haydel
  Chief Medical Officer . . . . Richard Seidman, MD, MPH
  CIO . . . . Tom Schwaninger

108   Lakeside Community Healthcare Network
191 S Buena Vista Street
Suite 240
Burbank, CA 91505
Phone: 818-557-7278
info@lakesidecommunityhealthcare.com
www.lakesidemed.com
For Profit Organization: Yes
Year Founded: 1997
Number of Primary Care Physicians: 300
Number of Referral/Specialty Physicians: 1,500
Total Enrollment: 250,000
State Enrollment: 250,000

Healthplan and Services Defined
  PLAN TYPE: HMO
  Model Type: IPA

Geographic Areas Served
  San Fernando, San Gabriel, and Santa Clarita Valleys. Parts of
  Ventura and San Bernadino counties

Key Personnel
  Dir., Network Management . . . . Julie Feind

109 Landmark Healthplan of California

P.O. Box 130028
Sacramento, CA 95853
Toll-Free: 800-298-4875
Fax: 800-547-9784
www.lhp-ca.com
For Profit Organization: Yes
Year Founded: 1985
Number of Referral/Specialty Physicians: 4,500
Total Enrollment: 150,000

Healthplan and Services Defined
  PLAN TYPE: HMO/PPO
  Model Type: IPA, Network
  Plan Specialty: Chiropractic, Acupuncture
  Benefits Offered: Chiropractic, Acupuncture

Type of Payment Plans Offered
  Combination FFS & DFFS

Geographic Areas Served
  Statewide

Network Qualifications
  Pre-Admission Certification: Yes

Peer Review Type
  Utilization Review: Yes
  Case Management: Yes

Key Personnel
  President/CEO . . . . George W. Vieth, Jr
  VP/CFO. . . . . Thomas P. Klammer
  VP, Sales . . . . Greg Clure
    800-298-4875
    Sales@LHP-CA.com

110 Liberty Dental Plan of California

340 Commerce
Suite 100
Irvine, CA 92602
Toll-Free: 888-703-6999
www.libertydentalplan.com
Mailing Address: P.O. Box 26110, Santa Ana, CA 92799-6110
For Profit Organization: Yes
Year Founded: 2001
Total Enrollment: 3,000,000

Healthplan and Services Defined
  PLAN TYPE: Dental
  Other Type: Dental HMO
  Plan Specialty: Dental
  Benefits Offered: Dental

Type of Coverage
  Commercial, Individual, Medicare, Medicaid, Medi-Cal

Geographic Areas Served
  Statewide

Accreditation Certification
  NCQA

Key Personnel
  Dir., Compliance SW Reg. . . . . Daniel Aguilar

111 Managed Health Network, Inc.

2370 Kerner Boulevard
San Rafael, CA 94901
Toll-Free: 800-327-2133
productinfo@mhn.com
www.mhn.com
Subsidiary of: Health Net, Inc.
For Profit Organization: Yes
Number of Affiliated Hospitals: 1,400
Number of Primary Care Physicians: 55,000
Total Enrollment: 7,300,000

Healthplan and Services Defined
  PLAN TYPE: Other
  Plan Specialty: Behavioral Health, Substance abuse and
    employee assistance programs (EAPs).
  Benefits Offered: Behavioral Health, Disease Management,
    Wellness, Work/life balance, employee productivity and
    organizational effectiveness.

Geographic Areas Served
  Nationwide

Accreditation Certification
  URAC

Key Personnel
  Psychologist Clinical Dir . . . . Nancy Mann
  Chief Medical Officer . . . . Ian Shaffer, MD

112 March Vision Care

6701 Center Drive W
Suite 790
Los Angeles, CA 90045
Toll-Free: 866-376-6780
Phone: 310-216-2300
marchinfo@marchvisioncare.com
www.marchvisioncare.com
For Profit Organization: Yes

Healthplan and Services Defined
  PLAN TYPE: Vision
  Plan Specialty: Vision
  Benefits Offered: Vision

Type of Coverage
  Commercial, Medicare, Medicaid

Geographic Areas Served
  Nationwide

Key Personnel
  Founder & CEO . . . . Glenville A March, Jr, MD
  Founder & CEO . . . . Cabrini T March, MD

113 Medcore Medical Group

2609 E Hammer Lane
Stockton, CA 95210
Toll-Free: 877-963-2673
Phone: 209-320-2650
Fax: 209-320-2644
medcoreipa.com
Year Founded: 1985

Healthplan and Services Defined
   PLAN TYPE: Other
   Model Type: Network

Geographic Areas Served
   San Joaquin County

Key Personnel
   Chief Operating Officer . . . . Maria Martinez

114 Medica HealthCare Plans, Inc

9100 S Dadeland Boulevard
Suite 1250
Miami, FL 33156
Toll-Free: 800-407-9069
Fax: 501-262-7070
MemberServices@uhcsouthflorida.com
www.medicaplans.com
Mailing Address: P.O. Box 29675, Hot Srpings, AR
   71903-9675
Total Enrollment: 12,000

Healthplan and Services Defined
   PLAN TYPE: Medicare
   Benefits Offered: Chiropractic, Dental, Disease Management,
      Inpatient SNF, Podiatry, Prescription, Psychiatric, Vision,
      Wellness

Type of Coverage
   Medicare, Supplemental Medicare

Geographic Areas Served
   Miami-Dade & Broward counties

115 Molina Healthcare

200 Oceangate
Suite 100
Long Beach, CA 90802
Toll-Free: 888-562-5442
Phone: 562-435-3666
www.molinahealthcare.com
For Profit Organization: Yes

Healthplan and Services Defined
   PLAN TYPE: Medicare
   Other Type: Madicaid
   Benefits Offered: Disease Management, Physical Therapy,
      Wellness

Type of Coverage
   Medicare, Supplemental Medicare, Medicaid

Geographic Areas Served
   California, Florida, Illinois, Michigan, Ohio, Puerto Rico,
   New Mexico, New York, South Carolina, Texas, Utah,
   Washington and Wisconsin

Key Personnel
   President/CEO . . . . Joseph Zubretsky
   Chief Financial Officer. . . . . Thomas Tran
   SVP/General Counsel . . . . Jeff D. Barlow, JD
   Health Plan Operations . . . . Pamela Sedmak
   EVP, Health Plan Services . . . . James Woys

116 Molina Healthcare of California

200 Oceangate
Suite 100
Long Beach, CA 90802
Toll-Free: 800-526-8196
www.molinahealthcare.com
Subsidiary of: Molina Healthcare, Inc.
For Profit Organization: Yes
Year Founded: 1980

Healthplan and Services Defined
   PLAN TYPE: Medicare
   Model Type: Network
   Plan Specialty: Dental, PBM, Vision, Integrated
      Medicare/Medicaid (Duals)
   Benefits Offered: Dental, Prescription, Vision, Wellness, Life

Type of Coverage
   Individual, Medicare, Supplemental Medicare, Medicaid

Geographic Areas Served
   Statewide

117 Molina Medicaid Solutions

200 Oceangate
Suite 100
Long Beach, CA 90802
Toll-Free: 888-562-5442
Phone: 562-435-3666
www.molinahealthcare.com
Subsidiary of: Molina Healthcare, Inc.
For Profit Organization: Yes
Year Founded: 2010

Healthplan and Services Defined
   PLAN TYPE: Medicare

Type of Coverage
   Medicaid information management sys

Geographic Areas Served
   Idaho, Louisiana, Maine, New Jersey, West Virginia

Key Personnel
   President/CEO . . . . Joseph Zubretsky
   Chief Financial Officer. . . . . Thomas Tran
   SVP/General Counsel . . . . Jeff D. Barlow, JD
   Health Plan Operations . . . . Pamela Sedmak
   EVP/Health Plan Services . . . . James Woys

118 On Lok Lifeways

1333 Bush Street
San Francisco, CA 94109
Phone: 415-292-8888
info@onlok.org
www.onlok.org
Non-Profit Organization: Yes
Year Founded: 1971
Number of Affiliated Hospitals: 7
Number of Primary Care Physicians: 10
Number of Referral/Specialty Physicians: 100
Total Enrollment: 1,000
State Enrollment: 942

Healthplan and Services Defined
  PLAN TYPE: HMO
  Model Type: Staff
  Benefits Offered: Dental, Home Care, Long-Term Care,
    Physical Therapy, Podiatry, Prescription, Vision, Wellness

Type of Coverage
  Medicaid
  Catastrophic Illness Benefit: Covered

Geographic Areas Served
  San Francisco, Fremont, Newark, Union City and Santa Clara
  County

Accreditation Certification
  TJC Accreditation, Medicare Approved, Utilization Review,
    Pre-Admission Certification, State Licensure, Quality
    Assurance Program

Key Personnel
  CEO . . . . Grace Li
  CFO . . . . Gary Campanella
  COO . . . . David C. Nolan
  Chief, Gov. Affairs . . . . Eileen Kunz, MPH
  CMO . . . . Jay Luxenberg, MD
  Chief Development Officer . . . . John V. Blazek

119 Optimum HealthCare, Inc
5403 North Church Avenue
Tampa, FL 33614
Toll-Free: 866-245-5360
Fax: 813-506-6150
www.youroptimumhealthcare.com
Mailing Address: P.O. Box 151137, Tampa, FL 33684

Healthplan and Services Defined
  PLAN TYPE: HMO

Type of Coverage
  Medicare, Medicaid

Geographic Areas Served
  Brevard, Broward, Charlotte, Citrus, Clay, Collier, Dade, De
  Soto, Duval, Escambia, Hernando, Hillsborough, Indian
  River, Lake, Lee, Manatee, Marion, Martin, Orange, Osceola,
  Palm Beach, Pasco, Pinellas, Polk, Sarasota, Seminole, St.
  Lucie, Sumter and Volusia counties

Accreditation Certification
  NCQA

120 Pacific Foundation for Medical Care
3510 Unocal Place
Suite 108
Santa Rosa, CA 95403
Toll-Free: 800-548-7677
Phone: 707-525-4281
Fax: 707-525-4311
jnacol@rhs.org
pfmc.org
Non-Profit Organization: Yes
Year Founded: 1957
Number of Primary Care Physicians: 34,000

Healthplan and Services Defined
  PLAN TYPE: Multiple
  Model Type: Network
  Plan Specialty: EPO, PPO, LOCO

Geographic Areas Served
  counties: Alameda, Butte, Colusa, Contra Costa, El Dorado,
  Glenn, Imperial, Lake, Lassen, Marin, Mendocino, Modoc,
  Napa, Nevada, Placer, Plumas, Sacramento, San Diego, San
  Francisco, Shasta, Sierra, Siskiyou, Solano, Sonoma, Sutter,
  Tehama, Trinity,Yolo, Yuba

Network Qualifications
  Pre-Admission Certification: Yes

Peer Review Type
  Utilization Review: Yes
  Second Surgical Opinion: Yes
  Case Management: Yes

Publishes and Distributes Report Card: No

Key Personnel
  President . . . . Dan Lightfoot, MD
  Medical Director . . . . William Pitt, MD
  Contact. . . . . Kathy Pass
    705-525-4281
    kpass@rhs.org

Specialty Managed Care Partners
  Enters into Contracts with Regional Business Coalitions: No

121 Pacific Health Alliance
1525 Rollins Road
Suite B
Burlingame, CA 94010
Toll-Free: 800-533-4742
Fax: 650-375-5820
pha@pacifichealthalliance.com
www.pacifichealthalliance.com
For Profit Organization: Yes
Year Founded: 1986
Number of Affiliated Hospitals: 400
Number of Primary Care Physicians: 50,000
Number of Referral/Specialty Physicians: 1,500
Total Enrollment: 338,000
State Enrollment: 197,000

Healthplan and Services Defined
  PLAN TYPE: PPO
  Model Type: Group
  Plan Specialty: Behavioral Health, Chiropractic, EPO, Lab,
    Worker's Compensation, UR
  Benefits Offered: Behavioral Health, Chiropractic, Dental,
    Home Care, Inpatient SNF, Long-Term Care, Physical
    Therapy, Podiatry, Psychiatric, Transplant, Vision, Worker's
    Compensation

Type of Coverage
  Commercial, Individual, Indemnity

Type of Payment Plans Offered
  DFFS, FFS

Geographic Areas Served
  Nationwide

Network Qualifications
Pre-Admission Certification: Yes

Peer Review Type
Utilization Review: Yes
Second Surgical Opinion: Yes
Case Management: Yes

Publishes and Distributes Report Card: No

Accreditation Certification
TJC Accreditation, Medicare Approved, Utilization Review, Pre-Admission Certification, State Licensure, Quality Assurance Program

Average Claim Compensation
Physician's Fees Charged: 70%
Hospital's Fees Charged: 75%

Specialty Managed Care Partners
Daughters of Charity, Saint Rose Hospital, San Monterry
Enters into Contracts with Regional Business Coalitions: No

---

122 Partnership HealthPlan of California

4665 Business Center Drive
Fairfield, CA 94534-1675
Toll-Free: 800-863-4155
Fax: 707-863-4117
www.partnershiphp.org
Secondary Address: 3688 Avtech Parkway, Redding, CA 96002, 855-798-8760
Non-Profit Organization: Yes
Year Founded: 1994
Total Enrollment: 560,000

Healthplan and Services Defined
PLAN TYPE: Other
Other Type: Medi-Cal
Benefits Offered: Behavioral Health, Chiropractic, Dental, Home Care, Inpatient SNF, Long-Term Care, Podiatry, Prescription, Vision, Durable Medical Equipment; Hospice; Prenatal Care; Substance Abuse; Transportation; Labs & Imaging; Pediatrics; and more

Type of Coverage
Individual, Medicare, Medicaid

Geographic Areas Served
counties: Del Norte, Humboldt, Lake, Lassen, Marin, Mendocino, Modoc, Napa, Shasta, Siskiyou, Solano, Sonoma, Trinity and Yolo

Accreditation Certification
NCQA

Key Personnel
Chief Executive Officer................... Liz Gibboney
Chief Operating Officer .... Sonja Bjork
Chief Financial Officer .... Patti McFarland
Administrative Officer...................... Sue Monez
Chief Information Officer................... Kirt Kemp
Chief Medical Officer............... Robert Moore, MD

---

123 Premier Access Insurance/Access Dental

P.O. Box 659010
Sacramento, CA 95865-9010
Toll-Free: 888-634-6074
Phone: 916-920-2500
Fax: 916-563-9000
info@premierlife.com
www.premierlife.com
Subsidiary of: Guardian Life Insurance Co.
For Profit Organization: Yes
Year Founded: 1989
Number of Primary Care Physicians: 1,000
Total Enrollment: 125,000

Healthplan and Services Defined
PLAN TYPE: PPO
Other Type: Dental
Model Type: Network
Plan Specialty: Dental
Benefits Offered: Dental

Type of Payment Plans Offered
FFS

Geographic Areas Served
California, Nevada, Utah, Arizona

Accreditation Certification
TJC Accreditation, Medicare Approved, Utilization Review, Pre-Admission Certification, State Licensure, Quality Assurance Program

Key Personnel
President & CEO .... Deanna M. Mulligan

---

124 Primecare Dental Plan

10700 Civic Center Drive
Suite 100-A
Rancho Cucamonga, CA 91730
Toll-Free: 800-937-3400
contact@primecaredental.net
www.primecaredental.net
For Profit Organization: Yes
Year Founded: 1983
Physician Owned Organization: Yes
Total Enrollment: 17,000

Healthplan and Services Defined
PLAN TYPE: Dental
Model Type: Staff
Plan Specialty: Dental
Benefits Offered: Dental
Offers Demand Management Patient Information Service: Yes

Type of Coverage
Commercial, Individual

Type of Payment Plans Offered
DFFS, Capitated

Geographic Areas Served
Alameda, Butte, Colusa, Contra Costa, El Dorado, Fresno, Glenn, Kern, Kings, Los Angeles, Madera, Mariposa, Merced Monterey, Napa, Nevada, Orange, Placer, Riverside, Sacramento, San Benito, San Bernardino, San Diego, San

Francisco, San Joaquin, San Luis Opispo, San Mateo, Santa Barbara, Santa Clara, Santa Cruz, Shasta, Siskiyou, Solano, Sonoma, Stanislaus, Sutter, Tehama, Tuolumne, Tulare, Ventura, Yolo, and Yuba counties

Network Qualifications
Pre-Admission Certification: Yes

Peer Review Type
Utilization Review: Yes

Publishes and Distributes Report Card: No

Accreditation Certification
URAC, NCQA
Utilization Review

Specialty Managed Care Partners
Enters into Contracts with Regional Business Coalitions: No

---

125 PTPN
26635 W Agoura Road
Suite 250
Calabasas, CA 91302
Toll-Free: 800-766-7876
info@ptpn.com
www.ptpn.com
Year Founded: 1985
Number of Primary Care Physicians: 3,500

Healthplan and Services Defined
PLAN TYPE: PPO
Other Type: Rehab Network
Model Type: Network
Plan Specialty: Outpatient Rehabilitation (Physical, Occupational and Speech Therapy)
Benefits Offered: Physical Therapy, Worker's Compensation, Occupational Therapy; Speech Therapy; Physical Therapy; Hand Therapy; Speech/Language Therapy; and Pediatric Therapy

Type of Payment Plans Offered
DFFS

Geographic Areas Served
Nationwide

Network Qualifications
Minimum Years of Practice: 3

Peer Review Type
Utilization Review: Yes

Accreditation Certification
NCQA

Key Personnel
President . . . . Michael Weinper
Vice President . . . . Nancy Rothenberg
Quality Assurance . . . . Michel Kaye

---

126 San Francisco Health Plan
50 Beale Street
12th Floor
San Francisco, CA 94119
Toll-Free: 800-288-5555
Phone: 415-547-7818
Fax: 415-547-7826
www.sfhp.org
Year Founded: 1994
Number of Affiliated Hospitals: 6
Number of Primary Care Physicians: 2,300
Total Enrollment: 55,000
State Enrollment: 55,000

Healthplan and Services Defined
PLAN TYPE: HMO
Benefits Offered: Dental, Disease Management, Prescription, Vision, Wellness

Type of Coverage
Medicare, Medicaid, Medi-Cal, Healthy Families, Healthy

Geographic Areas Served
San Francisco

Key Personnel
Chief Executive Officer . . . . John F Grgurina, Jr
Compliance Officer . . . . Nina Maruyama
Human Res Consultant . . . . Kate Gormley
Dir., System Development . . . . Cecil Newton
Dir, Business Services . . . . Van Wong

---

127 Santa Clara Family Health Foundations Inc
6201 San Ignacio Avenue
San Jose, CA 95119
Toll-Free: 800-260-2055
Phone: 408-376-2000
www.scfhp.com
Mailing Address: P.O. Box 18880, San Jose, CA 95158
Non-Profit Organization: Yes
Year Founded: 1997
Number of Affiliated Hospitals: 6
Number of Primary Care Physicians: 983
Number of Referral/Specialty Physicians: 3,356
Total Enrollment: 250,000
State Enrollment: 250,000

Healthplan and Services Defined
PLAN TYPE: HMO
Benefits Offered: Behavioral Health, Disease Management, Long-Term Care, Prescription, Wellness
Offers Demand Management Patient Information Service: Yes
DMPI Services Offered: 24 hour nurse advice line

Type of Coverage
Commercial, Medicaid, Medicare Advantage SNP, Medi-Cal, H

Geographic Areas Served
Santa Clara County

Subscriber Information
Average Monthly Fee Per Subscriber
(Employee + Employer Contribution):

Employee & 2 Family Members: $18 max per family

Key Personnel

Chief Executive Officer . . . . Christine M. Tomcala
Chief Information Officer . . . . Jonathan Tomayo
Chief Medical Officer . . . . Jeff Robertson
Chief Financial Officer . . . . Dave Cameron
Chief Compliance Officer. . . . . Robin L. Larmer
VP, Human Resources . . . . Sharon Valdez
Chief Operating Officer . . . . Christine K. Turner

Specialty Managed Care Partners
Medimpact

---

128 Sant, Community Physicians

7370 N Palm
Suite 101
Fresno, CA 93711
Toll-Free: 800-652-2900
Phone: 559-228-5400
Fax: 559-228-2958
www.santehealth.net
Year Founded: 1980
Number of Primary Care Physicians: 1,200
Total Enrollment: 120,000

Healthplan and Services Defined
PLAN TYPE: HMO/PPO
Model Type: IPA
Benefits Offered: Wellness

Type of Payment Plans Offered
FFS

Geographic Areas Served
Fresno, Madera and Kings counties

Network Qualifications
Pre-Admission Certification: Yes

Peer Review Type
Utilization Review: Yes
Case Management: Yes

Publishes and Distributes Report Card: Yes

Accreditation Certification
TJC Accreditation, Medicare Approved, Utilization Review,
Pre-Admission Certification, State Licensure, Quality
Assurance Program

Specialty Managed Care Partners
Enters into Contracts with Regional Business Coalitions: Yes

---

129 SCAN Health Plan

P.O. Box 22616
Long Beach, CA 90801-5616
Toll-Free: 800-559-3500
memberservices@scanhealthplan.com
www.scanhealthplan.com
Non-Profit Organization: Yes
Year Founded: 1977
Number of Affiliated Hospitals: 151
Number of Primary Care Physicians: 6,560
Number of Referral/Specialty Physicians: 17,186

Total Enrollment: 128,272
State Enrollment: 12,283

Healthplan and Services Defined
PLAN TYPE: HMO
Plan Specialty: Medicare
Benefits Offered: Vision

Type of Coverage
Medicare

Geographic Areas Served
California & Arizona

Subscriber Information
Average Annual Deductible Per Subscriber:
Medicare: $0
Average Subscriber Co-Payment:
Primary Care Physician: $0-$5
Hospital ER: $75
Home Health Care: $0
Nursing Home: $0
Nursing Home Max. Days/Visits Covered: 100

Key Personnel
Chief Executive Officer . . . . Christopher Wing
Chief Financial Officer . . . . Vinod Mohan
President . . . . Bill Roth
General Counsel . . . . Janet Kornblatt
Administrative Officer . . . . Nancy J. Monk
Chief Information Officer . . . . Josh Goode
Chief Pharmacy Officer . . . . Sharon K. Jhawar
SVP, National Sales. . . . . David Milligan
Chief Medical Executive. . . . . Romilla Batra

---

130 Sharp Health Plan

8520 Tech Way
Suite 200
San Diego, CA 92123
Toll-Free: 800-359-2002
Phone: 858-499-8300
customer.service@sharp.com
www.sharphealthplan.com
Subsidiary of: Sharp HealthCare
Non-Profit Organization: Yes
Year Founded: 1992
Total Enrollment: 49,000
State Enrollment: 49,000

Healthplan and Services Defined
PLAN TYPE: HMO
Model Type: Network
Benefits Offered: Prescription, Vision, Wellness

Type of Coverage
Medicare

Geographic Areas Served
San Diego and Southern Riverside counties

Key Personnel
President/CEO . . . . Melissa Hayden-Cook
VP/CFO . . . . Rita Datko
VP/COO . . . . Leslie Pels-Beck
VP Business Development. . . . . Michael Bryd

VP/CMO. . . . . Cary Shames

131   Stanislaus Foundation for Medical Care
2339 St Pauls Way
Modesto, CA 95355
Phone: 209-527-1704
Fax: 209-527-5861
sms@stanislausmedicalsociety.com
www.stanislausmedicalsociety.com
Non-Profit Organization: Yes
Year Founded: 1957
Physician Owned Organization: Yes
Number of Affiliated Hospitals: 400
Number of Primary Care Physicians: 27,000
Number of Referral/Specialty Physicians: 5,000

Healthplan and Services Defined
  PLAN TYPE: PPO
  Model Type: Network
  Benefits Offered: Dental, Prescription, Vision, Worker's
    Compensation
  Offers Demand Management Patient Information Service:
    Yes

Geographic Areas Served
  Stanislaus, Tuolumne counties

Network Qualifications
  Pre-Admission Certification: Yes

Publishes and Distributes Report Card: No

Key Personnel
  President of SFMC . . . . David Shiba, MD
  President of SMS . . . . Ronald Arakelian, MD
  Director . . . . Kathleen Eve, MD

Specialty Managed Care Partners
  Enters into Contracts with Regional Business Coalitions: No

132   Superior Vision
11101 White Rock Road
Rancho Cordova, CA 95670
Toll-Free: 800-507-3800
contactus@supervision.com
www.superiorvision.com
Secondary Address: Corporate Headquarters, 939 Elkridge
  Landing Road, Suite 200, Linthicum, MD 21090,
  800-243-1401
For Profit Organization: Yes
Year Founded: 1993

Healthplan and Services Defined
  PLAN TYPE: Vision
  Model Type: Group
  Plan Specialty: Vision
  Benefits Offered: Vision

Type of Coverage
  Commercial, Indemnity, Medicaid, Catastrophic

Geographic Areas Served
  Nationwide

Accreditation Certification
  AAPI, NCQA

Key Personnel
  Chief Executive Officer . . . . Kirk Rothrock
  Chief Information Officer. . . . . Greg Pontius
  Chief Financial Officer . . . . Brian Silverberg
  SVP, Operations. . . . . Glen McDonald
  VP, Provider Relations . . . . Zon Dunn
  VP, Marketing. . . . . Kathleen McMinn
  VP, Sales . . . . Thomas Luchetta

133   Taylor Benefits
4820 Harwood Road
Suite 130
San Jose, CA 95124
Toll-Free: 800-903-6066
Phone: 408-358-7502
Fax: 408-723-8201
taylorbenefitsinsurance.com
Year Founded: 1987

Healthplan and Services Defined
  PLAN TYPE: Multiple
  Benefits Offered: Behavioral Health, Dental, Inpatient SNF,
    Long-Term Care, Prescription, Vision, Wellness, Life,
    Short-and-long-term disability; Substance Abuse; Maternity
    & Newborn Care; Rehabiliation; Labs; Pediatrics

Geographic Areas Served
  Plans available for employers statewide

Key Personnel
  Principal. . . . . Todd Taylor
    todd@taylorbenefits.net
  Administrative Assistant . . . . Ronda Agpaoa
    ronda@taylorbenefits.net
  Principal . . . . Jennifer Taylor
    jennifer@taylorbenefits.net

134   Trinity Health of California
Saint Agnes Medical Center
1303 E Herndon Avenue
Fresno, CA 93720
Phone: 559-450-3000
www.trinity-health.org
Secondary Address: 20555 Victor Parkway, Livonia, MI
  48152-7018, 734-343-1000
Subsidiary of: Trinity Health
Non-Profit Organization: Yes
Year Founded: 2013
Total Enrollment: 30,000,000

Healthplan and Services Defined
  PLAN TYPE: Other
  Benefits Offered: Disease Management, Home Care,
    Long-Term Care, Psychiatric, Hospice programs, PACE
    (Program of All Inclusive Care for the Elderly)

Geographic Areas Served
  San Joaquin Valley

Key Personnel
President/CEO . . . . Nancy Hollingsworth, RN
Chief Financial Officer . . . . Michael Prusiatis
Chief Admin Officer . . . . Stacy Vaillancourt
Chief Operating Officer. . . . . Kim Meeker
Chief Medical Officer . . . . W. Eugene Egerton, MD

135 United Concordia of California

516 W Shaw Avenue
Suite 200
Fresno, CA 93704
Phone: 559-228-0400
www.unitedconcordia.com
For Profit Organization: Yes
Year Founded: 1971
Number of Primary Care Physicians: 96,000
Total Enrollment: 7,800,000

Healthplan and Services Defined
PLAN TYPE: Dental
Model Type: Network
Plan Specialty: Dental
Benefits Offered: Dental

Type of Coverage
Commercial, Individual, Military personnel & families

Geographic Areas Served
Nationwide

Accreditation Certification
URAC

136 UnitedHealthcare of Northern California

2300 Clayton Road
Suite 1000
Concord, CA 94520
Toll-Free: 888-545-5205
Phone: 925-246-1300
www.uhc.com
Subsidiary of: UnitedHealth Group
For Profit Organization: Yes

Healthplan and Services Defined
PLAN TYPE: HMO/PPO
Model Type: Network
Plan Specialty: Behavioral Health, Dental, Disease
   Management, PBM, Vision
Benefits Offered: Behavioral Health, Dental, Disease
   Management, Long-Term Care, Prescription, Vision,
   Wellness, Life, LTD, STD

Type of Coverage
Commercial, Individual, Medicare, Supplemental Medicare,
   Medicaid, Family, Group
Catastrophic Illness Benefit: Covered

Type of Payment Plans Offered
DFFS, Capitated

Geographic Areas Served
Statewide

Subscriber Information
Average Monthly Fee Per Subscriber
   (Employee + Employer Contribution):
      Employee Only (Self): Varies
      Employee & 1 Family Member: Varies
      Employee & 2 Family Members: Varies
      Medicare: Varies
Average Annual Deductible Per Subscriber:
      Employee Only (Self): Varies
      Employee & 1 Family Member: Varies
      Employee & 2 Family Members: Varies
      Medicare: Varies

Publishes and Distributes Report Card: Yes

Accreditation Certification
NCQA
TJC Accreditation, Utilization Review, State Licensure

Key Personnel
CEO, UHCC California. . . . . Kevin Kandalaft
SVP. . . . . Mark Knutson

Specialty Managed Care Partners
Enters into Contracts with Regional Business Coalitions: Yes

137 UnitedHealthcare of Southern California

2401 E Katella Avenue
Anaheim, CA 92806
Toll-Free: 888-835-9637
www.uhc.com
Subsidiary of: UnitedHealth Group
For Profit Organization: Yes

Healthplan and Services Defined
PLAN TYPE: HMO/PPO
Model Type: Network
Plan Specialty: Behavioral Health, Dental, Disease
   Management, PBM, Vision
Benefits Offered: Behavioral Health, Dental, Disease
   Management, Long-Term Care, Prescription, Vision,
   Wellness, Life, LTD, STD

Type of Coverage
Commercial, Individual, Medicare, Supplemental Medicare,
   Medicaid, Family, Group
Catastrophic Illness Benefit: Unlimited

Type of Payment Plans Offered
POS

Geographic Areas Served
Statewide

Network Qualifications
Pre-Admission Certification: Yes

Peer Review Type
Utilization Review: Yes
Second Surgical Opinion: Yes
Case Management: Yes

Publishes and Distributes Report Card: Yes

Accreditation Certification
NCQA

TJC Accreditation, Medicare Approved, Utilization Review, Pre-Admission Certification, State Licensure, Quality Assurance Program

Key Personnel
CEO, UHCC California . . . . Kevin Kandalaft
SVP . . . . Mark Knutson

Specialty Managed Care Partners
Enters into Contracts with Regional Business Coalitions: Yes

---

138 University HealthCare Alliance

7999 Gateway Boulevard
Suite 200
Newark, CA 95460
uha_communications@stanfordhealthcare.org
universityhealthcarealliance.org
For Profit Organization: Yes
Year Founded: 1996

Healthplan and Services Defined
PLAN TYPE: PPO
Model Type: Network

Geographic Areas Served
San Francisco Bay area

Key Personnel
Chief Medical Officer . . . . Bryan Bohman
Administrative Officer . . . . Catherine Krna
VP, Operations . . . . Gaguik Khachatourian

---

139 Ventura County Health Care Plan

2220 E Gonzales Rd
Suite 210 B
Oxnard, CA 93036
Toll-Free: 800-600-8247
Phone: 805-981-5050
www.vchealthcareplan.org
Non-Profit Organization: Yes
Year Founded: 1993

Healthplan and Services Defined
PLAN TYPE: HMO
Benefits Offered: Behavioral Health, Disease Management, Prescription, Wellness

Geographic Areas Served
Ventura County

Accreditation Certification
NCQA

---

140 Vision Plan of America

3255 Wilshire Boulevard
Suite 1610
Los Angeles, CA 90010
Toll-Free: 800-400-4872
Fax: 213-384-0084
info@visionplanofamerica.com
www.visionplanofamerica.com
For Profit Organization: Yes
Year Founded: 1986

Healthplan and Services Defined
PLAN TYPE: Vision
Model Type: IPA
Plan Specialty: Dental, Vision
Benefits Offered: Dental, Vision

Type of Coverage
Commercial, Individual

Type of Payment Plans Offered
POS, Capitated

Geographic Areas Served
Nationwide

Peer Review Type
Case Management: Yes

Key Personnel
President and CEO . . . . Stuart Needleman, OD
CFO . . . . Phillip Needleman
Manager . . . . Milori Lopez Duarte
Optometric Director . . . . Adolphus Lages, OD
Provider Relations . . . . Mayra Castillo

---

141 VSP Vision Care

3333 Quality Drive
Rancho Cordova, CA 95670
Toll-Free: 800-877-7195
vsp.com
Year Founded: 1955

Healthplan and Services Defined
PLAN TYPE: Vision
Plan Specialty: Vision
Benefits Offered: Vision

Geographic Areas Served
Nationwide, Canada, Australia, and the UK

Key Personnel
Chief Executive Officer . . . . Robert Lynch
President . . . . Kate Renwick-Espinosa

---

142 Western Dental Services

530 South Main Street
Orange, CA 92868
Toll-Free: 800-579-3783
corporate@westerndental.com
www.westerndental.com
Year Founded: 1903
Number of Primary Care Physicians: 1,700
Number of Referral/Specialty Physicians: 1,400
Total Enrollment: 315,440

Healthplan and Services Defined
PLAN TYPE: Dental
Other Type: Dental HMO
Model Type: Staff, IPA
Plan Specialty: Dental
Benefits Offered: Dental

Type of Coverage
Indemnity

Type of Payment Plans Offered
POS, Combination FFS & DFFS

Geographic Areas Served
California, Arizona, and Nevada

Subscriber Information
Average Monthly Fee Per Subscriber
(Employee + Employer Contribution):
Employee Only (Self): $9.25
Employee & 1 Family Member: $10.50
Employee & 2 Family Members: $12.00

Network Qualifications
Pre-Admission Certification: Yes

Peer Review Type
Utilization Review: Yes
Second Surgical Opinion: Yes
Case Management: Yes

Publishes and Distributes Report Card: No

Accreditation Certification
Utilization Review

Key Personnel
CEO/Chairman . . . . Daniel D. Crowley
SVP/CFO . . . . Bill Dembereckyj
VP/Chief Strategy Officer . . . . Lisa Dawe
SVP/General Counsel . . . . Jeffrey Miller
SVP, Specialty . . . . Zhi Meng
Chief Dental Officer. . . . . John Luther
Chief Marketing Officer . . . . Leslie Gibbs
CIO . . . . Preet M. Takkar

Average Claim Compensation
Physician's Fees Charged: 80%

Specialty Managed Care Partners
Enters into Contracts with Regional Business Coalitions: No

Key Personnel
President/CEO . . . . Garry Maisel
Chief Financial Officer. . . . . Rita Ruecker
Chief Legal Officer . . . . Rebecca Downing
Chief Marketing/Branding . . . . Rick Heron
Chief Medical Officer. . . . . Don Hufford
Chief Client Services . . . . Glenn Hamburg
Chief Information Officer. . . . . Ali Darugar
Chief Sales Officer. . . . . Bill Figenshu

---

143 Western Health Advantage

2349 Gateway Oaks Drive
Suite 100
Sacramento, CA 95833
Toll-Free: 888-227-5942
Phone: 916-563-2250
Fax: 916-568-0126
memberservices@westernhealth.com
www.westernhealth.com
Non-Profit Organization: Yes
Year Founded: 1996
Total Enrollment: 92,000
State Enrollment: 92,000

Healthplan and Services Defined
PLAN TYPE: HMO
Model Type: Network
Benefits Offered: Disease Management, Prescription,
Wellness, 24/7 Nurse hotline, 24/7 Travel Assistance

Geographic Areas Served
Sacramento, Yolo, Solano, western El Dorado, western Placer
counties

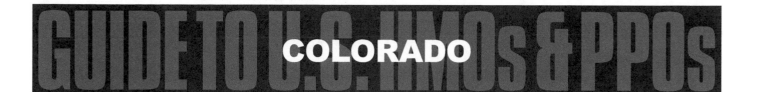

Health Insurance Coverage Status and Type of Coverage by Age

Category	All Persons		Under 18 years		Under 65 years	
	Number	%	Number	%	Number	%
Total population	5,514	-	1,334	-	4,755	-
Covered by some type of health insurance	5,100 (13)	92.5 (0.2)	1,277 (7)	95.7 (0.4)	4,347 (13)	91.4 (0.3)
Covered by private health insurance	3,862 (24)	70.0 (0.4)	847 (14)	63.5 (1.0)	3,418 (23)	71.9 (0.5)
Employer-based	3,054 (27)	55.4 (0.5)	700 (15)	52.5 (1.1)	2,828 (26)	59.5 (0.5)
Direct purchase	769 (19)	13.9 (0.3)	111 (8)	8.3 (0.6)	536 (17)	11.3 (0.4)
TRICARE	235 (11)	4.3 (0.2)	60 (6)	4.5 (0.5)	173 (11)	3.6 (0.2)
Covered by public health insurance	1,832 (25)	33.2 (0.4)	480 (16)	35.9 (1.2)	1,106 (24)	23.3 (0.5)
Medicaid	1,078 (25)	19.5 (0.5)	473 (15)	35.4 (1.2)	992 (25)	20.9 (0.5)
Medicare	830 (7)	15.1 (0.1)	10 (2)	0.8 (0.2)	105 (6)	2.2 (0.1)
VA Care	138 (6)	2.5 (0.1)	1 (1)	0.1 (0.1)	71 (5)	1.5 (0.1)
Not covered at any time during the year	414 (13)	7.5 (0.2)	57 (5)	4.3 (0.4)	408 (13)	8.6 (0.3)

Note: Numbers in thousands; Figures cover civilian noninstitutionalized population in 2017; N/A indicates that data was not available; Z represents or rounds to zero; Margin of error appears in parenthesis and is calculated using replicate weights.
Source: U.S. Census Bureau, American Community Survey, Table HIC-4_ACS. Health Insurance Coverage Status and Type of Coverage by State—All People: 2008 to 2017, Table HIC-5_ACS. Health Insurance Coverage Status and Type of Coverage by State—Children Under 18: 2008 to 2017, Table HIC-6_ACS. Health Insurance Coverage Status and Type of Coverage by State—Persons Under 65: 2008 to 2017

Colorado

144 Aetna Health of Colorado

151 Farmington Avenue
Hartford, CT 06156
Toll-Free: 800-872-3862
Phone: 860-273-0123
www.aetna.com
Subsidiary of: Aetna Inc.
For Profit Organization: Yes
Year Founded: 1987

Healthplan and Services Defined
PLAN TYPE: HMO/PPO
Other Type: POS
Model Type: Network
Plan Specialty: Behavioral Health, Vision
Benefits Offered: Behavioral Health, Dental, Disease
    Management, Home Care, Physical Therapy, Podiatry,
    Prescription, Vision, Worker's Compensation, Life

Type of Coverage
Commercial, Student health

Type of Payment Plans Offered
POS, Capitated, FFS, Combination FFS & DFFS

Geographic Areas Served
Statewide

Peer Review Type
Case Management: Yes

Publishes and Distributes Report Card: Yes

Accreditation Certification
TJC Accreditation, Medicare Approved, Utilization Review,
    Pre-Admission Certification, State Licensure, Quality
    Assurance Program

Key Personnel
Medicare Broker Manager . . . . Orlando Lopez
Sr. Network Manager . . . . David Jacobs

Specialty Managed Care Partners
Enters into Contracts with Regional Business Coalitions: Yes

145 American Dental Group

6755 Earl Drive
Suite 108
Colorado Springs, CO 80918
Toll-Free: 800-633-3010
Phone: 719-633-3000
adg@americandentalgroup.org
www.americandentalgroup.org
For Profit Organization: Yes
Year Founded: 1992
Physician Owned Organization: Yes

Healthplan and Services Defined
PLAN TYPE: Dental
Other Type: Vision
Model Type: Group
Plan Specialty: Dental, Vision
Benefits Offered: Dental, Vision

Type of Coverage
Commercial, Individual

Type of Payment Plans Offered
DFFS, FFS, Combination FFS & DFFS

Geographic Areas Served
Colorado, Maryland

Key Personnel
Chief Executive Officer. . . . . Don Whaley
VP, Operations . . . . Kathy Whaley
Marketing Director . . . . Leslie Massey

146 Anthem Blue Cross & Blue Shield of Colorado

700 Broadway
Denver, CO 80203
Phone: 303-831-2131
www.anthem.com
Subsidiary of: Anthem, Inc.
For Profit Organization: Yes
Year Founded: 1978

Healthplan and Services Defined
PLAN TYPE: HMO/PPO
Model Type: Network
Plan Specialty: Behavioral Health, Dental, Disease
    Management, Lab, PBM, Vision, Radiology
Benefits Offered: Behavioral Health, Dental, Disease
    Management, Inpatient SNF, Physical Therapy,
    Prescription, Psychiatric, Transplant, Vision, Wellness, Life,
    Benefits vary according to plan

Type of Coverage
Commercial, Individual, Medicare, Supplemental Medicare

Geographic Areas Served
Statewide

Accreditation Certification
URAC, NCQA

Key Personnel
President/GM Colorado. . . . . Mike Ramseier

147 Behavioral Healthcare

1290 Chambers Road
Aurora, CO 80011
Toll-Free: 844-818-2485
Phone: 303-361-8100
Fax: 303-364-2240
bhicares.org
Non-Profit Organization: Yes

Healthplan and Services Defined
PLAN TYPE: Other
Plan Specialty: Behavioral Health
Benefits Offered: Behavioral Health

Type of Coverage
Medicaid

Geographic Areas Served
Adams, Arapahoe and Douglas counties, and the city of
    Aurora

Key Personnel
Chief Executive Officer . . . . Pat Steadman
Chief Financial Officer . . . . Jennifer Lacov
Chief Medical Officer . . . . Ronald Morley
Quality Improvement . . . . Clara Cabanis
Clinical Services . . . . Katie Herrmann
Provider Relations . . . . Teresa Summers

148 Beta Health Association, Inc.

9725 E Hampden Avenue
Suite 400
Denver, CO 80231
Toll-Free: 800-807-0706
Phone: 303-744-3007
www.betadental.com
For Profit Organization: Yes
Year Founded: 1990
Physician Owned Organization: Yes

Healthplan and Services Defined
PLAN TYPE: Multiple
Plan Specialty: Dental, Vision
Benefits Offered: Dental, Vision, Life, LTD, STD

Type of Coverage
Commercial, Individual, Indemnity
Catastrophic Illness Benefit: Unlimited

Geographic Areas Served
48 states

Publishes and Distributes Report Card: Yes

Accreditation Certification
State Dental Board

Key Personnel
President & CEO. Rod Henningsen

Specialty Managed Care Partners
Enters into Contracts with Regional Business Coalitions: Yes

149 Boulder Valley Individual Practice Association

6676 Gunpark Drive
Suite B
Boulder, CO 80301
Phone: 303-530-3405
Fax: 303-530-2441
info@bvipa.com
www.bvipa.com
Non-Profit Organization: Yes
Year Founded: 1978
Physician Owned Organization: Yes
Number of Affiliated Hospitals: 4
Number of Primary Care Physicians: 487
Number of Referral/Specialty Physicians: 190
Total Enrollment: 60,000

Healthplan and Services Defined
PLAN TYPE: PPO
Model Type: IPA
Offers Demand Management Patient Information Service:
Yes

Type of Payment Plans Offered
POS

Geographic Areas Served
Boulder, Lafayette, Longmont & Louisville

Network Qualifications
Pre-Admission Certification: Yes

Peer Review Type
Utilization Review: Yes
Second Surgical Opinion: Yes
Case Management: Yes

Publishes and Distributes Report Card: No

Accreditation Certification
TJC Accreditation, Utilization Review, State Licensure

Key Personnel
President. . . . . Susan Roach, MD
Vice President . . . . Drigan Weider, MD

Specialty Managed Care Partners
Enters into Contracts with Regional Business Coalitions: No

150 Bright Health Colorado

219 N 2nd Street
Suite 310
Minneapolis, MN 55401
Phone: 844-691-6143
brighthealthplan.com
Year Founded: 2016
Number of Primary Care Physicians: 5,000

Healthplan and Services Defined
PLAN TYPE: HMO
Benefits Offered: Prescription, Wellness

Geographic Areas Served
Statewide

Key Personnel
Chief Executive Officer . . . . Bob Sheehy
Chief Medical Officer . . . . Tom Valdivia
President. . . . . Kyle Rolfing

151 Cigna HealthCare of Colorado

Denver Centerpoint I
3900 E Mexico Avenue
Denver, CO 80210
Phone: 303-782-1500
www.cigna.com
For Profit Organization: Yes
Number of Affiliated Hospitals: 80

Healthplan and Services Defined
PLAN TYPE: HMO
Other Type: POS
Plan Specialty: Behavioral Health, Dental, Vision
Benefits Offered: Behavioral Health, Dental, Disease
Management, Prescription, Vision, Wellness, Life, LTD,
STD
Offers Demand Management Patient Information Service: Yes

Type of Coverage
Commercial, Individual

Catastrophic Illness Benefit: Covered

Type of Payment Plans Offered
POS, Combination FFS & DFFS

Network Qualifications
Pre-Admission Certification: Yes

Peer Review Type
Utilization Review: Yes
Second Surgical Opinion: Yes
Case Management: Yes

Publishes and Distributes Report Card: Yes

Accreditation Certification
NCQA
TJC Accreditation, Medicare Approved, Utilization Review, Pre-Admission Certification, State Licensure, Quality Assurance Program

Key Personnel
Pres., Mountain States . . . . John Roble

Specialty Managed Care Partners
Enters into Contracts with Regional Business Coalitions: Yes

---

152 Colorado Access
11100 E Bethany Drive
Aurora, CO 80014
Toll-Free: 800-511-5010
customer.service@coaccess.com
www.coaccess.com
Non-Profit Organization: Yes
Year Founded: 1994

Healthplan and Services Defined
PLAN TYPE: HMO
Benefits Offered: Behavioral Health, Dental, Disease Management, Psychiatric, Wellness

Type of Coverage
Medicaid

Geographic Areas Served
Statewide

Key Personnel
President/CEO. . . . . Marshall Thomas, MD
CFO . . . . Philip J Reed
COO. . . . . April Abrahamson
VP of Legal Services . . . . Ann Edelman
Chief Medical Officer/SVP. . . . . Alexis Giese, MD
CIO . . . . Don Couch

---

153 Colorado Health Partnerships
9925 Federal Drive
Suite 100
Colorado Springs, CO 80921
Toll-Free: 800-804-5008
BHOMemberMailing@beaconhealthoptions.com
www.coloradohealthpartnerships.com
Non-Profit Organization: Yes
Year Founded: 1995
Number of Affiliated Hospitals: 8
Total Enrollment: 326,000

Healthplan and Services Defined
PLAN TYPE: HMO
Plan Specialty: Behavioral Health
Benefits Offered: Behavioral Health

Type of Coverage
Medicaid

Geographic Areas Served
Alamosa, Archuleta, Baca, Bent, Chaffee, Conejos, Costilla, Crowley, Custer, Delta, Dolores, Eagle, El Paso, Fremont, Garfield, Grand, Gunnison, Hinsdale, Huerfano, Jackson, Kiowa, Lake, La Plata, Las Animas, Mesa, Mineral, Moffat, Montezuma, Montrose, Otero, Ouray, Park, Pitkin, Pueblo, Prowers, Rio Blanco, Rio Grande, Routt, Saguache, San Juan, San Miguel, Summit and Teller counties

Accreditation Certification
URAC

Key Personnel
Executive Director. . . . . Arnold Salazar
719-587-0899
Quality Assurance . . . . Erica Arnold-Miller
719-538-1430
Medical Director . . . . Dr. Peter Brodrick
719-538-1430
Provider Relations . . . . Alma Mejorado
719-538-1430
Clinical Director . . . . Tamara Ballard, LPC
719-538-1430
Long Term Support/Service . . . . Jen Hale-Coulson
719-538-1430

---

154 Coventry Health Care of Colorado
337 Wright Street
Lakewood, CO 80228
www.coventryhealthcare.com
Subsidiary of: Aetna Inc.
For Profit Organization: Yes

Healthplan and Services Defined
PLAN TYPE: HMO/PPO
Model Type: Network
Plan Specialty: Behavioral Health, Dental, Worker's Compensation
Benefits Offered: Behavioral Health, Dental, Prescription, Wellness, Worker's Compensation

Type of Coverage
Commercial, Medicare, Medicaid

Geographic Areas Served
Statewide

---

155 Delta Dental of Colorado
4582 S Ulster Street
Suite 800
Denver, CO 80237
Toll-Free: 800-233-0860
Phone: 303-741-9300
customer_service@ddpco.com
www.deltadentalco.com

Non-Profit Organization: Yes
Year Founded: 1958
Number of Primary Care Physicians: 3,200
State Enrollment: 1,000,000

Healthplan and Services Defined
  PLAN TYPE: Dental
  Model Type: Network
  Plan Specialty: Dental
  Benefits Offered: Dental

Type of Coverage
  Commercial, Individual

Type of Payment Plans Offered
  DFFS

Geographic Areas Served
  Statewide

Publishes and Distributes Report Card: Yes

Key Personnel
  President & CEO . . . . Helen Drexler
  Chief Financial Officer . . . . Greg Vochis
  Network/Clinical Mgmt. . . . . Cheryl Lerner, MD
  General Counsel . . . . Dave Gerbus, JD
  VP, Marketing/Member Exp. . . . . Kathy Jacoby

156   Denver Health Medical Plan

777 Bannock Street
MC6000
Denver, CO 80204
Phone: 303-602-2100
www.denverhealthmedicalplan.com
Non-Profit Organization: Yes
Year Founded: 1997
Total Enrollment: 15,000

Healthplan and Services Defined
  PLAN TYPE: HMO
  Benefits Offered: Chiropractic, Home Care, Inpatient SNF,
    Physical Therapy, Podiatry, Psychiatric, Transplant, Vision,
    Wellness

Type of Coverage
  Commercial, Medicare, Medicare Advantage, CHP+

Key Personnel
  Chief Executive Officer . . . . Robin D. Wittenstein
  Marketing/PR Officer . . . . Rob Borland
  Chief Nursing Officer . . . . Kathy Boyle
  Chief Financial Officer . . . . Peg Burnett
  Director of Public Health . . . . Bill Burman
  Chief Operating Officer . . . . Timothy J. Harlin

157   Friday Health Plans

700 Main Street
Suite 100
Alamosa, CO 81101
Toll-Free: 800-475-8466
www.fridayhealthplans.com
Non-Profit Organization: Yes
Year Founded: 1972
Total Enrollment: 5,000

Healthplan and Services Defined
  PLAN TYPE: HMO
  Benefits Offered: Dental, Disease Management, Home Care,
    Inpatient SNF, Podiatry, Prescription, Vision, Wellness, Life

Type of Coverage
  Commercial, Individual, Medicare

Geographic Areas Served
  Southern Colorado, San Luis Valley, Arkansas Valley,
  Durango, Pueblo, Colorado Springs, Denver

Key Personnel
  Co-Founder/CEO . . . . Salvatore Gentile
  Co-Founder/President . . . . David Pinkert
  Chief Operating Officer . . . . Jennifer Mueller
  Chief Marketing Officer . . . . Tracy Faigin
    303-888-4803
    tracy.faigin@fridayhealthplans.com

158   Humana Health Insurance of Colorado

8033 N Academy Boulevard
Colorado Springs, CO 80920
Toll-Free: 800-871-6270
Phone: 719-532-7700
Fax: 719-531-7089
www.humana.com
Secondary Address: 6300 S Syracuse Way, Suite 555,
  Centennial, CO 80111, 866-355-6152
For Profit Organization: Yes
Year Founded: 1987

Healthplan and Services Defined
  PLAN TYPE: HMO/PPO
  Plan Specialty: Dental, Vision
  Benefits Offered: Dental, Disease Management, Transplant,
    Vision

Type of Coverage
  Commercial, Individual, Group, Medicare

Geographic Areas Served
  Statewide

Accreditation Certification
  URAC, NCQA

Key Personnel
  Sales Representative . . . . Glenn Berkley

159   Kaiser Permanente Northern Colorado

2950 E Harmony Road
Suite 190
Fort Collins, CO 80528
Toll-Free: 800-218-1059
thrive.kaiserpermanente.org/care-near-northern-colorado
Subsidiary of: Kaiser Permanente
Non-Profit Organization: Yes
Year Founded: 1969
Number of Primary Care Physicians: 1,121
Total Enrollment: 11,800,000
State Enrollment: 675,279

Healthplan and Services Defined
  PLAN TYPE: HMO

Model Type: Network
Benefits Offered: Disease Management, Home Care,
  Inpatient SNF, Long-Term Care, Physical Therapy,
  Podiatry, Prescription, Psychiatric, Transplant, Vision,
  Wellness, Benefits vary according to plan

Type of Coverage
Commercial, Individual, Medicare, Supplemental Medicare,
  Medicaid

Geographic Areas Served
Denver, Boulder, Fort Collins, Loveland, Greeley and
  surrounding areas

Accreditation Certification
NCQA

Key Personnel
Executive Med. Director . . . . Margaret Ferguson, MD
President, Colorado Area . . . . Roland Lyon

---

160   **Kaiser Permanente Southern Colorado**
1975 Research Parkway
Suite 250
Colorado Springs, CO 80920
Phone: 719-867-2100
thrive.kaiserpermanente.org/care-near-southern-colorado
Subsidiary of: Kaiser Permanente
Non-Profit Organization: Yes
Year Founded: 1969
Number of Primary Care Physicians: 1,121
Total Enrollment: 11,800,000
State Enrollment: 675,279

Healthplan and Services Defined
 PLAN TYPE: HMO/PPO
 Model Type: Network
 Benefits Offered: Disease Management, Home Care,
  Inpatient SNF, Long-Term Care, Physical Therapy,
  Podiatry, Prescription, Psychiatric, Transplant, Vision,
  Wellness, Benefits vary according to plan

Type of Coverage
Commercial, Individual, Medicare, Supplemental Medicare,
  Medicaid

Geographic Areas Served
Colorado Springs, Pueblo

Accreditation Certification
NCQA

Key Personnel
President, Colorado Area . . . . Roland Lyon
Executive Med. Director . . . . Margaret Ferguson, MD

---

161   **Pueblo Health Care**
400 W 16th Street
Pueblo, CO 81003
Phone: 719-584-4000
www.pueblohealthcare.com
Number of Primary Care Physicians: 270

Healthplan and Services Defined
 PLAN TYPE: PPO

Model Type: Network

Geographic Areas Served
Pueblo Market Area

Key Personnel
Executive Director . . . . Ann Bellah
  719-584-4371
  ann_bellah@parkviewmc.com
Provider Relations . . . . Sandra Proud
  719-584-4642
  sandra_proud@parkviewmc.com
President . . . . Bruce Johnson, MD
  719-566-3535

---

162   **Rocky Mountain Health Plans**
2775 Crossroads Boulevard
Grand Junction, CO 81506
Toll-Free: 800-346-4643
Phone: 970-243-7050
www.rmhp.org
Mailing Address: P.O. Box 10600, Grand Junction, CO
  81502-5600
Subsidiary of: Rocky Mountain Health Maintenance
  Organization
Non-Profit Organization: Yes
Year Founded: 1974
Owned by an Integrated Delivery Network (IDN): Yes
Number of Affiliated Hospitals: 107
Number of Primary Care Physicians: 2,630
Number of Referral/Specialty Physicians: 6,866
Total Enrollment: 236,962
State Enrollment: 236,962

Healthplan and Services Defined
 PLAN TYPE: HMO/PPO
 Other Type: HSA
 Model Type: Mixed
 Benefits Offered: Disease Management, Home Care,
  Prescription, Wellness

Type of Coverage
Commercial, Individual, Medicare, Supplemental Medicare
Catastrophic Illness Benefit: Unlimited

Type of Payment Plans Offered
FFS

Geographic Areas Served
Statewide

Network Qualifications
Minimum Years of Practice: 3
Pre-Admission Certification: Yes

Peer Review Type
Utilization Review: Yes
Second Surgical Opinion: Yes
Case Management: Yes

Publishes and Distributes Report Card: Yes

Accreditation Certification
NCQA
Medicare Approved, Utilization Review, Pre-Admission
  Certification, State Licensure, Quality Assurance Program

Key Personnel

President/CEO	Steven ErkenBrack
COO	Laurel Walters
CFO	Pat Duncan
VP, Human Resources	Jan Rohr
VP, Legal & Govt Affairs	Mike Huotari
Chief Marketing Officer	Neil Waldron
Chief Medical Officer	Kevin R Fitzgerald, MD

Specialty Managed Care Partners

Delta Dental, Landmark Chiropractic, Vision Service Plan, Life Strategies

---

163 United Concordia of Colorado

4401 Deer Path Road
Harrisburg, PA 17110
Phone: 717-260-6800
www.unitedconcordia.com
For Profit Organization: Yes
Year Founded: 1971
Number of Primary Care Physicians: 96,000

Healthplan and Services Defined

PLAN TYPE: Dental
Model Type: Network
Plan Specialty: Dental
Benefits Offered: Dental

Type of Coverage

Commercial, Individual, Military personnel & families

Geographic Areas Served

Nationwide

Accreditation Certification

URAC

---

164 UnitedHealthcare of Colorado

6465 S Greenwood Plaza Boulevard
Suite 300
Centennial, CO 80111
Toll-Free: 800-516-3344
www.uhc.com
Subsidiary of: UnitedHealth Group

Healthplan and Services Defined

PLAN TYPE: HMO/PPO
Model Type: Network
Plan Specialty: Behavioral Health, Dental, Disease Management, MSO, PBM, Vision
Benefits Offered: Behavioral Health, Chiropractic, Complementary
Medicine, Dental, Disease Management, Home Care, Inpatient SNF, Long-Term Care, Physical Therapy, Podiatry, Prescription, Psychiatric, Transplant, Vision, Wellness, AD&D, Life, Benefits vary according to plan

Type of Coverage

Commercial, Individual, Medicare, Medicaid, Family, Military, Veterans, Group,

Type of Payment Plans Offered

DFFS, FFS, Combination FFS & DFFS

Geographic Areas Served

HMO: Front Range Colorado; PPO/POS: Statewide

Subscriber Information

Average Monthly Fee Per Subscriber
(Employee + Employer Contribution):
Employee Only (Self): Varies

Network Qualifications

Pre-Admission Certification: Yes

Peer Review Type

Case Management: Yes

Publishes and Distributes Report Card: Yes

Accreditation Certification

URAC, NCQA
State Licensure, Quality Assurance Program

Key Personnel

VP, Network Management	Rob Rush
CEO, Medicare Health Plan	George Young
Dir., Public Relations	Will Shanley

Average Claim Compensation

Physician's Fees Charged: 70%
Hospital's Fees Charged: 55%

Specialty Managed Care Partners

United Behavioral Health
Enters into Contracts with Regional Business Coalitions: No

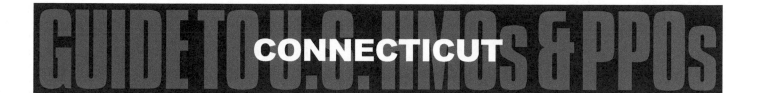

Health Insurance Coverage Status and Type of Coverage by Age

Category	All Persons		Under 18 years		Under 65 years	
	Number	%	Number	%	Number	%
Total population	3,537	-	793	-	2,957	-
Covered by some type of health insurance	3,343 *(12)*	94.5 *(0.3)*	769 *(6)*	96.9 *(0.5)*	2,767 *(12)*	93.6 *(0.4)*
Covered by private health insurance	2,524 *(21)*	71.4 *(0.6)*	526 *(9)*	66.4 *(1.2)*	2,169 *(20)*	73.3 *(0.7)*
Employer-based	2,124 *(20)*	60.1 *(0.6)*	473 *(10)*	59.6 *(1.3)*	1,909 *(19)*	64.6 *(0.6)*
Direct purchase	470 *(11)*	13.3 *(0.3)*	55 *(5)*	6.9 *(0.6)*	292 *(10)*	9.9 *(0.3)*
TRICARE	46 *(5)*	1.3 *(0.1)*	11 *(2)*	1.4 *(0.3)*	30 *(4)*	1.0 *(0.1)*
Covered by public health insurance	1,243 *(21)*	35.2 *(0.6)*	275 *(11)*	34.6 *(1.3)*	691 *(20)*	23.4 *(0.7)*
Medicaid	724 *(21)*	20.5 *(0.6)*	273 *(11)*	34.4 *(1.3)*	639 *(20)*	21.6 *(0.7)*
Medicare	628 *(6)*	17.8 *(0.2)*	3 *(1)*	0.4 *(0.2)*	76 *(5)*	2.6 *(0.2)*
VA Care	53 *(3)*	1.5 *(0.1)*	Z *(Z)*	Z *(Z)*	17 *(2)*	0.6 *(0.1)*
Not covered at any time during the year	194 *(12)*	5.5 *(0.3)*	24 *(4)*	3.1 *(0.5)*	190 *(12)*	6.4 *(0.4)*

Note: Numbers in thousands; Figures cover civilian noninstitutionalized population in 2017; N/A indicates that data was not available; Z represents or rounds to zero; Margin of error appears in parenthesis and is calculated using replicate weights.

Source: U.S. Census Bureau, American Community Survey, Table HIC-4_ACS. Health Insurance Coverage Status and Type of Coverage by State—All People: 2008 to 2017, Table HIC-5_ACS. Health Insurance Coverage Status and Type of Coverage by State—Children Under 18: 2008 to 2017, Table HIC-6_ACS. Health Insurance Coverage Status and Type of Coverage by State—Persons Under 65: 2008 to 2017

Connecticut

165   Aetna Health of Connecticut

151 Farmington Avenue
Hartford, CT 06156-3475
Toll-Free: 800-872-3862
www.aetna.com
Subsidiary of: Aetna Inc.
For Profit Organization: Yes
Year Founded: 1853

Healthplan and Services Defined
PLAN TYPE: HMO/PPO
Other Type: POS
Model Type: Network
Plan Specialty: Behavioral Health, Dental, EPO, Lab, PBM,
    Vision, Radiology
Benefits Offered: Behavioral Health, Dental, Disease
    Management, Long-Term Care, Physical Therapy,
    Podiatry, Prescription, Psychiatric, Vision, Wellness, Life,
    LTD, STD

Type of Coverage
Commercial, Medicare, Medicaid, Student health

Geographic Areas Served
Statewide

166   Aetna Inc.

151 Farmington Avenue
Hartford, CT 06156
Toll-Free: 800-872-3862
www.aetna.com
For Profit Organization: Yes
Year Founded: 1853
Number of Affiliated Hospitals: 5,667
Number of Primary Care Physicians: 664,301
Total Enrollment: 46,700,000

Healthplan and Services Defined
PLAN TYPE: Multiple
Other Type: POS
Model Type: Network
Plan Specialty: Behavioral Health, Dental, Lab, PBM, Vision,
    Radiology
Benefits Offered: Behavioral Health, Dental, Disease
    Management, Long-Term Care, Physical Therapy,
    Podiatry, Prescription, Psychiatric, Vision, Wellness, Life,
    LTD, STD

Type of Coverage
Commercial, Medicare, Medicaid, Public sector, Retirees,
    Part-time,

Type of Payment Plans Offered
FFS

Geographic Areas Served
Nationwide

Key Personnel
Chairman/CEO . . . . Mark T. Bertolini
President . . . . Karen S. Lynch
EVP/CFO/Enterprise Risk . . . . Shawn M. Guertin

EVP/Enterprise Strategy . . . . Rick M. Jelinek
EVP, Operations . . . . Meg McCarthy
EVP/CMO . . . . Harold L. Paz
EVP/General Counsel . . . . Thomas J. Sabatino, Jr.
EVP/Government Services . . . . Fran S. Soistman
EVP/Chief HR Officer . . . . Thomas W. Weidenkopf

167   Aetna Medicare

P.O. Box 14088
Lexington, KY 40512
Toll-Free: 800-282-5366
www.aetnamedicare.com
Subsidiary of: Aetna Inc.
For Profit Organization: Yes

Healthplan and Services Defined
PLAN TYPE: Medicare
Model Type: Network
Benefits Offered: Chiropractic, Dental, Disease Management,
    Home Care, Inpatient SNF, Physical Therapy, Prescription,
    Psychiatric, Vision, Wellness

Type of Coverage
Individual, Medicare, Supplemental Medicare

Geographic Areas Served
Available in multiple states

Subscriber Information
Average Monthly Fee Per Subscriber
    (Employee + Employer Contribution):
        Employee Only (Self): Varies
        Medicare: Varies
Average Annual Deductible Per Subscriber:
        Employee Only (Self): Varies
        Medicare: Varies
Average Subscriber Co-Payment:
        Primary Care Physician: Varies
        Non-Network Physician: Varies
        Prescription Drugs: Varies
        Hospital ER: Varies
        Home Health Care: Varies
        Home Health Care Max. Days/Visits Covered: Varies

Key Personnel
CEO . . . . Mark Bertolini

168   Aetna Student Health

151 Farmington Avenue
Hartford, CT 06156
Toll-Free: 877-437-6535
www.aetnastudenthealth.com
Subsidiary of: Aetna Inc.
For Profit Organization: Yes

Healthplan and Services Defined
PLAN TYPE: HMO/PPO
Other Type: POS
Model Type: Network
Plan Specialty: Disease Management, Vision
Benefits Offered: Dental, Prescription, Vision, Wellness, Life

Type of Coverage
Individual

Geographic Areas Served
Nationwide

169 Anthem Blue Cross & Blue Shield of Connecticut

108 Leigus Road
Wallingford, CT 06492
Toll-Free: 800-922-4670
www.anthem.com
Subsidiary of: Anthem, Inc.
For Profit Organization: Yes

Healthplan and Services Defined
  PLAN TYPE: HMO/PPO
  Model Type: Network
  Plan Specialty: Behavioral Health, Dental, Disease
    Management, Lab, PBM, Vision, Radiology
  Benefits Offered: Behavioral Health, Dental, Disease
    Management, Inpatient SNF, Physical Therapy,
    Prescription, Psychiatric, Transplant, Vision, Wellness, Life

Type of Coverage
  Commercial, Individual, Medicare, Supplemental Medicare,
    Catastrophic

Geographic Areas Served
  Statewide

Accreditation Certification
  URAC, NCQA

Key Personnel
  President/General Manager . . . . Jill Hummel

170 CareCentrix

20 Church Street
12th Floor
Hartford, CT 06103
Toll-Free: 800-808-1902
carecentrix.com
Secondary Address: 100 First Stamford Place, 2nd Floor W,
  Stamford, CT 06902
Year Founded: 1996
Number of Primary Care Physicians: 8,000

Healthplan and Services Defined
  PLAN TYPE: HMO
  Benefits Offered: Home Care, Physical Therapy, Durable
    Medical Equipment; Occupational & Respiratory Therapy;
    Orthotics; Prosthetics

Geographic Areas Served
  Arizona, Connecticut, Florida, Georgia, Kansas, and New
  York

Key Personnel
  Chief Executive Officer . . . . John Driscoll
  President/COO. Laizer Kornwasser
  Chief Medical Officer. . . . . Dr. Michael Cantor
  Chief Compliance Officer. . . . . Gisele Molloy
  Chief Customer Officer . . . . Tom Gaffney

Chief Legal Officer . . . . Alison Gilligan
Chief Financial Officer . . . . Steve Horowitz

171 Cigna Corporation

900 Cottage Grove Road
Bloomfield, CT 06002
Toll-Free: 800-244-6224
www.cigna.com
Secondary Address: Two Liberty Place, 1601 Chestnut Street,
  Philadelphia, PA 19192
For Profit Organization: Yes
Year Founded: 1982

Healthplan and Services Defined
  PLAN TYPE: Multiple
  Benefits Offered: Behavioral Health, Dental, Disease
    Management, Prescription, Vision, Wellness, AD&D, Life,
    LTD, STD

Type of Coverage
  Commercial, Individual, Medicare, Supplemental Medicare,
    Medicaid, Part-time and hourly workers; Union

Geographic Areas Served
  Nationwide

Accreditation Certification
  URAC, NCQA

Key Personnel
  President/CEO . . . . David M. Cordani
  EVP/Marketing Officer . . . . Lisa Bacus
  EVP/CIO . . . . Mark Boxer
  Pres., Gov. Business . . . . Brian Evanko
  EVP/General Counsel . . . . Nicole Jones
  EVP/CFO . . . . Eric Palmer
  President, US Markets . . . . Mike Triplett

172 Cigna-HealthSpring Medicare

900 Cottage Grove Road
Bloomfield, CT 06002
Toll-Free: 800-668-3813
cigna.com/medicare
For Profit Organization: Yes

Healthplan and Services Defined
  PLAN TYPE: Medicare
  Benefits Offered: Prescription

Type of Coverage
  Medicare, Supplemental Medicare

Geographic Areas Served
  Nationwide

Key Personnel
  Chairman & CEO . . . . David M. Cordani

173 ConnectiCare

175 Scott Swamp Road
P.O. Box 4050
Farmington, CT 06034-4050
Toll-Free: 800-251-7722
Phone: 860-674-5757
info@connecticare.com
www.connecticare.com
For Profit Organization: Yes
Year Founded: 1981
Owned by an Integrated Delivery Network (IDN): Yes

Healthplan and Services Defined
  PLAN TYPE: HMO/PPO
  Other Type: POS
  Model Type: IPA, HMO, POS
  Plan Specialty: Disease Management, Vision, UR
  Benefits Offered: Behavioral Health, Chiropractic,
    Complementary Medicine, Dental, Disease Management,
    Home Care, Inpatient SNF, Physical Therapy, Podiatry,
    Prescription, Psychiatric, Transplant, Vision, Wellness

Type of Coverage
  Commercial, Individual, Medicare, Medicare Advantage
  Catastrophic Illness Benefit: Unlimited

Type of Payment Plans Offered
  Capitated, FFS

Geographic Areas Served
  Statewide

Peer Review Type
  Utilization Review: Yes
  Second Surgical Opinion: Yes
  Case Management: Yes

Publishes and Distributes Report Card: Yes

Accreditation Certification
  TJC, NCQA
  Utilization Review, Pre-Admission Certification, State
    Licensure, Quality Assurance Program

Key Personnel
  President & CoO . . . . Eric Galvin
  SVP, Sales & Marketing . . . . Bert Wachtelhaussen
  SVP, Human Resources . . . . Cheryl Hutchinson
  Chief Medical Officer . . . . Wayne Rawlins

Average Claim Compensation
  Physician's Fees Charged: 100%
  Hospital's Fees Charged: 100%

Specialty Managed Care Partners
  United Behavioral Health, Express Scripts
  Enters into Contracts with Regional Business Coalitions: No

Employer References
  Federal Government, Hartford Insurance Company, United
    Technologies, State of Connecticut

174 Coventry Health Care of Connecticut

6720-B Rockledge Drive
Suite 800
Bethesda, MD 20817
Phone: 301-581-0600
www.coventryhealthcare.com
Subsidiary of: Aetna Inc.
For Profit Organization: Yes

Healthplan and Services Defined
  PLAN TYPE: HMO/PPO
  Model Type: Network
  Plan Specialty: Behavioral Health, Dental, Worker's
    Compensation
  Benefits Offered: Behavioral Health, Dental, Prescription,
    Vision, Wellness, Worker's Compensation

Type of Coverage
  Commercial, Medicare, Medicaid

Geographic Areas Served
  Statewide

175 Harvard Pilgrim Health Care Connecticut

City Place II
185 Asylum Street, 2nd Floor
Hartford, CT 06103
Toll-Free: 888-888-4742
www.harvardpilgrim.org
Non-Profit Organization: Yes
Year Founded: 1973
Number of Affiliated Hospitals: 179
Number of Referral/Specialty Physicians: 53,000

Healthplan and Services Defined
  PLAN TYPE: HMO
  Benefits Offered: Prescription

Geographic Areas Served
  Statewide

Peer Review Type
  Utilization Review: Yes
  Second Surgical Opinion: No
  Case Management: Yes

Publishes and Distributes Report Card: No

Accreditation Certification
  TJC Accreditation, Medicare Approved, Utilization Review,
    Pre-Admission Certification, State Licensure, Quality
    Assurance Program

Key Personnel
  VP, Regional Market . . . . Jason Madrak

Specialty Managed Care Partners
  Enters into Contracts with Regional Business Coalitions: No

176   Humana Health Insurance of Connecticut

125 Wolf Road
Suite 501
Albany, NY 12205
Toll-Free: 800-967-2370
Fax: 518-435-0412
www.humana.com
Subsidiary of: Humana
For Profit Organization: Yes

Healthplan and Services Defined
  PLAN TYPE: HMO/PPO
  Model Type: Network
  Plan Specialty: Dental, Vision
  Benefits Offered: Dental, Vision, Life, LTD, STD

Type of Coverage
  Commercial

Geographic Areas Served
  Connecticut is covered by the New York branch

Accreditation Certification
  URAC, NCQA, CORE

177   Oxford Health Plans

48 Monroe Turnpike
Trumbull, CT 06611
Toll-Free: 800-444-6222
Phone: 203-459-9100
www.oxhp.com
For Profit Organization: Yes
Year Founded: 1984
Owned by an Integrated Delivery Network (IDN): Yes

Healthplan and Services Defined
  PLAN TYPE: HMO/PPO
  Model Type: IPA, Network, POS
  Benefits Offered: Behavioral Health, Chiropractic,
    Complementary Medicine, Dental, Disease Management,
    Home Care, Inpatient SNF, Podiatry, Prescription,
    Psychiatric, Transplant, Vision, Wellness
  Offers Demand Management Patient Information Service:
    Yes

Type of Coverage
  Commercial, Individual, Indemnity, Medicare, Catastrophic
  Catastrophic Illness Benefit: Varies per case

Type of Payment Plans Offered
  FFS

Geographic Areas Served
  Connecticut: Fairfield, New Haven, Litchfield, Hartford,
  Middlesex, New London, Tolland & Windham counties; New
  Jersey: Essex, Hudson, Middlesex, Monmouth, Morris,
  Ocean, Passaic & Somerset counties; New York: Bronx,
  Dutchess, Kings, Nassau, New York, Putnam, Queens,
  Richmond, Rockland, Suffolk, & Westchester counties

Peer Review Type
  Utilization Review: Yes
  Second Surgical Opinion: Yes
  Case Management: Yes

Publishes and Distributes Report Card: Yes

Accreditation Certification
  NCQA
  TJC Accreditation, Medicare Approved, Utilization Review,
    Pre-Admission Certification, State Licensure, Quality
    Assurance Program

Key Personnel
  Chief Executive Officer . . . . David S. Wichmann
  Chief Operating Officer . . . . Dan Schumacher
  Chief Strategy Officer . . . . John Cosgriff
  Communications Officer . . . . Kirsten Gorsuch
  Chief Medical Officer. . . . . Sam Ho
  Chief Legal Officer . . . . Thad Johnson
  Chief Information Officer . . . . Phil McKoy
  Chief Financial Officer. . . . . Jeff Putnam

Specialty Managed Care Partners
  Enters into Contracts with Regional Business Coalitions: Yes

178   Trinity Health of Connecticut

1000 Asylum Avenue
5th Floor
Hartford, CT 06105
Phone: 860-714-1900
www.trinity-health.org
Secondary Address: Mercy Community, 2021 Albany Avenue,
  West Hartford, CT 06117, 860-570-8400
Subsidiary of: Trinity Health
Non-Profit Organization: Yes
Year Founded: 2013
Number of Affiliated Hospitals: 3
Number of Primary Care Physicians: 900
Total Enrollment: 30,000,000

Healthplan and Services Defined
  PLAN TYPE: Other
  Benefits Offered: Disease Management, Home Care,
    Long-Term Care, Psychiatric, Hospice programs, PACE
    (Program of All Inclusive Care for the Elderly)

Key Personnel
  President/CEO . . . . Dr. Reginald J. Eadie

179   UnitedHealthcare of Connecticut

185 Asylum Street
Hartford, CT 06103
Phone: 860-702-5000
www.uhc.com
Subsidiary of: UnitedHealth Group
For Profit Organization: Yes
Year Founded: 1991

Healthplan and Services Defined
  PLAN TYPE: HMO/PPO
  Model Type: Network
  Plan Specialty: Behavioral Health, Dental, Disease
    Management, PBM, Vision
  Benefits Offered: Behavioral Health, Dental, Disease
    Management, Long-Term Care, Prescription, Vision,
    Wellness, Life, LTD, STD

Type of Coverage
   Individual, Medicare, Supplemental Medicare, Medicaid,
      Catastrophic, Family, Military, Veterans, Group,

Geographic Areas Served
   Statewide

Key Personnel
   CEO, New England. Stephen Farrell

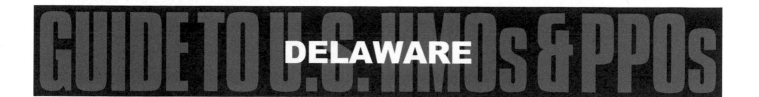
Health Insurance Coverage Status and Type of Coverage by Age

Category	All Persons		Under 18 years		Under 65 years	
	Number	%	Number	%	Number	%
Total population	947	-	218	-	778	-
Covered by some type of health insurance	896 *(6)*	94.6 *(0.6)*	211 *(2)*	96.5 *(1.0)*	728 *(5)*	93.6 *(0.7)*
Covered by private health insurance	697 *(12)*	73.6 *(1.3)*	145 *(6)*	66.6 *(2.6)*	584 *(11)*	75.1 *(1.4)*
Employer-based	590 *(13)*	62.3 *(1.4)*	130 *(6)*	59.7 *(2.7)*	518 *(12)*	66.6 *(1.5)*
Direct purchase	118 *(7)*	12.5 *(0.7)*	13 *(2)*	5.8 *(1.1)*	65 *(6)*	8.4 *(0.8)*
TRICARE	35 *(4)*	3.7 *(0.4)*	8 *(2)*	3.5 *(0.9)*	22 *(4)*	2.9 *(0.5)*
Covered by public health insurance	345 *(11)*	36.5 *(1.2)*	77 *(6)*	35.4 *(2.6)*	181 *(11)*	23.3 *(1.4)*
Medicaid	175 *(10)*	18.5 *(1.1)*	77 *(6)*	35.1 *(2.6)*	160 *(10)*	20.6 *(1.3)*
Medicare	190 *(4)*	20.1 *(0.5)*	2 *(1)*	1.1 *(0.7)*	26 *(4)*	3.3 *(0.5)*
VA Care	22 *(3)*	2.3 *(0.3)*	Z *(Z)*	0.2 *(0.2)*	10 *(2)*	1.2 *(0.3)*
Not covered at any time during the year	51 *(5)*	5.4 *(0.6)*	8 *(2)*	3.5 *(1.0)*	50 *(5)*	6.4 *(0.7)*

Note: Numbers in thousands; Figures cover civilian noninstitutionalized population in 2017; N/A indicates that data was not available; Z represents or rounds to zero; Margin of error appears in parenthesis and is calculated using replicate weights.
Source: U.S. Census Bureau, American Community Survey, Table HIC-4_ACS. Health Insurance Coverage Status and Type of Coverage by State—All People: 2008 to 2017, Table HIC-5_ACS. Health Insurance Coverage Status and Type of Coverage by State—Children Under 18: 2008 to 2017, Table HIC-6_ACS. Health Insurance Coverage Status and Type of Coverage by State—Persons Under 65: 2008 to 2017

Delaware

180 Delta Dental of Delaware

One Delta Drive
Mechanicsburg, PA 17055-6999
Toll-Free: 800-932-0783
www.deltadentalins.com
Mailing Address: P.O. Box 1803, Alpharetta, GA 30023
Non-Profit Organization: Yes

Healthplan and Services Defined
  PLAN TYPE: Dental
  Other Type: Dental PPO
  Plan Specialty: Dental
  Benefits Offered: Dental

Type of Coverage
  Commercial, Individual

Geographic Areas Served
  Statewide

Key Personnel
  President/CEO........................... Tony Barth
  Chief Financial Officer .... Michael Castro
  Chief Legal Officer .... Michael Hankinson
  EVP, Sales & Marketing .... Belinda Martinez
  Chief Operating Officer .... Nilesh Patel

181 Highmark BCBS Delaware

P.O. Box 1991
Wilmington, DE 19899-1991
Toll-Free: 800-633-2563
www.highmarkbcbsde.com
Non-Profit Organization: Yes
Year Founded: 1935

Healthplan and Services Defined
  PLAN TYPE: HMO/PPO
  Model Type: IPA, Network
  Benefits Offered: Dental, Disease Management, Prescription,
    Vision, Wellness

Type of Coverage
  Commercial, Individual, Medicare, Supplemental Medicare

Type of Payment Plans Offered
  Combination FFS & DFFS

Geographic Areas Served
  Statewide

Key Personnel
  Customer Service .... Becca Bartlett
  Manager, Underwriting .... Tim Rzepski
  Market Facing Analytics.................... Dave Stuart

182 Humana Health Insurance of Delaware

4191 Innslake Drive
Suite 100
Glen Allen, VA 23060
Toll-Free: 800-350-7213
Phone: 804-253-0060
Fax: 804-217-6514
www.humana.com
Subsidiary of: Humana
For Profit Organization: Yes

Healthplan and Services Defined
  PLAN TYPE: HMO/PPO
  Model Type: Network
  Plan Specialty: Dental, Vision
  Benefits Offered: Dental, Vision, Life, LTD, STD

Type of Coverage
  Commercial

Geographic Areas Served
  Statewide. Delaware is covered by the Virginia branch

Accreditation Certification
  URAC, NCQA, CORE

Key Personnel
  Market Manager .... Jose L. Cabrera, Jr.

183 Mid-Atlantic Behavioral Health

910 S Chapel Street
Suite 102
Newark, DE 19713
Phone: 302-224-1400
www.midatlanticbh.com
Secondary Address: 3521 Silverside Road, Suite 2F1,
  Wilmington, DE 19810, 302-224-1400

Healthplan and Services Defined
  PLAN TYPE: Multiple
  Plan Specialty: Behavioral Health
  Benefits Offered: Behavioral Health, Psychiatric

Type of Payment Plans Offered
  FFS

Geographic Areas Served
  Maryland, Virginia, West Virginia, North Carolina,
  Pennsylvania, Delaware & Washington DC

Network Qualifications
  Minimum Years of Practice: 2
  Pre-Admission Certification: Yes

Peer Review Type
  Utilization Review: No
  Second Surgical Opinion: No
  Case Management: No

Publishes and Distributes Report Card: No

Accreditation Certification
  TJC Accreditation, Medicare Approved, Utilization Review,
    Pre-Admission Certification, State Licensure, Quality
    Assurance Program

Key Personnel
  Practive Director .... Traci Bolander, Psy. D

Specialty Managed Care Partners
Enters into Contracts with Regional Business Coalitions: No

---

184   Trinity Health of Delaware
St. Francis Healthcare
701 North Clayton Street
Wilmington, DE 19805
Phone: 302-421-4100
www.trinity-health.org
Subsidiary of: Trinity Health
Non-Profit Organization: Yes
Year Founded: 2013
Total Enrollment: 30,000,000

Healthplan and Services Defined
PLAN TYPE: Other
Benefits Offered: Disease Management, Home Care,
Long-Term Care, Psychiatric, Hospice programs, PACE
(Program of All Inclusive Care for the Elderly)

Key Personnel
President/CEO . . . . Dan Sinnott
Vice President, Finance . . . . Mary Finn
Chief HR Officer . . . . Donna L. Campbell
General Counsel. . . . . John E. Newton
Regional CIO . . . . Terry O'Neil
VP, Medical Affairs/CMO . . . . Michael Polnerow
VP, Patient Servces/CAO . . . . Jennifer M. Kirby

---

185   UnitedHealthcare Community Plan
Delaware
UnitedHealthcare Customer Service
P.O. Box 29675
Hot Springs, AR 71903-9802
Toll-Free: 877-877-8159
www.uhccommunityplan.com/de.html
Subsidiary of: UnitedHealth Group

Healthplan and Services Defined
PLAN TYPE: HMO
Benefits Offered: Dental, Home Care, Long-Term Care,
Physical Therapy, Prescription, Vision, Wellness, Hearing,
Labs & X-rays, Diabetic Support

Type of Coverage
Medicaid

Geographic Areas Served
Statewide

Key Personnel
Chief Executive Officer . . . . Steve Nelson
Chief Operating Officer . . . . Dan Schumacher
Chief Strategy Officer . . . . John Cosgriff
Communications Officer . . . . Kirsten Gorsuch
Chief Medical Officer. . . . . Sam Ho
Chief Legal Officer . . . . Thad Johnson
Chief Information Officer . . . . Phil McKoy

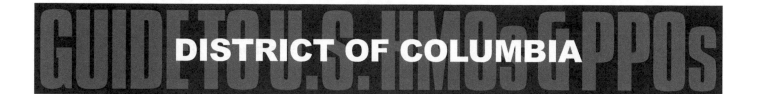

Health Insurance Coverage Status and Type of Coverage by Age

Category	All Persons		Under 18 years		Under 65 years	
	Number	%	Number	%	Number	%
Total population	684	-	134	-	602	-
Covered by some type of health insurance	658 (4)	96.2 (0.6)	132 (2)	98.8 (0.7)	577 (4)	95.8 (0.7)
Covered by private health insurance	479 (8)	70.1 (1.2)	74 (4)	55.2 (2.8)	426 (8)	70.7 (1.3)
Employer-based	398 (10)	58.2 (1.5)	57 (4)	42.4 (3.3)	357 (10)	59.3 (1.6)
Direct purchase	105 (7)	15.4 (1.1)	16 (3)	11.9 (2.5)	86 (6)	14.2 (1.1)
TRICARE	15 (3)	2.3 (0.5)	4 (2)	3.0 (1.3)	11 (3)	1.9 (0.5)
Covered by public health insurance	247 (7)	36.1 (1.1)	64 (4)	48.3 (2.8)	171 (7)	28.4 (1.2)
Medicaid	185 (8)	27.0 (1.1)	64 (4)	47.9 (2.8)	162 (7)	26.9 (1.2)
Medicare	93 (3)	13.6 (0.4)	2 (1)	1.4 (1.1)	17 (3)	2.9 (0.5)
VA Care	10 (2)	1.4 (0.2)	Z (Z)	0.1 (0.1)	5 (1)	0.9 (0.2)
Not covered at any time during the year	26 (4)	3.8 (0.6)	2 (1)	1.2 (0.7)	26 (4)	4.2 (0.7)

Note: Numbers in thousands; Figures cover civilian noninstitutionalized population in 2017; N/A indicates that data was not available; Z represents or rounds to zero; Margin of error appears in parenthesis and is calculated using replicate weights.
Source: U.S. Census Bureau, American Community Survey, Table HIC-4_ACS. Health Insurance Coverage Status and Type of Coverage by State—All People: 2008 to 2017, Table HIC-5_ACS. Health Insurance Coverage Status and Type of Coverage by State—Children Under 18: 2008 to 2017, Table HIC-6_ACS. Health Insurance Coverage Status and Type of Coverage by State—Persons Under 65: 2008 to 2017

District of Columbia

186 Aetna Health of District of Columbia
151 Farmington Avenue
Hartford, CT 06156
Toll-Free: 800-872-3862
www.aetnadcgov.com
Subsidiary of: Aetna Inc.
For Profit Organization: Yes

Healthplan and Services Defined
PLAN TYPE: HMO/PPO
Other Type: POS
Model Type: Network
Plan Specialty: Behavioral Health, EPO, Lab, PBM, Radiology
Benefits Offered: Behavioral Health, Dental, Disease Management, Long-Term Care, Physical Therapy, Podiatry, Prescription, Psychiatric, Vision, Wellness, Life, LTD, STD

Type of Coverage
Commercial, Student health

Geographic Areas Served
Statewide

Key Personnel
SVP, Government Affairs................. Jim Ricciuti
Project Manager................... Christopher Amidei

187 AmeriHealth Caritas District of Columbia
1120 Vermont Avenue NW
Suite 200
Washington, DC 20005
Toll-Free: 800-408-7511
Phone: 202-408-4720
www.amerihealthcaritasdc.com
For Profit Organization: Yes
Year Founded: 1987

Healthplan and Services Defined
PLAN TYPE: Other
Plan Specialty: Behavioral Health, Dental
Benefits Offered: Prescription

Type of Coverage
Medicaid

Geographic Areas Served
District of Columbia

Publishes and Distributes Report Card: Yes

Accreditation Certification
NCQA

Key Personnel
Market President .... Karen M. Dale
Finance Director .... Terrence J. Cunningham
Compliance Director.................. Brian Geesaman
Local Operations Director .... James R. Christian
Dental Director...................... Nathan Fletcher
Chief Medical Officer .... Lavdena Adams, MD

Specialty Managed Care Partners
Enters into Contracts with Regional Business Coalitions: Yes

188 Delta Dental of the District of Columbia
One Delta Drive
Mechanicsburg, PA 17055-6999
Toll-Free: 800-932-0783
www.deltadentalins.com
Non-Profit Organization: Yes

Healthplan and Services Defined
PLAN TYPE: Dental
Other Type: Dental PPO
Plan Specialty: Dental
Benefits Offered: Dental

Type of Coverage
Commercial, Individual

Geographic Areas Served
District of Columbia

Key Personnel
President & CEO......................... Tony Barth
Chief Financial Officer .... Michael Castro
Chief Legal Officer .... Michael Hankinson
EVP, Sales & Marketing .... Belinda Martinez
Chief Operating Officer .... Nilesh Patel

189 Quality Plan Administrators
7824 Eastern Avenue NW
Suite 100
Washington, DC 20012
Toll-Free: 800-900-4112
Phone: 202-722-2744
Fax: 202-291-5703
quality@qpatpa.com
qualityplanadmin.com
For Profit Organization: Yes
Year Founded: 1986
Number of Primary Care Physicians: 175
Total Enrollment: 90,000

Healthplan and Services Defined
PLAN TYPE: HMO/PPO
Plan Specialty: Dental, Vision
Benefits Offered: Dental, Vision

Type of Coverage
Commercial, Government, municipalities, correct

Key Personnel
President/CEO................... Milton Bernard, DDS

190 UnitedHealthcare Community Plan Capital Area
P.O. Box 29675
Hot Springs, AR 71903-9802
Toll-Free: 866-790-9424
www.uhccommunityplan.com/dc.html
Subsidiary of: UnitedHealth Group

Healthplan and Services Defined
 PLAN TYPE: PPO
 Model Type: Network
 Benefits Offered: Dental, Podiatry, Prescription, Vision, 24hr
 Nurse Line

Type of Coverage
 Medicare, Supplemental Medicare, Medicaid

Geographic Areas Served
 District of Columbia

---

191   UnitedHealthcare of the District of Columbia
1333 N Street NW
Washington, DC 20005
Toll-Free: 888-545-5205
Phone: 202-568-6332
www.uhc.com
Subsidiary of: UnitedHealth Group
Non-Profit Organization: Yes
Year Founded: 1976

Healthplan and Services Defined
 PLAN TYPE: HMO/PPO
 Model Type: Network
 Benefits Offered: Disease Management, Prescription,
 Wellness

Geographic Areas Served
 Statewide. The District of Columbia is covered by the
 Maryland branch

Subscriber Information
 Average Monthly Fee Per Subscriber
  (Employee + Employer Contribution):
   Employee Only (Self): $104.00-135.00
   Employee & 1 Family Member: $143.00-184.00
   Employee & 2 Family Members: $331.00-440.00
   Medicare: $112.00-156.00
 Average Annual Deductible Per Subscriber:
   Employee Only (Self): $100.00-250.00
   Employee & 1 Family Member: $500.00-1500.00
   Employee & 2 Family Members: $200.00-500.00
   Medicare: $0
 Average Subscriber Co-Payment:
   Primary Care Physician: $5.00/10.00
   Non-Network Physician: Deductible
   Prescription Drugs: $5.00/10.00
   Hospital ER: $25.00/50.00
   Home Health Care: $5.00/10.00

Network Qualifications
 Pre-Admission Certification: Yes

Peer Review Type
 Utilization Review: Yes
 Second Surgical Opinion: Yes
 Case Management: Yes

Publishes and Distributes Report Card: Yes

Accreditation Certification
 TJC Accreditation, Medicare Approved, Utilization Review,
  Pre-Admission Certification, State Licensure, Quality
  Assurance Program

Specialty Managed Care Partners
 Enters into Contracts with Regional Business Coalitions: Yes

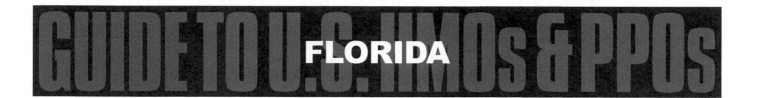
Health Insurance Coverage Status and Type of Coverage by Age

Category	All Persons		Under 18 years		Under 65 years	
	Number	%	Number	%	Number	%
Total population	20,679	-	4,450	-	16,532	-
Covered by some type of health insurance	18,003 *(43)*	87.1 *(0.2)*	4,126 *(17)*	92.7 *(0.3)*	13,905 *(43)*	84.1 *(0.3)*
Covered by private health insurance	12,835 *(61)*	62.1 *(0.3)*	2,334 *(27)*	52.5 *(0.6)*	10,731 *(57)*	64.9 *(0.3)*
Employer-based	9,310 *(61)*	45.0 *(0.3)*	1,838 *(27)*	41.3 *(0.6)*	8,293 *(58)*	50.2 *(0.4)*
Direct purchase	3,540 *(40)*	17.1 *(0.2)*	434 *(16)*	9.8 *(0.4)*	2,377 *(37)*	14.4 *(0.2)*
TRICARE	749 *(21)*	3.6 *(0.1)*	131 *(9)*	2.9 *(0.2)*	451 *(19)*	2.7 *(0.1)*
Covered by public health insurance	7,710 *(43)*	37.3 *(0.2)*	1,935 *(28)*	43.5 *(0.6)*	3,738 *(42)*	22.6 *(0.3)*
Medicaid	3,850 *(41)*	18.6 *(0.2)*	1,916 *(28)*	43.0 *(0.6)*	3,249 *(41)*	19.7 *(0.2)*
Medicare	4,494 *(16)*	21.7 *(0.1)*	33 *(5)*	0.7 *(0.1)*	529 *(13)*	3.2 *(0.1)*
VA Care	628 *(14)*	3.0 *(0.1)*	5 *(2)*	0.1 *(Z)*	258 *(10)*	1.6 *(0.1)*
Not covered at any time during the year	2,676 *(43)*	12.9 *(0.2)*	325 *(15)*	7.3 *(0.3)*	2,627 *(43)*	15.9 *(0.3)*

Note: Numbers in thousands; Figures cover civilian noninstitutionalized population in 2017; N/A indicates that data was not available; Z represents or rounds to zero; Margin of error appears in parenthesis and is calculated using replicate weights.

Source: U.S. Census Bureau, American Community Survey, Table HIC-4_ACS. Health Insurance Coverage Status and Type of Coverage by State—All People: 2008 to 2017, Table HIC-5_ACS. Health Insurance Coverage Status and Type of Coverage by State—Children Under 18: 2008 to 2017, Table HIC-6_ACS. Health Insurance Coverage Status and Type of Coverage by State—Persons Under 65: 2008 to 2017

Florida

192 Aetna Health of Florida

1340 Concord Terrace
Sunrise, CT 33323
Toll-Free: 800-441-5501
Fax: 877-542-6958
www.aetnabetterhealth.com/florida
Mailing Address: P.O. Box 63578, Phoenix, AZ 85082-1925
Subsidiary of: Aetna Inc.
For Profit Organization: Yes

Healthplan and Services Defined
PLAN TYPE: HMO/PPO
Other Type: POS
Model Type: Network
Plan Specialty: Behavioral Health, Dental, EPO, Lab, PBM, Vision, Radiology
Benefits Offered: Behavioral Health, Dental, Disease Management, Long-Term Care, Physical Therapy, Podiatry, Prescription, Psychiatric, Wellness, Life, LTD, STD

Type of Coverage
Commercial, Medicare, Medicaid, Catastrophic, Student health

Geographic Areas Served
Statewide

Key Personnel
President, Florida Market . . . . Richard Weiss

193 Amerigroup Florida

604 Courtland Street
Orlando, FL 32804
Toll-Free: 800-600-4441
Phone: 407-647-1710
www.myamerigroup.com/fl
Subsidiary of: Anthem, Inc.
For Profit Organization: Yes

Healthplan and Services Defined
PLAN TYPE: Other
Model Type: Network
Plan Specialty: Behavioral Health, Dental, Disease Management, Lab, Vision, Managed health care for people in public programs. Mental health and substance abuse services.
Benefits Offered: Behavioral Health, Dental, Disease Management, Long-Term Care, Podiatry, Prescription, Vision, Wellness, Transportation; Art Therapy; Hearing Aids Batteires

Type of Coverage
Medicaid

Key Personnel
Information Technology . . . . Jeff Schrecengost

194 AvMed

9400 S Dadeland Boulevard
Miami, FL 33156
Toll-Free: 800-477-8768
Phone: 305-671-5437
www.avmed.org
Subsidiary of: SantaFe HealthCare, Inc.
Non-Profit Organization: Yes
Year Founded: 1969
Total Enrollment: 340,000
State Enrollment: 340,000

Healthplan and Services Defined
PLAN TYPE: Medicare
Plan Specialty: Dental, Nurse On Call Program
Benefits Offered: Behavioral Health, Dental, Prescription, Wellness

Type of Coverage
Medicare

Type of Payment Plans Offered
POS

Geographic Areas Served
Miami-Dade counties

Subscriber Information
Average Annual Deductible Per Subscriber:
Employee Only (Self): $0
Employee & 1 Family Member: $0
Employee & 2 Family Members: $0
Medicare: $0

Accreditation Certification
NCQA

Key Personnel
President & CEO . . . . Michael P. Gallagher
President & COO . . . . James M. Repp
SVP, Human Resources . . . . Kay Ayers
SVP, Information Officer . . . . Jim Simpson
SVP, Financial Officer . . . . Randall L. Stuart
SVP, Medical Officer . . . . Ann O. Wehr, MD, FACP
SVP, General Counsel. . . . . Steven M. Ziegler

Specialty Managed Care Partners
Enters into Contracts with Regional Business Coalitions: No

195 AvMed Ft. Lauderdale

13450 W Sunrise Boulevard
Suite 370
Ft. Lauderdale, FL 33323
Toll-Free: 800-477-8768
Phone: 954-462-2520
www.avmed.org
Non-Profit Organization: Yes
Year Founded: 1973
Federally Qualified: Yes
Total Enrollment: 340,000
State Enrollment: 340,000

Healthplan and Services Defined
PLAN TYPE: Medicare
Model Type: IPA

Plan Specialty: Nurse On Call Program
Benefits Offered: Behavioral Health, Dental, Disease
Management, Prescription, Wellness

Type of Coverage
Medicare

Geographic Areas Served
Broward County

Accreditation Certification
TJC, NCQA

196 AvMed Gainesville

4300 NW 89th Boulevard
Gainesville, FL 32606
Toll-Free: 800-477-8768
Phone: 352-372-8400
www.avmed.org
Non-Profit Organization: Yes
Year Founded: 1986
Total Enrollment: 340,000
State Enrollment: 340,000

Healthplan and Services Defined
PLAN TYPE: HMO
Model Type: IPA
Plan Specialty: Nurse On Call Program
Benefits Offered: Behavioral Health, Dental, Disease
Management, Prescription, Wellness

Type of Coverage
Commercial, Individual
Catastrophic Illness Benefit: Unlimited

Type of Payment Plans Offered
POS, DFFS, Combination FFS & DFFS

Geographic Areas Served
Alachua, Bradford, Citrus, Columbia, Dixie, Gilchrist,
Hamilton, Levy, Marion, Suwannee and Union counties

Accreditation Certification
NCQA

Average Claim Compensation
Physician's Fees Charged: 85%
Hospital's Fees Charged: 70%

Specialty Managed Care Partners
Enters into Contracts with Regional Business Coalitions: No

197 AvMed Orlando

1800 Pembrook Drive
Suite 190
Orlando, FL 32810
Toll-Free: 800-477-8767
Phone: 407-539-0007
www.avmed.org
Non-Profit Organization: Yes
Year Founded: 1988
Total Enrollment: 340,000
State Enrollment: 340,000

Healthplan and Services Defined
PLAN TYPE: HMO

Benefits Offered: Behavioral Health, Dental, Disease
Management, Prescription, Wellness

Type of Coverage
Commercial, Individual

Type of Payment Plans Offered
FFS, Combination FFS & DFFS

Geographic Areas Served
Orange, Osceola and Seminole counties

Accreditation Certification
NCQA

Specialty Managed Care Partners
Enters into Contracts with Regional Business Coalitions: Yes

198 Capital Health Plan

2140 Centerville Place
Tallahassee, FL 32308
Toll-Free: 877-247-6512
Phone: 850-383-3311
memberservices@chp.org
www.capitalhealth.com
Mailing Address: P.O. Box 15349, Tallahassee, FL 32317-5349
Subsidiary of: Blue Cross Blue Shield of Florida
Non-Profit Organization: Yes
Year Founded: 1982
Owned by an Integrated Delivery Network (IDN): Yes
Number of Primary Care Physicians: 150
Number of Referral/Specialty Physicians: 400
Total Enrollment: 125,000
State Enrollment: 125,000

Healthplan and Services Defined
PLAN TYPE: HMO
Model Type: Staff, Mixed Model
Plan Specialty: Chiropractic, Lab, Vision, Radiology, UR
Benefits Offered: Behavioral Health, Chiropractic, Disease
Management, Home Care, Inpatient SNF, Physical Therapy,
Podiatry, Prescription, Psychiatric, Transplant, Vision,
Wellness

Type of Coverage
Commercial, Medicare, Supplemental Medicare, Catastrophic
Catastrophic Illness Benefit: Unlimited

Geographic Areas Served
Calhoun, Franklin, Gadsden, Jefferson, Leon, Liberty and
Wakulla counties

Peer Review Type
Second Surgical Opinion: Yes

Publishes and Distributes Report Card: Yes

Accreditation Certification
NCQA

Key Personnel
President & CEO . . . . John Hogan

Specialty Managed Care Partners
Enters into Contracts with Regional Business Coalitions: Yes

199 CareCentrix: Florida
9119 Corporate Lake Drive
Suite 300
Tampa, FL 33634
Toll-Free: 800-808-1902
carecentrix.com
Year Founded: 1996
Number of Primary Care Physicians: 8,000

Healthplan and Services Defined
PLAN TYPE: HMO
Benefits Offered: Home Care, Physical Therapy, Durable
Medical Equipment; Occupational & Respiratory Therapy;
Orthotics; Prosthetics

Key Personnel
Area VP, IT . . . . Fran Lanham

200 CarePlus Health Plans
11430 NW 20th Street
Suite 300
Miami, FL 33172
Toll-Free: 800-794-5907
cphp_memberservices@careplus-hp.com
www.careplushealthplans.com
Subsidiary of: Humana
Year Founded: 2003
Total Enrollment: 111,000
State Enrollment: 111,000

Healthplan and Services Defined
PLAN TYPE: Medicare
Benefits Offered: Prescription

Type of Coverage
Medicare

Geographic Areas Served
Miami-Dade, Broward, Palm Beach, Hillsborough, Pinellas,
Pasco, Polk, Lake, Marion, Sumter, Orange, Osceola,
Seminole, Brevard, Indian River, Martin, Okeechobee, St.
Lucie and Duval counties

Accreditation Certification
AAAHC

Key Personnel
President/CEO . . . . Bruce Dale Broussard
Director/CFO . . . . Brian Andrew Kane

201 Cigna Healthcare Florida
2701 North Rocky Point Drive
Suite 800
Tampa, FL 33607
Toll-Free: 800-832-3211
Phone: 813-637-1200
Fax: 813-637-1223
www.cigna.com
For Profit Organization: Yes
Year Founded: 1982

Healthplan and Services Defined
PLAN TYPE: Multiple

Benefits Offered: Behavioral Health, Dental, Disease
Management, Prescription, Vision, Wellness, AD&D, Life,
LTD, STD

Type of Coverage
Commercial, Individual, Medicare, Supplemental Medicare,
Medicaid, Part-time and hourly workers; Union

Geographic Areas Served
Statewide

Key Personnel
VP, Select Sales . . . . Tracy Carter-Hayes
VP, Provider Network . . . . Diane Wilkosz
Senior Client Manager . . . . Brian C. McNeil

202 Cigna HealthCare of Florida
900 Cottage Grove Road
Bloomfield, CT 06002
Toll-Free: 800-244-6224
www.cigna.com
For Profit Organization: Yes

Healthplan and Services Defined
PLAN TYPE: HMO
Other Type: POS
Model Type: Network
Benefits Offered: Dental, Disease Management, Prescription,
Transplant, Vision, Wellness, Life, LTD, STD

Type of Coverage
Commercial, Individual

Type of Payment Plans Offered
POS, DFFS, FFS, Combination FFS & DFFS

Network Qualifications
Minimum Years of Practice: 3

Peer Review Type
Second Surgical Opinion: Yes
Case Management: Yes

Publishes and Distributes Report Card: Yes

Accreditation Certification
NCQA
TJC Accreditation, Medicare Approved, Utilization Review,
Pre-Admission Certification, State Licensure, Quality
Assurance Program

Key Personnel
Regional Vice President . . . . Andrew Crooks

203 Coventry Health Care of Florida
1340 Concord Terrace
Sunrise, FL 33323
Toll-Free: 866-847-8235
coventryhealthcare.com
Subsidiary of: Aetna Inc.
For Profit Organization: Yes
Total Enrollment: 5,000,000
State Enrollment: 375,000

Healthplan and Services Defined
PLAN TYPE: HMO/PPO
Model Type: Network

Plan Specialty: Behavioral Health, Dental, Worker's
Compensation
Benefits Offered: Behavioral Health, Dental, Prescription,
Wellness, Worker's Compensation

Type of Coverage
Individual, Medicare, Medicaid

Type of Payment Plans Offered
POS

Geographic Areas Served
Greater Miami area, Greater Fort Lauderdale area, Boca
Raton, Boynton Beach, Clearwater, Gainesville, Ocala,
Pensacola, Port Saint Lucie, St. Petersburg, Tallahassee,
Tampa, Wellington, West Palm Beach

Accreditation Certification
URAC

Key Personnel
Manager of Sales. . . . . George Tsitouris

204 DentalPlans.com Inc.
8100 SW 10th Street
Suite 2000
Plantation, FL 33324
Toll-Free: 800-494-9294
Phone: 855-232-3467
Fax: 954-923-2694
members@dentalplans.com
www.dentalplans.com
For Profit Organization: Yes
Year Founded: 1999

Healthplan and Services Defined
PLAN TYPE: Dental
Plan Specialty: Dental
Benefits Offered: Dental

Geographic Areas Served
Statewide

Key Personnel
Chief Commercial Officer . . . . Jennifer Stoll
Chief Technology Officer . . . . Barry Newman
SVP, Marketing. . . . . Bill Chase
VP, Network Development . . . . Marge Keen
VP, Finance. . . . . Tara Rivera
VP, Call Center Sales . . . . Mark Powell

205 Dimension Health
5881 NW 151st Street
Suite 201
Hialeah, FL 33014
Toll-Free: 800-483-4992
Phone: 305-823-7664
info@dimensionhealth.com
www.dimensionhealth.com
Year Founded: 1985
Number of Affiliated Hospitals: 51

Healthplan and Services Defined
PLAN TYPE: PPO
Model Type: Network

Benefits Offered: Disease Management, Wellness, Worker's
Compensation

Type of Coverage
Commercial

Type of Payment Plans Offered
POS, DFFS, Capitated, FFS, Combination FFS & DFFS

Network Qualifications
Pre-Admission Certification: Yes

Peer Review Type
Utilization Review: Yes
Second Surgical Opinion: Yes
Case Management: Yes

Publishes and Distributes Report Card: No

Key Personnel
President & CEO. . . . . Charles A. Lindgren
VP, Network Development . . . . Creta Diehs
Office Manager . . . . Rosemary Osorio
rosorio@dimensionhealth.com

Average Claim Compensation
Physician's Fees Charged: 110%

Specialty Managed Care Partners
Enters into Contracts with Regional Business Coalitions: No

206 Florida Blue
PO Box 1798
Jacksonville, FL 32231-0014
Toll-Free: 877-352-5830
www.floridablue.com
Subsidiary of: Blue Cross and Blue Shield of Florida, Inc.
Non-Profit Organization: Yes
Year Founded: 1985
Owned by an Integrated Delivery Network (IDN): Yes

Healthplan and Services Defined
PLAN TYPE: HMO
Plan Specialty: Dental
Benefits Offered: Behavioral Health, Chiropractic,
Complementary Medicine, Dental, Disease Management,
Home Care, Inpatient SNF, Physical Therapy, Podiatry,
Prescription, Psychiatric, Transplant, Wellness, AD&D,
Life, Critical illness
Offers Demand Management Patient Information Service: Yes
DMPI Services Offered: Nurse Line 24x7x365, Health
Coaching, Support for Chronic Conditions, Health Risk
Assessments, Web Tools & Resources

Type of Coverage
Commercial, Individual, Indemnity, Medicare

Type of Payment Plans Offered
FFS

Geographic Areas Served
Statewide

Subscriber Information
Average Subscriber Co-Payment:
Primary Care Physician: Varies
Non-Network Physician: Varies
Prescription Drugs: Varies

Hospital ER: Varies
Home Health Care: Varies
Nursing Home: Varies

Network Qualifications
Pre-Admission Certification: Yes

Peer Review Type
Utilization Review: Yes

Publishes and Distributes Report Card: No

Accreditation Certification
Utilization Review

Key Personnel
CEO .... Patrick Geraghty
Chairman........................ Steven T. Halverson
Chief Operating Officer .... Catherine P. Bessant

Specialty Managed Care Partners
Prime Therapeutics, LLC-PBM and Mental Health Network
(MHnet), Health Dialog, Accordant and Quest Diagnostics
Enters into Contracts with Regional Business Coalitions: Yes

Employer References
State of Florida, Gevity HR (formerly Staff Leasing), Publix,
Lincare, Miami Dade County

207   Florida Health Care Plans

1340 Ridgewood Avenue
Holly Hill, FL 32117
Toll-Free: 800-352-9824
Fax: 386-676-7119
www.fhcp.com
Subsidiary of: Blue Cross Blue Shield of Florida
Non-Profit Organization: Yes
Year Founded: 1974
Owned by an Integrated Delivery Network (IDN): Yes
Federally Qualified: Yes

Healthplan and Services Defined
PLAN TYPE: HMO
Benefits Offered: Behavioral Health, Chiropractic, Dental,
Disease Management, Home Care, Inpatient SNF, Podiatry,
Prescription, Psychiatric, Transplant, Vision, Wellness

Type of Coverage
Commercial, Individual, Medicare, Supplemental Medicare
Catastrophic Illness Benefit: Varies per case

Geographic Areas Served
Volusia, Flagler, Brevard and Seminole counties

Publishes and Distributes Report Card: Yes

Accreditation Certification
TJC, NCQA

Key Personnel
President & CEO .... Wendy Myers, MD
Chief Financial Officer................ David Schandel
Chief Medical Officer .... Joseph Zuckerman, MD
Chief Information Officer .... Tim Moylan
Compliance Officer.................... Robert Gilliland
Quality Management .... Joann Adams
Legal Counsel...................... Pamerla Thomas

Specialty Managed Care Partners
Enters into Contracts with Regional Business Coalitions: Yes

208   Freedom Health

5403 N Church Avenue
Tampa, FL 33614
Toll-Free: 800-401-2740
Fax: 813-506-6150
www.freedomhealth.com
Mailing Address: P.O. Box 151137, Tampa, FL 33684
Physician Owned Organization: Yes

Healthplan and Services Defined
PLAN TYPE: Medicare
Benefits Offered: Prescription, Wellness

Type of Coverage
Supplemental Medicare, Medicaid

Geographic Areas Served
Brevard, Broward, Charlotte, Citrus, Collier, Hernando,
Hillsborough, Indian River, Lake, Lee, Manatee, Marion,
Martin, Miami-Dade, Orange, Osceola, Palm Beach, Pasco,
Pinellas, Polk, Sarasota, Seminole, St. Lucie, Sumter and
Volusia counties

Accreditation Certification
NCQA

Key Personnel
CEO .... Rupesh Shah

209   Health First Health Plans

6450 US Highway 1
Rockledge, FL 32955
Toll-Free: 800-716-7737
www.healthfirsthealthplans.org
Non-Profit Organization: Yes
Year Founded: 1995
Number of Affiliated Hospitals: 8
Number of Referral/Specialty Physicians: 3,000

Healthplan and Services Defined
PLAN TYPE: Medicare
Benefits Offered: Behavioral Health, Chiropractic, Disease
Management, Home Care, Inpatient SNF, Long-Term Care,
Physical Therapy, Podiatry, Prescription, Psychiatric,
Transplant, Vision, Wellness

Type of Coverage
Commercial, Medicare
Catastrophic Illness Benefit: Covered

Type of Payment Plans Offered
FFS

Geographic Areas Served
Brevard and Indian River counties

Peer Review Type
Utilization Review: Yes
Second Surgical Opinion: Yes
Case Management: Yes

Accreditation Certification
NCQA

Key Personnel

President & CEO. Steven P. Johnson
Chief Strategy Officer. . . . . Drew Rector
Chief Physician Officer . . . . Jeffrey Stalnaker
Chief Financial Officer . . . . Joe Felkner
Chief Information Officer . . . . Alex Popowycz

Average Claim Compensation

Physician's Fees Charged: 110%

Specialty Managed Care Partners

SXC, Ameripharm

Employer References

Boeing/McDonnell Douglas Corp., ITT, Computer Science
Raytheon, Intersil Corp.

210 Health First Medicare Plans

6450 US Highway 1
Rockledge, FL 32955
Toll-Free: 800-716-7737
www.health-first.org/health_plans/medicare
Subsidiary of: Health First
Year Founded: 1997
Number of Referral/Specialty Physicians: 1,100

Healthplan and Services Defined
PLAN TYPE: Medicare
Other Type: HMO-POS

Type of Coverage
Medicare

Geographic Areas Served
Brevard and Indian River counties

Key Personnel
President & CEO. Steven P. Johnson
Chief Strategy Officer. . . . . Drew Rector
Chief Financial Officer . . . . Joe Felkner
Chief Physician Officer . . . . Jeffrey Stalnaker
Chief Information Officer . . . . Alex Popowycz

211 Healthchoice

55 W Gore Street
Orlando, FL 32801
Toll-Free: 800-635-4345
Phone: 407-481-7100
Fax: 407-481-7190
hcweb@orlandohealth.com
www.healthchoiceorlando.org
Subsidiary of: Orlando Health
For Profit Organization: Yes
Year Founded: 1984
Number of Affiliated Hospitals: 9

Healthplan and Services Defined
PLAN TYPE: PPO
Plan Specialty: Behavioral Health, Worker's Compensation,
UR, Pediatrics
Benefits Offered: Behavioral Health, Disease Management

Type of Coverage
Commercial
Catastrophic Illness Benefit: Varies per case

Type of Payment Plans Offered
FFS

Geographic Areas Served
Central Florida

Peer Review Type
Utilization Review: Yes
Second Surgical Opinion: Yes
Case Management: Yes

Publishes and Distributes Report Card: Yes

Accreditation Certification
AAAHC
TJC Accreditation, Medicare Approved, Utilization Review,
Pre-Admission Certification, State Licensure, Quality
Assurance Program

Specialty Managed Care Partners
Enters into Contracts with Regional Business Coalitions: Yes

212 HealthNetwork

301 Clematis Street
Suite 3000
West Palm Beach, FL 33401
Toll-Free: 800-200-9416
healthnetwork.com
For Profit Organization: Yes

Healthplan and Services Defined
PLAN TYPE: Multiple
Plan Specialty: Dental, Vision
Benefits Offered: Dental, Prescription, Vision, Wellness,
Short-term,

Type of Coverage
Commercial, Individual, Medicare

Key Personnel
Chief Executive Officer . . . . Jeremy Kayne
General Counsel/COO . . . . Erika Sullivan
Creative Director . . . . Janna Gilleland
Chief Technology Officer . . . . James Beams

213 HealthSun

3250 Mary Street
Suite 400
Coconut Grove, FL 33133
Phone: 305-234-9292
www.healthsun.com
Subsidiary of: Anthem, Inc.
Year Founded: 2005
Number of Affiliated Hospitals: 19

Healthplan and Services Defined
PLAN TYPE: Medicare
Benefits Offered: Prescription, Transportation Services

Type of Coverage
Medicare

Geographic Areas Served
Miami-Dade and Broward counties

Key Personnel
Chief Executive Officer. . . . . Ron Schutzen

214 Humana Health Insurance of Florida

9965 San Jose Boulevard
Suite 12
Jacksonville, FL 32257
Toll-Free: 800-639-1133
Phone: 904-376-1234
Fax: 904-376-1270
www.humana.com
Secondary Address: Carollwood Center, 10037 N Dale Mabry
   Highway, Tampa, FL 33618, 813-463-4221
Subsidiary of: Humana
For Profit Organization: Yes
Year Founded: 1962

Healthplan and Services Defined
   PLAN TYPE: HMO/PPO
   Model Type: IPA
   Plan Specialty: Dental, Vision
   Benefits Offered: Dental, Disease Management, Prescription,
      Vision, Wellness, Life, LTD, STD

Type of Coverage
   Commercial, Individual

Type of Payment Plans Offered
   POS

Geographic Areas Served
   Statewide

Subscriber Information
   Average Annual Deductible Per Subscriber:
      Employee Only (Self): $0
      Medicare: $0
   Average Subscriber Co-Payment:
      Primary Care Physician: $10.00
      Prescription Drugs: $7.00
      Hospital ER: $25.00

Network Qualifications
   Pre-Admission Certification: Yes

Peer Review Type
   Utilization Review: Yes
   Second Surgical Opinion: Yes
   Case Management: Yes

Publishes and Distributes Report Card: Yes

Accreditation Certification
   URAC, NCQA, CORE
   TJC Accreditation, Medicare Approved, Utilization Review,
      Pre-Admission Certification, State Licensure, Quality
      Assurance Program

Key Personnel
   Market Vice President . . . . Al Hernandez

Specialty Managed Care Partners
   Enters into Contracts with Regional Business Coalitions: Yes

215 Leon Medical Centers Health Plan

8600 NW 41st Street
Suite 201
Doral, FL 33166
Toll-Free: 866-393-5366
Phone: 305-229-7461
membersupport@lmchealthplans.com
www.lmchealthplans.com
Subsidiary of: HealthSpring, Inc.
For Profit Organization: Yes
Year Founded: 1996
Number of Affiliated Hospitals: 5
Number of Primary Care Physicians: 1,200
Total Enrollment: 27,000

Healthplan and Services Defined
   PLAN TYPE: HMO
   Benefits Offered: Chiropractic, Dental, Inpatient SNF,
      Podiatry, Prescription, Psychiatric, Vision, Wellness

Type of Coverage
   Supplemental Medicare, Medicare Advantage

Geographic Areas Served
   Miami-Dade County

Key Personnel
   President/CEO . . . . Henry Hernandez
      henry.hernandez@lmchealthplans.com
   Vice President, IT . . . . Jennifer Velasquez
      jennifer.velasquez@lmchealthplans.com
   COO . . . . Guillermo Gurdian
      guillermo.gurdian@lmchealthplans.com
   VP, Claims . . . . Luis Fernandez
      luis.fernandez@lmchealthplans.com
   Director of Finance . . . . Mercy Kirkpatrick
      mercy.kirpatrick@lmchealthplans.com
   Medical Director . . . . Alina Campos, MD
      alina.campos@lmchealthplans.com

216 Liberty Dental Plan of Florida

PO Box 15149
Tampa, FL 33684-5149
Toll-Free: 877-877-1893
www.libertydentalplan.com
For Profit Organization: Yes
Total Enrollment: 2,000,000

Healthplan and Services Defined
   PLAN TYPE: Dental
   Other Type: Dental HMO
   Plan Specialty: Dental
   Benefits Offered: Dental

Type of Coverage
   Commercial, Medicare, Medicaid, Unions

Geographic Areas Served
   Statewide

Accreditation Certification
   NCQA

217   Magellan Complete Care of Florida

4800 North Scottdale Road
Suite 4400
Scottsdale, AZ 85251
Toll-Free: 800-327-8613
www.magellancompletecareoffl.com
For Profit Organization: Yes

Healthplan and Services Defined
  PLAN TYPE: Other
  Benefits Offered: Psychiatric

Type of Coverage
  Medicaid, Specialty plan for individuals with

Geographic Areas Served
  Statewide

Key Personnel
  Chairman & CEO . . . . Barry M. Smith
  Chief Financial Officer . . . . Jonathan N. Rubin
  General Counsel . . . . Daniel N. Gregoire
  Human Resources. . . . . Caskie Lewis-Clapper
  Chief Medical Officer . . . . Karen Amstutz
  Chief Information Officer . . . . Srini Koushik

218   Molina Healthcare of Florida

8300 NW 33rd Street
Suite 400
Miami, FL 33122
Toll-Free: 866-422-2541
www.molinahealthcare.com
Subsidiary of: Molina Healthcare, Inc.
For Profit Organization: Yes

Healthplan and Services Defined
  PLAN TYPE: Medicare
  Model Type: Network
  Plan Specialty: Dental, PBM, Vision, Integrated
    Medicare/Medicaid (Duals)
  Benefits Offered: Dental, Prescription, Vision, Wellness, Life

Type of Coverage
  Individual, Medicare, Supplemental Medicare, Medicaid

Geographic Areas Served
  Statewide

Key Personnel
  Plan President . . . . Mike Jones
  Chief Medical Officer. . . . . Mark Bloom, MD

219   Neighborhood Health Partnership

Miami, FL 33126
Toll-Free: 877-972-8845
www.uhc.com/nhpfl
Subsidiary of: UnitedHealthcare
For Profit Organization: Yes
Year Founded: 1993
Number of Primary Care Physicians: 1,282
Total Enrollment: 108,000
State Enrollment: 141,178

Healthplan and Services Defined
  PLAN TYPE: HMO
  Other Type: POS
  Plan Specialty: Behavioral Health, Chiropractic
  Benefits Offered: Disease Management, Home Care,
    Prescription, Transplant, Wellness, Durable Medical
    Equipment

Type of Coverage
  Commercial, Medicare

Type of Payment Plans Offered
  Capitated

Geographic Areas Served
  Orange, Seminole, Osceola, Flagler, Lake, Volusia,
  Hillsborough, Pasco, Pinellas, Sarasota, Polk, Hernando, and
  Lee counties

Peer Review Type
  Utilization Review: Yes

Publishes and Distributes Report Card: Yes

Accreditation Certification
  NCQA

Key Personnel
  President & CEO . . . . David Wichmann
  Chief Operating Officer . . . . Dan Schumacher
  Chief Strategy Officer . . . . John Cosgriff
  Communications Officer . . . . Kirsten Gorsuch
  Chief Medical Officer. . . . . Sam Ho
  Chief Legal Officer . . . . Thad Johnson
  Chief Information Officer . . . . Phil McKoy

220   One Call Care Management

841 Prudential Drive
Suite 900
Jacksonville, FL 32207
Toll-Free: 800-848-1989
www.onecallcm.com
Secondary Address: 8501 Fallbrook Avenue, West Hills, CA
91304
For Profit Organization: Yes
Year Founded: 1993

Healthplan and Services Defined
  PLAN TYPE: Other
  Plan Specialty: Worker's Compensation
  Benefits Offered: Worker's Compensation

Type of Payment Plans Offered
  POS, DFFS, FFS, Combination FFS & DFFS

Geographic Areas Served
  Nationwide

Network Qualifications
  Pre-Admission Certification: Yes

Publishes and Distributes Report Card: No

Accreditation Certification
  Utilization Review, Quality Assurance Program

Key Personnel
  President & CEO. . . . . Dale Wolf
  Chief Financial Officer . . . . Rick McCook

Chief Operating Officer . . . . Chris Watson
Sales & Marketing Officer. . . . . Robert Zeccardi
Chief Product Officer. Will Smith
Chief Strategy Officer. . . . . Pat Rowland

Specialty Managed Care Partners
Enters into Contracts with Regional Business Coalitions: No

221   Preferred Care Partners
9100 S Dadeland Boulevard
Suite 1250
Miami, FL 33156
Toll-Free: 866-231-7201
Fax: 501-262-7070
MemberServices@uhcsouthflorida.com
www.mypreferredcare.com
Mailing Address: P.O. Box 29675, Hot Springs, AR
  71903-9675
Number of Affiliated Hospitals: 27
Number of Primary Care Physicians: 1,500
Total Enrollment: 45,000

Healthplan and Services Defined
  PLAN TYPE: Multiple
  Benefits Offered: Dental, Prescription, Vision, Hearing,
    Transportation, Fitness Programs

Type of Coverage
  Supplemental Medicare

Geographic Areas Served
  Miami-Dade, Broward, and Palm Beach counties

Accreditation Certification
  URAC

Key Personnel
  President. . . . . Justo Pozo
  CEO . . . . Joseph Caruncho

222   Trinity Health of Florida
BayCare Health System
2985 Drew Street
Clearwater, FL 33759
Toll-Free: 800-229-2273
www.trinity-health.org
Secondary Address: Holy Cross Hospital, 4725 N Federal
  Highway, Fort Lauderdale, FL 33308
Subsidiary of: Trinity Health
Non-Profit Organization: Yes
Year Founded: 2013
Total Enrollment: 30,000,000

Healthplan and Services Defined
  PLAN TYPE: Other
  Benefits Offered: Disease Management, Home Care,
    Long-Term Care, Psychiatric, Hospice programs, PACE
    (Program of All Inclusive Care for the Elderly)

Geographic Areas Served
  South Florida

Key Personnel
  President/CEO . . . . Tommy Inzina
  EVP/CMO. . . . . Dr. Bruce Flareau

EVP/COO . . . . Glenn Waters
EVP/CFO . . . . Janice Polo

223   United Concordia of Florida
8932 Chambore Dr
Jacksonville, FL 32256
Phone: 904-998-7244
www.unitedconcordia.com
For Profit Organization: Yes
Year Founded: 1971
Total Enrollment: 7,800,000

Healthplan and Services Defined
  PLAN TYPE: Dental
  Plan Specialty: Dental
  Benefits Offered: Dental

Type of Coverage
  Commercial, Individual, Military personnel & families

Geographic Areas Served
  Nationwide

Accreditation Certification
  URAC

Key Personnel
  Senior Dental Network Svc . . . . Cynthia Byndas
  Contact. . . . . Beth Rutherford
    717-260-7659
    beth.rutherford@ucci.com

224   UnitedHealthcare of Florida
495 N Keller Road
Maitland, FL 32751
Toll-Free: 800-899-6500
www.uhc.com
Subsidiary of: UnitedHealth Group
For Profit Organization: Yes
Owned by an Integrated Delivery Network (IDN): Yes

Healthplan and Services Defined
  PLAN TYPE: HMO/PPO
  Model Type: Network
  Plan Specialty: Behavioral Health, Dental, Disease
    Management, PBM, Vision
  Benefits Offered: Behavioral Health, Chiropractic, Dental,
    Disease Management, Home Care, Inpatient SNF, Physical
    Therapy, Podiatry, Prescription, Psychiatric, Transplant,
    Vision, Wellness, AD&D, Life, LTD, STD

Type of Coverage
  Commercial, Individual, Medicare, Supplemental Medicare,
    Medicaid, Catastrophic, Family, Military, Veterans, Group,

Geographic Areas Served
  Statewide

Subscriber Information
  Average Monthly Fee Per Subscriber
    (Employee + Employer Contribution):
      Employee Only (Self): Varies

Peer Review Type
  Case Management: Yes

Accreditation Certification
TJC, NCQA

Key Personnel
Dir., Business . . . . David Price

Specialty Managed Care Partners
Own Network
Enters into Contracts with Regional Business Coalitions: Yes

225 UnitedHealthcare of South Florida

3100 SW 145th Avenue
Miramar, FL 33027
Toll-Free: 800-310-7622
www.uhc.com
Subsidiary of: UnitedHealth Group
For Profit Organization: Yes
Year Founded: 1970

Healthplan and Services Defined
PLAN TYPE: HMO/PPO
Model Type: Network
Plan Specialty: ASO, Behavioral Health, Chiropractic,
Dental, Disease Management, PBM, Vision
Benefits Offered: Behavioral Health, Chiropractic,
Complementary Medicine, Dental, Disease Management,
Long-Term Care, Physical Therapy, Podiatry, Prescription,
Psychiatric, Vision, Wellness, AD&D, Life, LTD, STD

Type of Coverage
Commercial, Individual, Medicare, Supplemental Medicare,
Medicaid, Catastrophic, Family, Military, Veterans, Group,
Catastrophic Illness Benefit: Varies per case

Type of Payment Plans Offered
POS, DFFS, Capitated, FFS, Combination FFS & DFFS

Geographic Areas Served
Palm Beach, Broward & Dade counties

Subscriber Information
Average Subscriber Co-Payment:
Primary Care Physician: $5.00-15.00
Non-Network Physician: Varies
Prescription Drugs: $5.00-10.00
Hospital ER: $100.00

Network Qualifications
Pre-Admission Certification: Yes

Peer Review Type
Utilization Review: Yes
Second Surgical Opinion: Yes
Case Management: Yes

Publishes and Distributes Report Card: Yes

Accreditation Certification
AAAHC, URAC, NCQA
TJC Accreditation, Medicare Approved, Utilization Review,
Pre-Admission Certification, State Licensure, Quality
Assurance Program

Key Personnel
President . . . . Nick Zaffiris

Specialty Managed Care Partners
Enters into Contracts with Regional Business Coalitions: No

226 WellCare Health Plans

8735 Henderson Road
Tampa, FL 33634
Toll-Free: 800-960-2530
www.wellcare.com
Mailing Address: P.O. Box 31370, Tampa, FL 33631-3372
For Profit Organization: Yes
Total Enrollment: 3,700,000

Healthplan and Services Defined
PLAN TYPE: Medicare
Model Type: Network
Plan Specialty: Dental, PBM, Vision, Integrated
Medicare/Medicaid (Duals)
Benefits Offered: Dental, Prescription, Vision, Wellness, Life

Type of Coverage
Individual, Medicare, Supplemental Medicare, Medicaid

Geographic Areas Served
Nationwide

Accreditation Certification
URAC

Key Personnel
Chief Executive Officer. . . . . Kenneth A. Burdick
Chief Financial Officer. . . . . Drew Asher
Chief Information Officer. . . . . Darren Ghanayem
General Counsel/Secretary. . . . . Anat Hakim
Chief Medical Officer . . . . Mark Lennay
SVP, Public Affairs . . . . Rhonda Mims

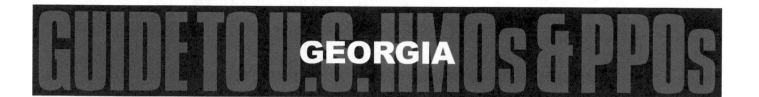
Health Insurance Coverage Status and Type of Coverage by Age

Category	All Persons		Under 18 years		Under 65 years	
	Number	%	Number	%	Number	%
Total population	10,242	-	2,671	-	8,869	-
Covered by some type of health insurance	8,866 *(29)*	86.6 *(0.3)*	2,471 *(13)*	92.5 *(0.4)*	7,505 *(29)*	84.6 *(0.3)*
Covered by private health insurance	6,774 *(46)*	66.1 *(0.5)*	1,511 *(24)*	56.6 *(0.9)*	5,983 *(44)*	67.5 *(0.5)*
Employer-based	5,497 *(44)*	53.7 *(0.4)*	1,294 *(24)*	48.5 *(0.9)*	5,043 *(42)*	56.9 *(0.5)*
Direct purchase	1,275 *(28)*	12.4 *(0.3)*	173 *(10)*	6.5 *(0.4)*	900 *(25)*	10.1 *(0.3)*
TRICARE	416 *(16)*	4.1 *(0.2)*	102 *(8)*	3.8 *(0.3)*	303 *(14)*	3.4 *(0.2)*
Covered by public health insurance	3,146 *(32)*	30.7 *(0.3)*	1,044 *(25)*	39.1 *(0.9)*	1,824 *(32)*	20.6 *(0.4)*
Medicaid	1,780 *(31)*	17.4 *(0.3)*	1,022 *(26)*	38.3 *(1.0)*	1,570 *(31)*	17.7 *(0.3)*
Medicare	1,591 *(13)*	15.5 *(0.1)*	27 *(4)*	1.0 *(0.2)*	271 *(11)*	3.1 *(0.1)*
VA Care	241 *(10)*	2.4 *(0.1)*	4 *(1)*	0.1 *(0.1)*	130 *(7)*	1.5 *(0.1)*
Not covered at any time during the year	1,375 *(29)*	13.4 *(0.3)*	200 *(12)*	7.5 *(0.4)*	1,365 *(29)*	15.4 *(0.3)*

Note: Numbers in thousands; Figures cover civilian noninstitutionalized population in 2017; N/A indicates that data was not available; Z represents or rounds to zero; Margin of error appears in parenthesis and is calculated using replicate weights.
Source: U.S. Census Bureau, American Community Survey, Table HIC-4_ACS. Health Insurance Coverage Status and Type of Coverage by State—All People: 2008 to 2017, Table HIC-5_ACS. Health Insurance Coverage Status and Type of Coverage by State—Children Under 18: 2008 to 2017, Table HIC-6_ACS. Health Insurance Coverage Status and Type of Coverage by State—Persons Under 65: 2008 to 2017

Georgia

227 Aetna Health of Georgia
151 Farmington Avenue
Hartford, CT 06156
Toll-Free: 800-872-3862
www.aetna.com
Subsidiary of: Aetna Inc.
For Profit Organization: Yes

Healthplan and Services Defined
PLAN TYPE: HMO/PPO
Other Type: POS
Model Type: Network
Plan Specialty: Behavioral Health, Dental, EPO, Lab, PBM, Vision, Radiology
Benefits Offered: Behavioral Health, Dental, Disease Management, Long-Term Care, Physical Therapy, Podiatry, Prescription, Psychiatric, Vision, Wellness, Life, LTD, STD

Type of Coverage
Commercial, Medicare, Supplemental Medicare, Medicaid, Catastrophic, Student health

Geographic Areas Served
Statewide

Key Personnel
Health Plan CFO, GA . . . . Greg Arnold
Medical Director. . . . . David Epstein
Reg. VP, Bus. Development . . . . R.J. Briscione
Dir., Health Care Quality . . . . Jacqueline Collins

228 Alliant Health Plans
P.O. Box 2667
Dalton, GA 30722
Toll-Free: 800-811-4793
Fax: 866-634-8917
information@alliantplans.com
www.alliantplans.com
Non-Profit Organization: Yes
Year Founded: 1998
Physician Owned Organization: Yes
Number of Affiliated Hospitals: 9,999
Number of Primary Care Physicians: 500,000
Total Enrollment: 15,000
State Enrollment: 15,000

Healthplan and Services Defined
PLAN TYPE: HMO/PPO
Model Type: PSHCC

Type of Coverage
Commercial, Individual

Geographic Areas Served
Statewide

Key Personnel
Chief Executive Officer . . . . Mark Mixer
Chief Operating Officer . . . . Amanda Reed
Chief Financial Officer . . . . Joe Caldwell, RN

229 Amerigroup Georgia
303 Perimeter Center North
Suite 400
Atlanta, GA 30346
Toll-Free: 800-600-4441
Phone: 678-587-4840
GAmembers@amerigroup.com
www.myamerigroup.com/ga
Subsidiary of: Anthem, Inc.
For Profit Organization: Yes
Year Founded: 2006

Healthplan and Services Defined
PLAN TYPE: HMO
Benefits Offered: Prescription

Type of Coverage
Medicaid, PeachCare for Kids, Planning for He

Accreditation Certification
NCQA

230 Anthem Blue Cross & Blue Shield of Georgia
3350 Peachtree Road
Atlanta, GA 30326
Phone: 404-842-8000
www.anthem.com
For Profit Organization: Yes

Healthplan and Services Defined
PLAN TYPE: HMO/PPO
Model Type: Network
Plan Specialty: ASO, Behavioral Health, Chiropractic, Dental, Disease Management, Lab, PBM, Vision, Radiology, Worker's Compensation, UR
Benefits Offered: Behavioral Health, Chiropractic, Dental, Disease Management, Home Care, Inpatient SNF, Physical Therapy, Podiatry, Prescription, Psychiatric, Transplant, Vision, Wellness, Worker's Compensation, Life

Type of Coverage
Commercial, Individual, Medicare, Supplemental Medicare, Medicaid, Catastrophic

Geographic Areas Served
Statewide

Accreditation Certification
URAC, NCQA

Key Personnel
President . . . . Jeff Fusile
Dir., Group Sales . . . . Sharon Winn
Dir., Provider Management . . . . Chris Goins
Marketing Director . . . . Samantha Bontrager

231 Blue Cross Blue Shield of Georgia
3350 Peachtree Road
Atlanta, GA 30326
Phone: 404-842-8000
www.bcbsga.com
Secondary Address: 6087 Technology Parkway, Suite 2000, Columbus, GA 31907, 706-286-8470
Subsidiary of: Anthem, Inc.

Healthplan and Services Defined
 PLAN TYPE: HMO/PPO
 Model Type: Network
 Plan Specialty: Behavioral Health, Dental, Disease
  Management, Lab, PBM, Vision, Radiology
 Benefits Offered: Behavioral Health, Dental, Disease
  Management, Inpatient SNF, Physical Therapy,
  Prescription, Psychiatric, Transplant, Vision, Wellness, Life

Type of Coverage
 Commercial, Individual, Medicare, Supplemental Medicare,
  Catastrophic

Geographic Areas Served
 Statewide

Accreditation Certification
 URAC

Key Personnel
 President . . . . Jeff Fusile
 Dir., Group Sales . . . . Sharon Winn
 Dir., Provider Management . . . . Chris Goins
 Marketing Director . . . . Samantha Bontrager

---

232   Cigna HealthCare of Georgia

3500 Piedmont Road NE
Atlanta, GA 30305
Toll-Free: 800-244-6224
Phone: 404-443-8800
www.cigna.com
For Profit Organization: Yes

Healthplan and Services Defined
 PLAN TYPE: HMO/PPO
 Plan Specialty: Behavioral Health, Dental, Vision
 Benefits Offered: Behavioral Health, Dental, Disease
  Management, Prescription, Vision, AD&D, Life, LTD,
  STD

Type of Coverage
 Commercial, Individual

Type of Payment Plans Offered
 POS

Accreditation Certification
 URAC, NCQA

Key Personnel
 VP, National Account Exec . . . . Jennifer Fann-Tucker

---

233   CompBenefits Corporation

100 Mansell Court East
Suite 400
Roswell, GA 30076
Toll-Free: 800-295-6279
Phone: 404-365-0074
Fax: 404-233-2366
www.compbenefits.com
Subsidiary of: Humana
Year Founded: 1978
Owned by an Integrated Delivery Network (IDN): Yes

Healthplan and Services Defined
 PLAN TYPE: HMO/PPO
 Model Type: Network, HMO, PPO, POS, TPA
 Plan Specialty: ASO, Dental, Vision
 Benefits Offered: Dental, Vision

Type of Coverage
 Commercial, Individual

Type of Payment Plans Offered
 DFFS, Capitated, FFS

Publishes and Distributes Report Card: Yes

Key Personnel
 President & CEO . . . . Bruce D. Broussard
 Chief Medical Officer . . . . Roy A. Beveridge
 Chief Consumer Officer . . . . Jody L. Bilney
 Human Resources . . . . Tim Huval
 Chief Financial Officer . . . . Brian Kane
 Chief Information Officer . . . . Brian LeClaire
 General Counsel . . . . Christopher M. Todoroff

Specialty Managed Care Partners
 Enters into Contracts with Regional Business Coalitions: Yes

Employer References
 Royal Caribbean Cruise Line, Tupperware

---

234   Coventry Health Care of Georgia

55 Pharr Road NW
Atlanta, GA 30305
Toll-Free: 800-395-2545
Phone: 770-667-8954
coventryhealthcare.com
Subsidiary of: Aetna Inc.
For Profit Organization: Yes
Year Founded: 1994
Number of Affiliated Hospitals: 111
Number of Primary Care Physicians: 31,000
Total Enrollment: 5,000,000
State Enrollment: 200,000

Healthplan and Services Defined
 PLAN TYPE: HMO/PPO
 Other Type: POS
 Model Type: Network
 Plan Specialty: Behavioral Health, Dental, Worker's
  Compensation
 Benefits Offered: Behavioral Health, Dental, Prescription,
  Wellness, Worker's Compensation

Type of Coverage
 Commercial, Individual, Medicare, Supplemental Medicare,
  Medicaid

Type of Payment Plans Offered
 POS

Geographic Areas Served
 Serves more than 100 counties in Georgia including Greater
  Atlanta, Augusta, Brunswick, Columbia, Columbus, Macon,
  Savannah and Valdosta

Publishes and Distributes Report Card: Yes

Accreditation Certification
AAAHC, URAC

Key Personnel
VP, Sales & Marketing . . . . Cory Scott
Senior Provider Relations . . . . LiGlenda Goggins

Specialty Managed Care Partners
Enters into Contracts with Regional Business Coalitions: Yes

235   Delta Dental Insurance Company

1130 Sanctuary Parkway
Suite 600
Alpharetta, GA 30009
Toll-Free: 800-521-2651
www.deltadentalins.com
Mailing Address: P.O. Box 1809, Alpharetta, GA 30023-1809
Non-Profit Organization: Yes

Healthplan and Services Defined
PLAN TYPE: Dental
Plan Specialty: Dental
Benefits Offered: Dental

Type of Coverage
Commercial, Individual

Type of Payment Plans Offered
POS, DFFS, FFS

Geographic Areas Served
Alabama, Florida, Georgia, Louisiana, Mississippi, Montana,
Nevada, Texas and Utah

Key Personnel
Dir., Application Dev. Navin Prabhu

236   Humana Health Insurance of Georgia

1200 Ashwood Parkway
Suite 250
Atlanta, GA 30338
Toll-Free: 800-986-9527
Phone: 770-508-2388
Fax: 770-391-1423
www.humana.com
Secondary Address: 100 Mansell Court East, Suite 125,
Roswell, GA 30076, 800-671-4055
Subsidiary of: Humana
For Profit Organization: Yes
Year Founded: 1961

Healthplan and Services Defined
PLAN TYPE: HMO/PPO
Model Type: Network
Plan Specialty: Dental, Vision
Benefits Offered: Behavioral Health, Chiropractic, Dental,
Disease Management, Prescription, Psychiatric, Transplant,
Vision, Wellness, Worker's Compensation, Life, LTD, STD

Type of Coverage
Commercial, Individual, Medicare, Supplemental Medicare

Geographic Areas Served
Statewide

Accreditation Certification
URAC, NCQA, CORE

Key Personnel
Market VP, GA/AL . . . . John Dammann

237   Kaiser Permanente Georgia

2525 Cumberland Parkway SE
Atlanta, GA 30305
Toll-Free: 800-611-1811
thrive.kaiserpermanente.org/care-near-georgia
Subsidiary of: Kaiser Permanente
Non-Profit Organization: Yes
Year Founded: 1985
Number of Primary Care Physicians: 450
State Enrollment: 269,962

Healthplan and Services Defined
PLAN TYPE: HMO
Model Type: Network
Benefits Offered: Disease Management, Prescription, Vision,
Wellness

Type of Coverage
Commercial, Individual, Medicare, Supplemental Medicare,
Medicaid

Geographic Areas Served
Atlanta, Athens

Key Personnel
National Dir., Members . . . . Tim Abbott
Natioanl VP, Pharmacy IT . . . . James Crawford
VP, Public Affairs . . . . Beverly Thomas

238   Northeast Georgia Health Partners

465 EE Butler Parkway
Gainesville, GA 30501
Phone: 770-219-6600
Fax: 770-219-6609
www.healthpartnersnetwork.com
Non-Profit Organization: Yes
Number of Affiliated Hospitals: 6
Number of Primary Care Physicians: 750
Number of Referral/Specialty Physicians: 75

Healthplan and Services Defined
PLAN TYPE: PPO
Benefits Offered: Behavioral Health, Home Care, Physical
Therapy, Podiatry, Prescription, Psychiatric, Wellness, Labs;
Occupational & Speech Therapy; Durable Medical
Equipment; Hearing Center

Type of Coverage
Commercial

Geographic Areas Served
Banks, Barrow, Dawson, Forsyth, Gwinnett (City of Buford
only), Habersham, Hall, Jackson, Lumpkin, Rabun, Stephens,
Towns, Union and White counties

Accreditation Certification
NCQA

Key Personnel
Vice President . . . . Steven McNeilly
Executive Director . . . . Wanda Katich
Operations Manager . . . . Kathryn Riner
Project Manager . . . . Jennifer Nicholson

239 Secure Health PPO Newtork

577 Mulberry Street
Suite 1000
Macon, GA 31201
Toll-Free: 800-648-7563
Phone: 478-314-2400
www.shpg.com
Mailing Address: P.O. Box 4088, Macon, GA 31028
For Profit Organization: Yes
Year Founded: 1992
Physician Owned Organization: Yes
Number of Affiliated Hospitals: 16
Number of Primary Care Physicians: 950
Total Enrollment: 68,000
State Enrollment: 68,000

Healthplan and Services Defined
 PLAN TYPE: PPO
 Other Type: TPA
 Benefits Offered: Disease Management, Prescription,
  Wellness, EAP

Type of Coverage
 Commercial

Geographic Areas Served
 Statewide

Peer Review Type
 Utilization Review: Yes
 Case Management: Yes

Accreditation Certification
 URAC

Key Personnel
 President/CEO . . . . Albert Ertel

240 Trinity Health of Georgia

Saint Mary's Health Care System
1230 Baxter Street
Athens, GA 30606
Phone: 706-389-3000
www.trinity-health.org
Secondary Address: Saint Joseph's Health System, 424
 Decatur Street SE, Atlanta, GA 30312, 678-843-8500
Subsidiary of: Trinity Health
Non-Profit Organization: Yes
Year Founded: 2013
Total Enrollment: 30,000,000

Healthplan and Services Defined
 PLAN TYPE: Other
 Benefits Offered: Disease Management, Home Care,
  Long-Term Care, Psychiatric, Hospice programs, PACE
  (Program of All Inclusive Care for the Elderly)

Geographic Areas Served
 Atlanta and Southeast Georgia

Key Personnel
 President/CEO . . . . Montez Carter
 Chief of Staff . . . . Andrew Leach

241 United Concordia of Georgia

9635 Ventana Way
Suite 100
Alpharetta, GA 30022
Phone: 678-893-8650
www.unitedconcordia.com
For Profit Organization: Yes
Year Founded: 1971
Total Enrollment: 7,800,000

Healthplan and Services Defined
 PLAN TYPE: Dental
 Plan Specialty: Dental
 Benefits Offered: Dental

Type of Coverage
 Commercial, Individual, Military personnel & families

Geographic Areas Served
 Nationwide

Accreditation Certification
 URAC

Key Personnel
 Sales Manager . . . . Donyale Drawdy
 Contact. . . . . Beth Rutherford
  717-260-7659
  beth.rutherford@ucci.com

242 UnitedHealthcare of Georgia

3720 Davinci Court
Suite 300
Norcross, GA 30092
Toll-Free: 888-545-5205
Phone: 770-628-7004
www.uhc.com
Subsidiary of: UnitedHealth Group
For Profit Organization: Yes
Year Founded: 1980

Healthplan and Services Defined
 PLAN TYPE: HMO/PPO
 Model Type: Network
 Plan Specialty: Behavioral Health, Dental, Disease
  Management, PBM, Vision
 Benefits Offered: Behavioral Health, Dental, Disease
  Management, Long-Term Care, Physical Therapy,
  Prescription, Vision, Wellness, Life, LTD, STD

Type of Coverage
 Individual, Medicare, Supplemental Medicare, Medicaid,
  Catastrophic, Family, Military, Veterans, Group,
  Catastrophic Illness Benefit: Unlimited

Type of Payment Plans Offered
 POS, FFS

Geographic Areas Served
Statewide

Network Qualifications
Pre-Admission Certification: Yes

Peer Review Type
Utilization Review: Yes
Case Management: Yes

Publishes and Distributes Report Card: Yes

Accreditation Certification
NCQA
TJC Accreditation, Medicare Approved, Utilization Review,
Pre-Admission Certification, State Licensure, Quality
Assurance Program

Key Personnel
VP, Account Management . . . . David Sturkey

Specialty Managed Care Partners
Enters into Contracts with Regional Business Coalitions: Yes

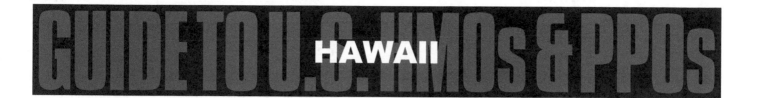

Health Insurance Coverage Status and Type of Coverage by Age

Category	All Persons		Under 18 years		Under 65 years	
	Number	%	Number	%	Number	%
Total population	1,373	-	321	-	1,124	-
Covered by some type of health insurance	1,320 *(5)*	96.2 *(0.4)*	314 *(2)*	97.8 *(0.5)*	1,072 *(5)*	95.4 *(0.4)*
Covered by private health insurance	1,057 *(13)*	77.0 *(0.9)*	223 *(6)*	69.6 *(1.9)*	880 *(12)*	78.3 *(1.0)*
Employer-based	870 *(15)*	63.3 *(1.0)*	177 *(6)*	55.2 *(1.9)*	742 *(13)*	66.0 *(1.2)*
Direct purchase	167 *(8)*	12.2 *(0.6)*	21 *(3)*	6.5 *(0.9)*	105 *(7)*	9.3 *(0.6)*
TRICARE	124 *(7)*	9.0 *(0.5)*	43 *(3)*	13.5 *(1.1)*	100 *(7)*	8.9 *(0.6)*
Covered by public health insurance	483 *(10)*	35.2 *(0.7)*	107 *(6)*	33.5 *(1.8)*	246 *(10)*	21.9 *(0.9)*
Medicaid	245 *(10)*	17.9 *(0.7)*	106 *(6)*	33.1 *(1.8)*	220 *(10)*	19.5 *(0.9)*
Medicare	255 *(3)*	18.6 *(0.2)*	1 *(1)*	0.4 *(0.2)*	19 *(2)*	1.7 *(0.2)*
VA Care	37 *(3)*	2.7 *(0.2)*	1 *(Z)*	0.2 *(0.1)*	17 *(2)*	1.6 *(0.2)*
Not covered at any time during the year	53 *(5)*	3.8 *(0.4)*	7 *(2)*	2.2 *(0.5)*	52 *(5)*	4.6 *(0.4)*

Note: Numbers in thousands; Figures cover civilian noninstitutionalized population in 2017; N/A indicates that data was not available; Z represents or rounds to zero; Margin of error appears in parenthesis and is calculated using replicate weights.
Source: U.S. Census Bureau, American Community Survey, Table HIC-4_ACS. Health Insurance Coverage Status and Type of Coverage by State—All People: 2008 to 2017, Table HIC-5_ACS. Health Insurance Coverage Status and Type of Coverage by State—Children Under 18: 2008 to 2017, Table HIC-6_ACS. Health Insurance Coverage Status and Type of Coverage by State—Persons Under 65: 2008 to 2017

Hawaii

243 AlohaCare

1357 Kapiolani Boulevard
Suite 1250
Honolulu, HI 96814
Toll-Free: 877-973-0712
Phone: 808-973-0712
www.alohacare.org
Secondary Address: 210 Imi Kala Street, Suite 206, Wailuku, HI 96793
Non-Profit Organization: Yes
Year Founded: 1994
Number of Primary Care Physicians: 3,500
Total Enrollment: 70,000

Healthplan and Services Defined
 PLAN TYPE: HMO
 Benefits Offered: Dental, Prescription, Vision, Wellness, Hearing; X-rays & Labs; Acupuncture; 24-hour Nurse Advice Line

Type of Coverage
 Medicare, Supplemental Medicare

Geographic Areas Served
 Oahu, Kauai, Molokai, Lanai, Maui, Hawaii

Peer Review Type
 Case Management: Yes

Publishes and Distributes Report Card: Yes

Key Personnel
 CEO . . . . Laura Esslinger
 CMO . . . . Gary Okamoto
 CFO. . . . . Bruce Lane
 CCO. . . . . Francoise Culley-Trotman
 CIO . . . . Todd Morgan

244 AlohaCare Advantage Plus

1357 Kapiolani Boulevard
Suite 1250
Honolulu, HI 96814
Toll-Free: 866-973-6395
Phone: 808-973-1657
www.alohacare.org
Non-Profit Organization: Yes
Year Founded: 1994

Healthplan and Services Defined
 PLAN TYPE: Medicare
 Other Type: HMO SNP
 Benefits Offered: Prescription

Type of Coverage
 Medicare, Part A, B, and D

Geographic Areas Served
 Oahu, Kauai, Molokai, Lanai, Maui, Hawaii

Key Personnel
 Chairman. . . . . Richard Bettini
 Vice Chair. . . . . Emmanuel Kintu
 Treasure. . . . . Richard Taafee

Secretary . . . . David Derauf

245 Coventry Health Care of Hawaii

6720-B Rockledge Drive
Suite 800
Bethesda, MD 20817
Phone: 301-581-0600
www.coventryhealthcare.com
Subsidiary of: Aetna Inc.
For Profit Organization: Yes

Healthplan and Services Defined
 PLAN TYPE: HMO/PPO
 Model Type: Network
 Plan Specialty: Behavioral Health, Dental, Worker's Compensation
 Benefits Offered: Behavioral Health, Dental, Prescription, Wellness, Worker's Compensation

Type of Coverage
 Commercial, Medicare, Medicaid

Geographic Areas Served
 Statewide

246 Hawaii Medical Assurance Association

737 Bishop Street
Suite 1200
Honolulu, HI 96813
Toll-Free: 800-621-6998
Phone: 808-591-0088
Fax: 808-591-0463
www.hmaa.com
Secondary Address: Customer Service Center , 888-941-4622
For Profit Organization: Yes
Year Founded: 1989

Healthplan and Services Defined
 PLAN TYPE: PPO
 Benefits Offered: Chiropractic, Dental, Prescription, Vision, Wellness, AD&D, Life, Acupuncture

Type of Coverage
 Commercial

Accreditation Certification
 URAC

Key Personnel
 Chairman, COO, CFO . . . . John Henry Felix
 Director. . . . . Gail Mukaihata Hannemann
 Director . . . . Dennis Y.C. Kwan
 Director . . . . Warren Price III
 President & CEO . . . . William C. McCorriston

247 Hawaii Medical Service Association

HMSA Building
818 Keeaumoku Street
Honolulu, HI 96814
hmsa.com
Secondary Address: HMSA, P.O. Box 860, Honolulu, HI 96808
State Enrollment: 700,000

Healthplan and Services Defined
PLAN TYPE: HMO/PPO
Benefits Offered: Dental, Prescription, Vision, Wellness

Type of Coverage
Commercial, Individual, Medicare, Medicaid

Key Personnel
President & CEO . . . . Michael A. Gold
Chief Operating Officer . . . . Michael B. Stollar
Chief Health Officer. . . . . Mark M. Mugiishi
Chief Information Officer . . . . Dick Escue
Chief Financial Officer . . . . Gina L. Marting
General Counsel . . . . Jennifer A. Walker

---

248 Humana Health Insurance of Hawaii
733 Bishop Street
Suite 2100
Honolulu, HI 96813
Phone: 808-540-2570
Fax: 808-548-7618
www.humana.com
Subsidiary of: Humana
For Profit Organization: Yes

Healthplan and Services Defined
PLAN TYPE: HMO/PPO
Model Type: Network
Plan Specialty: Dental, Vision
Benefits Offered: Dental, Vision, Life, LTD, STD

Type of Coverage
Commercial

Geographic Areas Served
Statewide

Accreditation Certification
URAC, NCQA, CORE

Key Personnel
Provider Engagement Exec. . . . . Jade Martinez
Medicare Sales/Enrollment . . . . Herman Hoi

---

249 Kaiser Permanente Hawaii
1010 Pensacola Street
Honolulu, HI 96814
Toll-Free: 808-432-2000
www.kpinhawaii.org
Subsidiary of: Kaiser Permanente
Non-Profit Organization: Yes
Year Founded: 1958
Number of Primary Care Physicians: 500
State Enrollment: 242,978

Healthplan and Services Defined
PLAN TYPE: HMO
Model Type: Group
Plan Specialty: Obstetrics/gynecology, orthopedics,
cardiothoracic and vascular surgery, neurosurgery,
oncology, gastroenterology
Benefits Offered: Chiropractic, Complementary Medicine,
Disease Management, Prescription, Vision, Wellness,
Worker's Compensation

Offers Demand Management Patient Information Service: Yes

Type of Coverage
Commercial, Individual, Medicare, Medicaid
Catastrophic Illness Benefit: Unlimited

Type of Payment Plans Offered
POS, Capitated, FFS

Geographic Areas Served
Big Island, Maui, Molokai & Lanai, Oahu, Kauai

Subscriber Information
Average Subscriber Co-Payment:
Home Health Care Max. Days/Visits Covered: Unlimited
Nursing Home: Skilled nursing fac.
Nursing Home Max. Days/Visits Covered: Skilled nursing
fac.

Network Qualifications
Pre-Admission Certification: No

Peer Review Type
Utilization Review: Yes
Case Management: Yes

Publishes and Distributes Report Card: Yes

Accreditation Certification
NCQA, UNICEF/WHO Baby Friendly
TJC Accreditation, Medicare Approved, Utilization Review,
State Licensure, Quality Assurance Program

Key Personnel
Sr. Consultant, Sales . . . . Bernie Boglioli
Associate Account Manager . . . . Marihoi Lee

Specialty Managed Care Partners
Enters into Contracts with Regional Business Coalitions: Yes

---

250 UnitedHealthcare of Hawaii
5901 Lincoln Drive
Minneapolis, MN 55436
Toll-Free: 877-842-3210
www.uhc.com
Subsidiary of: UnitedHealth Group
For Profit Organization: Yes
Year Founded: 1986

Healthplan and Services Defined
PLAN TYPE: HMO/PPO
Model Type: Network
Plan Specialty: Behavioral Health, Dental, Disease
Management, PBM, Vision
Benefits Offered: Behavioral Health, Dental, Disease
Management, Long-Term Care, Prescription, Vision,
Wellness, Life, LTD, STD

Type of Coverage
Medicare, Supplemental Medicare, Medicaid, Catastrophic,
Family, Military, Veterans, Group,
Catastrophic Illness Benefit: Covered

Type of Payment Plans Offered
DFFS, Capitated

Geographic Areas Served
Statewide. Hawaii is covered by the Minnesota branch

Subscriber Information

Average Monthly Fee Per Subscriber
  (Employee + Employer Contribution):
    Employee Only (Self): $120.00
    Employee & 1 Family Member: $240.00
    Employee & 2 Family Members: $375.00
Average Annual Deductible Per Subscriber:
    Employee & 2 Family Members: Varies
Average Subscriber Co-Payment:
    Primary Care Physician: $5.00-10.00
    Prescription Drugs: $5.00/10.00/25.00
    Hospital ER: $50.00
    Nursing Home Max. Days/Visits Covered: 120 per year

Publishes and Distributes Report Card: Yes

Accreditation Certification

NCQA
TJC Accreditation, Utilization Review, State Licensure

Key Personnel

VP, Quality . . . . Kie Kawano

Specialty Managed Care Partners

Enters into Contracts with Regional Business Coalitions: Yes

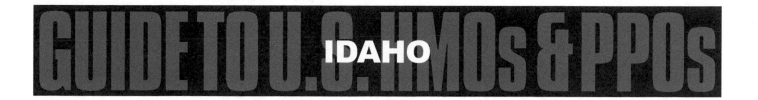

Health Insurance Coverage Status and Type of Coverage by Age

Category	All Persons		Under 18 years		Under 65 years	
	Number	%	Number	%	Number	%
Total population	1,695	-	472	-	1,437	-
Covered by some type of health insurance	1,523 *(9)*	89.9 *(0.5)*	450 *(5)*	95.4 *(0.7)*	1,265 *(9)*	88.1 *(0.6)*
Covered by private health insurance	1,184 *(14)*	69.8 *(0.8)*	293 *(9)*	62.0 *(1.8)*	1,020 *(14)*	71.0 *(0.9)*
Employer-based	895 *(19)*	52.8 *(1.1)*	244 *(9)*	51.8 *(2.0)*	831 *(18)*	57.9 *(1.2)*
Direct purchase	288 *(12)*	17.0 *(0.7)*	43 *(5)*	9.0 *(1.1)*	184 *(10)*	12.8 *(0.7)*
TRICARE	59 *(6)*	3.5 *(0.4)*	11 *(4)*	2.4 *(0.7)*	35 *(5)*	2.5 *(0.4)*
Covered by public health insurance	567 *(13)*	33.5 *(0.8)*	182 *(9)*	38.6 *(1.9)*	315 *(13)*	22.0 *(0.9)*
Medicaid	306 *(12)*	18.0 *(0.7)*	181 *(9)*	38.3 *(1.9)*	276 *(12)*	19.2 *(0.9)*
Medicare	295 *(4)*	17.4 *(0.3)*	3 *(1)*	0.7 *(0.2)*	43 *(4)*	3.0 *(0.3)*
VA Care	53 *(4)*	3.2 *(0.2)*	1 *(1)*	0.3 *(0.2)*	25 *(3)*	1.7 *(0.2)*
Not covered at any time during the year	172 *(9)*	10.1 *(0.5)*	22 *(3)*	4.6 *(0.7)*	171 *(9)*	11.9 *(0.6)*

Note: Numbers in thousands; Figures cover civilian noninstitutionalized population in 2017; N/A indicates that data was not available; Z represents or rounds to zero; Margin of error appears in parenthesis and is calculated using replicate weights.
Source: U.S. Census Bureau, American Community Survey, Table HIC-4_ACS. Health Insurance Coverage Status and Type of Coverage by State—All People: 2008 to 2017, Table HIC-5_ACS. Health Insurance Coverage Status and Type of Coverage by State—Children Under 18: 2008 to 2017, Table HIC-6_ACS. Health Insurance Coverage Status and Type of Coverage by State—Persons Under 65: 2008 to 2017

Idaho

251   Aetna Health of Idaho

151 Farmington Avenue
Hartford, CT 06156
Toll-Free: 800-872-3862
Phone: 860-273-0123
www.aetna.com
Subsidiary of: Aetna Inc.
For Profit Organization: Yes

Healthplan and Services Defined
PLAN TYPE: PPO
Other Type: POS
Model Type: Network
Plan Specialty: Behavioral Health, EPO, Lab, PBM,
    Radiology
Benefits Offered: Behavioral Health, Dental, Disease
    Management, Long-Term Care, Physical Therapy,
    Podiatry, Prescription, Psychiatric, Vision, Wellness, Life,
    LTD, STD

Type of Coverage
Commercial, Student health

Type of Payment Plans Offered
POS, FFS

Geographic Areas Served
Statewide

Key Personnel
Medicare Broker Manager . . . . Michael Beam

252   Blue Cross of Idaho Health Service, Inc.

3000 East Pine Avenue
Meridian, ID 83642
Toll-Free: 800-274-4018
Phone: 208-345-4550
Fax: 208-331-7311
www.bcidaho.com
Mailing Address: P.O. Box 7408, Boise, ID 83707
Subsidiary of: Blue Cross and Blue Shield Association
Non-Profit Organization: Yes
Year Founded: 1945
Number of Affiliated Hospitals: 44
Number of Primary Care Physicians: 1,631
Total Enrollment: 563,000
State Enrollment: 563,000

Healthplan and Services Defined
PLAN TYPE: HMO/PPO
Model Type: IPA, Group, Network
Plan Specialty: ASO, Chiropractic, Dental, Disease
    Management
Benefits Offered: Chiropractic, Dental, Disease Management,
    Prescription, Vision, Wellness

Type of Coverage
Commercial, Individual, Indemnity, Medicare, Supplemental
    Medicare

Type of Payment Plans Offered
POS, DFFS, FFS

Geographic Areas Served
Statewide

Subscriber Information
Average Subscriber Co-Payment:
    Prescription Drugs: Varies
    Hospital ER: Varies
    Home Health Care: Varies
    Nursing Home: Varies

Network Qualifications
Pre-Admission Certification: Yes

Peer Review Type
Utilization Review: Yes
Case Management: Yes

Publishes and Distributes Report Card: Yes

Accreditation Certification
TJC Accreditation, Pre-Admission Certification, State
    Licensure

Key Personnel
President & CEO . . . . Charlene Maher
Chief Financial Officer. . . . . Ralph Woodard
General Counsel . . . . Steven Tobiason
SVP, Compliance Officer . . . . Valerie A. Reardon
EVP, Strategy/Innovation . . . . David Jeppesen
Chief Medical Officer . . . . Rhonda Robinson-Beale, MD
VP, Sales. . . . . Peter Morrissey
Media Contact . . . . Bret Rumbeck
    208-387-6921
    bret.rumbeck@bcidaho.com

Specialty Managed Care Partners
Wellpoint Pharmacy Management, Dental through Blue Cross
    of Idaho, Vision through VSP, Life Insurance, EAP through
    Business Psychology Associates
Enters into Contracts with Regional Business Coalitions: No

253   Delta Dental of Idaho

555 East Parkcenter Boulevard
Boise, ID 83706
Toll-Free: 800-356-7586
Phone: 208-489-3580
customerservice@deltadentalid.com
www.deltadentalid.com
Non-Profit Organization: Yes
Year Founded: 1971

Healthplan and Services Defined
PLAN TYPE: Dental
Other Type: Dental PPO
Model Type: Network
Plan Specialty: Dental
Benefits Offered: Dental

Type of Coverage
Commercial, Individual, Medicare

Type of Payment Plans Offered
DFFS

Geographic Areas Served
Statewide

Network Qualifications
Pre-Admission Certification: Yes

Publishes and Distributes Report Card: Yes

Key Personnel
Chair/CEO . . . . Jon Jurevic
Director of Sales . . . . Don Murray
dmurray@deltadentalid.com

254 Humana Health Insurance of Idaho

1505 South Eagle Road
Suite 120
Meridian, ID 83642
Phone: 208-319-3400
Fax: 208-888-7298
www.humana.com
Subsidiary of: Humana
For Profit Organization: Yes

Healthplan and Services Defined
PLAN TYPE: HMO/PPO
Model Type: Network
Plan Specialty: Dental, Vision
Benefits Offered: Dental, Vision, Life, LTD, STD

Type of Coverage
Commercial

Geographic Areas Served
Statewide

Accreditation Certification
URAC, NCQA, CORE

Key Personnel
Market VP, UT/ID/WA/OR . . . . Catherine Field

255 Molina Healthcare of Idaho

7050 Union Park Center
Suite 200
Midvale, ID 84047
Phone: 844-879-4400
www.molinahealthcare.com
Secondary Address: Molina Medicaid Solutions, 9415 W
Golden Trout, Boise, ID 83704, 208-373-1300
Subsidiary of: Molina Healthcare, Inc.
For Profit Organization: Yes

Healthplan and Services Defined
PLAN TYPE: Medicare

Type of Coverage
Medicaid information management sys

Geographic Areas Served
Statewide

Key Personnel
President, ID/UT . . . . Brandon Hendrickson
Regional VP, WA/ID/UT . . . . Peter Adler
Mgr., Provider Services . . . . Jessica Pool

256 Primary Health Medical Group

10482 W Carlton Bay Drive
Garden City, ID 83714
Toll-Free: 800-481-9777
Phone: 208-955-6500
Fax: 208-955-6502
information@primaryhealth.com
www.primaryhealth.com
Year Founded: 1996
Physician Owned Organization: Yes

Healthplan and Services Defined
PLAN TYPE: Multiple
Model Type: IPA
Plan Specialty: ASO
Benefits Offered: Behavioral Health, Chiropractic, Dental,
Disease Management, Home Care, Inpatient SNF, Physical
Therapy, Podiatry, Prescription, Psychiatric, Transplant,
Vision, Wellness, AD&D, Life

Type of Coverage
Commercial, Individual, Indemnity

Type of Payment Plans Offered
POS, DFFS

Geographic Areas Served
Southwest Idaho

Accreditation Certification
NCQA

Key Personnel
Chief Operating Officer . . . . Steve Judy
Director of Information . . . . Paul Castronova

257 Regence BlueShield of Idaho

P.O. Box 1106
Lewiston, ID 83501
Toll-Free: 888-367-2117
www.regence.com
Secondary Address: Regence Corporate, P.O. Box 1071,
Portland, OR 97207
Subsidiary of: Regence
Non-Profit Organization: Yes
Total Enrollment: 2,400,000
State Enrollment: 160,000

Healthplan and Services Defined
PLAN TYPE: Multiple
Model Type: Network
Benefits Offered: Dental, Prescription, Vision, Wellness, Life,
Preventive Care

Type of Coverage
Commercial, Individual, Supplemental Medicare

Accreditation Certification
URAC

Key Personnel
President . . . . Sean Robbins

258 Trinity Health of Idaho

Saint Adolphus Health System
1055 N Curtis Road
Boise, ID 83706
Phone: 208-367-2121
www.trinity-health.org
Subsidiary of: Trinity Health
Non-Profit Organization: Yes
Year Founded: 2013
Number of Affiliated Hospitals: 4
Number of Primary Care Physicians: 1,400
Total Enrollment: 30,000,000
State Enrollment: 700,000

Healthplan and Services Defined
PLAN TYPE: Other
Benefits Offered: Disease Management, Home Care,
Long-Term Care, Psychiatric, Hospice programs, PACE
(Program of All Inclusive Care for the Elderly)

Geographic Areas Served
Boise and Nampa, Idaho and Ontario and Baker City, and
Oregon

Key Personnel
Chief Executive Officer . . . . Richard J. Gilfillan
Chief Financial Officer . . . . Lannie Checketts
Chief Nursing Officer . . . . Shelley Harris
Chief HR Officer. Heather Sprague
Chief Compliance Officer. . . . . Jennifer Johnson
VP/General Counsel . . . . Stephanie Westermeier
Interim CMO. . . . . Charles Davis

259 UnitedHealthcare of Idaho

Meridian, ID 83642
Toll-Free: 888-545-5205
www.uhc.com
Subsidiary of: UnitedHealth Group
For Profit Organization: Yes
Year Founded: 1986

Healthplan and Services Defined
PLAN TYPE: HMO/PPO
Model Type: Network
Plan Specialty: Behavioral Health, Dental, Disease
Management, PBM, Vision
Benefits Offered: Behavioral Health, Dental, Disease
Management, Long-Term Care, Prescription, Vision,
Wellness, Life, LTD, STD

Type of Coverage
Individual, Medicare, Supplemental Medicare, Medicaid,
Catastrophic, Family, Military, Veterans, Group,
Catastrophic Illness Benefit: Covered

Type of Payment Plans Offered
DFFS, Capitated

Geographic Areas Served
Statewide

Subscriber Information
Average Monthly Fee Per Subscriber
(Employee + Employer Contribution):
Employee Only (Self): $120.00
Employee & 1 Family Member: $240.00
Employee & 2 Family Members: $375.00
Average Annual Deductible Per Subscriber:
Employee & 2 Family Members: Varies
Average Subscriber Co-Payment:
Primary Care Physician: $5.00-10.00
Prescription Drugs: $5.00/10.00/25.00
Hospital ER: $50.00
Nursing Home Max. Days/Visits Covered: 120 per year

Publishes and Distributes Report Card: Yes

Accreditation Certification
NCQA
TJC Accreditation, Utilization Review, State Licensure

Key Personnel
VP, Sales . . . . Richard Jones

Specialty Managed Care Partners
Enters into Contracts with Regional Business Coalitions: Yes

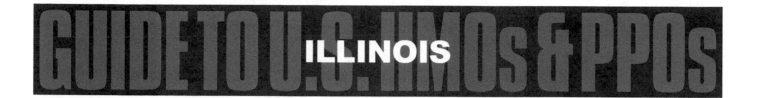
Health Insurance Coverage Status and Type of Coverage by Age

Category	All Persons		Under 18 years		Under 65 years	
	Number	%	Number	%	Number	%
Total population	12,620	-	3,069	-	10,739	-
Covered by some type of health insurance	11,761 *(23)*	93.2 *(0.2)*	2,980 *(9)*	97.1 *(0.2)*	9,898 *(22)*	92.2 *(0.2)*
Covered by private health insurance	8,822 *(49)*	69.9 *(0.4)*	1,918 *(23)*	62.5 *(0.7)*	7,670 *(48)*	71.4 *(0.4)*
Employer-based	7,404 *(51)*	58.7 *(0.4)*	1,752 *(21)*	57.1 *(0.7)*	6,789 *(49)*	63.2 *(0.5)*
Direct purchase	1,655 *(21)*	13.1 *(0.2)*	180 *(8)*	5.9 *(0.3)*	1,008 *(18)*	9.4 *(0.2)*
TRICARE	143 *(8)*	1.1 *(0.1)*	25 *(4)*	0.8 *(0.1)*	93 *(7)*	0.9 *(0.1)*
Covered by public health insurance	4,315 *(38)*	34.2 *(0.3)*	1,160 *(23)*	37.8 *(0.8)*	2,525 *(38)*	23.5 *(0.3)*
Medicaid	2,521 *(38)*	20.0 *(0.3)*	1,152 *(23)*	37.5 *(0.8)*	2,307 *(38)*	21.5 *(0.4)*
Medicare	2,049 *(10)*	16.2 *(0.1)*	12 *(2)*	0.4 *(0.1)*	261 *(8)*	2.4 *(0.1)*
VA Care	210 *(6)*	1.7 *(Z)*	2 *(1)*	0.1 *(Z)*	84 *(4)*	0.8 *(Z)*
Not covered at any time during the year	859 *(23)*	6.8 *(0.2)*	89 *(7)*	2.9 *(0.2)*	841 *(23)*	7.8 *(0.2)*

Note: Numbers in thousands; Figures cover civilian noninstitutionalized population in 2017; N/A indicates that data was not available; Z represents or rounds to zero; Margin of error appears in parenthesis and is calculated using replicate weights.
Source: U.S. Census Bureau, American Community Survey, Table HIC-4_ACS. Health Insurance Coverage Status and Type of Coverage by State—All People: 2008 to 2017, Table HIC-5_ACS. Health Insurance Coverage Status and Type of Coverage by State—Children Under 18: 2008 to 2017, Table HIC-6_ACS. Health Insurance Coverage Status and Type of Coverage by State—Persons Under 65: 2008 to 2017

Illinois

260 Aetna Health of Illinois

333 W Wacker Drive
Suite 2100
Chicago, IL 60606
Toll-Free: 866-600-2139
www.aetnabetterhealth.com/Illinois
Subsidiary of: Aetna Inc.
For Profit Organization: Yes

Healthplan and Services Defined
PLAN TYPE: HMO/PPO
Other Type: POS
Model Type: Network
Plan Specialty: Behavioral Health, Dental, EPO, Lab, PBM,
   Vision, Radiology
Benefits Offered: Behavioral Health, Dental, Disease
   Management, Long-Term Care, Physical Therapy,
   Podiatry, Prescription, Psychiatric, Vision, Wellness, Life,
   LTD, STD

Type of Coverage
Commercial, Student health

Geographic Areas Served
Statewide

Key Personnel
CEO. . . . . David Livingston
Quality Care Consultant. . . . . Delphia McWoodson

261 Aetna of Illinois

Toll-Free: 855-339-9731
www.aetnastateofillinois.com
For Profit Organization: Yes
Year Founded: 1984

Healthplan and Services Defined
PLAN TYPE: HMO
Model Type: Network
Plan Specialty: Behavioral Health, Dental, Worker's
   Compensation
Benefits Offered: Behavioral Health, Dental, Wellness,
   Worker's Compensation

Type of Coverage
Commercial, Individual, Medicare, Supplemental Medicare,
   Medicaid

Type of Payment Plans Offered
POS, DFFS, Capitated, FFS, Combination FFS & DFFS

Geographic Areas Served
Bond, Boone, Calhoun, Champaign, Christian, Clark,
   Clinton, Coles, Crawford, Cumberland, DeWitt, Douglas,
   Edgar, Effingham, Fayette, Ford, Greene, Iroquois, Jasper,
   Jersey, Kankakee, LaSalle, Lee, Logan, Macon, Macoupin,
   Madison, Marshall, McLean, Menard, Monroe, Montgomery,
   Morgan, Moultrie, Ogle, Peoria, Piatt, Sangaman, Saint Clair,
   Shelby, Stark, Stephenson, Tazewell, Vermilion, Washington,
   Whiteside, Will, Winnebago, Woodford counties

Network Qualifications
Pre-Admission Certification: Yes

Peer Review Type
Utilization Review: Yes
Second Surgical Opinion: Yes
Case Management: Yes

Accreditation Certification
NCQA
TJC Accreditation, Medicare Approved, Utilization Review,
   Pre-Admission Certification, State Licensure, Quality
   Assurance Program

Key Personnel
CEO. . . . . David Livingston
Dir., Clinical Services. . . . . Mimi Fairley
VP, Government Programs . . . . Michael Kavouras, Esq.
Dir., Info Management . . . . Rhiannon Yandell

Employer References
Horace Mann, Verizon, Pepsi, Sarah Bush Lincoln Health,
   Walgreen's

262 Blue Cross & Blue Shield of Illinois

300 East Randolph Street
Chicago, IL 60601-5099
Toll-Free: 800-654-7385
www.bcbsil.com
Subsidiary of: Health Care Service Corporation
Year Founded: 1936
Total Enrollment: 8,100,000
State Enrollment: 8,100,000

Healthplan and Services Defined
PLAN TYPE: HMO/PPO
Benefits Offered: Disease Management, Physical Therapy,
   Prescription, Wellness

Type of Coverage
Commercial, Individual, Supplemental Medicare, Medicaid,
   Healthy Kids, Healthy Families

Type of Payment Plans Offered
POS, FFS

Geographic Areas Served
Statewide

Key Personnel
President BCBS Illinois. . . . . Maurice Smith
Medica Contact . . . . Dana Holmes
   312-653-1266
   Dana_L_Holmes@bcbsil.com
Media Contact . . . . Colleen Miller
   312-653-6904
   colleen_miller@bcbsil.com

Specialty Managed Care Partners
Prime Therapeutics

263 BlueCross BlueShield Association

225 North Michigan Avenue
Chicago, IL 60601
Toll-Free: 888-630-2583
www.bcbs.com
Secondary Address: 1310 G Street NW, Washington, DC
   20005

Total Enrollment: 105,000,000

Healthplan and Services Defined
PLAN TYPE: Medicare
Benefits Offered: Chiropractic, Disease Management, Home Care, Inpatient SNF, Physical Therapy, Podiatry, Prescription, Psychiatric, Wellness

Type of Coverage
Individual, Medicare

Geographic Areas Served
Nationwide, including the District of Columbia and Puerto Rico

Subscriber Information
Average Monthly Fee Per Subscriber
(Employee + Employer Contribution):
Employee Only (Self): Varies
Medicare: Varies
Average Annual Deductible Per Subscriber:
Employee Only (Self): Varies
Medicare: Varies
Average Subscriber Co-Payment:
Primary Care Physician: Varies
Non-Network Physician: Varies
Prescription Drugs: Varies
Hospital ER: Varies
Home Health Care: Varies
Home Health Care Max. Days/Visits Covered: Varies
Nursing Home: Varies
Nursing Home Max. Days/Visits Covered: Varies

Key Personnel
President/CEO . . . . Scott P. Serota
Chief Financial Officer . . . . Robert Kolodgy
EVP/Chief of Staff. Jennifer Vachon
SVP, Government Program. . . . . William A. Breskin
Chief Medical Officer. . . . . Trent Haywood
SVP/General Counsel. Scott Nehs
Strategy/Innovation. . . . . Maureen E. Sullivan

---

264   Celtic Insurance Company
77 W Wacker
Suite 1200
Chicago, OH 60601
Toll-Free: 800-477-7870
Phone: 312-619-3000
Fax: 800-749-3340
info@celtic-net.com
www.celtic-net.com
Subsidiary of: Centene Corporation
Year Founded: 1978

Healthplan and Services Defined
PLAN TYPE: PPO

Geographic Areas Served
All states except NY

Key Personnel
VP, HR/CIO . . . . Barbara Basham

---

265   Cigna Healthcare Illinois
525 W Monroe Street
Chicago, IL 60661
Phone: 312-648-2460
www.cigna.com
Secondary Address: 206208 W Prairie Street, Marengo, IL 60152, 815-255-6424
For Profit Organization: Yes
Year Founded: 1982

Healthplan and Services Defined
PLAN TYPE: Multiple
Benefits Offered: Behavioral Health, Dental, Disease Management, Prescription, Vision, Wellness, AD&D, Life, LTD, STD

Type of Coverage
Commercial, Individual, Medicare, Supplemental Medicare, Medicaid, Part-time and hourly workers; Union

Geographic Areas Served
Statewide

Key Personnel
President, Midwest . . . . Michael Phillips
Product Manager. . . . . Michele Nawara
Sales Manager . . . . Brent Smith

---

266   CNA
CNA Center
333 S Wabash Avenue
Chicago, IL 60604
Toll-Free: 877-262-2727
Phone: 312-822-5000
www.cna.com
Year Founded: 1987
Owned by an Integrated Delivery Network (IDN): Yes

Healthplan and Services Defined
PLAN TYPE: Other
Model Type: Network
Plan Specialty: Dental, Disease Management, Lab, MSO, Vision, Radiology, Worker's Compensation, UR
Benefits Offered: Behavioral Health, Chiropractic, Dental, Disease Management, Home Care, Inpatient SNF, Long-Term Care, Physical Therapy, Podiatry, Prescription, Psychiatric, Transplant, Vision, Wellness, Worker's Compensation, AD&D, Life, LTD, STD

Type of Coverage
Commercial, Individual, Indemnity, Medicaid, Catastrophic

Type of Payment Plans Offered
POS

Network Qualifications
Pre-Admission Certification: Yes

Peer Review Type
Utilization Review: Yes
Case Management: Yes

Publishes and Distributes Report Card: Yes

Accreditation Certification
URAC

TJC Accreditation, Pre-Admission Certification

Key Personnel

Chairman & CEO . . . . Thomas F. Motamed

Specialty Managed Care Partners

Enters into Contracts with Regional Business Coalitions: Yes

---

267 CoreSource

400 Field Drive
Lake Forest, IL 60045
Toll-Free: 800-832-3332
Phone: 847-604-9200
www.coresource.com
Subsidiary of: Trustmark
Year Founded: 1980
Total Enrollment: 1,100,000

Healthplan and Services Defined
PLAN TYPE: PPO
Other Type: TPA
Model Type: Network
Plan Specialty: Benefits Administration
Benefits Offered: Behavioral Health, Dental, Home Care,
Prescription, Transplant, Vision, Wellness

Type of Coverage
Commercial

Geographic Areas Served
Nationwide

Accreditation Certification
URAC
Utilization Review, Pre-Admission Certification

Key Personnel
President/CEO . . . . Nancy Eckrich
Chief Clinical Leader. . . . . Meera Atkins
Chief Operating Officer. . . . . Lloyd Sarrel
Chief Financial Officer. . . . . Clare Smith
Chief Information Officer . . . . Brooke Terry
VP, Marketing. . . . . Steve Horvath
VP, Human Resources . . . . Dave Kenney

---

268 Delta Dental of Illinois

111 Shuman Boulevard
Naperville, IL 60563
Toll-Free: 800-335-8215
Phone: 630-718-4700
askdelta@deltadentalil.com
www.deltadentalil.com
Non-Profit Organization: Yes
Year Founded: 1967
State Enrollment: 2,000,000

Healthplan and Services Defined
PLAN TYPE: Dental
Other Type: Dental PPO
Model Type: Network
Plan Specialty: Dental
Benefits Offered: Dental

Type of Coverage
Commercial, Individual

Geographic Areas Served
Statewide

Peer Review Type
Utilization Review: Yes

Key Personnel
President & CEO . . . . Bernard Glossy
Dental Network Admin. . . . . Lynne Williams
Corp. Communications. . . . . Lyndsay Bradshaw
VP, Service Operations . . . . Terry Maddox
Underwriting Manager. . . . . Laurend Doumba
IT Project Manager . . . . Eita Harshman
Small Bus. Sales Manager . . . . Steve Soyke
Director, Compliance . . . . Carolyn Shanahan
Corporate Counsel. . . . . Alexandra Kotelon

---

269 Dental Network of America

701 East 22nd Street
Suite 300
Lombard, IL 60148
Toll-Free: 800-972-7565
Phone: 630-691-1133
general_inquiry@dnoa.com
www.dnoa.com
Subsidiary of: Health Care Service Corporation
For Profit Organization: Yes
Year Founded: 1985
Federally Qualified: Yes
Number of Primary Care Physicians: 80,000
Total Enrollment: 6,200,000

Healthplan and Services Defined
PLAN TYPE: Dental
Other Type: TPA, Dental PPO
Plan Specialty: ASO, Dental, Dental, Fully Insured
Benefits Offered: Dental

Type of Coverage
Commercial, Individual, Indemnity, Group

Type of Payment Plans Offered
Capitated

Geographic Areas Served
Nationwide

Network Qualifications
Pre-Admission Certification: Yes

Peer Review Type
Utilization Review: Yes

Key Personnel
Dental Director. . . . . Timothy Custer

---

270 Health Alliance

301 S Vine Street
Urbana, IL 61801
Toll-Free: 877-686-1168
www.healthalliance.org
For Profit Organization: Yes
Year Founded: 1980
Physician Owned Organization: Yes
Federally Qualified: Yes

Healthplan and Services Defined
  PLAN TYPE: HMO/PPO
  Plan Specialty: Dental, Vision
  Benefits Offered: Dental, Disease Management, Vision,
    Wellness

Type of Coverage
  Commercial, Individual, Medicare, Medicaid

Geographic Areas Served
  Illinois and Central Iowa

Publishes and Distributes Report Card: Yes

Accreditation Certification
  NCQA

271 Health Alliance Medicare

3310 Fields South Drive
Champaign, IL 61822
Toll-Free: 887-686-1168
memberservices@healthalliance.org
www.healthalliance.org
Year Founded: 1997
Number of Primary Care Physicians: 3,000
Total Enrollment: 255,494

Healthplan and Services Defined
  PLAN TYPE: Medicare
  Other Type: HMO/PPO
  Benefits Offered: Prescription

Type of Coverage
  Medicare, Supplemental Medicare

Accreditation Certification
  NCQA

272 Health Care Service Corporation

300 E Randolph Street
Chicago, IL 60601
Toll-Free: 800-654-7385
www.hcsc.com
For Profit Organization: Yes
Year Founded: 1975
Total Enrollment: 15,000,000
State Enrollment: 15,000,000

Healthplan and Services Defined
  PLAN TYPE: HMO/PPO
  Model Type: Network
  Plan Specialty: Chiropractic, Dental, Disease Management,
    Lab, Vision, Radiology, UR
  Benefits Offered: Chiropractic, Dental, Disease Management,
    Home Care, Inpatient SNF, Physical Therapy, Podiatry,
    Prescription, Psychiatric, Transplant, Vision, Wellness,
    AD&D, Life, LTD, STD

Type of Coverage
  Commercial, Individual, Indemnity, Supplemental Medicare,
    Catastrophic

Geographic Areas Served
  Illinois, Montana, New Mexico, Oklahoma, Texas

Peer Review Type
  Second Surgical Opinion: Yes

Accreditation Certification
  NCQA

Key Personnel
  President/CEO . . . . Paula Steiner
  SVP/CIO . . . . Steve Betts
  SVP/CFO. . . . . Eric Feldstein
  SVP/CCO . . . . Thomas Lubben
  SVP/Chief HR Officer. . . . . Nazneen Razi
  SVP/Chief Legal Officer. . . . . Blair Todt

273 Humana Health Insurance of Illinois

2301 W 22nd Street
Suite 301
Oak Brook, IL 60523
Toll-Free: 800-569-2492
Phone: 630-794-5950
Fax: 630-794-0107
www.humana.com
Secondary Address: 2601 West Lake Avenue, Suite A3-5,
  Peoria, IL 61615-1677
For Profit Organization: Yes
Year Founded: 1972

Healthplan and Services Defined
  PLAN TYPE: HMO/PPO
  Model Type: Network
  Plan Specialty: Behavioral Health, Chiropractic, Dental,
    Disease Management, Lab, PBM, Vision, Worker's
    Compensation, UR
  Benefits Offered: Behavioral Health, Chiropractic,
    Complementary Medicine, Dental, Disease Management,
    Home Care, Inpatient SNF, Long-Term Care, Physical
    Therapy, Prescription, Psychiatric, Transplant, Vision,
    Wellness, Worker's Compensation, AD&D, Life, LTD, STD

Type of Coverage
  Commercial, Individual, Indemnity, Medicare, Supplemental
    Medicare, Medicaid, Catastrophic

Type of Payment Plans Offered
  POS, DFFS, Capitated, FFS

Geographic Areas Served
  Statewide

Network Qualifications
  Pre-Admission Certification: Yes

Peer Review Type
  Utilization Review: Yes
  Second Surgical Opinion: Yes
  Case Management: Yes

Publishes and Distributes Report Card: Yes

Accreditation Certification
  URAC, NCQA, CORE
  TJC Accreditation, Medicare Approved, Utilization Review,
    Pre-Admission Certification, State Licensure, Quality
    Assurance Program

Key Personnel
  Regional VP, Health Svcs. . . . . Neal C. Fischer, MD

Specialty Managed Care Partners
Behavioral Health, Disease Management, PBM, Worker's
Compensation
Enters into Contracts with Regional Business Coalitions: Yes
Midwest Business Group on Health, Mercer Coalition

274   Liberty Dental Plan of Illinois

P.O. Box 26110
Santa Ana, CA 92799-6110
Toll-Free: 877-558-6489
www.libertydentalplan.com
For Profit Organization: Yes
Total Enrollment: 2,000,000

Healthplan and Services Defined
PLAN TYPE: Dental
Other Type: Dental HMO
Plan Specialty: Dental
Benefits Offered: Dental

Type of Coverage
Commercial, Medicare, Medicaid, Unions

Geographic Areas Served
Statewide

Accreditation Certification
NCQA

Key Personnel
Network Manager........................ Daniel Flott

275   Meridian Health Plan of Illinois

333 S Wabash Avenue
Suite 2900
Chicago, IL 60604
Toll-Free: 866-606-3700
memberservices.il@mhplan.com
www.mhplan.com
Total Enrollment: 750,000
State Enrollment: 240,000

Healthplan and Services Defined
PLAN TYPE: Medicare

Type of Coverage
Medicare, Medicaid

Geographic Areas Served
Statewide

Accreditation Certification
URAC, NCQA

Key Personnel
President .... Karen Brach

276   Molina Healthcare of Illinois

1520 Kensington Road
Suite 212
Oak Brook, IL 60523
Toll-Free: 888-858-2156
www.molinahealthcare.com
Secondary Address: 1 West Old State Capital Plaza, Suite 300,
Springfield, IL 62701

Subsidiary of: Molina Healthcare, Inc.
For Profit Organization: Yes

Healthplan and Services Defined
PLAN TYPE: Medicare
Model Type: Network
Plan Specialty: Dental, PBM, Vision, Integrated
Medicare/Medicaid (Duals)
Benefits Offered: Dental, Prescription, Vision, Wellness, Life

Type of Coverage
Individual, Medicare, Supplemental Medicare, Medicaid

Geographic Areas Served
Statewide

Key Personnel
Plan President......................... Pam Sanborn
Medical Director .... E. Chris Eze, MD
Provider Network Manager .... Marietta Miner

277   OptumRx

1600 McConnor Parkway
Schaumburg, IL 60173-6801
Toll-Free: 800-788-4863
Phone: 224-231-1000
www.catamaranrx.com
Secondary Address: 2300 Main Street, Irvine, CA 92614

Healthplan and Services Defined
PLAN TYPE: Other
Other Type: PBM
Benefits Offered: Prescription

Key Personnel
CEO, OptumRx......................... John Prince

278   OSF Healthcare

800 NE Glen Oak Avenue
Peoria, IL 61603-3200
Toll-Free: 800-421-5700
www.osfhealthcare.org
Subsidiary of: Sisters of the Third Order of St Francis
Non-Profit Organization: Yes
Number of Affiliated Hospitals: 11
Number of Primary Care Physicians: 700
Number of Referral/Specialty Physicians: 50
Total Enrollment: 1,500,000

Healthplan and Services Defined
PLAN TYPE: HMO
Model Type: Network
Plan Specialty: Integrated Healthcare Network of Facilities
Benefits Offered: Disease Management, Wellness

Geographic Areas Served
Illinois and Michigan

Key Personnel
Chief Executive Officer.................. Bob Sehring
Media Relations .... Shelli Dankoff
shelli.j.dankoff@osfhealthcare.org

279 Preferred Network Access

1510 W 75th Street
Suite 250
Darien, IL 60561
Phone: 630-493-0905
www.pna-usa.net
For Profit Organization: Yes
Year Founded: 1995
Number of Affiliated Hospitals: 113
Number of Primary Care Physicians: 34,000
Number of Referral/Specialty Physicians: 250
Total Enrollment: 316,000
State Enrollment: 316,000

Healthplan and Services Defined
PLAN TYPE: PPO
Plan Specialty: Group, Health
Benefits Offered: Home Care, Physical Therapy, Wellness,
Worker's Compensation, Occupational Health

Type of Coverage
Commercial

Geographic Areas Served
Illinois, Indiana, Wisconsin

Key Personnel
President.......................... Joseph M Zerega

280 Trinity Health of Illinois

Mercy Health System
2525 S Michigan Avenue
Chicago, IL 60616
Phone: 312-567-2000
www.trinity-health.org
Secondary Address: Layola University Medical Center, 2160
S First Avenue, Maywood, IL 60153, 888-584-7888
Subsidiary of: Trinity Health
Non-Profit Organization: Yes
Year Founded: 2013
Total Enrollment: 30,000,000

Healthplan and Services Defined
PLAN TYPE: Other
Benefits Offered: Disease Management, Home Care,
Long-Term Care, Psychiatric, Hospice programs, PACE
(Program of All Inclusive Care for the Elderly)

Geographic Areas Served
Greater Chicago

Key Personnel
President.................... Carol L. Garikes Schneider
Chief Medical Officer............... Michael Davenport
Chief HR Officer.................... Diane Hargreaves
Chief Operating Officer .... Joan Ormsby

281 Trustmark Companies

400 Field Drive
Lake Forest, IL 60045
Phone: 847-615-1500
Fax: 847-615-3910
customercare@trustmarksolutions.com

www.trustmarkcompanies.com
For Profit Organization: Yes
Year Founded: 1913
Federally Qualified: Yes
Total Enrollment: 475,000

Healthplan and Services Defined
PLAN TYPE: PPO
Other Type: Self-funded
Model Type: Network
Plan Specialty: Behavioral Health, Dental, Lab
Benefits Offered: Behavioral Health, Dental, Disease
Management, Prescription, Vision, Wellness, AD&D, Life,
LTD, STD, Major Medical, Nurse Line, Health Advocacy
Service

Type of Coverage
Commercial, Indemnity

Type of Payment Plans Offered
FFS

Geographic Areas Served
Nationwide

Network Qualifications
Pre-Admission Certification: Yes

Peer Review Type
Utilization Review: Yes
Second Surgical Opinion: Yes

Accreditation Certification
TJC Accreditation, Utilization Review, State Licensure

Key Personnel
President/CEO .... Joe Pray
SVP/General Counsel .... Steve Auburn
SVP/CFO/Treasurer .... Phil Goss
SVP, Human Resources............... Kristin Zelkowitz

282 UniCare Illinois

233 S Wacker Drive
Chicago, IL 60606
Phone: 312-234-8000
www.unicare.com
Subsidiary of: Anthem, Inc.
For Profit Organization: Yes
Year Founded: 1995

Healthplan and Services Defined
PLAN TYPE: HMO/PPO
Model Type: Network
Benefits Offered: Behavioral Health, Chiropractic,
Complementary
Medicine, Dental, Disease Management, Home Care,
Inpatient SNF, Long-Term Care, Physical Therapy,
Podiatry, Prescription, Psychiatric, Transplant,
Vision, Wellness, Worker's Compensation, AD&D,
Life, LTD, STD

Type of Coverage
Commercial, Individual, Medicare, Supplemental Medicare

Type of Payment Plans Offered
POS

Geographic Areas Served
Statewide

Network Qualifications
Pre-Admission Certification: Yes

Peer Review Type
Utilization Review: Yes
Second Surgical Opinion: Yes

Accreditation Certification
URAC, NCQA
TJC Accreditation, State Licensure

Specialty Managed Care Partners
Enters into Contracts with Regional Business Coalitions: Yes

---

283   UnitedHealthcare of Illinois

Chicago, IL 60601
Toll-Free: 888-545-5205
www.uhc.com
Subsidiary of: UnitedHealth Group
For Profit Organization: Yes

Healthplan and Services Defined
PLAN TYPE: HMO/PPO
Model Type: Network
Plan Specialty: Behavioral Health, Dental, Disease
    Management, PBM, Vision
Benefits Offered: Behavioral Health, Chiropractic, Dental,
    Disease Management, Home Care, Inpatient SNF,
    Long-Term Care, Podiatry, Prescription, Psychiatric,
    Transplant, Vision, Wellness, Life, LTD, STD

Type of Coverage
Individual, Medicare, Supplemental Medicare, Medicaid,
    Catastrophic, Family, Military, Veterans, Group,

Geographic Areas Served
Statewide

Key Personnel
President	David Wichmann
Chief Operating Officer	Dan Schumacher
Chief Strategy Officer	John Cosgriff
Communications Officer	Kirsten Gorsuch
Chief Medical Officer	Sam Ho
Chief Legal Officer	Thad Johnson
Chief Information Officer	Phil McKoy
Chief Financial Officer	Jeff Putnam

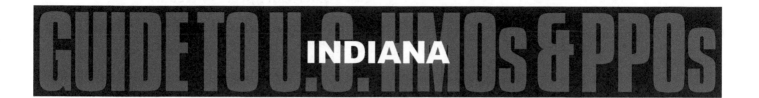
Health Insurance Coverage Status and Type of Coverage by Age

Category	All Persons		Under 18 years		Under 65 years	
	Number	%	Number	%	Number	%
Total population	6,568	-	1,670	-	5,581	-
Covered by some type of health insurance	6,032 *(18)*	91.8 *(0.3)*	1,565 *(9)*	93.7 *(0.5)*	5,050 *(18)*	90.5 *(0.3)*
Covered by private health insurance	4,644 *(31)*	70.7 *(0.5)*	1,056 *(16)*	63.2 *(1.0)*	4,014 *(30)*	71.9 *(0.5)*
Employer-based	3,876 *(33)*	59.0 *(0.5)*	961 *(17)*	57.5 *(1.0)*	3,579 *(32)*	64.1 *(0.6)*
Direct purchase	882 *(17)*	13.4 *(0.3)*	100 *(7)*	6.0 *(0.4)*	498 *(15)*	8.9 *(0.3)*
TRICARE	101 *(7)*	1.5 *(0.1)*	20 *(3)*	1.2 *(0.2)*	64 *(6)*	1.1 *(0.1)*
Covered by public health insurance	2,198 *(26)*	33.5 *(0.4)*	576 *(16)*	34.5 *(0.9)*	1,239 *(26)*	22.2 *(0.5)*
Medicaid	1,181 *(25)*	18.0 *(0.4)*	571 *(16)*	34.2 *(0.9)*	1,086 *(25)*	19.5 *(0.4)*
Medicare	1,141 *(9)*	17.4 *(0.1)*	9 *(3)*	0.5 *(0.2)*	183 *(8)*	3.3 *(0.2)*
VA Care	151 *(6)*	2.3 *(0.1)*	1 *(1)*	0.1 *(Z)*	67 *(4)*	1.2 *(0.1)*
Not covered at any time during the year	536 *(18)*	8.2 *(0.3)*	106 *(8)*	6.3 *(0.5)*	531 *(17)*	9.5 *(0.3)*

Note: Numbers in thousands; Figures cover civilian noninstitutionalized population in 2017; N/A indicates that data was not available; Z represents or rounds to zero; Margin of error appears in parenthesis and is calculated using replicate weights.
Source: U.S. Census Bureau, American Community Survey, Table HIC-4_ACS. Health Insurance Coverage Status and Type of Coverage by State—All People: 2008 to 2017, Table HIC-5_ACS. Health Insurance Coverage Status and Type of Coverage by State—Children Under 18: 2008 to 2017, Table HIC-6_ACS. Health Insurance Coverage Status and Type of Coverage by State—Persons Under 65: 2008 to 2017

Indiana

284 Aetna Health of Indiana

151 Farmington Avenue
Hartford, CT 06156
Toll-Free: 800-872-3862
Phone: 860-273-0123
www.aetna.com
Subsidiary of: Aetna Inc.
For Profit Organization: Yes
Year Founded: 1995

Healthplan and Services Defined
  PLAN TYPE: HMO/PPO
  Other Type: POS
  Model Type: Network
  Plan Specialty: Dental, Vision
  Benefits Offered: Chiropractic, Complementary Medicine,
    Dental, Home Care, Inpatient SNF, Long-Term Care,
    Podiatry, Prescription, Psychiatric, Transplant, Vision,
    Wellness

Type of Coverage
  Commercial, Student health

Geographic Areas Served
  Statewide

Key Personnel
  Network Manager . . . . Jennifer Jordan

285 American Health Network

10689 N Pennsylvania Street
Suite 200
Indianapolis, IN 46280
Toll-Free: 888-255-2246
Phone: 317-580-6309
www.ahni.com
Secondary Address: 2500 Corporate Exchange, Suite 100,
  Columbus, OH 43229, 800-880-5896
Year Founded: 1994
Number of Primary Care Physicians: 200

Healthplan and Services Defined
  PLAN TYPE: PPO
  Plan Specialty: Lab, Vision, Family medicine, general
    surgery, pain management, pediatrics
  Benefits Offered: Physical Therapy

Type of Payment Plans Offered
  Capitated

Geographic Areas Served
  Indiana and Ohio

Accreditation Certification
  TJC Accreditation, State Licensure

Key Personnel
  President. . . . . Ben Park, MD

286 American Specialty Health

12800 N Meridian Street
Carmel, IN 46032
Toll-Free: 800-848-3555
Phone: 855-328-2746
Fax: 619-237-3859
www.ashcompanies.com
For Profit Organization: Yes
Year Founded: 1987
Number of Primary Care Physicians: 60,000

Healthplan and Services Defined
  PLAN TYPE: HMO
  Model Type: Network
  Plan Specialty: Chiropractic
  Benefits Offered: Chiropractic, Complementary Medicine,
    Acupuncture

Type of Coverage
  Commercial, Supplemental Medicare

Geographic Areas Served
  Nationwide

Key Personnel
  Co-Founder/Chairman/CEO . . . . George T. DeVries, III
  President/COO. . . . . Robert White
  EVP/CFO/Treasurer . . . . William Comer
  EVP/CIO . . . . Kevin Kujawa
  EVP/Technical Officer . . . . Jerome Bonhomme
  EVP/Health Services. . . . . Douglas Metz

287 Anthem Blue Cross & Blue Shield of Indiana

4681 Masons Ridge Road
Lafayette, IN 47909
Phone: 317-315-5448
www.anthem.com
Subsidiary of: Anthem, Inc.
For Profit Organization: Yes
Year Founded: 1990
Number of Affiliated Hospitals: 105
Number of Primary Care Physicians: 3,532
Number of Referral/Specialty Physicians: 8,475
Total Enrollment: 900,000

Healthplan and Services Defined
  PLAN TYPE: HMO/PPO
  Model Type: Network
  Benefits Offered: Behavioral Health, Chiropractic,
    Complementary Medicine, Dental, Disease Management,
    Home Care, Inpatient SNF, Physical Therapy, Podiatry,
    Prescription, Psychiatric, Transplant, Vision, Wellness

Type of Coverage
  Medicare, Supplemental Medicare

Type of Payment Plans Offered
  DFFS, FFS, Combination FFS & DFFS

Geographic Areas Served
  Statewide

Subscriber Information
  Average Annual Deductible Per Subscriber:
    Employee Only (Self): Varies $250-$5000

Employee & 2 Family Members: Varies $2500-$10000
Average Subscriber Co-Payment:
  Primary Care Physician: Varies $25/20%
  Non-Network Physician: 20%
  Prescription Drugs: Varies $15/$30/$0
  Hospital ER: 20%
  Home Health Care: 20%
  Home Health Care Max. Days/Visits Covered: 100 days
  Nursing Home Max. Days/Visits Covered: 60 days

Network Qualifications
Pre-Admission Certification: Yes

Peer Review Type
Utilization Review: Yes
Second Surgical Opinion: No
Case Management: Yes

Publishes and Distributes Report Card: Yes

Accreditation Certification
URAC, NCQA
TJC Accreditation, Medicare Approved, Utilization Review,
  Pre-Admission Certification, State Licensure, Quality
  Assurance Program

Key Personnel
Director of Sales . . . . David Watt
Regional VP of Sales. . . . . Rick Rhodes

288 Anthem, Inc.
120 Monument Circle
Indianapolis, IN 46204
Toll-Free: 800-331-1476
www.antheminc.com
For Profit Organization: Yes
Year Founded: 2004

Healthplan and Services Defined
PLAN TYPE: HMO/PPO
Model Type: Network
Plan Specialty: Behavioral Health, Dental, Vision
Benefits Offered: Behavioral Health, Dental, Vision, Life,
  LTD, STD

Type of Coverage
Commercial, Individual, Medicare, Supplemental Medicare,
  Medicaid, Federal employee program

Key Personnel
President/CEO. . . . . Gail K. Boudreaux
EVP/CFO . . . . John E. Gallina
EVP/CAO. . . . . Gloria McCarthy
EVP/General Counsel . . . . Thomas C. Zielinski

289 Ascension At Home
St Vincent Home Health & Hospice
2015 Jackson Street
Anderson, IN 46016
Phone: 765-646-8179
Fax: 765-648-3805
ascensionathome.com
Subsidiary of: Ascension
Non-Profit Organization: Yes

Healthplan and Services Defined
PLAN TYPE: Other
Plan Specialty: Disease Management
Benefits Offered: Dental, Disease Management, Home Care,
  Wellness, Abulance & Transportation; Nursing Service;
  Short-and-long-term care management planning; Hospice

Geographic Areas Served
Texas, Alabama, Indiana, Kansas, Michigan, Mississipi,
  Oklahoma, Wisconsin

Key Personnel
President. . . . . Kirk Allen
Dir., Home Health Service . . . . Darcy Burthay

290 CareSource Indiana
P.O. Box 8738
Dayton, OH 45401-8738
Toll-Free: 877-806-9284
www.caresource.com
Non-Profit Organization: Yes
Total Enrollment: 1,000,000

Healthplan and Services Defined
PLAN TYPE: Medicare
Benefits Offered: Dental, Disease Management, Prescription,
  Vision, 24-hour Nurse Advice Line; Durable Medical
  Equipment

Type of Coverage
Medicare, Medicaid

Geographic Areas Served
Statewide

Key Personnel
President, INdiana Market . . . . Steve Smitherman

291 Cigna Healthcare Indiana
11595 N Meridian Street
Suite 500
Carmel, IN 46032
Phone: 317-208-3230
www.cigna.com
Secondary Address: 347 West Berry Street, Suite 200, Fort
  Wayne, IN 46802, 888-705-2933
For Profit Organization: Yes
Year Founded: 1982

Healthplan and Services Defined
PLAN TYPE: Multiple
Benefits Offered: Behavioral Health, Dental, Disease
  Management, Prescription, Vision, Wellness, AD&D, Life,
  LTD, STD

Type of Coverage
Commercial, Individual, Medicare, Supplemental Medicare,
  Medicaid

Geographic Areas Served
Statewide

292 Coventry Health Care of Indiana
46802, 2763 Smith Street
Fort Wayne, IN 46806
Phone: 260-408-4629
www.coventryhealthcare.com
Subsidiary of: Aetna Inc.
For Profit Organization: Yes

Healthplan and Services Defined
PLAN TYPE: HMO/PPO
Model Type: Network
Plan Specialty: Behavioral Health, Dental, Worker's
   Compensation
Benefits Offered: Behavioral Health, Dental, Prescription,
   Wellness, Worker's Compensation

Type of Coverage
Commercial, Medicare, Medicaid

Geographic Areas Served
Statewide

293 Deaconess Health Plans
600 Mary St Evanville
Evansville, IN 47747
Phone: 812-450-5000
www.deaconess.com
Year Founded: 1892
Physician Owned Organization: Yes
Number of Affiliated Hospitals: 6

Healthplan and Services Defined
PLAN TYPE: PPO
Model Type: Network
Plan Specialty: Behavioral Health, Chiropractic
Benefits Offered: Disease Management, Wellness

Type of Coverage
Individual

Geographic Areas Served
Illinois, Indiana, Kentucky

Peer Review Type
Utilization Review: Yes
Second Surgical Opinion: No
Case Management: Yes

Accreditation Certification
TJC Accreditation, Medicare Approved, Utilization Review,
   Pre-Admission Certification, State Licensure, Quality
   Assurance Program

Key Personnel
President . . . . James R. Porter
Chief Executive Officer . . . . Shawn McCoy
Chief Financial Officer . . . . Cheryl Wathen
Chief Operating Officer . . . . Lynn Lingafelter

Average Claim Compensation
Physician's Fees Charged: 1%
Hospital's Fees Charged: 1%

294 Encore Health Network
8520 Allison Pointe Boulevard
Suite 200
Indianapolis, IN 46250-4299
Toll-Free: 888-574-8180
Phone: 317-621-4250
Fax: 317-621-2388
encoreconnect.com
Subsidiary of: The HealthCare Group, LLC
Year Founded: 1986

Healthplan and Services Defined
PLAN TYPE: PPO
Benefits Offered: Worker's Compensation

Type of Coverage
Commercial, Individual

Geographic Areas Served
Select Indiana markets

Key Personnel
President . . . . Bruce Smiley

295 Golden Rule Insurance
7440 Woodland Drive
Indianapolis, IN 46278
Toll-Free: 800-444-8990
www.uhc.com
Subsidiary of: UnitedHealthcare

Healthplan and Services Defined
PLAN TYPE: HMO/PPO

Geographic Areas Served
Available in 40 states and the District of Columbia

Key Personnel
Chief Executive Officer . . . . Steve Nelson

296 Healthy Indiana Plan
Toll-Free: 877-438-4479
www.in.gov/fssa/hip
Year Founded: 2007

Healthplan and Services Defined
PLAN TYPE: HMO
Benefits Offered: Behavioral Health, Disease Management,
   Home Care, Inpatient SNF, Prescription, Wellness

Type of Coverage
Individual

Geographic Areas Served
Statewide

297 Humana Health Insurance of Indiana
7035 E 96th Street
Suite F
Indianapolis, IN 46250
Toll-Free: 866-355-6170
Phone: 317-558-5670
Fax: 502-508-8169
www.humana.com

Secondary Address: 7525 E Virginia Street, Suite 430, Evansville, IN 47715, 888-652-9151

For Profit Organization: Yes

Year Founded: 1986

Healthplan and Services Defined
PLAN TYPE: HMO/PPO
Model Type: IPA
Benefits Offered: Disease Management, Wellness

Type of Coverage
Commercial, Individual, Medicare, Medicaid

Geographic Areas Served
(Southern Indiana) Boone, Clark, Crawford, Delaware, Dubois, Floyd, Gibson, Hamilton, Hancock, Harrison, Hendricks, Howard, Jackson, Jefferson, Jennings, Johnson, Knox, Lake, LaPorte, Madison, Marrion, Morgan, Orange, Pike, Porter, Posey, Scott, Shelby, Spencer, Tipton, Vanderburgh, Warrick, Washington

Accreditation Certification
URAC, NCQA, CORE

Key Personnel
Sales Manager . . . . Charles Woelfert

---

298 MDwise

1200 Madison Avenue
Suite 400
Indianapolis, IN 46225
Toll-Free: 800-356-1204
Phone: 317-630-2831
www.mdwise.org
Subsidiary of: McLaren Health Care
Non-Profit Organization: Yes
Year Founded: 1994

Healthplan and Services Defined
PLAN TYPE: Multiple

Type of Coverage
Individual, Medicare, Medicaid

Geographic Areas Served
Idiana

Key Personnel
President/CEO . . . . Bruce Hayes, CPA
VP/General Counsel . . . . Patricia Hebenstreit, JD
VP, Operations. . . . . Lindsey Lux
VP, Business Information . . . . Brian Arrowood
VP, Health Services . . . . Chris Callahan, PharmD

---

299 Mid America Health

1499 Windhorst Way
Suite 100
Greenwood, IN 46143
Toll-Free: 888-309-8239
Fax: 317-972-7969
mahweb.com
For Profit Organization: Yes
Year Founded: 1986

Healthplan and Services Defined
PLAN TYPE: Multiple
Plan Specialty: Behavioral Health, Dental, Vision

Geographic Areas Served
Correctional facilities, county jails, military installations and long-term care facilities nationwide

Key Personnel
President. . . . . Patrick Murphy
   patrick@mahweb.com
VP of Operations . . . . Jose Lopez
   jlopez@mahweb.com
Marketing/Sales Director. . . . . Elizabeth McClure
   emcclure@mahweb.com

---

300 Parkview Total Health

Toll-Free: 800-666-4449
Phone: 260-266-5510
www.parkviewtotalhealth.com
Non-Profit Organization: Yes
Year Founded: 1992

Healthplan and Services Defined
PLAN TYPE: PPO
Benefits Offered: Disease Management, Wellness

Type of Coverage
Commercial

Geographic Areas Served
Indiana & Northwestern Ohio

Network Qualifications
Pre-Admission Certification: Yes

Peer Review Type
Utilization Review: Yes
Second Surgical Opinion: No
Case Management: Yes

Accreditation Certification
TJC Accreditation, Medicare Approved, Utilization Review, Pre-Admission Certification, State Licensure, Quality Assurance Program

Key Personnel
Wellness Coordinator . . . . Courntey Drummond

Employer References
Parkview Hospitals, East Allen County Schools, Guardian Industries, Chore Timer Brook, Tomkins

---

301 Physicians Health Plan of Northern Indiana

8101 W Jefferson Boulevard
Fort Wayne, IN 46804
Toll-Free: 800-982-6257
Phone: 260-432-6690
Fax: 260-432-0493
custsvc@phpni.com
www.phpni.com
Non-Profit Organization: Yes
Year Founded: 1983
Physician Owned Organization: Yes
Federally Qualified: Yes

Healthplan and Services Defined
  PLAN TYPE: HMO
  Model Type: IPA, POS
  Benefits Offered: Behavioral Health, Dental, Disease
    Management, Home Care, Physical Therapy, Podiatry,
    Prescription, Psychiatric, Transplant, Vision, Wellness,
    AD&D, Life, LTD, STD
  Offers Demand Management Patient Information Service:
    Yes

Type of Coverage
  Commercial, Individual
  Catastrophic Illness Benefit: Unlimited

Type of Payment Plans Offered
  POS, DFFS, FFS, Combination FFS & DFFS

Geographic Areas Served
  40 Northern Indiana counties

Peer Review Type
  Utilization Review: Yes
  Case Management: Yes

Publishes and Distributes Report Card: Yes

Accreditation Certification
  Utilization Review, Pre-Admission Certification, State
    Licensure, Quality Assurance Program

Key Personnel
  Chairman . . . . James C. Stevens
  Vice-Chairwoman . . . . Theresa A. Gutierrez
  Secretary. . . . . Karl R. LePan
  Treasurer . . . . Michael R. DeWald

Specialty Managed Care Partners
  Enters into Contracts with Regional Business Coalitions: Yes

---

302   Renaissance Dental
P.O. Box 1596
Indianapolis, IN 46206-4596
Toll-Free: 800-963-4596
Fax: 800-963-4597
renaissancedental.com

Healthplan and Services Defined
  PLAN TYPE: Dental
  Plan Specialty: Dental
  Benefits Offered: Dental

Type of Coverage
  Supplemental Medicare

Geographic Areas Served
  Georgia, Indiana, Kentucky, Michigan, New Mexico, New
    York, North Carolina, Ohio, and Tennessee

Key Personnel
  President & CEO. . . . . Robert P. Mulligan

---

303   Sagamore Health Network
11595 N Meridian Street
Suite 600
Carmel, IN 46032
Toll-Free: 800-364-3469
Phone: 317-573-2900
www.sagamorehn.com
Subsidiary of: Cigna
Year Founded: 1985

Healthplan and Services Defined
  PLAN TYPE: PPO
  Model Type: IPA

Geographic Areas Served
  Entire state of Indiana, Kentucky, Illinois, Michigan and Ohio

Accreditation Certification
  URAC
  TJC Accreditation, Medicare Approved, Utilization Review,
    Pre-Admission Certification, State Licensure, Quality
    Assurance Program

---

304   SIHO Insurance Services
417 Washington Street
Columbus, IN 47201
Toll-Free: 800-443-2980
Phone: 812-378-7070
memberservices@siho.org
www.siho.org
Mailing Address: P.O. Box 1787, Columbus, IN 47202-1787
Non-Profit Organization: Yes
Year Founded: 1987
Physician Owned Organization: Yes

Healthplan and Services Defined
  PLAN TYPE: HMO
  Model Type: IPA, Network, POS
  Plan Specialty: ASO, Dental, Disease Management, Vision
  Benefits Offered: Behavioral Health, Chiropractic, Dental,
    Disease Management, Home Care, Inpatient SNF,
    Long-Term Care, Physical Therapy, Prescription,
    Transplant, Vision, Wellness, AD&D, Life, STD

Type of Coverage
  Individual, Indemnity, Medicaid
  Catastrophic Illness Benefit: Unlimited

Type of Payment Plans Offered
  POS, DFFS, FFS

Geographic Areas Served
  Bloomington, Columbus, Evansville, Indianapolis and
    Seymour

Network Qualifications
  Pre-Admission Certification: Yes

Peer Review Type
  Utilization Review: Yes
  Case Management: Yes

Publishes and Distributes Report Card: Yes

Accreditation Certification

TJC Accreditation, Utilization Review, Pre-Admission
Certification, State Licensure

Key Personnel

Chief Executive Officer. . . . . Dave Barker
VP of Medical Management . . . . Hoskins Mary

Specialty Managed Care Partners

Caremark Rx
Enters into Contracts with Regional Business Coalitions: Yes

Employer References

Columbus Regional Hospital, Enkei America, Seymour
Memorial Hospital, Seymour Tubing

---

305   Trinity Health of Indiana

Saint Joseph Health System
5215 Holy Cross Parkway
Mishawaka, IN 46545
Phone: 574-335-5000
www.trinity-health.org
Subsidiary of: Trinity Health
Non-Profit Organization: Yes
Year Founded: 2013
Total Enrollment: 30,000,000

Healthplan and Services Defined
PLAN TYPE: Other

Benefits Offered: Disease Management, Home Care,
Long-Term Care, Psychiatric, Hospice programs, PACE
(Program of All Inclusive Care for the Elderly)

Geographic Areas Served

North Central Indiana

Key Personnel

Chief Executive Officer . . . . Chad W. Towner
Chief Financial Officer . . . . Kevin Higdon
Chief HR Officer . . . . Kurt Meyer
General Counsel. . . . . Jason Schultz
Chief Nursing Officer . . . . Loretta Schmidt
Chief Medical Officer . . . . Genevieve Lankowicz

---

306   UnitedHealthcare of Indiana

7440 Woodland Drive
Indianapolis, IN 46278
Toll-Free: 800-444-8990
www.uhc.com
Subsidiary of: UnitedHealth Group
For Profit Organization: Yes
Year Founded: 1986

Healthplan and Services Defined
PLAN TYPE: HMO/PPO

Model Type: Network
Plan Specialty: Behavioral Health, Dental, Disease
Management, PBM, Vision
Benefits Offered: Behavioral Health, Chiropractic, Dental,
Disease Management, Home Care, Inpatient SNF,
Long-Term Care, Podiatry, Prescription, Psychiatric,
Transplant, Vision, Wellness, Life, LTD, STD

Type of Coverage

Commercial, Individual, Medicare, Supplemental Medicare,
Medicaid, Catastrophic, Family, Military, Veterans, Group,

Type of Payment Plans Offered

POS

Geographic Areas Served

Statewide

Subscriber Information

Average Monthly Fee Per Subscriber
(Employee + Employer Contribution):
Employee Only (Self): Varies per plan
Employee & 2 Family Members: Variers per plan
Average Annual Deductible Per Subscriber:
Employee Only (Self): Varies per plan
Employee & 2 Family Members: Varies per plan
Average Subscriber Co-Payment:
Primary Care Physician: Varies per plan

Accreditation Certification

TJC

Key Personnel

CEO, IN/KY . . . . Dan Krajnovich

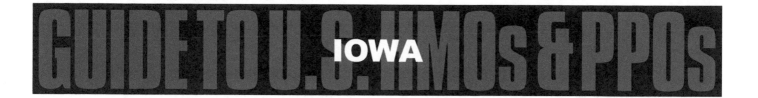
Health Insurance Coverage Status and Type of Coverage by Age

Category	All Persons		Under 18 years		Under 65 years	
	Number	%	Number	%	Number	%
Total population	3,102	-	776	-	2,602	-
Covered by some type of health insurance	2,956 *(8)*	95.3 *(0.3)*	752 *(5)*	96.9 *(0.4)*	2,458 *(8)*	94.5 *(0.3)*
Covered by private health insurance	2,351 *(17)*	75.8 *(0.5)*	538 *(9)*	69.4 *(1.2)*	2,013 *(16)*	77.4 *(0.6)*
Employer-based	1,885 *(19)*	60.8 *(0.6)*	478 *(9)*	61.6 *(1.1)*	1,764 *(19)*	67.8 *(0.7)*
Direct purchase	523 *(11)*	16.9 *(0.4)*	61 *(4)*	7.8 *(0.5)*	282 *(10)*	10.8 *(0.4)*
TRICARE	52 *(5)*	1.7 *(0.2)*	13 *(3)*	1.6 *(0.4)*	33 *(4)*	1.3 *(0.2)*
Covered by public health insurance	1,050 *(14)*	33.9 *(0.5)*	263 *(9)*	33.9 *(1.2)*	562 *(14)*	21.6 *(0.5)*
Medicaid	562 *(14)*	18.1 *(0.5)*	262 *(9)*	33.7 *(1.2)*	515 *(13)*	19.8 *(0.5)*
Medicare	552 *(5)*	17.8 *(0.2)*	2 *(1)*	0.3 *(0.1)*	64 *(4)*	2.5 *(0.2)*
VA Care	74 *(4)*	2.4 *(0.1)*	1 *(Z)*	0.1 *(0.1)*	26 *(2)*	1.0 *(0.1)*
Not covered at any time during the year	146 *(8)*	**4.7** *(0.3)*	24 *(3)*	3.1 *(0.4)*	144 *(8)*	5.5 *(0.3)*

Note: Numbers in thousands; Figures cover civilian noninstitutionalized population in 2017; N/A indicates that data was not available; Z represents or rounds to zero; Margin of error appears in parenthesis and is calculated using replicate weights.
Source: U.S. Census Bureau, American Community Survey, Table HIC-4_ACS. Health Insurance Coverage Status and Type of Coverage by State—All People: 2008 to 2017, Table HIC-5_ACS. Health Insurance Coverage Status and Type of Coverage by State—Children Under 18: 2008 to 2017, Table HIC-6_ACS. Health Insurance Coverage Status and Type of Coverage by State—Persons Under 65: 2008 to 2017

Iowa

307 Amerigroup Iowa

P.O. Box 71099
Clive, IA 50325
Toll-Free: 800-338-8366
www.myamerigroup.com/ia
Subsidiary of: Anthem, Inc.
For Profit Organization: Yes
Year Founded: 2016

Healthplan and Services Defined
PLAN TYPE: HMO
Model Type: Network
Plan Specialty: Behavioral Health, Disease Management,
  Lab, Vision, Managed health care for people in public
  programs. Mental health and substance abuse services.
Benefits Offered: Behavioral Health, Disease Management,
  Physical Therapy, Podiatry, Prescription, Vision, Wellness

Type of Coverage
Medicaid

Key Personnel
Dir., Long Term Services . . . . Kelly Espeland
Director, Operations . . . . Jill Cook
Dir., Provider Solutions. . . . . Bailey Forrest
Mgr., Provider Relations. . . . . Gloria J. Scholl

308 Coventry Health Care of Iowa

4320 114th Street
Urbandale, IA 50322-5408
Toll-Free: 800-470-6352
Phone: 515-225-1234
www.coventryhealthcare.com
Subsidiary of: Aetna Inc.
For Profit Organization: Yes

Healthplan and Services Defined
PLAN TYPE: HMO/PPO
Model Type: Network
Plan Specialty: Behavioral Health, Dental, Worker's
  Compensation
Benefits Offered: Behavioral Health, Dental, Prescription,
  Wellness, Worker's Compensation

Type of Coverage
Commercial, Individual, Medicare, Medicaid

Geographic Areas Served
Central Iowa & South Dakota

Key Personnel
Sr. Provider Relations. . . . . Paula Ironside

309 Delta Dental of Iowa

P.O. Box 9010
Johnston, IA 50131-9010
Toll-Free: 800-544-0718
IndividualProduct@deltadentalia.com
www.deltadentalia.com
Non-Profit Organization: Yes
Year Founded: 1970

Healthplan and Services Defined
PLAN TYPE: Dental
Other Type: Dental PPO
Model Type: Network
Plan Specialty: Dental
Benefits Offered: Dental

Type of Coverage
Commercial

Type of Payment Plans Offered
DFFS

Geographic Areas Served
Statewide

Publishes and Distributes Report Card: Yes

Key Personnel
President & CEO. . . . . Jeff Russell
VP, Operations . . . . Liz Myers
VP & Dental Director . . . . Jeffrey Chaffin
VP, Finance & Controller. . . . . Sherry Perkins
VP, Marketing . . . . April Schmaltz
VP, Technology . . . . Todd Herren

310 hawk-i Healthy and Well Kids in Iowa

Toll-Free: 800-257-8563
Fax: 515-457-7701
hawk-i@dhs.state.ia.us
www.hawk-i.org

Healthplan and Services Defined
PLAN TYPE: HMO
Plan Specialty: Chiropractic, Dental, Vision
Benefits Offered: Behavioral Health, Chiropractic, Dental,
  Home Care, Prescription, Vision, Wellness

Geographic Areas Served
Statewide

311 Humana Health Insurance of Iowa

1415 Kimberly Road
Bettendorf, IA 52722
Toll-Free: 866-653-7275
Phone: 563-344-1242
Fax: 563-355-0730
www.humana.com
For Profit Organization: Yes
Year Founded: 1961
Federally Qualified: Yes

Healthplan and Services Defined
PLAN TYPE: HMO/PPO
Model Type: Staff
Plan Specialty: Dental
Benefits Offered: Behavioral Health, Chiropractic, Dental,
  Disease Management, Prescription, Psychiatric, Wellness,
  Worker's Compensation, Life, LTD, STD

Type of Coverage
Commercial, Individual, Supplemental Medicare

Geographic Areas Served
Statewide

Accreditation Certification
URAC, NCQA, CORE

---

312 Medical Associates
1500 Associates Drive
Dubuque, IA 52002
Toll-Free: 800-648-6868
Phone: 563-584-3000
www.mahealthcare.com
Non-Profit Organization: Yes
Year Founded: 1982
Physician Owned Organization: Yes
Number of Primary Care Physicians: 170
Number of Referral/Specialty Physicians: 1,000
Total Enrollment: 45,000

Healthplan and Services Defined
PLAN TYPE: HMO
Model Type: Group
Plan Specialty: EPO
Benefits Offered: Behavioral Health, Chiropractic,
    Complementary Medicine, Home Care, Inpatient SNF,
    Physical Therapy, Podiatry, Prescription, Psychiatric,
    Transplant, Vision, Wellness

Type of Coverage
Commercial, Indemnity, Medicare, Supplemental Medicare

Type of Payment Plans Offered
POS

Geographic Areas Served
Iowa-Wisconsin-Illinois tri-state area

Accreditation Certification
NCQA

Key Personnel
Chief Executive Officer . . . . John Tallent
Director of Finance . . . . Jill Mitchell
Chief Operating Officer . . . . Zach Keeling

---

313 Mercy Health Network
1755 59th Place
West Des Moines, IA 50266
Phone: 515-358-8027
Fax: 515-358-8931
mhninfo@mercydesmoines.org
www.mercyhealthnetwork.com
Year Founded: 1998
Number of Affiliated Hospitals: 15

Healthplan and Services Defined
PLAN TYPE: HMO
Plan Specialty: Lab, Cardiac Care
Benefits Offered: Disease Management, Home Care, Physical
    Therapy, Prescription, Wellness

Type of Coverage
Individual

Geographic Areas Served
Clinton, Des Moines, Dubuque, North Iowa, Sioux City

Key Personnel
Chief Executive Officer . . . . Bob Ritz
SVP, Human Resources . . . . Barbara Gessel
    bgessel@mercydesmoines.org
VP of Marketing . . . . Janell Pittman
    jpittman@mercydesmoines.org
VP, General Counsel . . . . Marcia Smith

---

314 Sanford Health Plan
300 Cherapa Place
Suite 201
Sioux Falls, SD 57103
Toll-Free: 877-305-5463
Phone: 605-328-6868
memberservices@sanfordhealth.org
www.sanfordhealthplan.org
Mailing Address: P.O. Box 91110, Sioux Falls, SD 57109-1110
Non-Profit Organization: Yes
Year Founded: 1996
Number of Affiliated Hospitals: 349
Total Enrollment: 50,000

Healthplan and Services Defined
PLAN TYPE: HMO
Model Type: IPA
Plan Specialty: Commercial Group
Benefits Offered: Disease Management, Home Care,
    Long-Term Care, Prescription, Wellness

Type of Coverage
Commercial, Individual, Medicare, Supplemental Medicare,
    Sec 125, TPA, Individual, Lg Group

Geographic Areas Served
Northwest Iowa, Southwest Minnesota, South Dakota

Accreditation Certification
NCQA

---

315 Trinity Health of Iowa
Mercy Health Network
1755 59th Place
West Des Moines, IA 50266
Phone: 515-358-8027
Fax: 515-358-8931
MHNinfo@mercydesmoines.org
www.trinity-health.org/iowa
Non-Profit Organization: Yes
Year Founded: 2013
Number of Affiliated Hospitals: 40

Healthplan and Services Defined
PLAN TYPE: Other
Benefits Offered: Disease Management, Home Care,
    Long-Term Care, Physical Therapy, Psychiatric, Hospice
    programs, Senior Living

Geographic Areas Served
Iowa, Nebraska, and South Dakota

Key Personnel
CEO . . . . Bob Ritz

VP, Quality & Safety . . . . Dave Hickman
   dhickman@mercydesmoines.org
VP, Marketing/Comm. . . . . Janell Pittman
   jpittman@mercydesmoines.org
VP/General Counsel . . . . Marcia Smith
VP, Network Affiliates . . . . Mike Trachta
   mtrachta@mercydesmoines.org
SVP, Operations/CFO . . . . Mike Wegner

316   UnitedHealthcare of Iowa

1089 Jordan Creek Parkway
Suite 320
West Des Moines, IA 50266
Toll-Free: 888-545-5205
www.uhc.com
Subsidiary of: UnitedHealth Group
For Profit Organization: Yes
Year Founded: 1984

Healthplan and Services Defined
  PLAN TYPE: HMO/PPO
  Model Type: Network
  Plan Specialty: Behavioral Health, Dental, Disease
    Management, PBM, Vision
  Benefits Offered: Behavioral Health, Dental, Disease
    Management, Long-Term Care, Prescription, Vision,
    Wellness, Life, LTD, STD

Type of Coverage
  Commercial, Individual, Indemnity, Medicare, Supplemental
    Medicare, Medicaid, Catastrophic, Family, Military,
    Veterans, Group,

Type of Payment Plans Offered
  POS, DFFS, FFS

Geographic Areas Served
  Statewide

Network Qualifications
  Pre-Admission Certification: Yes

Peer Review Type
  Utilization Review: Yes
  Second Surgical Opinion: Yes
  Case Management: Yes

Publishes and Distributes Report Card: Yes

Accreditation Certification
  TJC Accreditation, Medicare Approved, Utilization Review,
    Pre-Admission Certification, State Licensure, Quality
    Assurance Program

Key Personnel
  CFO, Community Plan Iowa . . . . Alissa Weber

317   Wellmark Blue Cross Blue Shield

1331 Grand Avenue
Des Moines, IA 50309
Toll-Free: 800-524-9242
Phone: 515-376-4500
www.wellmark.com
Secondary Address: 600 3rd Avenue SE, Suite 200, Cedar
  Rapids, IA 52401, 319-294-5950

Year Founded: 1939

Healthplan and Services Defined
  PLAN TYPE: HMO
  Model Type: IPA
  Plan Specialty: ASO, Chiropractic, Disease Management,
    Lab, Vision, Radiology, UR
  Benefits Offered: Chiropractic, Disease Management, Home
    Care, Inpatient SNF, Physical Therapy, Podiatry,
    Prescription, Psychiatric, Transplant, Vision, Wellness
  Offers Demand Management Patient Information Service: Yes

Type of Coverage
  Commercial, Individual, Indemnity, Medicare, Supplemental
    Medicare, Medicaid

Type of Payment Plans Offered
  POS, Capitated

Geographic Areas Served
  Statewide except Alamakee, Winneshiek, Fayette, Des Moines
  and Dubuque counties

Network Qualifications
  Pre-Admission Certification: Yes

Peer Review Type
  Utilization Review: Yes

Publishes and Distributes Report Card: Yes

Accreditation Certification
  URAC, NCQA
  TJC Accreditation, Medicare Approved, Utilization Review,
    Pre-Admission Certification, State Licensure, Quality
    Assurance Program

Key Personnel
  Chairman & CEO . . . . John D. Forsyth
  EVP/CFO/Treasurer . . . . David Brown
  EVP/CIO . . . . Paul Eddy
  SVP/Chief Legal Officer . . . . John T. Clendenin
  EVP/COO . . . . Cory R. Harris

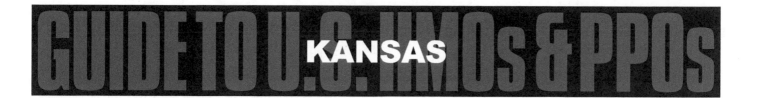
Health Insurance Coverage Status and Type of Coverage by Age

Category	All Persons		Under 18 years		Under 65 years	
	Number	%	Number	%	Number	%
Total population	2,855	-	755	-	2,427	-
Covered by some type of health insurance	2,606 *(11)*	91.3 *(0.4)*	716 *(6)*	94.8 *(0.6)*	2,179 *(11)*	89.8 *(0.4)*
Covered by private health insurance	2,129 *(16)*	74.5 *(0.6)*	505 *(9)*	66.9 *(1.2)*	1,842 *(15)*	75.9 *(0.6)*
Employer-based	1,672 *(16)*	58.6 *(0.6)*	430 *(10)*	56.9 *(1.2)*	1,569 *(16)*	64.6 *(0.7)*
Direct purchase	476 *(11)*	16.7 *(0.4)*	61 *(5)*	8.1 *(0.6)*	276 *(10)*	11.4 *(0.4)*
TRICARE	112 *(7)*	3.9 *(0.2)*	33 *(4)*	4.4 *(0.5)*	84 *(6)*	3.5 *(0.3)*
Covered by public health insurance	844 *(10)*	29.6 *(0.4)*	239 *(8)*	31.7 *(1.1)*	427 *(10)*	17.6 *(0.4)*
Medicaid	401 *(11)*	14.1 *(0.4)*	236 *(8)*	31.2 *(1.1)*	359 *(11)*	14.8 *(0.4)*
Medicare	484 *(5)*	16.9 *(0.2)*	5 *(2)*	0.7 *(0.2)*	67 *(4)*	2.8 *(0.2)*
VA Care	77 *(4)*	2.7 *(0.1)*	1 *(1)*	0.2 *(0.1)*	37 *(3)*	1.5 *(0.1)*
Not covered at any time during the year	249 *(11)*	8.7 *(0.4)*	39 *(4)*	5.2 *(0.6)*	248 *(11)*	10.2 *(0.4)*

Note: Numbers in thousands; Figures cover civilian noninstitutionalized population in 2017; N/A indicates that data was not available; Z represents or rounds to zero; Margin of error appears in parenthesis and is calculated using replicate weights.
Source: U.S. Census Bureau, American Community Survey, Table HIC-4_ACS. Health Insurance Coverage Status and Type of Coverage by State—All People: 2008 to 2017, Table HIC-5_ACS. Health Insurance Coverage Status and Type of Coverage by State—Children Under 18: 2008 to 2017, Table HIC-6_ACS. Health Insurance Coverage Status and Type of Coverage by State—Persons Under 65: 2008 to 2017

Kansas

318 Advance Insurance Company of Kansas
1133 SW Topeka Boulevard
Topeka, KS 66629
Toll-Free: 800-530-5989
Phone: 785-273-9804
Fax: 785-290-0727
claims@advanceinsurance.com
www.advanceinsurance.com
Subsidiary of: Blue Cross & Blue Shield of Kansas
For Profit Organization: Yes
Total Enrollment: 134,000

Healthplan and Services Defined
  PLAN TYPE: Multiple
  Benefits Offered: AD&D, Life, LTD, STD

Key Personnel
  President . . . . Treena Mason
  VP/COO . . . . Mike Eichten

319 Aetna Health of Kansas
151 Farmington Avenue
Hartford, CT 06156
Toll-Free: 866-851-0754
www.aetnastateofkansas.com
Subsidiary of: Aetna Inc.
For Profit Organization: Yes

Healthplan and Services Defined
  PLAN TYPE: HMO/PPO
  Other Type: POS
  Model Type: Network
  Plan Specialty: Behavioral Health, Dental, EPO, Lab, PBM,
    Vision, Radiology
  Benefits Offered: Behavioral Health, Dental, Disease
    Management, Long-Term Care, Physical Therapy,
    Podiatry, Prescription, Psychiatric, Vision, Wellness, Life,
    LTD, STD

Type of Coverage
  Commercial, Student health

Type of Payment Plans Offered
  POS, FFS

Geographic Areas Served
  Statewide

Key Personnel
  Sales Director . . . . Syd Warner

320 Aetna Health of Kansas
1999 N 63rd Drive
Kansas City, KS 66102
Toll-Free: 866-581-0754
Phone: 913-214-9536
www.aetnastateofkansas.com
Subsidiary of: Aetna Inc.
For Profit Organization: Yes

Healthplan and Services Defined
  PLAN TYPE: HMO/PPO
  Other Type: POS
  Model Type: Network
  Plan Specialty: Behavioral Health, Dental, EPO, Lab, PBM,
    Vision, Radiology
  Benefits Offered: Behavioral Health, Dental, Disease
    Management, Long-Term Care, Physical Therapy, Podiatry,
    Prescription, Psychiatric, Vision, Wellness, Life, LTD, STD

Type of Coverage
  Commercial, Medicare, Medicaid, Student health

Geographic Areas Served
  Statewide

Key Personnel
  Provider Network Manager . . . . Irene Hermreck

321 Ascension At Home
Via Christi Home Health
555 S Washington, Suite 103
Wichita, KS 67211
Phone: 316-268-8588
Fax: 316-264-1265
ascensionathome.com
Non-Profit Organization: Yes

Healthplan and Services Defined
  PLAN TYPE: Other
  Plan Specialty: Disease Management
  Benefits Offered: Dental, Disease Management, Home Care,
    Wellness, Ambulance & Transportation; Nursing Service;
    Short-and-long-term care management planning; Hospice

Geographic Areas Served
  Texas, Alabama, Indiana, Kansas, Michigan, Mississippi,
  Oklahoma, Wisconsin

Key Personnel
  President . . . . Kirk Allen
  Dir., Home Health Service . . . . Darcy Burthay

322 Blue Cross and Blue Shield of Kansas
1133 SW Topeka Boulevard
Topeka, KS 66629
Toll-Free: 800-432-3990
Phone: 785-291-4180
www.bcbsks.com
For Profit Organization: Yes
Year Founded: 1942
State Enrollment: 880,000

Healthplan and Services Defined
  PLAN TYPE: HMO
  Model Type: Staff
  Benefits Offered: Chiropractic, Disease Management,
    Inpatient SNF, Podiatry, Psychiatric, Wellness

Type of Coverage
  Commercial, Individual

Geographic Areas Served
  All counties in Kansas except Johnson and Wyandotte

Subscriber Information
Average Annual Deductible Per Subscriber:
Employee Only (Self): $1,000
Employee & 2 Family Members: $2,000
Average Subscriber Co-Payment:
Primary Care Physician: $15.00
Prescription Drugs: $5.00
Hospital ER: $50.00

Accreditation Certification
TJC, URAC

Key Personnel
President/CEO . . . . Matt All
VP, Finance . . . . Ron Simmons
VP, Operations . . . . Rusty Doty
VP, Medical Affairs . . . . Michael Atwood, MD
SVP, Provider/Gov Affairs . . . . Fredrick D. Palenske
VP, IT Services . . . . Keith Kapp
VP, Legal Services . . . . Scott Raymond
VP, Sales/Markteting . . . . Treena Mason

323 CareCentrix: Kansas
6130 Sprint Parkway
Suite 200
Overland Park, KS 66211
Toll-Free: 800-808-1902
carecentrix.com
Year Founded: 1996
Number of Primary Care Physicians: 8,000

Healthplan and Services Defined
PLAN TYPE: HMO
Benefits Offered: Home Care, Physical Therapy, Durable
Medical Equipment; Occupational & Respiratory Therapy;
Orthotics; Prosthetics

324 Coventry Health Care of Kansas
8535 East 21st Street N
Wichita, KS 67206
Toll-Free: 800-289-0345
Phone: 316-634-1222
www.coventryhealthcare.com
Secondary Address: 9401 Indian Creek Parkway, Suite 1300,
Overland Park, KS 66210, 800-969-3343
Subsidiary of: Aetna Inc.
For Profit Organization: Yes
Year Founded: 1976

Healthplan and Services Defined
PLAN TYPE: HMO/PPO
Other Type: POS
Plan Specialty: Behavioral Health, Dental, Worker's
Compensation
Benefits Offered: Behavioral Health, Dental, Prescription,
Wellness, Worker's Compensation, Alternative and
complementary care services include discounts on massage
therapy, acupuncture and chiropractic services.

Type of Coverage
Commercial, Individual, Medicare, Supplemental Medicare,
Medicaid

Catastrophic Illness Benefit: Covered

Type of Payment Plans Offered
DFFS

Geographic Areas Served
Kansas, Missouri, Oklahoma

Subscriber Information
Average Monthly Fee Per Subscriber
(Employee + Employer Contribution):
Employee Only (Self): Varies
Average Annual Deductible Per Subscriber:
Employee & 2 Family Members: None
Average Subscriber Co-Payment:
Primary Care Physician: $10.00
Prescription Drugs: $5.00/15.00
Hospital ER: $50
Home Health Care: None
Nursing Home: None

Peer Review Type
Second Surgical Opinion: Yes
Case Management: Yes

Publishes and Distributes Report Card: Yes

Accreditation Certification
URAC, NCQA
Medicare Approved, Utilization Review, Pre-Admission
Certification, State Licensure, Quality Assurance Program

Specialty Managed Care Partners
Enters into Contracts with Regional Business Coalitions: Yes

325 Delta Dental of Kansas
1619 N Waterfront Parkway
P.O. Box 789769
Wichita, KS 67278-9769
Toll-Free: 800-733-5823
Phone: 316-264-1099
Fax: 316-462-3393
moreinfo@deltadentalks.com
www.deltadentalks.com
Secondary Address: 11300 Tomahawk Creek Parkway,
Pinnacle Corporate Centre, Suite 350, Leawood, KS 66211,
913-381-4928
Non-Profit Organization: Yes
Year Founded: 1972

Healthplan and Services Defined
PLAN TYPE: Dental
Other Type: Dental PPO
Model Type: Network
Plan Specialty: Dental
Benefits Offered: Dental

Type of Coverage
Commercial, Individual

Type of Payment Plans Offered
DFFS

Geographic Areas Served
Statewide

Network Qualifications
Pre-Admission Certification: Yes

Publishes and Distributes Report Card: Yes

Key Personnel
President & CEO . . . . Michael Herbert
EVP & Managing Director . . . . Dean Newton
Chief Financial Officer. . . . . Michael Ellis
Chief Operating Officer . . . . Patrick Tuttle
In-House Counsel . . . . Jennifer Bauer
VP, Information . . . . Bob Ebenkamp
Controller . . . . Bryce Dougherty

326 Health Partners of Kansas

550 N Lorraine Street
Wichita, KS 67214
Phone: 316-652-1327
www.hpkansas.com
Subsidiary of: Wesley Medical Center
For Profit Organization: Yes
Year Founded: 1987
Number of Affiliated Hospitals: 149
Number of Primary Care Physicians: 1,000
Number of Referral/Specialty Physicians: 6,000
Total Enrollment: 95,000
State Enrollment: 95,000

Healthplan and Services Defined
 PLAN TYPE: PPO
 Model Type: IPA, Network
 Benefits Offered: Worker's Compensation, Network Rental,
  Provider Servicing, Provider Credentialing

Type of Coverage
 Catastrophic Illness Benefit: Maximum $1M

Type of Payment Plans Offered
 POS, DFFS, Capitated, FFS, Combination FFS & DFFS

Geographic Areas Served
 Statewide

Network Qualifications
 Pre-Admission Certification: Yes

Peer Review Type
 Utilization Review: Yes
 Second Surgical Opinion: Yes
 Case Management: Yes

Key Personnel
 President . . . . Gaylee Dolloff
 Vice President . . . . Teresa Montenegro

Specialty Managed Care Partners
 Enters into Contracts with Regional Business Coalitions: No

327 Humana Health Insurance of Kansas

7311 W 132nd Street
Suite 200
Overland Park, KS 66213
Toll-Free: 800-842-6188
Phone: 913-217-3300
Fax: 913-217-3245
www.humana.com
For Profit Organization: Yes
Year Founded: 1985

Healthplan and Services Defined
 PLAN TYPE: HMO/PPO
 Model Type: IPA
 Plan Specialty: Dental, Vision
 Benefits Offered: Dental, Disease Management, Prescription,
  Vision, Wellness, Life, LTD, STD

Type of Coverage
 Commercial, Individual

Geographic Areas Served
 Kansas City metro area

Subscriber Information
 Average Monthly Fee Per Subscriber
  (Employee + Employer Contribution):
   Employee Only (Self): $150.44
   Employee & 1 Family Member: $354.06
   Employee & 2 Family Members: $354.06
   Medicare: $196.48
 Average Subscriber Co-Payment:
   Primary Care Physician: $5.00
   Non-Network Physician: Not covered
   Prescription Drugs: $5.00
   Hospital ER: $25.00
   Home Health Care: $0
   Nursing Home: $0
   Nursing Home Max. Days/Visits Covered: 60 days

Accreditation Certification
 URAC, NCQA, CORE

Key Personnel
 Regional President . . . . Jeremy L. Gaskill

Average Claim Compensation
 Physician's Fees Charged: 70%
 Hospital's Fees Charged: 60%

Specialty Managed Care Partners
 Enters into Contracts with Regional Business Coalitions: Yes

328 Mercy Clinic Kansas

220 N Pennsylvania Avenue
Columbus, KS 66725
Phone: 620-429-2545
mercy.net
Subsidiary of: IBM Watson Health
Non-Profit Organization: Yes
Number of Affiliated Hospitals: 44
Number of Primary Care Physicians: 700
Number of Referral/Specialty Physicians: 2,000

Healthplan and Services Defined
PLAN TYPE: HMO
Benefits Offered: Behavioral Health, Disease Management, Home Care, Physical Therapy, Podiatry, Vision, Wellness, Non-Surgical Weight Loss; Urgent Care; Dermatology; Rehabilitation; Breast Cancer; Orthopedics; Ostoclerosis; Pediatrics

Geographic Areas Served
Arkansas, Kansas, Missouri, and Oklahoma

Key Personnel
President, Joplin/Kansas . . . . Tracy Godfrey, MD

329 PCC Preferred Chiropractic Care
555 North McLean Boulevard
Suite 301
Wichita, KS 67203
Toll-Free: 800-611-3048
Phone: 316-263-7800
Fax: 316-263-7814
providerrelations@pccnetwork.com
www.pccnetwork.com
For Profit Organization: Yes
Year Founded: 1984
Physician Owned Organization: No
Federally Qualified: No
Number of Primary Care Physicians: 3,500
Total Enrollment: 5,000,000

Healthplan and Services Defined
PLAN TYPE: PPO
Model Type: Network
Plan Specialty: Chiropractic
Benefits Offered: Chiropractic, Disease Management, Wellness, Worker's Compensation
Offers Demand Management Patient Information Service: Yes
DMPI Services Offered: Chiropractic, Physical Therapy

Type of Coverage
Medicaid

Type of Payment Plans Offered
POS, DFFS, Capitated, FFS, Combination FFS & DFFS

Geographic Areas Served
Nationwide

Network Qualifications
Pre-Admission Certification: No

Peer Review Type
Utilization Review: Yes
Second Surgical Opinion: Yes
Case Management: No

Publishes and Distributes Report Card: No

Accreditation Certification
URAC, NCQA

Key Personnel
President and CEO . . . . Brad Dopps

Average Claim Compensation
Physician's Fees Charged: 80%

Specialty Managed Care Partners
Enters into Contracts with Regional Business Coalitions: Yes

Employer References
Preferred Health Systems, fiserv, Health Partners of Kansas

330 Preferred Mental Health Management
7309 E 21st N Street
Suite 110
Wichita, KS 67206
Toll-Free: 800-819-9571
Phone: 316-262-0444
providerrelations@pmhm.com
www.pmhm.com
Subsidiary of: Family Health America
Year Founded: 1987
Number of Affiliated Hospitals: 1,900
Number of Primary Care Physicians: 10,500
Number of Referral/Specialty Physicians: 4,000
Total Enrollment: 400,000

Healthplan and Services Defined
PLAN TYPE: Multiple
Model Type: Network
Plan Specialty: Mental Health
Benefits Offered: Behavioral Health, Prescription, Psychiatric, Substance Abuse
Offers Demand Management Patient Information Service: Yes

Type of Coverage
Work

Geographic Areas Served
Nationwide including Puerto Rico

Network Qualifications
Minimum Years of Practice: 6
Pre-Admission Certification: Yes

Peer Review Type
Utilization Review: Yes

Publishes and Distributes Report Card: Yes

Accreditation Certification
URAC, NCQA
TJC Accreditation, Utilization Review, Pre-Admission Certification, State Licensure, Quality Assurance Program

Key Personnel
President/CEO . . . . Les Ruthven, PhD
316-262-0444

Specialty Managed Care Partners
Enters into Contracts with Regional Business Coalitions: No

331 Preferred Vision Care
P.O. Box 26025
Overland Park, KS 66225-6025
Phone: 913-451-1672
Fax: 913-451-1704
customerservice@preferredvisioncare.com
preferredvisioncare.com
For Profit Organization: Yes
Owned by an Integrated Delivery Network (IDN): Yes

Healthplan and Services Defined
PLAN TYPE: Vision
Other Type: PPO
Model Type: Network
Plan Specialty: Vision
Benefits Offered: Vision

Type of Coverage
Commercial
Catastrophic Illness Benefit: Unlimited

Type of Payment Plans Offered
POS, DFFS

Network Qualifications
Pre-Admission Certification: No

Peer Review Type
Utilization Review: Yes
Second Surgical Opinion: Yes
Case Management: Yes

Publishes and Distributes Report Card: Yes

Accreditation Certification
URAC
Quality Assurance Program

Key Personnel
CEO . . . . Michele G. Disser, RN

Specialty Managed Care Partners
Enters into Contracts with Regional Business Coalitions: Yes

---

332 ProviDRs Care Network
1102 S Hillside
Wichita, KS 67211
Toll-Free: 800-801-9772
Phone: 316-683-4111
customerservice@providrscare.net
www.providrscare.net
Subsidiary of: Medical Society Medical Review Foundation
For Profit Organization: Yes
Year Founded: 1985
Physician Owned Organization: Yes
Number of Affiliated Hospitals: 157
Number of Primary Care Physicians: 11,000
Number of Referral/Specialty Physicians: 700
Total Enrollment: 152,000

Healthplan and Services Defined
PLAN TYPE: PPO
Model Type: Group
Benefits Offered: Behavioral Health, Chiropractic, Home
Care, Physical Therapy, Podiatry, Psychiatric, Transplant,
Worker's Compensation

Type of Coverage
Commercial, Individual

Type of Payment Plans Offered
POS

Geographic Areas Served
Kansas, Southwest Missouri; parts of Oklahoma and
Nebraska; 1 county in Colorado

Subscriber Information
Average Monthly Fee Per Subscriber
(Employee + Employer Contribution):
Employee Only (Self): $3.00
Employee & 1 Family Member: $3.00
Employee & 2 Family Members: $3.00
Average Annual Deductible Per Subscriber:
Employee Only (Self): Varies
Employee & 1 Family Member: Varies
Average Subscriber Co-Payment:
Primary Care Physician: Varies
Non-Network Physician: Varies
Prescription Drugs: Varies
Hospital ER: Varies

Network Qualifications
Pre-Admission Certification: Yes

Peer Review Type
Utilization Review: Yes
Second Surgical Opinion: Yes
Case Management: No

Publishes and Distributes Report Card: No

Accreditation Certification
URAC
TJC Accreditation, Medicare Approved, Utilization Review,
Pre-Admission Certification, State Licensure, Quality
Assurance Program

Key Personnel
Chief Executive Officer . . . . Karen Cox
316-683-0665
karencox@providrscare.net
Dir., Network Innovations . . . . Justin Leitzen
316-683-0604
justinleitzen@providrscare.net
Claims Manager . . . . Jeanne Hingst
316-683-4111
jeannehingst@providrscare.net
Director of Claims/Info . . . . Nikki Sade
316-683-0805
nikkisade@providrscare.net

Specialty Managed Care Partners
Enters into Contracts with Regional Business Coalitions: No

Employer References
Western Resources, Kansas Health Insurance Association,
Medicalodges, County of Reno Kansas, National
Cooperative of Refineries Association

---

333 UniCare Kansas
825 Kansas Avenue
Suite 101
Topeka, KS 66608-1210
Toll-Free: 877-864-2273
www.unicare.com
Secondary Address: 327 North Hillside Road, Wichita, KS
67214
Subsidiary of: Anthem, Inc.
For Profit Organization: Yes
Year Founded: 1995

Healthplan and Services Defined
PLAN TYPE: HMO/PPO
Model Type: Network
Benefits Offered: Behavioral Health, Chiropractic,
   Complementary Medicine, Dental, Disease Management,
   Home Care, Inpatient SNF, Long-Term Care, Physical
   Therapy, Podiatry, Prescription, Psychiatric, Transplant,
   Vision, Wellness, Life, LTD, STD

Type of Coverage
Commercial, Individual, Medicare, Supplemental Medicare,
   Medicaid

Type of Payment Plans Offered
POS

Geographic Areas Served
Illinois: Cook, DuPage, Kane, Kankakee, Kendall, Lake,
   McHenry, Will counties. Indiana: Lake, Porter counties

Network Qualifications
Pre-Admission Certification: Yes

Peer Review Type
Utilization Review: Yes
Second Surgical Opinion: Yes
Case Management: Yes

Publishes and Distributes Report Card: Yes

Accreditation Certification
URAC, NCQA
TJC Accreditation, Utilization Review, Pre-Admission
   Certification, State Licensure, Quality Assurance Program

Specialty Managed Care Partners
WellPoint Pharmacy Management, WellPoint Dental
   Services, WellPoint Behavioral Health
Enters into Contracts with Regional Business Coalitions: Yes

334   UnitedHealthcare of Kansas
9900 W 109th Street
Overland Park, KS 66210
Toll-Free: 888-545-5205
www.uhc.com
Subsidiary of: UnitedHealth Group
For Profit Organization: Yes

Healthplan and Services Defined
PLAN TYPE: HMO/PPO
Model Type: Network
Plan Specialty: Behavioral Health, Dental, Disease
   Management, PBM, Vision
Benefits Offered: Behavioral Health, Dental, Disease
   Management, Long-Term Care, Prescription, Vision,
   Wellness, Life, LTD, STD

Type of Coverage
Individual, Medicare, Supplemental Medicare, Medicaid,
   Catastrophic, Family, Military, Veterans, Group,

Geographic Areas Served
Statewide

Key Personnel
CEO, IA/KS/NE . . . . Rob Broomfield

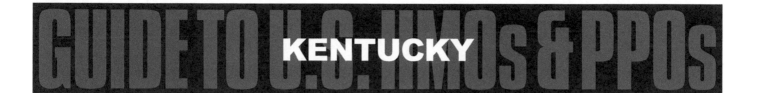

KENTUCKY

Health Insurance Coverage Status and Type of Coverage by Age

Category	All Persons		Under 18 years		Under 65 years	
	Number	%	Number	%	Number	%
Total population	4,371	-	1,079	-	3,686	-
Covered by some type of health insurance	4,136 *(13)*	94.6 *(0.3)*	1,038 *(8)*	96.2 *(0.6)*	3,452 *(13)*	93.7 *(0.3)*
Covered by private health insurance	2,821 *(29)*	64.5 *(0.7)*	608 *(14)*	56.4 *(1.3)*	2,398 *(26)*	65.1 *(0.7)*
Employer-based	2,328 *(26)*	53.3 *(0.6)*	538 *(13)*	49.9 *(1.2)*	2,098 *(23)*	56.9 *(0.6)*
Direct purchase	524 *(13)*	12.0 *(0.3)*	58 *(5)*	5.4 *(0.5)*	294 *(11)*	8.0 *(0.3)*
TRICARE	123 *(7)*	2.8 *(0.2)*	26 *(3)*	2.4 *(0.3)*	81 *(6)*	2.2 *(0.2)*
Covered by public health insurance	1,890 *(24)*	43.2 *(0.5)*	475 *(14)*	44.0 *(1.3)*	1,221 *(25)*	33.1 *(0.7)*
Medicaid	1,179 *(24)*	27.0 *(0.6)*	469 *(14)*	43.5 *(1.3)*	1,083 *(24)*	29.4 *(0.6)*
Medicare	853 *(8)*	19.5 *(0.2)*	12 *(2)*	1.1 *(0.2)*	184 *(7)*	5.0 *(0.2)*
VA Care	129 *(6)*	3.0 *(0.1)*	2 *(1)*	0.2 *(0.1)*	55 *(5)*	1.5 *(0.1)*
Not covered at any time during the year	235 *(12)*	5.4 *(0.3)*	41 *(7)*	3.8 *(0.6)*	234 *(12)*	6.3 *(0.3)*

Note: Numbers in thousands; Figures cover civilian noninstitutionalized population in 2017; N/A indicates that data was not available; Z represents or rounds to zero; Margin of error appears in parenthesis and is calculated using replicate weights.
Source: U.S. Census Bureau, American Community Survey, Table HIC-4_ACS. Health Insurance Coverage Status and Type of Coverage by State—All People: 2008 to 2017, Table HIC-5_ACS. Health Insurance Coverage Status and Type of Coverage by State—Children Under 18: 2008 to 2017, Table HIC-6_ACS. Health Insurance Coverage Status and Type of Coverage by State—Persons Under 65: 2008 to 2017

Kentucky

335 Aetna Better Health of Kentucky

9900 Corporate Campus Drive
Suite 1000
Louisville, KY 40223
Toll-Free: 855-300-5528
www.aetnabetterhealth.com/kentucky
Mailing Address: P.O. Box 65195, Phoenix, AZ 85082
Subsidiary of: Aetna, Inc.
Non-Profit Organization: Yes

Healthplan and Services Defined
PLAN TYPE: HMO/PPO
Other Type: MCO, POS
Benefits Offered: Behavioral Health, Dental, Disease
Management, Physical Therapy, Prescription, Wellness,
Worker's Compensation

Type of Coverage
Medicaid

Type of Payment Plans Offered
FFS

Geographic Areas Served
Statewide

Subscriber Information
Average Subscriber Co-Payment:
Primary Care Physician: Varies
Hospital ER: Varies
Home Health Care: Varies
Home Health Care Max. Days/Visits Covered: Varies
Nursing Home: Varies
Nursing Home Max. Days/Visits Covered: Varies

Key Personnel
CEO . . . . Jonathan Copley
VP, Health Services . . . . Rick Schultz
CMO/Sr. Medical Director . . . . Vaughn Payne
Behavioral Health Mgmt. . . . . Cathy Jones
Dir., Strategic Planning . . . . Paige Franklin Mankovich

336 Aetna Health of Kentucky

9900 Corporate Campus Drive
Suite 1000
Louisville, KY 40223
Toll-Free: 855-300-5528
www.aetnabetterhealth.com/kentucky
Mailing Address: P.O. Box 65195, Phoenix, AZ 85082
Subsidiary of: Aetna Inc.
For Profit Organization: Yes

Healthplan and Services Defined
PLAN TYPE: HMO/PPO
Other Type: POS
Model Type: Network
Plan Specialty: Behavioral Health, EPO, Lab, PBM,
Radiology
Benefits Offered: Behavioral Health, Dental, Disease
Management, Long-Term Care, Physical Therapy,
Podiatry, Prescription, Psychiatric, Vision, Wellness, Life,
LTD, STD

Type of Coverage
Commercial, Medicaid, Student health

Type of Payment Plans Offered
POS, FFS

Geographic Areas Served
Statewide

Key Personnel
VP, Health Services . . . . Rick Schultz
CMO/Sr. Medical Director . . . . Vaughn Payne, MD
Provider Network Manager . . . . Connie Edelen
Dir., Network Manager . . . . Pierre Gerald

337 Anthem Blue Cross & Blue Shield of Kentucky

1792 Alysheba Way
Suite 200
Lexington, KY 40509
Phone: 859-226-5300
www.anthem.com
Secondary Address: 13550 Triton Park Boulevard, Louisville,
KY 40223, 855-738-6671
Subsidiary of: Anthem, Inc.
For Profit Organization: Yes

Healthplan and Services Defined
PLAN TYPE: HMO/PPO
Model Type: Network
Plan Specialty: Behavioral Health, Dental, Disease
Management, Lab, PBM, Vision, Radiology
Benefits Offered: Behavioral Health, Dental, Disease
Management, Inpatient SNF, Physical Therapy,
Prescription, Psychiatric, Transplant, Vision, Wellness, Life

Type of Coverage
Commercial, Individual, Medicare, Supplemental Medicare,
Catastrophic

Geographic Areas Served
Statewide

Accreditation Certification
URAC, NCQA

Key Personnel
Regional Vice President . . . . Mike Lorch

338 Baptist Health Plan

651 Perimeter Drive
Suite 300
Lexington, KY 40517
Toll-Free: 800-787-2680
cservice@baptisthealthplan.com
www.baptisthealthplan.com
Subsidiary of: Baptist Health Care Systems
Non-Profit Organization: Yes
Year Founded: 1993
Number of Affiliated Hospitals: 40
Number of Primary Care Physicians: 764

Number of Referral/Specialty Physicians: 1,000
Total Enrollment: 136,472
State Enrollment: 65,428

Healthplan and Services Defined
PLAN TYPE: HMO/PPO
Other Type: POS
Model Type: Network
Plan Specialty: ASO, Behavioral Health, Dental, EPO, MSO, PBM, Vision
Benefits Offered: Chiropractic, Disease Management, Home Care, Inpatient SNF, Physical Therapy, Podiatry, Prescription, Transplant, Vision, Wellness, Occupational & Speech Therapy; Hospice; Durable Medical Equipment

Type of Coverage
Commercial, Medicare

Type of Payment Plans Offered
POS, Combination FFS & DFFS

Geographic Areas Served
Bullitt, Estill, Fayette, Garrard, Henry, Hopkins, Jefferson, Jessamine, Madison, Mercer, Oldham, Rockcastle, Shelby, Spencer, Trimble, Webster, Whitley, Woodford counties

Peer Review Type
Second Surgical Opinion: Yes
Case Management: Yes

Publishes and Distributes Report Card: Yes

Accreditation Certification
TJC Accreditation, Medicare Approved, Utilization Review, Pre-Admission Certification, State Licensure, Quality Assurance Program

Key Personnel
President................................ James S Fritz

339 CareSource Kentucky
10200 Forest Green Boulevard
Suite 400
Louisville, KY 40223
Phone: 502-213-4700
www.caresource.com
Non-Profit Organization: Yes
Total Enrollment: 1,000,000

Healthplan and Services Defined
PLAN TYPE: Medicare
Benefits Offered: Chiropractic, Dental, Podiatry, Prescription, Psychiatric, Vision

Type of Coverage
Medicare, Medicaid

Geographic Areas Served
Statewide

Key Personnel
Dir., Administration .... Samantha Harrison
Regulatory Contract Mgr............... Brian K. Staples
Quality Improvement Mgr................ Sanggil Tsai
Dir., Pharmacy Operations .... Joe Vennari

340 Delta Dental of Kentucky
10100 Linn Station Road
Louisville, KY 40223
Toll-Free: 800-955-2030
Fax: 877-224-0052
www.deltadentalky.com
Non-Profit Organization: Yes
Year Founded: 1966

Healthplan and Services Defined
PLAN TYPE: Dental
Other Type: Dental PPO
Model Type: IPA
Plan Specialty: Dental
Benefits Offered: Dental

Type of Coverage
Commercial, Individual

Type of Payment Plans Offered
DFFS

Geographic Areas Served
Statewide

Peer Review Type
Utilization Review: Yes
Second Surgical Opinion: Yes
Case Management: Yes

Publishes and Distributes Report Card: Yes

Key Personnel
President/CEO .... J. Jude Thompson
VP/Chief Finance Officer .... Russell Skaggs
VP/Adminstrative Officer .... Angie Zuvon Nenni
VP/General Counsel...................... John Weeks
VP/Chief Revenue Officer .... Brian Hart
VP/Information Officer..................... Ron Story

Specialty Managed Care Partners
Enters into Contracts with Regional Business Coalitions: Yes

341 Humana Inc.
1918 Hikes Lane
Suite 101
Louisville, KY 40218
Phone: 502-479-6580
www.humana.com
Secondary Address: 2530 Sir Barton Way, Suite 100, Lexington, KY 40509, 800-941-6172
For Profit Organization: Yes

Healthplan and Services Defined
PLAN TYPE: HMO/PPO
Model Type: Network
Plan Specialty: Dental, Vision
Benefits Offered: Dental, Prescription, Vision, Life, LTD, STD

Type of Coverage
Commercial, Individual, Medicare, Supplemental Medicare

Geographic Areas Served
Statewide

Accreditation Certification
URAC, NCQA

Key Personnel
President & CEO . . . . Bruce D. Broussard
Chief Financial Officer. . . . . Brian A. Kane
Chief Information Officer . . . . Brian LeClaire
Segment Pres., Health Svc. . . . . . . William Fleming, PharmD
Chief Legal Officer . . . . Christopher M. Todoroff
Chief Medical Officer . . . . Roy A. Beveridge, MD

342 Humana Medicare
Humana Correspondence Office
P.O. Box 14601
Lexington, KY 40512-4601
Toll-Free: 888-223-9950
Fax: 888-556-2128
www.humana.com/medicare
Subsidiary of: Humana
For Profit Organization: Yes

Healthplan and Services Defined
PLAN TYPE: Medicare
Benefits Offered: Chiropractic, Dental, Home Care, Inpatient SNF, Physical Therapy, Podiatry, Prescription, Psychiatric, Vision, Wellness

Type of Coverage
Individual, Medicare, Supplemental Medicare

Geographic Areas Served
Available in multiple states

Subscriber Information
Average Monthly Fee Per Subscriber
(Employee + Employer Contribution):
Employee Only (Self): Varies
Medicare: Varies
Average Annual Deductible Per Subscriber:
Employee Only (Self): Varies
Medicare: Varies
Average Subscriber Co-Payment:
Primary Care Physician: Varies
Non-Network Physician: Varies
Prescription Drugs: Varies
Hospital ER: Varies
Home Health Care: Varies
Home Health Care Max. Days/Visits Covered: Varies
Nursing Home: Varies
Nursing Home Max. Days/Visits Covered: Varies

Accreditation Certification
URAC, NCQA, CORE

Key Personnel
Segment President, Retail . . . . Alan Wheatley

343 Passport Health Plan
5100 Commerce Crossings Drive
Louisville, KY 40229
Toll-Free: 800-578-0603
Phone: 502-585-7900
www.passporthealthplan.com

Subsidiary of: AmeriHealth Mercy Health Plan
Non-Profit Organization: Yes
Year Founded: 1997
Total Enrollment: 170,000
State Enrollment: 170,000

Healthplan and Services Defined
PLAN TYPE: HMO

Geographic Areas Served
Jefferson, Oldham, Trimble, Carroll, Henry, Shelby, Spencer, Bullitt, Nelson, Washington, Marion, Larue, Hardin, Grayson, Meade, Breckinridge counties

Accreditation Certification
NCQA

Key Personnel
Chief Executive Officer. . . . . Mark B. Carter
Chief Financial Officer . . . . David A. Stanley
VP/Chief Medical Officer . . . . . . Stephen J. Houghland, MD
VP/Chief Communications . . . . Jill Joseph Bell
VP, Human Resources . . . . Gary Bensing
Chief Operations Officer . . . . Carl Felix

344 Rural Carrier Benefit Plan
P.O. Box 7404
London, KY 40742
Toll-Free: 800-638-8432
www.rcbphealth.com
Subsidiary of: Aetna

Healthplan and Services Defined
PLAN TYPE: PPO
Benefits Offered: Disease Management, Prescription, Vision, Wellness, Cancer Treatment; Kidney Dialysis; 24-hour Nurse Line; Travel Assistance Program; Healthy Maternity; Quest Lab Program

Type of Coverage
Commercial, Individual

Type of Payment Plans Offered
Capitated, FFS

Subscriber Information
Average Monthly Fee Per Subscriber
(Employee + Employer Contribution):
Employee Only (Self): $73.11
Employee & 2 Family Members: $119.87
Average Annual Deductible Per Subscriber:
Employee & 2 Family Members: $350.00
Average Subscriber Co-Payment:
Primary Care Physician: 10%
Prescription Drugs: $20 - $30
Hospital ER: $0

Key Personnel
Chief Executive Officer. . . . . Mark T. Bertolini
President. . . . . Karen S. Lynch
Chief Financial Officer . . . . Shawn M. Guertin
Operations & Technology . . . . Meg McCarthy
Chief Medical Officer . . . . Harold L. Paz
EVP, General Counsel . . . . Thomas J. Sabatino Jr.
Government Services . . . . Fran S. Soistman

345   UnitedHealthcare of Kentucky

3847 Cane Run Road
Louisville, KY 40211
Toll-Free: 888-835-9637
www.uhc.com
Subsidiary of: UnitedHealth Group
For Profit Organization: Yes
Year Founded: 1986

Healthplan and Services Defined
  PLAN TYPE: HMO/PPO
  Model Type: Network
  Plan Specialty: Behavioral Health, Dental, Disease
    Management, PBM, Vision
  Benefits Offered: Behavioral Health, Chiropractic, Dental,
    Disease Management, Long-Term Care, Prescription,
    Vision, Wellness, Life, LTD, STD

Type of Coverage
  Individual, Medicare, Supplemental Medicare, Medicaid,
    Catastrophic, Family, Military, Veterans, Group,
  Catastrophic Illness Benefit: Maximum $1M

Type of Payment Plans Offered
  POS

Geographic Areas Served
  Central Kentucky: 99 counties

Subscriber Information
  Average Monthly Fee Per Subscriber
    (Employee + Employer Contribution):
      Employee Only (Self): $139.00
      Employee & 1 Family Member: $282.00
      Employee & 2 Family Members: $445.00
      Medicare: $0
  Average Annual Deductible Per Subscriber:
      Employee Only (Self): $0
      Employee & 1 Family Member: $0
      Employee & 2 Family Members: $0
  Average Subscriber Co-Payment:
      Primary Care Physician: $10.00
      Non-Network Physician: Not covered
      Prescription Drugs: $7.00
      Hospital ER: $50.00
      Home Health Care: 20%
      Nursing Home: Not covered

Network Qualifications
  Pre-Admission Certification: Yes

Peer Review Type
  Utilization Review: Yes
  Second Surgical Opinion: No
  Case Management: Yes

Publishes and Distributes Report Card: Yes

Accreditation Certification
  TJC Accreditation, Utilization Review, Pre-Admission
    Certification, State Licensure, Quality Assurance Program

Key Personnel
  CEO, OH/KY . . . . Kurt Lewis

Average Claim Compensation
  Physician's Fees Charged: 1%

Hospital's Fees Charged: 1%

Specialty Managed Care Partners
  Enters into Contracts with Regional Business Coalitions: Yes

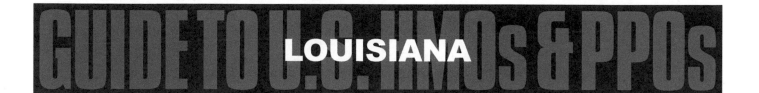
Health Insurance Coverage Status and Type of Coverage by Age

Category	All Persons		Under 18 years		Under 65 years	
	Number	%	Number	%	Number	%
Total population	4,580	-	1,175	-	3,905	-
Covered by some type of health insurance	4,198 *(13)*	91.6 *(0.3)*	1,139 *(7)*	96.9 *(0.4)*	3,526 *(13)*	90.3 *(0.3)*
Covered by private health insurance	2,760 *(30)*	60.3 *(0.7)*	578 *(15)*	49.2 *(1.2)*	2,392 *(28)*	61.3 *(0.7)*
Employer-based	2,247 *(27)*	49.1 *(0.6)*	501 *(14)*	42.7 *(1.2)*	2,037 *(26)*	52.2 *(0.7)*
Direct purchase	550 *(17)*	12.0 *(0.4)*	68 *(7)*	5.8 *(0.6)*	370 *(15)*	9.5 *(0.4)*
TRICARE	125 *(8)*	2.7 *(0.2)*	25 *(3)*	2.1 *(0.3)*	83 *(7)*	2.1 *(0.2)*
Covered by public health insurance	1,952 *(25)*	42.6 *(0.5)*	613 *(14)*	52.2 *(1.2)*	1,306 *(24)*	33.4 *(0.6)*
Medicaid	1,307 *(23)*	28.5 *(0.5)*	610 *(14)*	51.9 *(1.2)*	1,195 *(22)*	30.6 *(0.6)*
Medicare	796 *(8)*	17.4 *(0.2)*	7 *(1)*	0.6 *(0.1)*	150 *(7)*	3.8 *(0.2)*
VA Care	102 *(7)*	2.2 *(0.2)*	1 *(1)*	0.1 *(0.1)*	51 *(5)*	1.3 *(0.1)*
Not covered at any time during the year	383 *(13)*	8.4 *(0.3)*	36 *(5)*	3.1 *(0.4)*	379 *(13)*	9.7 *(0.3)*

Note: Numbers in thousands; Figures cover civilian noninstitutionalized population in 2017; N/A indicates that data was not available; Z represents or rounds to zero; Margin of error appears in parenthesis and is calculated using replicate weights.
Source: U.S. Census Bureau, American Community Survey, Table HIC-4_ACS. Health Insurance Coverage Status and Type of Coverage by State—All People: 2008 to 2017, Table HIC-5_ACS. Health Insurance Coverage Status and Type of Coverage by State—Children Under 18: 2008 to 2017, Table HIC-6_ACS. Health Insurance Coverage Status and Type of Coverage by State—Persons Under 65: 2008 to 2017

Louisiana

346   Aetna Health of Louisiana

2400 Veterans Memorial Boulevard
Suite 200
Kenner, LA 70062
Toll-Free: 855-242-0802
www.aetnabetterhealth.com/louisiana
Subsidiary of: Aetna Inc.
For Profit Organization: Yes

Healthplan and Services Defined
  PLAN TYPE: PPO
  Other Type: POS
  Model Type: Network
  Plan Specialty: Behavioral Health, Dental, EPO, Lab, PBM,
    Vision, Radiology
  Benefits Offered: Behavioral Health, Dental, Disease
    Management, Long-Term Care, Physical Therapy,
    Podiatry, Prescription, Psychiatric, Vision, Wellness, Life,
    LTD, STD

Type of Coverage
  Commercial, Medicaid, Student health

Type of Payment Plans Offered
  POS, FFS

Geographic Areas Served
  Statewide with some exceptions

Key Personnel
  CEO . . . . Rick Born
  COO . . . . Mark Grippi
  Dir., Quality Management . . . . Shelley Krawchuk
  Dir., Provider Experience . . . . Tabitha Marchand

347   Blue Cross and Blue Shield of Louisiana

5525 Reitz Avenue
Baton Rouge, LA 70809
Toll-Free: 800-495-2583
Phone: 225-295-2527
www.bcbsla.com
Secondary Address: 4508 Coliseum Boulevard, Suite A,
    Alexandria, LA 71303, 318-442-8107
For Profit Organization: Yes
Year Founded: 1934
Number of Affiliated Hospitals: 39
Number of Primary Care Physicians: 962
Number of Referral/Specialty Physicians: 2,219
Total Enrollment: 1,300,000
State Enrollment: 1,300,000

Healthplan and Services Defined
  PLAN TYPE: HMO/PPO
  Model Type: Network
  Benefits Offered: Behavioral Health, Disease Management,
    Prescription, Wellness

Type of Coverage
  Commercial, Individual, Medicare, Supplemental Medicare
  Catastrophic Illness Benefit: Maximum $2M

Type of Payment Plans Offered
  POS

Subscriber Information
  Average Subscriber Co-Payment:
      Primary Care Physician: 10%/20%
      Home Health Care: Varies

Network Qualifications
  Pre-Admission Certification: Yes

Peer Review Type
  Utilization Review: Yes

Publishes and Distributes Report Card: No

Accreditation Certification
  URAC, NCQA
  TJC Accreditation, Medicare Approved, Utilization Review,
    Pre-Admission Certification, State Licensure, Quality
    Assurance Program

Key Personnel
  President/CEO . . . . I. Steven Udvarhelyi
  Chair. . . . . J. Kevin McCotter
  Vice Chair . . . . Michael B. Bruno
  Chief HR Officer . . . . John E. Brown, Jr.
  Chief Information Officer . . . . Sue Kozik
  Chief Financial Officer. . . . . Bryan Camerlinck

Specialty Managed Care Partners
  Enters into Contracts with Regional Business Coalitions: Yes

348   Coventry Health Care of Louisiana

Shreveport, LA 71101
Toll-Free: 800-654-5988
Phone: 318-549-9823
www.coventryhealthcare.com
Subsidiary of: Aetna Inc.
For Profit Organization: Yes

Healthplan and Services Defined
  PLAN TYPE: HMO
  Benefits Offered: Behavioral Health, Dental, Disease
    Management, Physical Therapy, Prescription, Wellness

Geographic Areas Served
  New Orleans metropolitan area, Baton Rouge, Metairie,
  Shreveport, Slidell, Bayou Region

Accreditation Certification
  URAC

Key Personnel
  VP, Provider Network Dev. . . . . Thomas Groves
  Clinical Reviewer . . . . Julie M. Lockett
  Mgr., Quality Improvement . . . . Deborah Junot
  Account Manager. . . . . Janet McNulty

349 DINA Dental Plan

11969 Bricksome Avenue
Suite A
Baton Rouge, LA 70816
Toll-Free: 800-376-3462
Phone: 225-291-3172
Fax: 225-292-3075
info@dinadental.com
www.dinadental.com
For Profit Organization: Yes
Year Founded: 1978

Healthplan and Services Defined
PLAN TYPE: Dental
Model Type: Group
Plan Specialty: Dental
Benefits Offered: Dental

Type of Coverage
Commercial, Individual

Geographic Areas Served
Statewide

Peer Review Type
Second Surgical Opinion: Yes

Publishes and Distributes Report Card: No

Specialty Managed Care Partners
Enters into Contracts with Regional Business Coalitions: No

350 Humana Health Insurance of Louisiana

10330 Airline Highway
Baton Rouge, LA 70816
Phone: 225-442-6100
www.humana.com
Secondary Address: 1655 E Bert Kouns Industrial Loop, Suite 200, Shreveport, LA 71105, 318-383-5969
Subsidiary of: Humana
For Profit Organization: Yes
Year Founded: 1985
Physician Owned Organization: Yes
Federally Qualified: Yes

Healthplan and Services Defined
PLAN TYPE: HMO/PPO
Model Type: Network
Plan Specialty: Dental, Vision
Benefits Offered: Behavioral Health, Chiropractic, Dental, Disease Management, Home Care, Inpatient SNF, Physical Therapy, Podiatry, Prescription, Psychiatric, Transplant, Vision, Wellness, Life, LTD, STD

Type of Coverage
Commercial, Individual, Indemnity, Medicare
Catastrophic Illness Benefit: Unlimited

Type of Payment Plans Offered
POS, Combination FFS & DFFS

Geographic Areas Served
Statewide, excluding Monroe

Subscriber Information
Average Monthly Fee Per Subscriber
(Employee + Employer Contribution):
Employee Only (Self): $189.31
Employee & 1 Family Member: $378.62
Employee & 2 Family Members: $530.07
Average Subscriber Co-Payment:
Primary Care Physician: $15.00
Prescription Drugs: $10/$25/$40
Home Health Care Max. Days/Visits Covered: 60 days

Network Qualifications
Pre-Admission Certification: Yes

Peer Review Type
Utilization Review: Yes
Second Surgical Opinion: Yes
Case Management: Yes

Publishes and Distributes Report Card: Yes

Accreditation Certification
URAC, NCQA, CORE
Medicare Approved, Utilization Review, Pre-Admission Certification, State Licensure, Quality Assurance Program

Key Personnel
Market Vice President . . . . Rhonda Bagby

Specialty Managed Care Partners
CMS Healthcare, Medimpact
Enters into Contracts with Regional Business Coalitions: Yes
Chamber of Commerce

Employer References
State of Louisiana, Exxon-Mobil, Shell, Chevron, Sears

351 Molina Medicaid Solutions

8495 United Plaza Boulevard
Suite 110, 280
Baton Rouge, LA 70809
Phone: 225-216-6000
www.molinahealthcare.com
Subsidiary of: Molina Healthcare, Inc.
For Profit Organization: Yes

Healthplan and Services Defined
PLAN TYPE: Medicare

Type of Coverage
Medicaid information management sys

Geographic Areas Served
Statewide

352 Peoples Health

3838 N Causeway Boulevard
Suite 2200
Metairie, LA 70002
Toll-Free: 800-222-8600
Phone: 504-849-4685
www.peopleshealth.com
Secondary Address: 7434 Perkins Road, Suite 200, Baton Rouge, LA 70808, 225-346-5704
For Profit Organization: Yes

Year Founded: 1994
Total Enrollment: 50,000
State Enrollment: 4,707

Healthplan and Services Defined
PLAN TYPE: HMO
Plan Specialty: Lab, Radiology
Benefits Offered: Dental, Disease Management, Home Care, Prescription, Wellness

Type of Coverage
Commercial, Medicare

Geographic Areas Served
Statewide

Accreditation Certification
NCQA

Key Personnel
Chief Executive Officer .... Warren Murrell
VP, Finance/Controller .... Emmet Geary
Chief Financial Officer .... Kim Eller
Chief Information Officer.................. Colin Hulin
Marketing/Communications .... Nick Karl
VP, Health Services.................. Barbara Guerard
Chief Medical Officer .... Frank N. Deus
SVP, Network Development .... Janice Ortego

---

353   Starmount

8485 Goodwood Boulevard
Baton Rouge, LA 70806
Toll-Free: 888-400-9304
starmountlife.com
Mailing Address: P.O. Box 98100, Baton Rouge, LA 70898-9100

Healthplan and Services Defined
PLAN TYPE: Dental
Benefits Offered: Dental, Prescription, Vision, Life, Hearing aids

Geographic Areas Served
Available in 41 states

Key Personnel
Chief Executive Officer .... Erich Sternberg
President .... Deborah Sternberg

---

354   UnitedHealthcare of Louisiana

3838 N Causeway Boulevard
Suite 2600
Metairie, LA 70002
Toll-Free: 800-826-1981
www.uhc.com
Subsidiary of: UnitedHealth Group
For Profit Organization: Yes
Year Founded: 1986

Healthplan and Services Defined
PLAN TYPE: HMO/PPO
Model Type: Network
Plan Specialty: Behavioral Health, Dental, Disease Management, PBM, Vision

Benefits Offered: Behavioral Health, Dental, Disease Management, Long-Term Care, Prescription, Vision, Wellness, Life, LTD, STD

Type of Coverage
Individual, Medicare, Supplemental Medicare, Medicaid, Catastrophic, Family, Military, Veterans, Group,

Geographic Areas Served
Ascension, Assumption, East Baton Rouge, East Feliciana, Iberville, Jefferson, LaFourche, Livingston, Orleans, Plaquemines, Point Coupee, St. Bernard, St. Charles, St. Helena, St. James, St. Tammany, Tangipahoa, Terrabona, West Baton Rouge, West Feliciana

Subscriber Information
Average Monthly Fee Per Subscriber
(Employee + Employer Contribution):
Employee Only (Self): $129.45
Employee & 1 Family Member: $261.04
Employee & 2 Family Members: $422.40
Average Annual Deductible Per Subscriber:
Employee Only (Self): $5.00
Average Subscriber Co-Payment:
Primary Care Physician: $10.00
Prescription Drugs: $10.00
Hospital ER: $50.00

Network Qualifications
Pre-Admission Certification: Yes

Peer Review Type
Utilization Review: Yes

Publishes and Distributes Report Card: No

Accreditation Certification
TJC Accreditation, Medicare Approved, Utilization Review, Pre-Admission Certification, State Licensure, Quality Assurance Program

Key Personnel
President/CEO, Louisiana .... Allison Young

Specialty Managed Care Partners
Enters into Contracts with Regional Business Coalitions: No

---

355   Vantage Health Plan

130 DeSiard Street
Suite 300
Monroe, LA 71201
Toll-Free: 888-823-1910
Phone: 318-361-0900
www.vantagehealthplan.com
For Profit Organization: Yes
Year Founded: 1994
Number of Referral/Specialty Physicians: 7,000
Total Enrollment: 50,000
State Enrollment: 50,000

Healthplan and Services Defined
PLAN TYPE: HMO
Plan Specialty: Lab, Radiology
Benefits Offered: Behavioral Health, Chiropractic, Disease Management, Home Care, Inpatient SNF, Physical Therapy, Prescription, Wellness, Durable Medical Equipment

Type of Coverage
Medicare, Supplemental Medicare

Geographic Areas Served
Statewide

Network Qualifications
Pre-Admission Certification: Yes

Key Personnel
Executive Vice President. . . . . Mike Breard
Chief Financial Officer . . . . Rhonda Haygood
Chief Information Officer . . . . Landon Wright

Specialty Managed Care Partners
Caremark Rx

---

356 Vantage Medicare Advantage
122 St. John Street
Monroe, LA 71201
Toll-Free: 888-823-1910
Phone: 318-361-0900
www.vantagehealthplan.com
Secondary Address: 130 DeSiard Street, Suite 300, Monroe,
LA 71201, 318-361-0900
Year Founded: 1994
Total Enrollment: 14,000

Healthplan and Services Defined
PLAN TYPE: Medicare
Other Type: Medicare PPO
Plan Specialty: Dental, Vision
Benefits Offered: Home Care, Inpatient SNF, Prescription,
Vision

Type of Coverage
Medicare, Supplemental Medicare

Geographic Areas Served
Bossier, Caddo, Caldwell, Jackson, Lincoln, Morehouse,
Rapides, Ouachita, richland, and Union Parishes

Key Personnel
Executive Vice President. . . . . Mike Breard
Chief Financial Officer . . . . Rhonda Haygood
Chief Information Officer . . . . Landon Wright

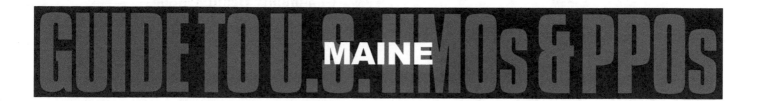

Health Insurance Coverage Status and Type of Coverage by Age

Category	All Persons		Under 18 years		Under 65 years	
	Number	%	Number	%	Number	%
Total population	1,322	-	272	-	1,062	-
Covered by some type of health insurance	1,215 (6)	91.9 (0.5)	258 (3)	95.1 (0.7)	955 (6)	90.0 (0.6)
Covered by private health insurance	932 (12)	70.5 (0.9)	183 (5)	67.3 (1.8)	772 (11)	72.7 (1.1)
Employer-based	729 (12)	55.2 (0.9)	160 (5)	58.9 (1.8)	653 (12)	61.5 (1.1)
Direct purchase	211 (8)	15.9 (0.6)	21 (3)	7.7 (1.0)	121 (6)	11.4 (0.6)
TRICARE	44 (4)	3.3 (0.3)	8 (2)	2.9 (0.7)	26 (4)	2.5 (0.3)
Covered by public health insurance	478 (9)	36.2 (0.7)	86 (5)	31.6 (1.8)	227 (9)	21.3 (0.8)
Medicaid	235 (9)	17.8 (0.7)	84 (5)	30.9 (1.8)	194 (9)	18.3 (0.8)
Medicare	300 (4)	22.7 (0.3)	2 (1)	0.9 (0.5)	49 (3)	4.6 (0.3)
VA Care	47 (3)	3.6 (0.2)	1 (Z)	0.2 (0.1)	19 (2)	1.8 (0.2)
Not covered at any time during the year	107 (6)	8.1 (0.5)	13 (2)	4.9 (0.7)	107 (6)	10.0 (0.6)

Note: Numbers in thousands; Figures cover civilian noninstitutionalized population in 2017; N/A indicates that data was not available; Z represents or rounds to zero; Margin of error appears in parenthesis and is calculated using replicate weights.
Source: U.S. Census Bureau, American Community Survey, Table HIC-4_ACS. Health Insurance Coverage Status and Type of Coverage by State—All People: 2008 to 2017, Table HIC-5_ACS. Health Insurance Coverage Status and Type of Coverage by State—Children Under 18: 2008 to 2017, Table HIC-6_ACS. Health Insurance Coverage Status and Type of Coverage by State—Persons Under 65: 2008 to 2017

Maine

357 Aetna Health of Maine
151 Farmington Avenue
Hartford, CT 06156
Toll-Free: 800-872-3862
Phone: 860-273-0123
www.aetna.com
Subsidiary of: Aetna Inc.
For Profit Organization: Yes

Healthplan and Services Defined
PLAN TYPE: HMO/PPO
Other Type: POS
Model Type: Network
Plan Specialty: Behavioral Health, Dental, EPO, Lab, PBM,
Vision, Radiology
Benefits Offered: Behavioral Health, Dental, Disease
Management, Long-Term Care, Physical Therapy,
Podiatry, Prescription, Psychiatric, Vision, Wellness, Life,
LTD, STD

Type of Coverage
Commercial, Medicare, Medicaid, Student health

Geographic Areas Served
Statewide

Key Personnel
Sr. Dir., Strategic Mkt. . . . . Christine Haslam
Director, Operations . . . . Matthew H. Orlando

358 Anthem Blue Cross & Blue Shield of Maine
2 Gannett Drive
South Portland, ME 04106
Phone: 207-822-7000
Fax: 207-822-7366
www.anthem.com
Subsidiary of: Anthem, Inc.
For Profit Organization: Yes

Healthplan and Services Defined
PLAN TYPE: HMO/PPO
Model Type: Network
Plan Specialty: Behavioral Health, Dental, Disease
Management, Lab, PBM, Vision, Radiology
Benefits Offered: Behavioral Health, Dental, Disease
Management, Inpatient SNF, Physical Therapy,
Prescription, Psychiatric, Transplant, Vision, Wellness, Life

Type of Coverage
Commercial, Individual, Medicare, Supplemental Medicare,
Catastrophic

Geographic Areas Served
Statewide

Accreditation Certification
URAC, NCQA

Key Personnel
VP, Sales . . . . William Whitmore

359 Community Health Options
150 Mill Street
Lewiston, ME 04240
Toll-Free: 855-624-6463
healthoptions.org
Secondary Address: Mail Stop 200, P.O. Box 1121, Lewiston,
ME 04243
Non-Profit Organization: Yes

Healthplan and Services Defined
PLAN TYPE: HMO/PPO

Geographic Areas Served
Maine and New Hampshire

Key Personnel
President & CEO. . . . . Kevin Lewis
SVP, Operations Officer . . . . Robert Hillman
SVP, Financial Officer . . . . Ed Vozzo
SVP, Medical Officer. . . . . John Yindra, MD
SVP, Information Officer . . . . Will Kilbreth
SVP, Human Resources . . . . Joyce McPhetres

360 Coventry Health Care of Maine
6720-B Rockledge Drive
Suite 800
Bethesda, MD 20817
Phone: 301-581-0600
www.coventryhealthcare.com
Subsidiary of: Aetna Inc.
For Profit Organization: Yes

Healthplan and Services Defined
PLAN TYPE: HMO/PPO
Model Type: Network
Plan Specialty: Behavioral Health, Dental, Worker's
Compensation
Benefits Offered: Behavioral Health, Dental, Prescription,
Wellness, Worker's Compensation

Type of Coverage
Commercial, Medicare, Medicaid

Geographic Areas Served
Statewide

Key Personnel
Chef . . . . Jorge Descart

361 Harvard Pilgrim Health Care Maine
1 Market Street
3rd Floor
Portland, ME 04101
Toll-Free: 888-888-4742
www.harvardpilgrim.org
Non-Profit Organization: Yes
Year Founded: 1977
Number of Affiliated Hospitals: 179
Number of Referral/Specialty Physicians: 53,000

Healthplan and Services Defined
PLAN TYPE: Multiple
Model Type: Network

Plan Specialty: ASO, Behavioral Health, Chiropractic, Dental, Disease Management, EPO, Lab, MSO, PBM, Vision, Radiology, Worker's Compensation, UR

Benefits Offered: Behavioral Health, Chiropractic, Disease Management, Home Care, Inpatient SNF, Long-Term Care, Physical Therapy, Podiatry, Prescription, Psychiatric, Transplant, Vision, Wellness

Type of Coverage
Commercial, Individual, Indemnity, Medicare, Supplemental Medicare, Medicaid

Geographic Areas Served
Statewide

Peer Review Type
Utilization Review: Yes
Second Surgical Opinion: Yes
Case Management: Yes

Publishes and Distributes Report Card: Yes

Accreditation Certification
NCQA
TJC Accreditation, Medicare Approved, Utilization Review, Pre-Admission Certification, State Licensure, Quality Assurance Program

Key Personnel
Vice President. . . . . Edward J. Kane
Client Manager. . . . . Steve Conley

Average Claim Compensation
Physician's Fees Charged: 51%
Hospital's Fees Charged: 40%

Specialty Managed Care Partners
Enters into Contracts with Regional Business Coalitions: No

---

362   Martin's Point HealthCare
331 Veranda Street
Portland, ME 04103
Toll-Free: 800-322-0280
Phone: 207-828-2402
www.martinspoint.org
Non-Profit Organization: Yes
Year Founded: 1981
Total Enrollment: 70,000

Healthplan and Services Defined
PLAN TYPE: Multiple
Benefits Offered: Disease Management, Prescription, Wellness, No co-pay for: routine physical exams/hearing tests/eye exams/mammograms/prostrate & pap exams/bone mass/flu vaccines.

Type of Coverage
Commercial, Medicare, Military

Geographic Areas Served
Maine, New Hampshire, Vermont, Northeastern New York

Subscriber Information
Average Monthly Fee Per Subscriber
(Employee + Employer Contribution):
Employee Only (Self): Varies
Medicare: Varies

Average Annual Deductible Per Subscriber:
Employee Only (Self): Varies
Medicare: Varies
Average Subscriber Co-Payment:
Primary Care Physician: Varies
Prescription Drugs: Varies
Hospital ER: Varies

Key Personnel
President/CEO. . . . . David Howes, MD
Chief Financial Officer. . . . . Dan Chojnowski
COO/Delivery System . . . . Sandra Monfiletto
Chief Human Resources . . . . Teresa Nizza
Chief Medical Officer. . . . . Jonathan Harvey, MD

---

363   Molina Medicaid Solutions
45 Commerce Drive
Augusta, ME 04330
Toll-Free: 888-562-5442
www.molinahealthcare.com
Subsidiary of: Molina Healthcare, Inc.
For Profit Organization: Yes

Healthplan and Services Defined
PLAN TYPE: Medicare

Type of Coverage
Medicaid information management sys

Geographic Areas Served
Statewide

Key Personnel
Claims Manager . . . . Wendy Eames
Director . . . . Doug Smith

---

364   Northeast Delta Dental Maine
1022 Portland Road
Suite 2
Saco, ME 04072-9674
Phone: 207-282-0404
Fax: 207-282-0505
nedelta@nedelta.com
www.nedelta.com
Non-Profit Organization: Yes
Year Founded: 1961

Healthplan and Services Defined
PLAN TYPE: Dental
Other Type: Dental PPO
Plan Specialty: ASO, Dental
Benefits Offered: Dental

Type of Coverage
Commercial, Individual

Geographic Areas Served
Maine, New Hampshire and Vermont

Key Personnel
President/CEO. . . . . Thomas Raffio
Chair . . . . Don Oakes
Vice Chair . . . . Kyra Chadbourne, DDS
Treasurer. . . . . Michael A. Bevilacqua
Clerk . . . . Benjamin E. Marcus, Esq.

Senior Vice President . . . . Francis Boucher

---

365   UnitedHealthcare of Maine
475 Kilvert Street
Warwick, RI 02886
Toll-Free: 888-545-5205
Phone: 401-737-6900
www.uhc.com
Subsidiary of: UnitedHealth Group
Year Founded: 1977

Healthplan and Services Defined
  PLAN TYPE: HMO/PPO
  Model Type: Network
  Plan Specialty: Behavioral Health, Dental, Disease
    Management, Lab, PBM, Vision, Radiology
  Benefits Offered: Behavioral Health, Chiropractic, Dental,
    Disease Management, Long-Term Care, Physical Therapy,
    Prescription, Vision, Wellness, AD&D, Life, LTD, STD

Type of Coverage
  Commercial, Individual, Indemnity, Medicare, Supplemental
    Medicare, Medicaid, Catastrophic, Family, Military,
    Veterans, Group,

Geographic Areas Served
  Statewide. Maine is covered by the Rhode Island branch

Network Qualifications
  Pre-Admission Certification: Yes

Peer Review Type
  Utilization Review: Yes
  Second Surgical Opinion: Yes
  Case Management: Yes

Publishes and Distributes Report Card: Yes

Accreditation Certification
  TJC, NCQA

Key Personnel
  CEO, CT/ME/MA/NH/RI . . . . Stephen Farrell

Specialty Managed Care Partners
  Enters into Contracts with Regional Business Coalitions: Yes

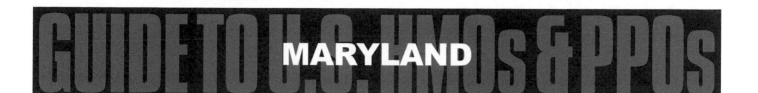

Health Insurance Coverage Status and Type of Coverage by Age

Category	All Persons		Under 18 years		Under 65 years	
	Number	%	Number	%	Number	%
Total population	5,958	-	1,420	-	5,079	-
Covered by some type of health insurance	5,592 (15)	93.9 (0.2)	1,365 (7)	96.2 (0.4)	4,721 (16)	93.0 (0.3)
Covered by private health insurance	4,428 (27)	74.3 (0.5)	945 (15)	66.6 (1.0)	3,806 (27)	74.9 (0.5)
Employer-based	3,784 (29)	63.5 (0.5)	840 (16)	59.2 (1.1)	3,344 (29)	65.8 (0.6)
Direct purchase	717 (16)	12.0 (0.3)	90 (6)	6.4 (0.4)	469 (14)	9.2 (0.3)
TRICARE	206 (11)	3.5 (0.2)	48 (5)	3.4 (0.4)	148 (10)	2.9 (0.2)
Covered by public health insurance	1,918 (25)	32.2 (0.4)	464 (16)	32.7 (1.1)	1,091 (25)	21.5 (0.5)
Medicaid	1,067 (26)	17.9 (0.4)	455 (15)	32.0 (1.1)	968 (25)	19.1 (0.5)
Medicare	956 (9)	16.0 (0.2)	12 (4)	0.9 (0.3)	129 (8)	2.5 (0.2)
VA Care	119 (5)	2.0 (0.1)	1 (1)	0.1 (Z)	61 (4)	1.2 (0.1)
Not covered at any time during the year	366 (15)	6.1 (0.2)	54 (6)	3.8 (0.4)	358 (15)	7.0 (0.3)

Note: Numbers in thousands; Figures cover civilian noninstitutionalized population in 2017; N/A indicates that data was not available; Z represents or rounds to zero; Margin of error appears in parenthesis and is calculated using replicate weights.
Source: U.S. Census Bureau, American Community Survey, Table HIC-4_ACS. Health Insurance Coverage Status and Type of Coverage by State—All People: 2008 to 2017, Table HIC-5_ACS. Health Insurance Coverage Status and Type of Coverage by State—Children Under 18: 2008 to 2017, Table HIC-6_ACS. Health Insurance Coverage Status and Type of Coverage by State—Persons Under 65: 2008 to 2017

Maryland

366 Aetna Health of Maryland

509 Progress Drive
Suite 117
Linthicum, MD 21090-2256
Toll-Free: 866-827-2710
Fax: 866-361-8495
www.aetnabetterhealth.com/maryland
Subsidiary of: Aetna Inc.
For Profit Organization: Yes

Healthplan and Services Defined
PLAN TYPE: HMO/PPO
Other Type: POS
Model Type: Network
Plan Specialty: Behavioral Health, EPO, Lab, PBM,
    Radiology
Benefits Offered: Behavioral Health, Disease Management,
    Long-Term Care, Physical Therapy, Podiatry, Prescription,
    Psychiatric, Vision, Wellness, Life, LTD, STD

Type of Coverage
Commercial, Student health

Type of Payment Plans Offered
DFFS, Capitated, FFS

Geographic Areas Served
Statewide

Key Personnel
Chief Medical Officer . . . . Nina F. Miles Everett

367 American Postal Workers Union (APWU) Health Plan

799 Cromwell Park Drive
Suite K-Z
Glen Burnie, MD 21061
Toll-Free: 800-222-2798
Fax: 410-424-1588
www.apwuhp.com
Year Founded: 1960
Number of Affiliated Hospitals: 6,000
Number of Primary Care Physicians: 600,000
Total Enrollment: 205,000
State Enrollment: 205,000

Healthplan and Services Defined
PLAN TYPE: PPO
Plan Specialty: Behavioral Health, Dental, Disease
    Management
Benefits Offered: Behavioral Health, Dental, Disease
    Management, Prescription, Wellness
Offers Demand Management Patient Information Service:
    Yes
DMPI Services Offered: 24 Hour Nurse Advisory Line

Type of Payment Plans Offered
FFS

Geographic Areas Served
Nationwide - APWU/The American Postal Workers Union
Health Plan is health insurance for federal employees and
retirees

Subscriber Information
Average Monthly Fee Per Subscriber
    (Employee + Employer Contribution):
        Employee Only (Self): $36.80-177.20 varies
        Employee & 2 Family Members: $82.80-398.66 varies
Average Annual Deductible Per Subscriber:
    Employee Only (Self): $250
Average Subscriber Co-Payment:
    Primary Care Physician: 15%
    Prescription Drugs: 25%
    Hospital ER: 15% - 30%
    Home Health Care Max. Days/Visits Covered: 10 - 30%

Key Personnel
President . . . . Mark Dimondstein
Director . . . . John L. Marcotte

368 Amerigroup Maryland

7550 Teague Road
Hanover, MD 21076
Toll-Free: 800-600-4441
Phone: 410-859-5800
www.myamerigroup.com/md
Subsidiary of: Anthem, Inc.
For Profit Organization: Yes
Year Founded: 1999

Healthplan and Services Defined
PLAN TYPE: HMO
Plan Specialty: Dental, Disease Management, Vision, Taking
    Care of Baby and Me program
Benefits Offered: Disease Management

Type of Coverage
Medicare, Medicaid

Accreditation Certification
NCQA

Key Personnel
Provider Network Director . . . . Tianna Goldring
VP, Finance . . . . Kevin Criswell
Market President, MD/DC . . . . Vincent Ancona
Quality Management . . . . Myron Arthur

369 Avesis: Maryland

10324 S Dolfield Road
Owings Mills, MD 21117
Toll-Free: 800-643-1132
www.avesis.com
Subsidiary of: Guardian Life Insurance Company
Year Founded: 1978
Number of Primary Care Physicians: 25,000
Total Enrollment: 3,500,000

Healthplan and Services Defined
PLAN TYPE: PPO
Other Type: Vision, Dental

Model Type: Network
Plan Specialty: Dental, Vision, Hearing
Benefits Offered: Dental, Vision

Type of Coverage
Commercial

Type of Payment Plans Offered
POS, Capitated, Combination FFS & DFFS

Geographic Areas Served
Nationwide and Puerto Rico

Publishes and Distributes Report Card: Yes

Accreditation Certification
AAAHC
TJC Accreditation

Key Personnel
Accountant . . . . Mary Griffin

370   CareFirst BlueCross BlueShield

Canton Tower
1501 S Clinton Street
Baltimore, MD 21224
Toll-Free: 800-544-8703
Phone: 410-581-3000
individual.carefirst.com
Secondary Address: Union Center Plaza, 840 First Street NE,
   Washington, DC 20065, 202-479-8000
Non-Profit Organization: Yes
Year Founded: 1984
Number of Primary Care Physicians: 5,000
Total Enrollment: 3,200,000

Healthplan and Services Defined
   PLAN TYPE: HMO/PPO
   Model Type: Network
   Benefits Offered: Dental, Prescription, Vision

Type of Coverage
Commercial, Individual, Medicare
Catastrophic Illness Benefit: Unlimited

Geographic Areas Served
Maryland, the District of Columbia and parts of Northern
Virginia

Accreditation Certification
NCQA
TJC Accreditation, Medicare Approved, Utilization Review,
   Pre-Admission Certification, State Licensure, Quality
   Assurance Program

Key Personnel
Preisdent/CEO . . . . Brian D. Pieninck
EVP/CFO . . . . G. Mark Chaney
VP/CMO . . . . Daniel Winn, MD
EVP/General Counsel . . . . Meryl Burgin
SVP/Chief Actuary . . . . Peter Berry
SVP/CIO . . . . Andy Fitzsimmons
SVP/App. Development . . . . Ken Sullivan

Specialty Managed Care Partners
Enters into Contracts with Regional Business Coalitions: Yes

371   Cigna HealthSpring Maryland

3601 O'Donnell Street
Baltimore, MD 21224
Toll-Free: 800-701-5909
www.cigna.com
For Profit Organization: Yes
Year Founded: 1982

Healthplan and Services Defined
   PLAN TYPE: Multiple
   Benefits Offered: Behavioral Health, Dental, Disease
      Management, Prescription, Vision, Wellness, AD&D, Life,
      LTD, STD

Type of Coverage
Commercial, Individual, Medicare, Supplemental Medicare,
   Medicaid, Part-time and hourly workers; Union

Geographic Areas Served
Statewide

Key Personnel
Assistant VP, Quality . . . . Valerie James

372   Coventry Health Care, Inc.

6720-B Rockledge Drive
Suite 800
Bethesda, MD 20817
Phone: 301-581-0600
coventryhealthcare.com
Subsidiary of: Aetna Inc.
For Profit Organization: Yes

Healthplan and Services Defined
   PLAN TYPE: HMO/PPO
   Model Type: Network
   Plan Specialty: Behavioral Health, Dental, Worker's
      Compensation
   Benefits Offered: Behavioral Health, Dental, Prescription,
      Wellness, Worker's Compensation

Type of Coverage
Commercial, Individual, Medicare, Medicaid

Geographic Areas Served
Nationwide, including the District of Columbia and Puerto
Rico

Key Personnel
President . . . . Karen S. Lynch

373   Denta-Chek of Maryland

10400 Little Patuxet Parkway
Suite 260
Columbia, MD 21044
Toll-Free: 888-478-8833
Phone: 410-997-3300
Fax: 410-997-3796
info@dentachek.com
www.dentachek.com
Non-Profit Organization: Yes
Year Founded: 1981
Number of Primary Care Physicians: 300
Number of Referral/Specialty Physicians: 200

Total Enrollment: 10,000

Healthplan and Services Defined
PLAN TYPE: Dental
Model Type: IPA
Plan Specialty: Dental
Benefits Offered: Dental

Type of Coverage
Catastrophic Illness Benefit: None

Type of Payment Plans Offered
POS, Combination FFS & DFFS

Geographic Areas Served
Statewide

Subscriber Information
Average Monthly Fee Per Subscriber
(Employee + Employer Contribution):
Employee Only (Self): $16.00
Employee & 1 Family Member: $22.00
Employee & 2 Family Members: $28.00
Medicare: $0
Average Annual Deductible Per Subscriber:
Employee Only (Self): $0
Employee & 1 Family Member: $0
Employee & 2 Family Members: $0
Medicare: $0
Average Subscriber Co-Payment:
Non-Network Physician: $0
Prescription Drugs: $0
Hospital ER: $0
Home Health Care: $0
Nursing Home: $0

Network Qualifications
Pre-Admission Certification: Yes

Peer Review Type
Utilization Review: Yes
Second Surgical Opinion: Yes
Case Management: Yes

Publishes and Distributes Report Card: No

Accreditation Certification
State Licensure, Quality Assurance Program

Specialty Managed Care Partners
Enters into Contracts with Regional Business Coalitions: No

---

374   Dental Benefit Providers

6220 Old Dobbin Lane
Columbia, MD 21045
Toll-Free: 800-307-7820
www.dbp.com
Secondary Address: 425 Market Street, 14th Floor, San
Francisco, CA 94105, 415-778-3800
Subsidiary of: UnitedHealth Group
For Profit Organization: Yes
Year Founded: 1984
Number of Primary Care Physicians: 125,000
Total Enrollment: 6,600,000

Healthplan and Services Defined
PLAN TYPE: Dental

Model Type: IPA
Plan Specialty: ASO, Dental, EPO, DHMO, PPO, CSO,
Preventive, Claims Repricing and Network Access
Benefits Offered: Dental

Type of Coverage
Indemnity, Medicare, Medicaid

Type of Payment Plans Offered
POS, DFFS, Capitated, FFS

Geographic Areas Served
48 states including District of Columbia, Puerto Rico and
Virgin Islands

Accreditation Certification
NCQA

Key Personnel
President, UH Dental . . . . Paul Hebert

---

375   First Health Part D

6730-B Rockledge Drive
Suite 700
Bethasda, MD 20817
Phone: 301-581-0600
coventry-medicare.com
Subsidiary of: Coventry Health Care
For Profit Organization: Yes

Healthplan and Services Defined
PLAN TYPE: Medicare
Benefits Offered: Prescription

Type of Coverage
Medicare, Medicare Part D

Geographic Areas Served
Nationwide

---

376   Jai Medical Systems

301 International Circle
Hunt Valley, MD 21030
Toll-Free: 888-524-1999
www.jaimedicalsystems.com
Subsidiary of: Managed Care Organization Inc.
For Profit Organization: Yes
Year Founded: 1997

Healthplan and Services Defined
PLAN TYPE: HMO
Plan Specialty: Dental, Lab, Radiology
Benefits Offered: Behavioral Health, Dental, Disease
Management, Home Care, Inpatient SNF, Prescription,
Vision, Substance abuse treatment, HIV/AIDS treatment,
Family planning services, Diabetes care

Type of Coverage
Individual

Geographic Areas Served
Statewide

Key Personnel
Chief Financial Officer . . . . Tim Barrett
Medical Director . . . . Aye Lwin
HR Manager. . . . . Landy Castillo

Medical Assistant . . . . Nessa Williams
Chief Information Officer . . . . Devon Bowers
Data Analyst . . . . Robert Frey

---

377 Kaiser Permanente Mid-Atlantic

2101 E Jefferson Street
Rockville, MD 20852
Toll-Free: 800-777-7904
thrive.kaiserpermanente.org/care-near-mid-atlantic
Subsidiary of: Kaiser Permanente
Non-Profit Organization: Yes
Year Founded: 1945
Number of Primary Care Physicians: 1,100
Total Enrollment: 614,350

Healthplan and Services Defined
 PLAN TYPE: Multiple
 Model Type: Network
 Benefits Offered: Disease Management, Prescription, Vision,
 Wellness

Type of Coverage
 Commercial, Individual, Medicare, Supplemental Medicare,
 Medicaid

Geographic Areas Served
 Virginia, Maryland and the District of Columbia

Key Personnel
 President, Mid-Atlantic . . . . Kim Horn
 Chief Executive Officer . . . . Richard Isaacs
 Executive Vice President . . . . Gregory A. Adams

---

378 Priority Partners Health Plans

6704 Curtis Court
Glen Burnie, MD 21060-9949
Toll-Free: 800-654-9728
ppcustomerservice@jhhc.com
www.ppmco.org
Subsidiary of: John Hopkins HealthCare LLC/Maryland
 Community Health System
Non-Profit Organization: Yes
Year Founded: 1996
Total Enrollment: 185,000
State Enrollment: 185,000

Healthplan and Services Defined
 PLAN TYPE: HMO
 Benefits Offered: Behavioral Health, Dental, Prescription,
 Vision

Type of Coverage
 Medicaid

Type of Payment Plans Offered
 Capitated, FFS

Geographic Areas Served
 Maryland

Peer Review Type
 Second Surgical Opinion: Yes

Publishes and Distributes Report Card: Yes

Accreditation Certification
 TJC, NCQA, JACHO, HMO

---

379 Spectera Eyecare Networks

6220 Old Dobbin Lane
Liberty 6, Suite 200
Columbia, MD 21045
Toll-Free: 800-638-3120
www.spectera.com
Mailing Address: P.O. Box 30978, Salt Lake City, UT 84130
Subsidiary of: UnitedHealth Group
For Profit Organization: Yes
Year Founded: 1964
Number of Primary Care Physicians: 24,000
Total Enrollment: 17,000,000

Healthplan and Services Defined
 PLAN TYPE: Multiple
 Model Type: Network
 Plan Specialty: Vision
 Benefits Offered: Disease Management, Vision

Type of Coverage
 Commercial, Individual

Type of Payment Plans Offered
 POS, DFFS, Capitated

Subscriber Information
 Average Monthly Fee Per Subscriber
  (Employee + Employer Contribution):
   Employee Only (Self): Varies
 Average Annual Deductible Per Subscriber:
   Employee & 2 Family Members: Varies
 Average Subscriber Co-Payment:
   Primary Care Physician: Varies

Network Qualifications
 Pre-Admission Certification: Yes

Publishes and Distributes Report Card: Yes

Key Personnel
 Mgr, Strategic Provider . . . . Kate O'Brien

Specialty Managed Care Partners
 United Heath Group
 Enters into Contracts with Regional Business Coalitions: No

---

380 Trinity Health of Maryland

Holy Cross Health
1500 Forest Glen Road
Silver Spring, MD 20910
Phone: 301-754-7000
www.trinity-health.org
Subsidiary of: Trinity Health
Non-Profit Organization: Yes
Year Founded: 2013
Total Enrollment: 30,000,000

Healthplan and Services Defined
 PLAN TYPE: Other

Benefits Offered: Disease Management, Home Care,
Long-Term Care, Psychiatric, Hospice programs, PACE
(Program of All Inclusive Care for the Elderly)

Geographic Areas Served
Montgomery, Prince Georges and Howard counties

Key Personnel
President/CEO .... Norvell V. Coots
Chief Medical Officer .... Blair M. Eig
Chief Strategy Officer................. Kristin Feliciano
Chief Financial Officer .... Anne Gillis
Chief Development Officer .... Wendy Friar
Chief Quality Officer .... Yancy Phillips
General Counsel .... Elizabeth Simpson

---

381 United Concordia of Maryland

11311 McCormick Ep 4 Road
Suite 170
Hunt Valley, MD 21031
Phone: 443-866-9500
www.unitedconcordia.com
For Profit Organization: Yes
Year Founded: 1971
Total Enrollment: 7,800,000

Healthplan and Services Defined
PLAN TYPE: Dental
Plan Specialty: Dental
Benefits Offered: Dental

Type of Coverage
Commercial, Individual, Military personnel & families

Geographic Areas Served
Nationwide

Accreditation Certification
URAC

Key Personnel
Professional Relations...................... Tim Dodd
Contact............................ Beth Rutherford
717-260-7659
beth.rutherford@ucci.com

---

382 UnitedHealthcare of Maryland

6220 Old Dobbin Lane
Suite 100
Columbia, MD 21045
Toll-Free: 888-545-5205
Phone: 443-201-1186
www.uhc.com
Subsidiary of: UnitedHealth Group
Non-Profit Organization: Yes
Year Founded: 1976

Healthplan and Services Defined
PLAN TYPE: HMO/PPO
Model Type: Network
Plan Specialty: Behavioral Health, Dental, Disease
Management, PBM, Vision

Benefits Offered: Behavioral Health, Dental, Disease
Management, Long-Term Care, Prescription, Vision,
Wellness, Life, LTD, STD

Type of Coverage
Individual, Medicare, Supplemental Medicare, Medicaid,
Catastrophic, Family, Military, Veterans, Group,

Geographic Areas Served
Maryland, Virginia, and the District of Columbia

Subscriber Information
Average Monthly Fee Per Subscriber
(Employee + Employer Contribution):
Employee Only (Self): $104.00-135.00
Employee & 1 Family Member: $143.00-184.00
Employee & 2 Family Members: $331.00-440.00
Medicare: $112.00-156.00
Average Annual Deductible Per Subscriber:
Employee Only (Self): $100.00-250.00
Employee & 1 Family Member: $500.00-1500.00
Employee & 2 Family Members: $200.00-500.00
Medicare: $0
Average Subscriber Co-Payment:
Primary Care Physician: $5.00/10.00
Non-Network Physician: Deductible
Prescription Drugs: $5.00/10.00
Hospital ER: $25.00/50.00
Home Health Care: $5.00/10.00

Network Qualifications
Pre-Admission Certification: Yes

Peer Review Type
Utilization Review: Yes
Second Surgical Opinion: Yes
Case Management: Yes

Publishes and Distributes Report Card: Yes

Accreditation Certification
TJC Accreditation, Medicare Approved, Utilization Review,
Pre-Admission Certification, State Licensure, Quality
Assurance Program

Specialty Managed Care Partners
Enters into Contracts with Regional Business Coalitions: Yes

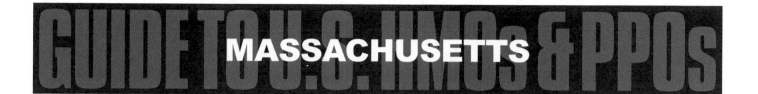
Health Insurance Coverage Status and Type of Coverage by Age

Category	All Persons		Under 18 years		Under 65 years	
	Number	%	Number	%	Number	%
Total population	6,786	-	1,479	-	5,714	-
Covered by some type of health insurance	6,596 *(10)*	97.2 *(0.1)*	1,457 *(5)*	98.5 *(0.2)*	5,528 *(10)*	96.7 *(0.2)*
Covered by private health insurance	5,009 *(29)*	73.8 *(0.4)*	1,030 *(14)*	69.7 *(0.8)*	4,300 *(28)*	75.2 *(0.5)*
Employer-based	4,261 *(29)*	62.8 *(0.4)*	936 *(13)*	63.3 *(0.9)*	3,823 *(28)*	66.9 *(0.5)*
Direct purchase	904 *(18)*	13.3 *(0.3)*	103 *(7)*	7.0 *(0.4)*	554 *(16)*	9.7 *(0.3)*
TRICARE	82 *(7)*	1.2 *(0.1)*	17 *(3)*	1.1 *(0.2)*	51 *(7)*	0.9 *(0.1)*
Covered by public health insurance	2,489 *(30)*	36.7 *(0.4)*	511 *(13)*	34.6 *(0.9)*	1,476 *(29)*	25.8 *(0.5)*
Medicaid	1,570 *(30)*	23.1 *(0.4)*	508 *(13)*	34.4 *(0.9)*	1,396 *(30)*	24.4 *(0.5)*
Medicare	1,150 *(8)*	16.9 *(0.1)*	6 *(2)*	0.4 *(0.1)*	137 *(7)*	2.4 *(0.1)*
VA Care	106 *(6)*	1.6 *(0.1)*	Z *(Z)*	Z *(Z)*	40 *(4)*	0.7 *(0.1)*
Not covered at any time during the year	190 *(10)*	2.8 *(0.1)*	22 *(3)*	1.5 *(0.2)*	186 *(9)*	3.3 *(0.2)*

Note: Numbers in thousands; Figures cover civilian noninstitutionalized population in 2017; N/A indicates that data was not available; Z represents or rounds to zero; Margin of error appears in parenthesis and is calculated using replicate weights.
Source: U.S. Census Bureau, American Community Survey, Table HIC-4_ACS. Health Insurance Coverage Status and Type of Coverage by State—All People: 2008 to 2017, Table HIC-5_ACS. Health Insurance Coverage Status and Type of Coverage by State—Children Under 18: 2008 to 2017, Table HIC-6_ACS. Health Insurance Coverage Status and Type of Coverage by State—Persons Under 65: 2008 to 2017

Massachusetts

383 Aetna Health of Massachusetts

151 Farmington Avenue
Hartford, CT 06156
Toll-Free: 800-872-3862
Phone: 860-273-0123
www.aetna.com
Subsidiary of: Aetna Inc.
For Profit Organization: Yes
Year Founded: 1987

Healthplan and Services Defined
PLAN TYPE: HMO/PPO
Other Type: POS
Model Type: IPA, Network
Plan Specialty: Behavioral Health, EPO, Lab, PBM,
   Radiology
Benefits Offered: Behavioral Health, Dental, Disease
   Management, Long-Term Care, Physical Therapy,
   Podiatry, Prescription, Psychiatric, Vision, Life, LTD, STD

Type of Coverage
Commercial, Student health
Catastrophic Illness Benefit: Covered

Geographic Areas Served
Statewide

Peer Review Type
Second Surgical Opinion: Yes
Case Management: Yes

Publishes and Distributes Report Card: Yes

Accreditation Certification
NCQA

384 Araz Group

7201 West 78th Street
Bloomington, MN 55439
Toll-Free: 800-444-3005
Phone: 952-896-1200
info@araz.com
www.araz.com
For Profit Organization: Yes
Year Founded: 1982
Number of Primary Care Physicians: 71,000
Total Enrollment: 250,000
State Enrollment: 160,000

Healthplan and Services Defined
PLAN TYPE: PPO
Plan Specialty: UR
Benefits Offered: Behavioral Health, Disease Management,
   Prescription, Worker's Compensation, AD&D, LTD, STD

Type of Coverage
Commercial, Medicare

Geographic Areas Served
Minnesota, Western Wisconsin, Northern Iowa, North and
South Dakota

Accreditation Certification
Pre-Admission Certification

Key Personnel
Founder & CEO . . . . Nazie Eftekhari
President . . . . Amir Eftekhari

Specialty Managed Care Partners
Intracorp

385 Avesis: Massachusetts

10324 S Dolfield Road
Owing Mills, MD 21117
Toll-Free: 800-643-1132
www.avesis.com
Subsidiary of: Guardian Life Insurance Co.
Year Founded: 1978
Number of Primary Care Physicians: 25,000
Total Enrollment: 3,500,000

Healthplan and Services Defined
PLAN TYPE: PPO
Other Type: Vision, Dental
Model Type: Network
Plan Specialty: Dental, Vision
Benefits Offered: Dental, Vision

Type of Coverage
Commercial

Type of Payment Plans Offered
POS, Capitated, Combination FFS & DFFS

Geographic Areas Served
Nationwide and Puerto Rico

Publishes and Distributes Report Card: Yes

Accreditation Certification
AAAHC
TJC Accreditation

Key Personnel
VP, Regional Sales . . . . Lawrence Ford

386 Blue Cross & Blue Shield of Massachusetts

101 Huntington Avenue
Suite 1300
Boston, MA 02199-7611
Toll-Free: 800-262-2583
www.bcbsma.com
Non-Profit Organization: Yes
Year Founded: 1937
Number of Affiliated Hospitals: 77
Number of Primary Care Physicians: 20,266
Total Enrollment: 3,000,000
State Enrollment: 3,000,000

Healthplan and Services Defined
PLAN TYPE: HMO
Model Type: Network
Plan Specialty: Dental, Group Medical
Benefits Offered: Behavioral Health, Chiropractic,
   Complementary Medicine, Dental, Disease Management,
   Home Care, Inpatient SNF, Long-Term Care, Physical

Therapy, Podiatry, Prescription, Psychiatric, Transplant, Vision, Wellness, AD&D, Life, LTD, STD
Offers Demand Management Patient Information Service: Yes
DMPI Services Offered: 24-Hour Nurse Care Line

Type of Coverage
Medicare, Group Insurance

Type of Payment Plans Offered
FFS

Geographic Areas Served
Massachusetts & Southern New Hampshire

Subscriber Information
Average Monthly Fee Per Subscriber
(Employee + Employer Contribution):
Employee Only (Self): Varies by plan

Network Qualifications
Pre-Admission Certification: Yes

Peer Review Type
Utilization Review: Yes

Accreditation Certification
NCQA
TJC Accreditation, Medicare Approved, Utilization Review, Pre-Admission Certification, State Licensure

Key Personnel
President/CEO .... Andrew Dreyfus
Chief Operating Officer .... Deborah Devaux
Chief Financial Officer .... Andreana Santangelo
Chief Legal Officer. .... Stephanie Lovell
SVP, Corp Communications .... Jay McQuaide
Chief Physician Executive .... Bruce Nash
EVP, Sales/Marketing. .... Patrick Gilligan

Specialty Managed Care Partners
Express Scripts

387 Dentaquest
465 Medford Street
Boston, MA 02129-1454
Toll-Free: 888-278-7310
www.dentaquest.com
Subsidiary of: DentaQuest Ventures
Year Founded: 1980
Number of Primary Care Physicians: 750
Total Enrollment: 14,000,000

Healthplan and Services Defined
   PLAN TYPE: Dental
   Plan Specialty: Dental
   Benefits Offered: Dental

Type of Coverage
Individual, Medicare, Medicaid

Geographic Areas Served
Arizona, California, Colorado, Florida, Georgia, Idaho, Illinois, Indiana, Kentucky, Louisiana, Maryland, Massachusetts, Michicgan, Minnesota, Mississippi, Missouri, New Hampshire, New Jersey, New Mexico, New York, Ohio,

Rhode Island, Pennsylvania, North Carolina, South Carolina, Tennessee, Texas, Utah, Virginia, Washington, Wisconsin

Key Personnel
President/CEO .... Steve Pollock
EVP/COO .... Alan Madison
SVP, Corporate Controller .... Jeff Brown
Chief Dental Officer .... Olivia Croom
Chief Legal Officer .... David Abelman
EVP, Chief Sales Officer .... Bob Lynn

388 Fallon Health
10 Chestnut Street
Worcester, MA 01608
Toll-Free: 800-333-2535
Phone: 508-799-2100
contactcustomerservice@fallonhealth.org
www.fchp.org
Non-Profit Organization: Yes
Year Founded: 1977

Healthplan and Services Defined
   PLAN TYPE: Multiple
   Benefits Offered: Behavioral Health, Chiropractic, Dental, Disease Management, Home Care, Inpatient SNF, Physical Therapy, Podiatry, Prescription, Psychiatric, Vision, Wellness

Type of Coverage
Individual, Medicare, Medicaid

Geographic Areas Served
Statewide

Key Personnel
President & CEO .... Richard P. Burke
Senior VP & CCO..................... James Gentile
Senior VP & COO........................ Emily West
Chief Legal Counsel .... Mark Mosby
Chief Medical Officer .... Thomas H. Ebert, MD
SVP & Chief Sales Officer .... David Przesiek
Director, Community Rel............... Kimberly Salmon
   508-368-9439
   kimberly.salmon@fallonhealth.org

389 Harvard Pilgrim Health Care Massachusetts
93 Worcester Street
Wellesley, MA 02481
Toll-Free: 888-888-4742
Phone: 617-509-1000
www.harvardpilgrim.org
Secondary Address: Landmark Center, 401 Park Drive, Suite 401, East Boston, MA 02215-3325
Non-Profit Organization: Yes
Year Founded: 1977
Number of Affiliated Hospitals: 179
Number of Referral/Specialty Physicians: 53,000

Healthplan and Services Defined
   PLAN TYPE: Multiple
   Model Type: Network

Plan Specialty: ASO, Behavioral Health, Chiropractic, Dental, Disease Management, EPO, Lab, MSO, PBM, Vision, Radiology, Worker's Compensation, UR

Benefits Offered: Behavioral Health, Chiropractic, Disease Management, Home Care, Inpatient SNF, Long-Term Care, Physical Therapy, Podiatry, Prescription, Psychiatric, Transplant, Vision, Wellness

Type of Coverage
Commercial, Individual, Indemnity, Medicare, Supplemental Medicare, Medicaid

Geographic Areas Served
Statewide

Peer Review Type
Utilization Review: Yes
Second Surgical Opinion: Yes
Case Management: Yes

Publishes and Distributes Report Card: Yes

Accreditation Certification
NCQA
TJC Accreditation, Medicare Approved, Utilization Review, Pre-Admission Certification, State Licensure, Quality Assurance Program

Average Claim Compensation
Physician's Fees Charged: 51%
Hospital's Fees Charged: 40%

Specialty Managed Care Partners
Enters into Contracts with Regional Business Coalitions: No

---

390 Health New England

One Monarch Place
Suite 1500
Springfield, MA 01144-1500
Toll-Free: 800-310-2835
Phone: 413-787-4004
healthnewengland.org
Non-Profit Organization: Yes
Year Founded: 1985
Number of Affiliated Hospitals: 22
Number of Primary Care Physicians: 4,300
Total Enrollment: 200,000
State Enrollment: 200,000

Healthplan and Services Defined
PLAN TYPE: HMO/PPO
Model Type: IPA
Plan Specialty: ASO, Disease Management
Benefits Offered: Behavioral Health, Chiropractic, Complementary Medicine, Dental, Disease Management, Home Care, Inpatient SNF, Physical Therapy, Podiatry, Prescription, Psychiatric, Transplant, Vision, Wellness

Type of Coverage
Commercial, Medicare, Medicaid, Catastrophic
Catastrophic Illness Benefit: Maximum $1M

Type of Payment Plans Offered
POS

Geographic Areas Served
Berkshire, Franklin, Hampden, Hampshire and Worcester counties in Massachusetts, and Hartford and Tolland counties in Connecticut

Peer Review Type
Utilization Review: Yes
Second Surgical Opinion: Yes
Case Management: Yes

Publishes and Distributes Report Card: Yes

Accreditation Certification
NCQA
TJC Accreditation, Medicare Approved, Utilization Review, Pre-Admission Certification, State Licensure, Quality Assurance Program

Key Personnel
Interim President/CEO. . . . . Jody Gross
VP, Sales & Marketing . . . . Ashley Allen
VP, Info Technology . . . . Ken Bernard
VP/CMO . . . . Laurie Gianturco, MD
VP/General Counsel. . . . . Susan O'Connor, Esq.
VP/CFO . . . . Steven J. Sigal, CPA

Average Claim Compensation
Physician's Fees Charged: 59%
Hospital's Fees Charged: 49%

Specialty Managed Care Partners
Enters into Contracts with Regional Business Coalitions: No

---

391 Health Plans, Inc.

1500 West Park Drive
Suite 330
Westborough, MA 01581
Toll-Free: 800-532-7575
Phone: 508-752-2480
Fax: 508-754-9664
www.healthplansinc.com
Subsidiary of: Harvard Pilgrim
Year Founded: 1981

Healthplan and Services Defined
PLAN TYPE: PPO
Other Type: TPA
Model Type: Network
Plan Specialty: ASO, Behavioral Health, Chiropractic, Dental, Disease Management, EPO, Lab, PBM, Vision, Radiology, UR
Benefits Offered: Home Care, Inpatient SNF, Long-Term Care, Physical Therapy, Podiatry, Prescription, Psychiatric, Transplant, Vision, Wellness, Worker's Compensation, AD&D, Life, LTD, STD

Geographic Areas Served
New England and South Carolina

Accreditation Certification
TJC Accreditation, Pre-Admission Certification

Key Personnel
President & CEO . . . . Deborah Hodges
Senior Vice President. Todd Bailey
Chief Information Officer . . . . Chuck Moulter

VP, Operations. . . . . Chris Parr
VP, Financial Operations . . . . Joan Recore

392 Humana Health Insurance of Massachusetts

125 Wolf Road
Suite 501
Albany, NY 12205
Toll-Free: 800-967-2370
Fax: 518-435-0412
www.humana.com
Subsidiary of: Humana
For Profit Organization: Yes

Healthplan and Services Defined
PLAN TYPE: HMO/PPO
Model Type: Network
Plan Specialty: Dental, Vision
Benefits Offered: Dental, Vision, Life, LTD, STD

Type of Coverage
Commercial

Geographic Areas Served
Massachusetts is covered by the New York branch

Accreditation Certification
URAC, NCQA, CORE

393 Medical Center Healthnet Plan

529 Main Street
Suite 500
Charlestown, MA 02129
Toll-Free: 800-792-4355
Phone: 617-748-6000
memberquestions@bmchp.org
www.bmchp.org
Non-Profit Organization: Yes
Year Founded: 1997
Number of Affiliated Hospitals: 60
Number of Primary Care Physicians: 3,000
Number of Referral/Specialty Physicians: 12,000
Total Enrollment: 240,890
State Enrollment: 240,890

Healthplan and Services Defined
PLAN TYPE: HMO
Benefits Offered: Disease Management, Prescription,
Wellness

Type of Coverage
Individual

Key Personnel
President . . . . Susan Coakley
Chief Financial Officer. . . . . Michael Guerriere
Chief Information Officer . . . . Kim Sinclair
Chief Medical Officer . . . . Jonathan Welch, MD
Chief Legal Officer . . . . Matt Herndon

394 Minuteman Health

38 Chauncy Street
Boston, MA 02111
Toll-Free: 855-644-1776
Fax: 857-263-8951
info@minutemanhealth.org
minutemanhealth.org
Non-Profit Organization: Yes
Number of Affiliated Hospitals: 44

Healthplan and Services Defined
PLAN TYPE: HMO
Benefits Offered: Behavioral Health, Chiropractic, Physical
Therapy, Prescription, Psychiatric, Wellness, Maternity;
Pediatric; Chemotherapy & Radiology; Hearing;
Short-Term Rehabilitation; Labs & Imaging; Speech
Therapy

Type of Coverage
Coverage varies per plan

Geographic Areas Served
Massachusetts & New Hampshire

Key Personnel
General Counsel & COO . . . . Susan E. Brown
Chief Medical Officer. . . . . Jan Cook
Media Contact. . . . . Kevin Beagan
617-521-7347
kevin.beagan@state.ma.us

395 Neighborhood Health Plan

399 Revolution Drive
Somerville, MA 02145
Toll-Free: 866-414-5533
memberservices@nhp.org
www.nhp.org
Subsidiary of: Partners HealthCare
Non-Profit Organization: Yes
Year Founded: 1986
Owned by an Integrated Delivery Network (IDN): Yes
Number of Affiliated Hospitals: 41
Number of Primary Care Physicians: 2,800
Number of Referral/Specialty Physicians: 10,400
Total Enrollment: 430,000
State Enrollment: 430,000

Healthplan and Services Defined
PLAN TYPE: HMO
Model Type: Network
Plan Specialty: ASO, Behavioral Health, Disease
Management, Medicaid Focus
Benefits Offered: Behavioral Health, Complementary
Medicine, Dental, Disease Management, Home Care,
Prescription, Vision, Wellness

Type of Coverage
Commercial, Medicaid
Catastrophic Illness Benefit: Covered

Geographic Areas Served
Most of Massachusetts counties

Network Qualifications
Pre-Admission Certification: Yes

Peer Review Type
Utilization Review: Yes
Second Surgical Opinion: Yes
Case Management: Yes

Publishes and Distributes Report Card: Yes

Accreditation Certification
State of Ma
TJC Accreditation, Medicare Approved, Utilization Review,
  Pre-Admission Certification, State Licensure, Quality
  Assurance Program

Key Personnel
President/CEO . . . . David Segal
Chief Operating Officer . . . . Mark McCormick
Chief Financial Officer . . . . Joseph C. Capezza
Chief, Stategy/Marketing . . . . Tim Walsh
Chief Medical Officer . . . . Anton B. Dodek, MD

Specialty Managed Care Partners
Beacon Health Strategies
Enters into Contracts with Regional Business Coalitions: No

---

396   Trinity Health of Massachusetts
1000 Asylum Avenue
5th Floor
Hartford, CT 06105
Phone: 860-714-1900
www.trinity-health.org
Secondary Address: Mercy Community, 2021 Albany Avenue,
  West Hartford, CT 06117, 860-570-8400
Subsidiary of: Trinity Health
Non-Profit Organization: Yes
Year Founded: 2013
Total Enrollment: 30,000,000

Healthplan and Services Defined
PLAN TYPE: Other
Benefits Offered: Disease Management, Home Care,
  Long-Term Care, Psychiatric, Hospice programs, PACE
  (Program of All Inclusive Care for the Elderly)

Geographic Areas Served
Western Massachusetts

Key Personnel
President/CEO . . . . Dr. Reginald J. Eadie

---

397   Tufts Health Medicare Plan
705 Mt Auburn Street
Watertown, MA 02472
Toll-Free: 800-890-6600
Phone: 617-972-9400
www.tuftshealthplan.com
Secondary Address: One Mercantile Street, Suite 130,
  Worcester, MA 01608
Non-Profit Organization: Yes
Year Founded: 1979

Healthplan and Services Defined
PLAN TYPE: Medicare

Benefits Offered: Chiropractic, Dental, Disease Management,
  Home Care, Inpatient SNF, Physical Therapy, Podiatry,
  Prescription, Psychiatric, Vision, Wellness

Type of Coverage
Individual, Medicare

Geographic Areas Served
Massachusetts, Connecticut, New Hampshire, Rhode Island
and Vermont

Subscriber Information
Average Monthly Fee Per Subscriber
  (Employee + Employer Contribution):
    Employee Only (Self): Varies
    Medicare: Varies
Average Annual Deductible Per Subscriber:
    Employee Only (Self): Varies
    Medicare: Varies
Average Subscriber Co-Payment:
    Primary Care Physician: Varies
    Non-Network Physician: Varies
    Prescription Drugs: Varies
    Hospital ER: Varies
    Home Health Care: Varies
    Home Health Care Max. Days/Visits Covered: Varies
    Nursing Home: Varies
    Nursing Home Max. Days/Visits Covered: Varies

Key Personnel
President/CEO . . . . Thomas A. Crowsell
Chief Operations Officer. . . . . Tricia Terbino
SVP/CIO . . . . Umesh Kurpad
SVP/Senior Products. . . . . Patty Blake
Chief Medical Officer . . . . Pual Kasuba, MD
Chief, Human Resources . . . . Lydia Greene

---

398   Tufts Health Plan
705 Mt Auburn Street
Watertown, MA 02472
Phone: 617-972-9400
www.tuftshealthplan.com
Secondary Address: One Mercantile Street, Suite 130,
  Worcester, MA 01608
Non-Profit Organization: Yes
Year Founded: 1979
Number of Affiliated Hospitals: 90
Number of Primary Care Physicians: 25,000
Number of Referral/Specialty Physicians: 12,500
Total Enrollment: 737,411

Healthplan and Services Defined
PLAN TYPE: Multiple
Other Type: POS
Model Type: IPA
Plan Specialty: ASO, Behavioral Health, Chiropractic,
  Disease Management, EPO, Lab, PBM, Vision, Radiology,
  UR, Pharmacy
Benefits Offered: Behavioral Health, Chiropractic,
  Complementary Medicine, Disease Management, Home
  Care, Inpatient SNF, Physical Therapy, Podiatry,
  Prescription, Psychiatric, Transplant, Vision, Wellness

Type of Coverage
Commercial, Individual, Medicare, Supplemental Medicare, Medicaid, HSA, HRA

Type of Payment Plans Offered
POS, DFFS, FFS, Combination FFS & DFFS

Geographic Areas Served
Massachusetts, New Hampshire and Rhode Island

Subscriber Information
Average Monthly Fee Per Subscriber
(Employee + Employer Contribution):
Employee Only (Self): $190.00-220.00
Employee & 2 Family Members: $800.00-950.00
Medicare: $150.00
Average Annual Deductible Per Subscriber:
Employee Only (Self): $1000.00
Employee & 1 Family Member: $500.00
Employee & 2 Family Members: $3000.00
Average Subscriber Co-Payment:
Primary Care Physician: $10.00
Non-Network Physician: 20%
Prescription Drugs: $10/20/35
Hospital ER: $50.00
Home Health Care: $0
Home Health Care Max. Days/Visits Covered: 120 days
Nursing Home: $0
Nursing Home Max. Days/Visits Covered: 120 days

Network Qualifications
Pre-Admission Certification: No

Peer Review Type
Utilization Review: Yes
Case Management: Yes

Publishes and Distributes Report Card: Yes

Accreditation Certification
TJC, AAPI, NCQA

Key Personnel
President/CEO . . . . Thomas A. Croswell
Chief Operations Officer. . . . . Tricia Terbino
Chief Financial Officer . . . . Umesh Kurpad
SVP/Chief Legal Officer . . . . Mary O'Toole Mahoney
Chief Medical Officer . . . . Paul Kasuba, MD
Chief, Human Resources . . . . Lydia Greene

Average Claim Compensation
Physician's Fees Charged: 75%
Hospital's Fees Charged: 70%

Specialty Managed Care Partners
Advance PCS, Private Healthe Care Systems

Employer References
Commonwealth of Massachuestts, Fleet Boston, Roman Catholic Archdiocese of Boston, City of Boston, State Street Corporation

---

399 UniCare Massachusetts
Brickstone Square
Eight Floor
Andover, MA 01810
Phone: 978-470-1795
www.unicare.com
Subsidiary of: Anthem, Inc.
Year Founded: 1985

Healthplan and Services Defined
PLAN TYPE: HMO/PPO
Model Type: Network
Benefits Offered: Behavioral Health, Chiropractic, Complementary
Medicine, Dental, Disease Management, Home Care, Inpatient SNF, Long-Term Care, Physical Therapy, Podiatry, Prescription, Psychiatric, Transplant, Vision, Wellness, Worker's Compensation, AD&D, Life, LTD, STD

Type of Coverage
Commercial, Individual, Indemnity, Medicare

Geographic Areas Served
Massachusetts, Southern New Hampshire & Rhode Island

Subscriber Information
Average Monthly Fee Per Subscriber
(Employee + Employer Contribution):
Employee Only (Self): Varies
Employee & 1 Family Member: Varies
Employee & 2 Family Members: Varies
Medicare: Varies
Average Annual Deductible Per Subscriber:
Employee Only (Self): Varies
Employee & 1 Family Member: Varies
Employee & 2 Family Members: Varies
Medicare: Varies
Average Subscriber Co-Payment:
Primary Care Physician: Varies
Non-Network Physician: Varies
Prescription Drugs: Varies
Hospital ER: Varies
Home Health Care: Varies
Home Health Care Max. Days/Visits Covered: Varies
Nursing Home: Varies
Nursing Home Max. Days/Visits Covered: Varies

Network Qualifications
Pre-Admission Certification: Yes

Peer Review Type
Utilization Review: Yes
Second Surgical Opinion: Yes
Case Management: Yes

Publishes and Distributes Report Card: No

Accreditation Certification
URAC
TJC Accreditation, Medicare Approved, Utilization Review, Pre-Admission Certification, State Licensure, Quality Assurance Program

400 UnitedHealthcare of Massachusetts

475 Kilvert Street
Warwick, RI 02886
Toll-Free: 888-545-5205
Phone: 401-737-6900
www.uhc.com
Subsidiary of: UnitedHealth Group
For Profit Organization: Yes

Healthplan and Services Defined
  PLAN TYPE: HMO/PPO
  Model Type: Network
  Plan Specialty: Behavioral Health, Dental, Disease
    Management, PBM, Vision
  Benefits Offered: Behavioral Health, Dental, Disease
    Management, Long-Term Care, Prescription, Vision,
    Wellness, Life, LTD, STD
  Offers Demand Management Patient Information Service:
    Yes

Type of Coverage
  Individual, Medicare, Supplemental Medicare, Medicaid,
    Catastrophic, Family, Military, Veterans, Group,
  Catastrophic Illness Benefit: None

Type of Payment Plans Offered
  POS, FFS

Geographic Areas Served
  Statewide. Massachusetts is covered by the Rhode Island
  branch

Subscriber Information
  Average Monthly Fee Per Subscriber
    (Employee + Employer Contribution):
      Employee Only (Self): $150.00
      Employee & 2 Family Members: $300.00

Network Qualifications
  Pre-Admission Certification: Yes

Peer Review Type
  Utilization Review: Yes
  Second Surgical Opinion: Yes
  Case Management: Yes

Publishes and Distributes Report Card: Yes

Accreditation Certification
  AAPI, NCQA
  TJC Accreditation, Medicare Approved, Utilization Review,
    Pre-Admission Certification, State Licensure, Quality
    Assurance Program

Key Personnel
  CEO, CT/ME/MA/NH/RI . . . . Stephen Farrell

Average Claim Compensation
  Physician's Fees Charged: 70%
  Hospital's Fees Charged: 80%

Specialty Managed Care Partners
  Enters into Contracts with Regional Business Coalitions: Yes

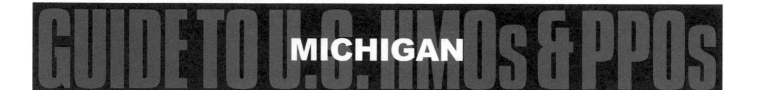
Health Insurance Coverage Status and Type of Coverage by Age

Category	All Persons		Under 18 years		Under 65 years	
	Number	%	Number	%	Number	%
Total population	9,853	-	2,313	-	8,227	-
Covered by some type of health insurance	9,344 *(15)*	94.8 *(0.2)*	2,244 *(7)*	97.0 *(0.2)*	7,724 *(14)*	93.9 *(0.2)*
Covered by private health insurance	7,038 *(32)*	71.4 *(0.3)*	1,467 *(13)*	63.4 *(0.6)*	5,860 *(29)*	71.2 *(0.4)*
Employer-based	5,979 *(36)*	60.7 *(0.4)*	1,344 *(14)*	58.1 *(0.6)*	5,218 *(33)*	63.4 *(0.4)*
Direct purchase	1,288 *(17)*	13.1 *(0.2)*	134 *(7)*	5.8 *(0.3)*	734 *(16)*	8.9 *(0.2)*
TRICARE	123 *(7)*	1.3 *(0.1)*	20 *(3)*	0.9 *(0.1)*	74 *(5)*	0.9 *(0.1)*
Covered by public health insurance	3,799 *(27)*	38.6 *(0.3)*	889 *(13)*	38.4 *(0.6)*	2,218 *(26)*	27.0 *(0.3)*
Medicaid	2,213 *(27)*	22.5 *(0.3)*	885 *(13)*	38.3 *(0.6)*	2,020 *(26)*	24.6 *(0.3)*
Medicare	1,874 *(10)*	19.0 *(0.1)*	8 *(1)*	0.4 *(0.1)*	294 *(9)*	3.6 *(0.1)*
VA Care	200 *(6)*	2.0 *(0.1)*	2 *(1)*	0.1 *(Z)*	85 *(4)*	1.0 *(Z)*
Not covered at any time during the year	510 *(15)*	5.2 *(0.2)*	69 *(6)*	3.0 *(0.2)*	502 *(15)*	6.1 *(0.2)*

Note: Numbers in thousands; Figures cover civilian noninstitutionalized population in 2017; N/A indicates that data was not available; Z represents or rounds to zero; Margin of error appears in parenthesis and is calculated using replicate weights.
Source: U.S. Census Bureau, American Community Survey, Table HIC-4_ACS. Health Insurance Coverage Status and Type of Coverage by State—All People: 2008 to 2017, Table HIC-5_ACS. Health Insurance Coverage Status and Type of Coverage by State—Children Under 18: 2008 to 2017, Table HIC-6_ACS. Health Insurance Coverage Status and Type of Coverage by State—Persons Under 65: 2008 to 2017

Michigan

401 Aetna Health of Michigan

1333 Gratiot Avenue
Suite 400
Detroit, MI 48207
Toll-Free: 866-316-3784
www.aetnabetterhealth.com/michigan
Mailing Address: P.O. Box 66215, Phoenix, AZ 85082-6215
Subsidiary of: Aetna Inc.
For Profit Organization: Yes

Healthplan and Services Defined
PLAN TYPE: HMO/PPO
Other Type: POS
Model Type: Network
Plan Specialty: Behavioral Health, EPO, Lab, PBM, Radiology
Benefits Offered: Behavioral Health, Dental, Disease Management, Long-Term Care, Physical Therapy, Podiatry, Prescription, Psychiatric, Vision, Wellness, Life, LTD, STD

Type of Coverage
Commercial, Catastrophic, Student health

Geographic Areas Served
Statewide

Key Personnel
Senior Health Care Exec. . . . . Jelka Petrovic

402 Ascension At Home

Crittenton Home Care
2251 Squirrel Road, Suite 320
Auburn Hills, MI 48326
Phone: 248-656-6757
Fax: 248-656-6758
ascensionathome.com
Subsidiary of: Ascension
Non-Profit Organization: Yes

Healthplan and Services Defined
PLAN TYPE: Other
Plan Specialty: Disease Management
Benefits Offered: Dental, Disease Management, Home Care, Wellness, Ambulance & Transportation; Nursing Service; Short-and-long-term care management planning; Hospice

Geographic Areas Served
Texas, Alabama, Indiana, Kansas, Michigan, Mississippi, Oklahoma, Wisconsin

Key Personnel
President. . . . . Kirk Allen
Dir., Home Health Service . . . . Darcy Burthay

403 Blue Care Network of Michigan

20500 Civic Center Drive
Southfield, MI 48076
Toll-Free: 800-662-6667
www.bcbsm.com
Subsidiary of: Blue Cross Blue Shield of Michigan

Non-Profit Organization: Yes
Year Founded: 1998
Federally Qualified: Yes
Number of Primary Care Physicians: 5,000
Number of Referral/Specialty Physicians: 17,000
Total Enrollment: 807,000

Healthplan and Services Defined
PLAN TYPE: HMO
Model Type: IPA, Network
Plan Specialty: Lab, Radiology
Benefits Offered: Behavioral Health, Disease Management, Prescription, Psychiatric, Wellness

Type of Coverage
Commercial, Individual, Medicare, Medicaid
Catastrophic Illness Benefit: Covered

Geographic Areas Served
Statewide

Peer Review Type
Case Management: Yes

Publishes and Distributes Report Card: Yes

Accreditation Certification
NCQA

Key Personnel
President & CEO . . . . Daniel J. Loepp
EVP, Financial Officer. . . . . Mark R. Bartlett
SVP, Information Officer . . . . William M. Fandrich
SVP, Medical Officer . . . . Thomas L. Simmer, MD

Specialty Managed Care Partners
Enters into Contracts with Regional Business Coalitions: Yes

Employer References
General Motors, Ford Motor Company, State of Michigan, Federal Employee Program, Daimler Chrysler

404 Blue Care Network of Michigan

20500 Civic Center Drive
Southfield, MI 48076
www.bcbsm.com
Non-Profit Organization: Yes
Year Founded: 1998
Federally Qualified: Yes
Number of Primary Care Physicians: 5,000
Number of Referral/Specialty Physicians: 17,000
State Enrollment: 807,000

Healthplan and Services Defined
PLAN TYPE: HMO
Model Type: Network
Plan Specialty: Dental, Lab, Vision, Radiology
Benefits Offered: Behavioral Health, Dental, Disease Management, Physical Therapy, Prescription, Psychiatric, Vision, Wellness

Type of Coverage
Commercial, Individual
Catastrophic Illness Benefit: Varies per case

Type of Payment Plans Offered
POS, Capitated, Combination FFS & DFFS

Geographic Areas Served
Muskegon, Newago, Oceana & Ottawa counties

Peer Review Type
Utilization Review: Yes
Second Surgical Opinion: Yes

Publishes and Distributes Report Card: Yes

Key Personnel
President and CEO. . . . . Daniel Loepp
Chief Financial Officer . . . . Mark Bartlett
Chief Medical Officer . . . . Thomas Simmer, MD

405   Blue Cross Blue Shield of Michigan

600 E Lafayette Boulevard
Detroit, MI 48226
Toll-Free: 855-237-3501
www.bcbsm.com
Year Founded: 1939
Number of Affiliated Hospitals: 153
Number of Primary Care Physicians: 30,000
Total Enrollment: 5,800,000
State Enrollment: 4,500,000

Healthplan and Services Defined
PLAN TYPE: Multiple
Model Type: Network
Benefits Offered: Chiropractic, Disease Management, Home
Care, Inpatient SNF, Physical Therapy, Podiatry,
Prescription, Psychiatric, Wellness

Type of Coverage
Commercial, Individual, Medicare, Supplemental Medicare,
Medicaid

Geographic Areas Served
Blue Care Network available in 26 counties in southeastern
Michigan. PPO plans available statewide

Subscriber Information
Average Monthly Fee Per Subscriber
(Employee + Employer Contribution):
Employee Only (Self): Varies
Medicare: Varies
Average Annual Deductible Per Subscriber:
Employee Only (Self): Varies
Medicare: Varies
Average Subscriber Co-Payment:
Primary Care Physician: Varies
Non-Network Physician: Varies
Prescription Drugs: Varies
Hospital ER: Varies
Home Health Care: Varies
Home Health Care Max. Days/Visits Covered: Varies
Nursing Home: Varies
Nursing Home Max. Days/Visits Covered: Varies

Key Personnel
President & CEO . . . . Daniel J. Loepp
Chief Financial Officer . . . . Mark R. Bartlett
EVP, Operations . . . . Darrell E. Middleton
EVP, Group Business . . . . Kenneth R. Dallafior
Chief Medical Officer. . . . . Thomas L. Simmer, MD
EVP, Strategy . . . . Lynda M. Rossi

VP & Treasurer. . . . . Carolynn Walton
Corporate Compliance. . . . . Michele A. Samuels

406   Cofinity

28588 Northwestern Highway
Suite 380
Southfield, MI 48034
Toll-Free: 800-831-1166
Fax: 888-499-3957
www.cofinity.net
Subsidiary of: Aetna, Inc.
For Profit Organization: Yes
Year Founded: 1979
Physician Owned Organization: Yes
Total Enrollment: 2,500,000

Healthplan and Services Defined
PLAN TYPE: PPO
Other Type: TPA
Model Type: Network
Plan Specialty: Behavioral Health, Chiropractic, Disease
Management, EPO, Lab, Vision, Radiology, Worker's
Compensation, UR, Medical Management, Medical
Networks, Out-of-Network Claims Mgmt, Fraud & Abuse
Mgmt, Credentialing Services
Benefits Offered: Dental, Prescription, Transplant, Worker's
Compensation

Type of Coverage
Catastrophic Illness Benefit: Varies per case

Type of Payment Plans Offered
FFS

Geographic Areas Served
Statewide

Network Qualifications
Pre-Admission Certification: Yes

Peer Review Type
Utilization Review: Yes
Second Surgical Opinion: Yes
Case Management: Yes

Publishes and Distributes Report Card: No

Accreditation Certification
TJC Accreditation, Medicare Approved, Utilization Review,
Pre-Admission Certification, State Licensure, Quality
Assurance Program

Key Personnel
Executive Director . . . . Paul Lavin
215-280-5986
plavin@ahhinc.com
VP, Business Development . . . . Kara Dornig
VP, Account Management . . . . Susan Korth
619-610-3982
SusanKorth@FirstHealth.com
Wholesale Operations . . . . Ron Gibb
614-933-7354
rgibb@ahhinc.com

Average Claim Compensation
Physician's Fees Charged: 1%

Hospital's Fees Charged: 1%

Specialty Managed Care Partners
Gentiva
Enters into Contracts with Regional Business Coalitions: No

407 ConnectCare

4000 Wellness Drive
Midland, MI 48670
Toll-Free: 888-646-2429
Phone: 989-839-1629
Fax: 989-389-1626
info@connectcare.com
www.connectcare.com
Subsidiary of: MidMichigan Health Network LLC
Non-Profit Organization: Yes
Year Founded: 1993
Physician Owned Organization: Yes
Owned by an Integrated Delivery Network (IDN): Yes
Federally Qualified: No
Number of Affiliated Hospitals: 5,000
Number of Referral/Specialty Physicians: 90,000
Total Enrollment: 17,000
State Enrollment: 36,000

Healthplan and Services Defined
PLAN TYPE: PPO
Model Type: Network
Benefits Offered: Behavioral Health, Dental, Home Care,
Inpatient SNF, Long-Term Care, Physical Therapy,
Podiatry, Prescription, Psychiatric, Wellness

Type of Coverage
Commercial, Indemnity

Type of Payment Plans Offered
POS, DFFS

Geographic Areas Served
Domiciled in central Michigan, with primary counties served
including Clare, Gladwin, Gratiot, Isabella, Midland,
Montcalm and Roscommon. Arrangement with national
PPO's for coverage of downstate and those enrollees residing
outside of Michigan

Subscriber Information
Average Annual Deductible Per Subscriber:
Employee Only (Self): $275.00
Employee & 2 Family Members: $550.00

Network Qualifications
Pre-Admission Certification: Yes

Peer Review Type
Utilization Review: Yes
Second Surgical Opinion: Yes
Case Management: Yes

Accreditation Certification
NCQA
Quality Assurance Program

408 Coventry Health Care of Michigan

1333 Brewery Park Boulevard
Suite 400
Detroit, MI 48207
Phone: 313-465-1500
www.coventryhealthcare.com
Subsidiary of: Aetna Inc.
For Profit Organization: Yes
Year Founded: 1975

Healthplan and Services Defined
PLAN TYPE: HMO/PPO
Model Type: Network
Plan Specialty: Behavioral Health, Dental, Worker's
Compensation
Benefits Offered: Behavioral Health, Dental, Prescription,
Wellness, Worker's Compensation

Type of Coverage
Commercial, Medicare, Medicaid

Geographic Areas Served
Statewide

Key Personnel
Medical Director . . . . Joseph L. Blount

409 Delta Dental of Michigan

4100 Okemos Road
Okemos, MI 48864
Toll-Free: 800-524-0149
www.deltadentalmi.com
Mailing Address: P.O. Box 9089, Farmington Hills, MI
48333-9089
Subsidiary of: Delta Dental Plans Association
Number of Primary Care Physicians: 5,000
Total Enrollment: 14,100,000

Healthplan and Services Defined
PLAN TYPE: Dental
Plan Specialty: Dental
Benefits Offered: Dental

Type of Coverage
Commercial, Individual

Geographic Areas Served
Michigan, Ohio, Indiana and Tennessee

Key Personnel
CEO, Effective Jan 2019 . . . . Goran Jurkovic

410 Dencap Dental Plans

45 E Milwaukee Street
Detroit, MI 48202
Toll-Free: 888-988-3384
Phone: 313-972-1400
Fax: 313-972-4662
info@dencap.com
www.dencap.com
Year Founded: 1984
Number of Primary Care Physicians: 200
State Enrollment: 20,000

Healthplan and Services Defined
PLAN TYPE: Dental
Model Type: Network
Plan Specialty: Dental
Benefits Offered: Dental

Type of Coverage
Commercial, Individual

Type of Payment Plans Offered
DFFS, FFS

Geographic Areas Served
Southeastern Michigan

Subscriber Information
Average Monthly Fee Per Subscriber
(Employee + Employer Contribution):
Employee Only (Self): Varies

Peer Review Type
Case Management: Yes

Publishes and Distributes Report Card: Yes

Accreditation Certification
Utilization Review, Quality Assurance Program

Key Personnel
CEO . . . . Joe Lentine, Jr
Provider Relations Dir . . . . Frank Berge

Specialty Managed Care Partners
Midwest and Dentals, Great Expression

---

411 DenteMax
25925 Telegraph Road
Suite 400
Southfield, MI 48033
Toll-Free: 800-752-1547
Fax: 888-586-0296
customerservices@dentemax.com
www.dentemax.com
Subsidiary of: Dental Network of America
For Profit Organization: Yes
Year Founded: 1985
Number of Primary Care Physicians: 113,000
Total Enrollment: 4,500,000

Healthplan and Services Defined
PLAN TYPE: Dental
Other Type: Dental PPO
Plan Specialty: Dental
Benefits Offered: Dental

Type of Coverage
Commercial, Individual
Catastrophic Illness Benefit: None

Type of Payment Plans Offered
DFFS

Geographic Areas Served
Nationwide

Subscriber Information
Average Monthly Fee Per Subscriber
(Employee + Employer Contribution):

Employee Only (Self): Varies by plan

Network Qualifications
Pre-Admission Certification: No

Peer Review Type
Utilization Review: Yes

Accreditation Certification
Quality Assurance Program

Key Personnel
President/CEO . . . . Melissa Wagner
VP, Dental Networks . . . . Mike Miller
VP, Sales & Marketing . . . . Kim Sharbatz
Regulatory Oversight . . . . Kathy Larking
Dental Director . . . . Dr. Timothy Custer
Network Development . . . . Ignacio Quiaro von Thun

---

412 Golden Dental Plans
29377 Hoover Road
Warren, MI 48093
Phone: 586-573-8118
www.goldendentalplans.com
Year Founded: 1984
Number of Primary Care Physicians: 3,200
Total Enrollment: 130,000

Healthplan and Services Defined
PLAN TYPE: Dental
Other Type: Dental HMO
Model Type: Network
Plan Specialty: Dental
Benefits Offered: Dental

Type of Coverage
Individual

Type of Payment Plans Offered
DFFS

Geographic Areas Served
Statewide

Accreditation Certification
Utilization Review, Pre-Admission Certification

---

413 HAP-Health Alliance Plan: Flint
2050 S Linden Road
Flint, MI 48532
Toll-Free: 800-422-4641
www.hap.org
Secondary Address: 2850 W Grand Boulevard, Detroit, MI
48202, 313-872-8100
Non-Profit Organization: Yes
Year Founded: 1979
Federally Qualified: Yes
Number of Affiliated Hospitals: 29
Number of Primary Care Physicians: 900
Number of Referral/Specialty Physicians: 1,800
Total Enrollment: 650,000
State Enrollment: 650,000

Healthplan and Services Defined
PLAN TYPE: HMO/PPO

Model Type: Network

Plan Specialty: Lab, Radiology

Benefits Offered: Behavioral Health, Chiropractic,
Complementary Medicine, Disease Management, Home
Care, Inpatient SNF, Long-Term Care, Physical Therapy,
Podiatry, Prescription, Psychiatric, Transplant, Vision,
Wellness, Women's Health

Offers Demand Management Patient Information Service:
Yes

Type of Coverage

Commercial, Individual, Medicare, Supplemental Medicare,
Medicaid, Catastrophic, TPA

Catastrophic Illness Benefit: Unlimited

Type of Payment Plans Offered

POS, DFFS, Capitated, Combination FFS & DFFS

Geographic Areas Served

Commercial Product: Bay, Genesee, Huron, Lapeer,
Livingston, Midland, Northern Oakland counties, Saginaw,
Sanilac, Shiawassee, Tuscola. Full counties: Arenac, Sanilac
and St Clair

Subscriber Information

Average Monthly Fee Per Subscriber
(Employee + Employer Contribution):
Employee Only (Self): Varies by plan

Network Qualifications

Pre-Admission Certification: Yes

Peer Review Type

Utilization Review: Yes

Second Surgical Opinion: Yes

Case Management: Yes

Publishes and Distributes Report Card: Yes

Accreditation Certification

NCQA

TJC Accreditation, Medicare Approved, Utilization Review,
Pre-Admission Certification, State Licensure, Quality
Assurance Program

Key Personnel

President/CEO . . . . Teresa Kline

Chief Financial Officer . . . . Richard Swift

VP, Human Resources . . . . Derek Adams

Chief Operating Officer . . . . Mike Treash

Chief Medical Officer . . . . Michael Genord, MD

Specialty Managed Care Partners

American Healthways

Enters into Contracts with Regional Business Coalitions: No

Employer References

General Motors, Delphi, Covenant Health Partners

**414   HAP-Health Alliance Plan: Senior Medicare
Plan**

2850 W Grand Boulevard

Detroit, MI 48202

Toll-Free: 800-422-4641

Phone: 313-872-8100

msweb1@hap.org

www.hap.org

Non-Profit Organization: Yes

Number of Affiliated Hospitals: 29

Number of Primary Care Physicians: 900

Number of Referral/Specialty Physicians: 1,800

Total Enrollment: 14,000

State Enrollment: 14,000

Healthplan and Services Defined

PLAN TYPE: Medicare

Benefits Offered: Chiropractic, Disease Management, Home
Care, Inpatient SNF, Physical Therapy, Podiatry,
Prescription, Psychiatric, Vision, Wellness

Type of Coverage

Individual, Medicare, MIChild

Geographic Areas Served

Health Plus Senior Medicare Coverage Plans available only
within Michigan

Subscriber Information

Average Monthly Fee Per Subscriber
(Employee + Employer Contribution):
Employee Only (Self): Varies
Medicare: Varies

Average Annual Deductible Per Subscriber:
Employee Only (Self): Varies
Medicare: Varies

Average Subscriber Co-Payment:
Primary Care Physician: Varies
Non-Network Physician: Varies
Prescription Drugs: Varies
Hospital ER: Varies
Home Health Care: Varies
Home Health Care Max. Days/Visits Covered: Varies
Nursing Home: Varies
Nursing Home Max. Days/Visits Covered: Varies

---

415   Health Alliance Medicare

2850 W Grand Boulevard

Detroit, MI 48202

Toll-Free: 800-422-4641

Phone: 313-872-8100

msweb1@hap.org

www.hap.org/medicare

Non-Profit Organization: Yes

Total Enrollment: 383,000

Healthplan and Services Defined

PLAN TYPE: Medicare

Other Type: HMO/PPO, POS

Benefits Offered: Chiropractic, Dental, Home Care, Inpatient
SNF, Physical Therapy, Podiatry, Prescription, Psychiatric,
Wellness, Worldwide Emergency, Fitness Benefits, Hearing
Exams, Preventive Services, Eye Exams & Eyeglasses,
Urgent Care, Hospice

Type of Coverage

Individual, Medicare, Group Medicare Plans

Geographic Areas Served

Statewide

Subscriber Information
Average Monthly Fee Per Subscriber
   (Employee + Employer Contribution):
      Employee Only (Self): Varies
      Medicare: Varies
Average Annual Deductible Per Subscriber:
      Employee Only (Self): Varies
      Medicare: Varies
Average Subscriber Co-Payment:
      Primary Care Physician: Varies
      Non-Network Physician: Varies
      Prescription Drugs: Varies
      Hospital ER: Varies
      Home Health Care: Varies
      Home Health Care Max. Days/Visits Covered: Varies
      Nursing Home: Varies
      Nursing Home Max. Days/Visits Covered: Varies

Key Personnel
President/CEO.......................... Teresa Kline

416 Health Alliance Plan
2850 W Grand Boulevard
Detroit, MI 48202
Toll-Free: 800-422-4641
Phone: 313-872-8100
www.hap.org
Non-Profit Organization: Yes
Year Founded: 1979
Number of Affiliated Hospitals: 157
Number of Primary Care Physicians: 18,000
Number of Referral/Specialty Physicians: 1,000
Total Enrollment: 650,000
State Enrollment: 650,000

Healthplan and Services Defined
PLAN TYPE: HMO/PPO
Other Type: EPO
Model Type: Staff
Benefits Offered: Dental, Disease Management, Prescription,
   Vision, Wellness, Alternative Medicine
Offers Demand Management Patient Information Service:
   Yes
DMPI Services Offered: Health Education Classes

Type of Coverage
Commercial, Individual, Medicare, Supplemental Medicare,
   Medicaid, Catastrophic

Type of Payment Plans Offered
POS, Capitated, FFS, Combination FFS & DFFS

Geographic Areas Served
Statewide

Network Qualifications
Pre-Admission Certification: Yes

Peer Review Type
Utilization Review: Yes
Second Surgical Opinion: No
Case Management: Yes

Publishes and Distributes Report Card: Yes

Accreditation Certification
NCQA
TJC Accreditation, Medicare Approved, Utilization Review,
   Pre-Admission Certification, State Licensure, Quality
   Assurance Program

Key Personnel
President/CEO.......................... Teresa Kline
Chief Financial Officer .... Richard Swift
VP, Human Resources .... Derick Adams, Esq.
Chief Operating Officer................... Mike Treash
Chief Medical Officer .... Michael Genord, MD

Specialty Managed Care Partners
Enters into Contracts with Regional Business Coalitions: Yes

417 Humana Health Insurance of Michigan
18610 Fenkell Street
Suite A
Detroit, MI 48223
Toll-Free: 800-649-0059
Phone: 313-437-6532
Fax: 313-273-8375
www.humana.com
For Profit Organization: Yes

Healthplan and Services Defined
PLAN TYPE: HMO/PPO
Plan Specialty: ASO
Benefits Offered: Disease Management, Prescription,
   Wellness

Type of Coverage
Commercial, Individual

Geographic Areas Served
Statewide

Accreditation Certification
URAC, NCQA, CORE

Specialty Managed Care Partners
Caremark Rx

Employer References
Tricare

418 McLaren Health Plan
G-3245 Beecher Road
Flint, MI 48532
Toll-Free: 888-327-0671
Fax: 877-502-1567
www.mclarenhealthplan.org
For Profit Organization: Yes
Year Founded: 2003
Number of Affiliated Hospitals: 14
Number of Primary Care Physicians: 490

Healthplan and Services Defined
PLAN TYPE: HMO
Benefits Offered: Home Care, Prescription, Hospice care

Type of Coverage
Commercial, Medicaid

Geographic Areas Served
Michigan and Indiana

Key Personnel
President/CEO . . . . Nancy Jenkins

---

419 Meridian Health Plan
1 Campus Martius
Suite 700
Detroit, MI 48226
Toll-Free: 888-437-0606
memberservices.mi@mhplan.com
www.mhplan.com
Total Enrollment: 750,000

Healthplan and Services Defined
PLAN TYPE: HMO

Geographic Areas Served
Michigan, Iowa, Illinois, Ohio, Indiana, Kentucky

Accreditation Certification
URAC, NCQA

Key Personnel
President/Chairman . . . . Jon Cotton

---

420 Molina Healthcare of Michigan
880 West Long Lake Road
Troy, MI 48098
Toll-Free: 866-449-6828
Phone: 248-925-1700
www.molinahealthcare.com
Subsidiary of: Molina Healthcare, Inc.
For Profit Organization: Yes
Year Founded: 1980
Physician Owned Organization: Yes

Healthplan and Services Defined
PLAN TYPE: Medicare
Model Type: Network
Plan Specialty: Integrated Medicare/Medicaid (Duals)
Benefits Offered: Chiropractic, Dental, Home Care, Inpatient
SNF, Long-Term Care, Podiatry, Vision

Type of Coverage
Commercial, Medicare, Supplemental Medicare, Medicaid

Accreditation Certification
URAC, NCQA

Key Personnel
Chief Operating Officer . . . . Tonya Wardena
Mgr., Provider Engagement . . . . Josiah Eberle
VP, Provider Network Mgmt . . . . Elyse Berry

---

421 Paramount Care of Michigan
106 Park Place
Dundee, MI 48131
Toll-Free: 888-241-5604
Phone: 734-529-7800
www.paramounthealthcare.com
Secondary Address: 1901 Indian Wood Circle, Maumee, OH
43537, 800-462-3589

Subsidiary of: ProMedica Health System
For Profit Organization: Yes
Year Founded: 1988
Number of Affiliated Hospitals: 34
Number of Primary Care Physicians: 1,900
Total Enrollment: 187,000

Healthplan and Services Defined
PLAN TYPE: HMO/PPO
Benefits Offered: Disease Management, Prescription,
Wellness

Type of Coverage
Commercial, Medicare

Geographic Areas Served
Southeast Michigan

Accreditation Certification
NCQA

Specialty Managed Care Partners
Express Scripts

---

422 Physicians Health Plan of Mid-Michigan
1400 East Michigan Avenue
Lansing, MI 48912
Toll-Free: 800-562-6197
Phone: 517-364-8400
Fax: 517-364-8460
www.phpmichigan.com
Mailing Address: P.O. Box 30377, Lansing, MI 48909-7877
Subsidiary of: Sparrow Health System
Non-Profit Organization: Yes
Year Founded: 1980
Owned by an Integrated Delivery Network (IDN): Yes
Number of Affiliated Hospitals: 31
Number of Primary Care Physicians: 3,100
Total Enrollment: 68,942
State Enrollment: 68,942

Healthplan and Services Defined
PLAN TYPE: HMO/PPO
Model Type: IPA
Plan Specialty: Behavioral Health, Chiropractic, Dental,
Disease Management, Lab, PBM, Vision, Radiology, UR
Benefits Offered: Behavioral Health, Chiropractic, Dental,
Disease Management, Home Care, Inpatient SNF, Physical
Therapy, Podiatry, Prescription, Psychiatric, Transplant,
Vision, Wellness, AD&D, Life, STD, FSA

Type of Coverage
Commercial, Medicaid, Catastrophic, PPO, TPA
Catastrophic Illness Benefit: Unlimited

Type of Payment Plans Offered
POS, DFFS

Geographic Areas Served
Clinton, Eaton, Gratiot, Ionia, Ingham, Isabella, Montcalm,
Saginaw and Shiawassee counties

Subscriber Information
Average Subscriber Co-Payment:
Primary Care Physician: $10.00
Non-Network Physician: 20%

Prescription Drugs: $10.00/25.00/40.00
Hospital ER: $50.00
Home Health Care: $0
Nursing Home: $0
Nursing Home Max. Days/Visits Covered: 100

Network Qualifications
Pre-Admission Certification: Yes

Peer Review Type
Utilization Review: Yes
Second Surgical Opinion: Yes
Case Management: Yes

Publishes and Distributes Report Card: No

Accreditation Certification
URAC, NCQA
Medicare Approved, Utilization Review, Pre-Admission
Certification, State Licensure, Quality Assurance Program

Key Personnel
President/CEO........................ Dennis J Reese
Chair .... James Butler, III

Specialty Managed Care Partners
United Behavioral Health
Enters into Contracts with Regional Business Coalitions: No

---

423   Priority Health
1231 E Beltline Avenue NE
Grand Rapids, MI 49525-4501
Toll-Free: 800-942-0954
Phone: 616-942-0954
www.priorityhealth.com
Non-Profit Organization: Yes
Year Founded: 1985
Physician Owned Organization: Yes
Owned by an Integrated Delivery Network (IDN): Yes
Federally Qualified: No
Number of Affiliated Hospitals: 5,000
Number of Referral/Specialty Physicians: 617,000
Total Enrollment: 596,220

Healthplan and Services Defined
PLAN TYPE: HMO
Model Type: IPA
Plan Specialty: ASO, Behavioral Health, Chiropractic,
Dental, Disease Management, EPO, Lab, MSO, PBM,
Vision, Radiology, UR
Benefits Offered: Behavioral Health, Chiropractic,
Complementary Medicine, Dental, Disease Management,
Home Care, Inpatient SNF, Long-Term Care, Physical
Therapy, Podiatry, Prescription, Psychiatric, Transplant,
Vision, Wellness, AD&D, Life, LTD, STD
Offers Demand Management Patient Information Service: No

Type of Coverage
Commercial, Individual, Indemnity, Medicare, Medicaid
Catastrophic Illness Benefit: Varies per case

Type of Payment Plans Offered
DFFS, Capitated, FFS, Combination FFS & DFFS

Geographic Areas Served
69 counties in Michigan

Subscriber Information
Average Monthly Fee Per Subscriber
(Employee + Employer Contribution):
Employee Only (Self): Varies
Employee & 1 Family Member: Varies
Employee & 2 Family Members: Varies
Medicare: Varies
Average Annual Deductible Per Subscriber:
Employee Only (Self): Varies
Employee & 1 Family Member: Varies
Employee & 2 Family Members: Varies
Medicare: Varies
Average Subscriber Co-Payment:
Primary Care Physician: Varies
Non-Network Physician: Varies
Prescription Drugs: Varies
Hospital ER: Varies
Home Health Care: Varies
Home Health Care Max. Days/Visits Covered: Varies
Nursing Home: Varies
Nursing Home Max. Days/Visits Covered: Varies

Network Qualifications
Pre-Admission Certification: No

Peer Review Type
Utilization Review: Yes
Case Management: Yes

Publishes and Distributes Report Card: No

Accreditation Certification
NCQA
Utilization Review, Pre-Admission Certification, State
Licensure, Quality Assurance Program

Key Personnel
President/CEO .... Joan Budden
SVP, Finance/Operations .... Mary Anne Jones
Chief Actuary .... Jian Yu
General Counsel .... Kimberly Thomas
Chief Medical Officer .... James D. Forshee, MD

Specialty Managed Care Partners
Enters into Contracts with Regional Business Coalitions: Yes
National Federation of Independent Business

---

424   PriorityHealth Medicare Plans
1231 E Beltline NE
Grand Rapids, MI 49525-4501
Toll-Free: 800-942-0954
Phone: 616-942-0954
www.priorityhealth.com/medicare
Subsidiary of: PriorityHealth

Healthplan and Services Defined
PLAN TYPE: Medicare
Benefits Offered: Chiropractic, Dental, Disease Management,
Home Care, Inpatient SNF, Physical Therapy, Podiatry,
Prescription, Psychiatric, Vision, Wellness

Type of Coverage
Individual, Medicare

Geographic Areas Served
Statewide

Subscriber Information
Average Monthly Fee Per Subscriber
(Employee + Employer Contribution):
Employee Only (Self): Varies
Medicare: Varies
Average Annual Deductible Per Subscriber:
Employee Only (Self): Varies
Medicare: Varies
Average Subscriber Co-Payment:
Primary Care Physician: Varies
Non-Network Physician: Varies
Prescription Drugs: Varies
Hospital ER: Varies
Home Health Care: Varies
Home Health Care Max. Days/Visits Covered: Varies
Nursing Home: Varies
Nursing Home Max. Days/Visits Covered: Varies

Accreditation Certification
NCQA

Key Personnel
President and CEO . . . . Joan Budden
Chief Financial Officer . . . . Mary Anne Jones
Chief Operating Officer . . . . Michael Koziara
VP, General Counsel. . . . . Kimberly Thomas

425 SVS Vision
118 Cass Avenue
Mount Clemens, MI 48043
Toll-Free: 800-787-4600
customerservice@svsvision.com
www.svsvision.com
For Profit Organization: Yes
Year Founded: 1974
Total Enrollment: 390,000

Healthplan and Services Defined
PLAN TYPE: Vision
Other Type: Vision Plan
Plan Specialty: Vision
Benefits Offered: Vision, Services limited to vision care

Type of Payment Plans Offered
DFFS

Geographic Areas Served
Michigan; Illinois; Ohio; Indiana; Kentucky; Missouri;
Georgia; New York

Subscriber Information
Average Monthly Fee Per Subscriber
(Employee + Employer Contribution):
Employee Only (Self): Varies by plan

Network Qualifications
Pre-Admission Certification: Yes

Peer Review Type
Utilization Review: Yes
Second Surgical Opinion: Yes
Case Management: Yes

Key Personnel
President/CFO . . . . Kenneth Stann
CEO . . . . Robert G. Farrell, Jr.
EVP/COO. . . . . Lisa Stann

426 Total Health Care
3011 W Grand Boulevard
Suite 1600
Detroit, MI 48202
Toll-Free: 800-826-2862
Phone: 313-871-2000
www.thcmi.com
Non-Profit Organization: Yes
Year Founded: 1973
Owned by an Integrated Delivery Network (IDN): Yes
Number of Affiliated Hospitals: 28
Total Enrollment: 90,000
State Enrollment: 90,000

Healthplan and Services Defined
PLAN TYPE: HMO
Other Type: PPN, POS
Model Type: Staff
Plan Specialty: Lab, Radiology
Benefits Offered: Behavioral Health, Chiropractic,
Complementary
Medicine, Disease Management, Home Care, Inpatient
SNF, Long-Term Care, Physical Therapy, Podiatry,
Prescription, Psychiatric, Transplant, Vision,
Wellness, Worker's Compensation, Alternative
Treatments, Durable Medical Equipment, Speech, OT
24-hour Nurse Advice Line
Offers Demand Management Patient Information Service: Yes
DMPI Services Offered: Educational Classes and Programs

Type of Coverage
Commercial, Individual, Medicare, Medicaid

Type of Payment Plans Offered
Combination FFS & DFFS

Subscriber Information
Average Monthly Fee Per Subscriber
(Employee + Employer Contribution):
Employee Only (Self): $67.12
Employee & 2 Family Members: $164.88
Average Subscriber Co-Payment:
Primary Care Physician: $10.00
Hospital ER: $40.00

Accreditation Certification
TJC, NCQA

Key Personnel
Chief Executive Officer. . . . . Randy Narowitz
Office Manager . . . . Nancy Kowal
Medical Director . . . . Robyn James Arrington Jr, MD

Specialty Managed Care Partners
RxAmerica

Employer References
Federal Government, State of Michigan, American Airlines,
Detroit Board of Education, Wayne County Employees

427   Trinity Health
20555 Victor Parkway
Livonia, MI 48152-7018
Phone: 734-343-1000
www.trinity-health.org
Subsidiary of: Trinity Health
Non-Profit Organization: Yes
Year Founded: 2013
Number of Affiliated Hospitals: 86
Number of Primary Care Physicians: 3,600
Total Enrollment: 30,000,000

Healthplan and Services Defined
 PLAN TYPE: Other
 Benefits Offered: Disease Management, Home Care,
  Long-Term Care, Psychiatric, Hospice programs, PACE
  (Program of All Inclusive Care for the Elderly)

Geographic Areas Served
 California, Connecticut, Delaware, Florida, Georgia, Idaho,
 Illinois, Indiana, Iowa, Nebraska, Maryland, Massachusetts,
 Michigan, New Jersey, New York, Ohio, and Pennsylvania

Key Personnel
 Chief Executive Officer . . . . Richard J. Gilfillan
 Chief Financial Officer. . . . . Benjamin R. Carter
 Human Resources. . . . . Edmund F. Hodge
 EVP, Chief Legal Officer. . . . . Paul G. Neumann
 Chief Clinical Officer . . . . Daniel J. Roth
 Chief Operating Officer . . . . Michael A. Slubowski

428   Trinity Health of Michigan
Saint Joseph Mercy Health System
5301 McAuley Drive
Ypsilanti, MI 48197
Phone: 734-712-3456
www.trinity-health.org
Secondary Address: Mercy Health, 200 Jefferson Avenue SE,
 Grand Rapids, MI 49503, 616-685-5000
Subsidiary of: Trinity Health
Non-Profit Organization: Yes
Year Founded: 2013
Total Enrollment: 30,000,000

Healthplan and Services Defined
 PLAN TYPE: Other
 Benefits Offered: Disease Management, Home Care,
  Long-Term Care, Psychiatric, Hospice programs, PACE
  (Program of All Inclusive Care for the Elderly)

Geographic Areas Served
 Statewide

Key Personnel
 President/CEO. . . . . Rob Casalou
 Chief Financial Officer . . . . Michael Gusho
 Chief HR Officer . . . . An, McNeil
 VP, Development. . . . . Fran Patonic
 Chief Marketing Officer. . . . . Michele Szczypka
 VP, Strategy. . . . . Steve Paulus

429   UniCare Michigan
3200 Greenfield Road
Dearborn, MI 48120
Phone: 313-336-5550
www.unicare.com
Subsidiary of: Anthem, Inc.
For Profit Organization: Yes
Year Founded: 1995

Healthplan and Services Defined
 PLAN TYPE: HMO
 Model Type: Network
 Benefits Offered: Behavioral Health, Chiropractic,
  Complementary Medicine, Dental, Disease Management,
  Home Care, Inpatient SNF, Long-Term Care, Physical
  Therapy, Podiatry, Prescription, Psychiatric, Transplant,
  Vision, Wellness, Life

Type of Coverage
 Commercial, Individual, Supplemental Medicare, Medicaid

Geographic Areas Served
 Statewide

Network Qualifications
 Pre-Admission Certification: Yes

Peer Review Type
 Utilization Review: Yes
 Second Surgical Opinion: Yes
 Case Management: Yes

Publishes and Distributes Report Card: Yes

Accreditation Certification
 URAC, NCQA
 TJC Accreditation, Utilization Review, Pre-Admission
  Certification, State Licensure, Quality Assurance Program

Specialty Managed Care Partners
 WellPoint Pharmacy Management, WellPoint Dental Services,
  WellPoint Behavioral Health
 Enters into Contracts with Regional Business Coalitions: Yes

430   United Concordia of Michigan
4401 Deer Path Road
Harrisburg, PA 17110
Phone: 717-260-6800
www.unitedconcordia.com
For Profit Organization: Yes
Year Founded: 1971
Total Enrollment: 7,800,000

Healthplan and Services Defined
 PLAN TYPE: Dental
 Plan Specialty: Dental
 Benefits Offered: Dental

Type of Coverage
 Commercial, Individual, Military personnel & families

Geographic Areas Served
 Nationwide

Accreditation Certification
 URAC

Key Personnel
Contact. . . . . Beth Rutherford
717-260-7659
beth.rutherford@ucci.com

---

431 UnitedHealthcare Great Lakes Health Plan
26957 Northwestern Highway
Suite 400
Southfield, MI 48033
www.glhp.com/mi.html
Subsidiary of: UnitedHealth Group
For Profit Organization: Yes
Year Founded: 1994
State Enrollment: 235,000

Healthplan and Services Defined
PLAN TYPE: HMO
Plan Specialty: Case Management
Benefits Offered: Disease Management, Home Care, Physical Therapy, Prescription, Vision, Wellness, Hearing, Labs & X-rays, Diabetic Support

Type of Coverage
Medicare, Medicaid, MIChild

Type of Payment Plans Offered
DFFS, Capitated

Geographic Areas Served
Allegan, Berrien, Branch, Calhoun, Cass, Hillsdale, Huron, Jackson, Kalamazoo, Kent, Lenawee, Livingston, Macomb, Monroe, Muskegon, Oakland, Oceana, Ottawa, Saginaw, Sanilac, St. Clair, St. Joseph, Tuscola, Van Buren and Wayne counties

Publishes and Distributes Report Card: No

Accreditation Certification
TJC
Utilization Review

Key Personnel
Chief Executive Officer. . . . . David Wichmann
Chief Operating Officer . . . . Dan Schumacher
Chief Strategy Officer . . . . John Cosgriff
Communications Officer . . . . Kirsten Gorsuch
Chief Medical Officer. . . . . Sam Ho
Chief Legal Officer . . . . Thad Johnson
Chief Information. . . . . Phil McKoy

Specialty Managed Care Partners
Rx America
Enters into Contracts with Regional Business Coalitions: No

---

432 UnitedHealthcare of Michigan
143 S Kalamazoo Mall
Kalamazoo, MI 49007
Toll-Free: 888-545-5205
Phone: 269-345-2561
www.uhc.com
Subsidiary of: UnitedHealth Group
Year Founded: 1977

Healthplan and Services Defined
PLAN TYPE: HMO/PPO

Model Type: Network
Plan Specialty: Behavioral Health, Dental, Disease Management, Lab, PBM, Vision, Radiology
Benefits Offered: Behavioral Health, Chiropractic, Dental, Disease Management, Physical Therapy, Prescription, Vision, Wellness, AD&D, Life, LTD, STD

Type of Coverage
Commercial, Individual, Indemnity, Medicare, Supplemental Medicare, Medicaid, Catastrophic, Family, Military, Veterans, Group,

Geographic Areas Served
Statewide

Network Qualifications
Pre-Admission Certification: Yes

Peer Review Type
Utilization Review: Yes
Second Surgical Opinion: Yes
Case Management: Yes

Publishes and Distributes Report Card: Yes

Accreditation Certification
TJC, NCQA

Key Personnel
President/CEO, WI/MI . . . . Dustin Hinton

Specialty Managed Care Partners
Enters into Contracts with Regional Business Coalitions: Yes

---

433 Upper Peninsula Health Plan
853 W Washington Street
Marquette, MI 49855
Toll-Free: 800-835-2556
Phone: 906-225-7500
Fax: 906-225-7690
uphpwebmaster@uphp.com
www.uphp.com
Year Founded: 1998
Total Enrollment: 47,000
State Enrollment: 47,000

Healthplan and Services Defined
PLAN TYPE: HMO

Type of Coverage
Medicaid

Accreditation Certification
NCQA

Key Personnel
Chief Executive Officer. . . . . Melissa Holmquist
Chief Quality Officer. . . . . Anne Levandoski
Corporate Communications . . . . Carly Harrington
906-225-7158
charrington@uphp.com

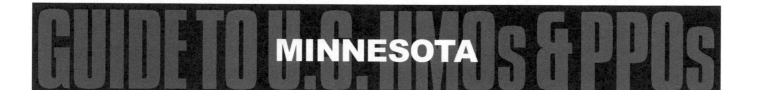
Health Insurance Coverage Status and Type of Coverage by Age

Category	All Persons		Under 18 years		Under 65 years	
	Number	%	Number	%	Number	%
Total population	5,519	-	1,373	-	4,690	-
Covered by some type of health insurance	5,277 *(11)*	95.6 *(0.2)*	1,326 *(5)*	96.6 *(0.3)*	4,450 *(10)*	94.9 *(0.2)*
Covered by private health insurance	4,193 *(19)*	76.0 *(0.3)*	973 *(10)*	70.9 *(0.7)*	3,612 *(19)*	77.0 *(0.4)*
Employer-based	3,455 *(19)*	62.6 *(0.3)*	889 *(9)*	64.7 *(0.7)*	3,239 *(17)*	69.1 *(0.4)*
Direct purchase	847 *(13)*	15.3 *(0.2)*	91 *(6)*	6.6 *(0.4)*	434 *(12)*	9.2 *(0.3)*
TRICARE	77 *(5)*	1.4 *(0.1)*	13 *(2)*	1.0 *(0.2)*	46 *(4)*	1.0 *(0.1)*
Covered by public health insurance	1,820 *(17)*	33.0 *(0.3)*	415 *(10)*	30.2 *(0.7)*	1,014 *(17)*	21.6 *(0.4)*
Medicaid	986 *(16)*	17.9 *(0.3)*	413 *(10)*	30.1 *(0.7)*	913 *(16)*	19.5 *(0.3)*
Medicare	912 *(5)*	16.5 *(0.1)*	4 *(1)*	0.3 *(0.1)*	107 *(5)*	2.3 *(0.1)*
VA Care	142 *(4)*	2.6 *(0.1)*	1 *(1)*	0.1 *(Z)*	51 *(4)*	1.1 *(0.1)*
Not covered at any time during the year	243 *(11)*	4.4 *(0.2)*	47 *(4)*	3.4 *(0.3)*	240 *(10)*	5.1 *(0.2)*

Note: Numbers in thousands; Figures cover civilian noninstitutionalized population in 2017; N/A indicates that data was not available; Z represents or rounds to zero; Margin of error appears in parenthesis and is calculated using replicate weights.
Source: U.S. Census Bureau, American Community Survey, Table HIC-4_ACS. Health Insurance Coverage Status and Type of Coverage by State—All People: 2008 to 2017, Table HIC-5_ACS. Health Insurance Coverage Status and Type of Coverage by State—Children Under 18: 2008 to 2017, Table HIC-6_ACS. Health Insurance Coverage Status and Type of Coverage by State—Persons Under 65: 2008 to 2017

Minnesota

434 Aetna Health of Minnesota

151 Farmington Avenue
Hartford, CT 06156
Toll-Free: 800-872-3862
Phone: 860-273-0123
www.aetna.com
Subsidiary of: Aetna Inc.
For Profit Organization: Yes

Healthplan and Services Defined
PLAN TYPE: PPO
Other Type: POS
Benefits Offered: Dental, Currently not marketing medical

Type of Coverage
Commercial, Student Health

Type of Payment Plans Offered
POS, DFFS, Combination FFS & DFFS

Geographic Areas Served
Statewide

Peer Review Type
Second Surgical Opinion: Yes
Case Management: Yes

Accreditation Certification
AAAHC, URAC
TJC Accreditation

435 Americas PPO

7201 W 78th Street
Suite 100
Bloomington, MN 55439
Phone: 952-806-1200
www.americasppo.com
Subsidiary of: Araz Group Inc
For Profit Organization: Yes
Year Founded: 1982
Physician Owned Organization: No
Number of Affiliated Hospitals: 260
Number of Primary Care Physicians: 18,000
Number of Referral/Specialty Physicians: 71,000
State Enrollment: 245,000

Healthplan and Services Defined
PLAN TYPE: PPO
Model Type: Staff, Group
Benefits Offered: Behavioral Health, Wellness, Worker's
    Compensation, Maternity
Offers Demand Management Patient Information Service: No

Type of Coverage
Commercial, Individual, Medicaid
Catastrophic Illness Benefit: Maximum $1M

Type of Payment Plans Offered
DFFS, Capitated

Geographic Areas Served
Minnesota, South Dakota, North Dakota, Western Wisconsin

Subscriber Information
Average Monthly Fee Per Subscriber
    (Employee + Employer Contribution):
        Employee Only (Self): Varies by plan
Average Annual Deductible Per Subscriber:
    Employee Only (Self): $500.00
    Employee & 1 Family Member: $500.00
    Employee & 2 Family Members: $750.00
Average Subscriber Co-Payment:
    Primary Care Physician: $15.00
    Non-Network Physician: $500.00-1000.00
    Prescription Drugs: $10.00/15.00
    Hospital ER: $150.00
    Nursing Home: Varies

Network Qualifications
Pre-Admission Certification: Yes

Peer Review Type
Utilization Review: Yes
Case Management: Yes

Publishes and Distributes Report Card: No

Accreditation Certification
URAC
TJC Accreditation, Utilization Review, Pre-Admission
    Certification, State Licensure, Quality Assurance Program

Key Personnel
President . . . . Amir Eftekhari
Founder and CEO. . . . . Nazie Eftekhari

Specialty Managed Care Partners
Enters into Contracts with Regional Business Coalitions: Yes

436 Avesis: Minnesota

904 Oak Pond Court
Sartell, MN 56377
Toll-Free: 888-363-1377
www.avesis.com
Subsidiary of: Guardian Life Insurance Co.
Year Founded: 1978
Number of Primary Care Physicians: 25,000
Total Enrollment: 3,500,000

Healthplan and Services Defined
PLAN TYPE: PPO
Other Type: Vision, Dental
Model Type: Network
Plan Specialty: Dental, Vision, Hearing
Benefits Offered: Dental, Vision

Type of Coverage
Commercial

Type of Payment Plans Offered
POS, Capitated, Combination FFS & DFFS

Geographic Areas Served
Nationwide and Puerto Rico

Publishes and Distributes Report Card: Yes

Accreditation Certification
AAAHC
TJC Accreditation

Key Personnel
VP, Regional Sales. . . . . James Wegleitner

437 Blue Cross & Blue Shield of Minnesota

3433 Broadway St NE
Suite 500
Minneapolis, MN 55413
Toll-Free: 800-382-2000
Phone: 651-662-8000
www.bluecrossmn.com
Mailing Address: P.O. Box 64560, St. Paul, MN 55164-0560
Subsidiary of: Blue Cross Blue Shield
Non-Profit Organization: Yes
Year Founded: 1933
Owned by an Integrated Delivery Network (IDN): Yes
Number of Affiliated Hospitals: 30
Number of Primary Care Physicians: 8,000
Total Enrollment: 2,700,000
State Enrollment: 2,700,000

Healthplan and Services Defined
PLAN TYPE: HMO
Model Type: Network
Plan Specialty: Medical
Benefits Offered: Disease Management, Prescription,
Wellness, Life

Type of Coverage
Individual, Medicare, Supplemental Medicare

Geographic Areas Served
Statewide

Network Qualifications
Pre-Admission Certification: Yes

Peer Review Type
Utilization Review: Yes
Second Surgical Opinion: Yes

Publishes and Distributes Report Card: Yes

Accreditation Certification
URAC, NCQA

Key Personnel
President & CEO . . . . Craig E. Samitt
SVP, Health Services . . . . Garrett Black
SVP, Chief Legal Officer . . . . Scott Lynch
EVP/COO. . . . . Cain A. Hayes
SVP, Government Programs . . . . Kurt C. Small
SVP, Chief Financial Offc . . . . Jay Matushak
SVP/CMO . . . . Glenn Pomerantz
Chief Strategy Officer . . . . Rochelle Myers
SVP, Human Resources. . . . . Ruth Hafoka
SVP, Operations . . . . Ellen Vonderhaar

Specialty Managed Care Partners
Enters into Contracts with Regional Business Coalitions: No

Employer References
General Mills/Pillsbury, Northwest Airlines, Target

438 Coventry Health Care of Minnesota

6720-B Rockledge Drive
Suite 800
Bethesda, MD 20817
Phone: 301-581-0600
www.coventryhealthcare.com
Subsidiary of: Aetna Inc.
For Profit Organization: Yes

Healthplan and Services Defined
PLAN TYPE: HMO/PPO
Model Type: Network
Plan Specialty: Behavioral Health, Dental, Worker's
Compensation
Benefits Offered: Behavioral Health, Dental, Prescription,
Wellness, Worker's Compensation

Type of Coverage
Commercial, Medicare, Medicaid

Geographic Areas Served
Statewide

439 Delta Dental of Minnesota

500 Washington Avenue S
Minneapolis, MN 55415
Toll-Free: 800-553-9536
www.deltadentalmn.org
Non-Profit Organization: Yes
Year Founded: 1969

Healthplan and Services Defined
PLAN TYPE: Dental
Other Type: Dental PPO
Model Type: Network
Plan Specialty: ASO, Dental
Benefits Offered: Dental

Type of Coverage
Commercial, Individual, Group
Catastrophic Illness Benefit: None

Geographic Areas Served
Minnesota and North Dakota

Key Personnel
President/CEO . . . . Rodney Young
SVP/CFO. . . . . Tamera Robinson
SVP/COO/CIO . . . . Michael McGuire
VP/General Counsel . . . . Stephanie Albert
VP, Sales . . . . David Anderson
VP, Medical Services . . . . Eileen Crespo, MD
VP, Marketing. . . . . Sarah Leeth
VP, Human Resources . . . . Judy Peterson
Media Contact . . . . Clarise Tushie-Lessard
612-224-3341
ctushie-lessard@deltadentalmn.org

440 HealthEZ

7201 West 78th Street
Bloomington, MN 55439
Toll-Free: 800-948-9450
Phone: 952-896-1208
service@healthez.com
www.healthez.com
For Profit Organization: Yes
Year Founded: 1982
Number of Primary Care Physicians: 71,000

Healthplan and Services Defined
 PLAN TYPE: PPO
 Other Type: Dental, Vision, Life
 Benefits Offered: Dental, Disease Management, Prescription,
 Psychiatric, Vision, Wellness, Life, HSA, Case
 management, High-risk maternity management

Type of Coverage
 Individual

Geographic Areas Served
 Minnesota, North Dakota, and South Dakota

Key Personnel
 President . . . . Amir Eftekhari
 952-896-1204
 amir.eftekhari@healthez.com
 Founder/CEO . . . . Nazie Eftekhari
 VP, Care Management. . . . . Joann Damawand
 Mgr., Claims/Operations . . . . Dawn Potter
 VP, Medical Affairs. . . . . Brian Ebeling, MD
 Medical Director . . . . Maria A. Shah, MD
 Provider Relations . . . . Matthew Parker

441 HealthPartners

8170 33rd Avenue S
Bloomington, MN 55425
Toll-Free: 800-883-2177
Phone: 952-883-6000
www.healthpartners.com
Non-Profit Organization: Yes
Year Founded: 1957
Owned by an Integrated Delivery Network (IDN): Yes

Healthplan and Services Defined
 PLAN TYPE: HMO
 Model Type: Staff, Network
 Benefits Offered: Behavioral Health, Chiropractic, Dental,
 Disease Management, Home Care, Inpatient SNF, Physical
 Therapy, Prescription, Psychiatric, Transplant, Vision,
 Worker's Compensation

Type of Coverage
 Commercial, Individual, Indemnity, Medicare, Supplemental
 Medicare, Medicaid
 Catastrophic Illness Benefit: Unlimited

Type of Payment Plans Offered
 POS, Combination FFS & DFFS

Geographic Areas Served
 Minnesota and 8 counties in Northwestern Wisconsin

Peer Review Type
 Utilization Review: Yes
 Case Management: Yes

Accreditation Certification
 URAC, NCQA

Key Personnel
 President & CEO. . . . . Andrea Walsh
 EVP, Chief Admin Officer . . . . Kathy Cooney
 SVP, General Counsel . . . . Barb Tretheway
 Chief Operating Officer . . . . Nance McClure
 Co-Medical Officer. . . . . Steven Connelly
 Co-Medical Officer. . . . . Brian Rank
 SVP, Human Resources. . . . . Calvin Allen

Specialty Managed Care Partners
 Alere, Accordant, RMS
 Enters into Contracts with Regional Business Coalitions: Yes

Employer References
 University of MN, St Paul Public Schools, The College of St
 Catherine

442 Hennepin Health

Minneapolis Grain Exchange Building
400 South Fourth Street, Suite 201
Minneapolis, MN 55415
Phone: 612-596-1036
hennepinhealth@hennepin.us
www.hennepinhealth.org
Non-Profit Organization: Yes
Year Founded: 2012
Total Enrollment: 10,500

Healthplan and Services Defined
 PLAN TYPE: HMO
 Model Type: Network
 Benefits Offered: Behavioral Health, Chiropractic, Dental,
 Disease Management, Home Care, Podiatry, Prescription,
 Psychiatric, Vision, Substance Abuse Care; Hearing;
 Durable Medical Equipment; Family Planning

Type of Coverage
 Medicaid

Type of Payment Plans Offered
 Combination FFS & DFFS

Geographic Areas Served
 Hennepin County

Subscriber Information
 Average Subscriber Co-Payment:
  Primary Care Physician: $0
  Non-Network Physician: $0
  Home Health Care: $0
  Nursing Home: $0

Peer Review Type
 Utilization Review: Yes
 Case Management: Yes

Key Personnel
 Chief Executive Officer . . . . Shannon Mayer
 Chief Financial Officer. . . . . Abdirahman Abdi
 Medical Director . . . . Marc Manley

443 Humana Health Insurance of Minnesota

12600 Whitewater Drive
Suite 150
Minnetonka, MN 55343
Toll-Free: 877-367-6990
Phone: 952-253-3540
Fax: 952-938-2787
www.humana.com
Subsidiary of: Humana
For Profit Organization: Yes

Healthplan and Services Defined
  PLAN TYPE: HMO/PPO
  Model Type: Network
  Plan Specialty: Dental, Vision
  Benefits Offered: Dental, Vision, Life, LTD, STD

Type of Coverage
  Commercial, Individual

Geographic Areas Served
  Statewide

Accreditation Certification
  URAC, NCQA, CORE

Key Personnel
  Market Sales Director . . . . Jan Mudd

444 Medica

401 Carlson Parkway
Minnetonka, MN 55305
Toll-Free: 800-952-3455
Phone: 952-945-8000
www.medica.com
Subsidiary of: Medica Holding Company
Non-Profit Organization: Yes
Year Founded: 1975
Total Enrollment: 1,700,000

Healthplan and Services Defined
  PLAN TYPE: HMO
  Model Type: IPA
  Benefits Offered: Behavioral Health, Disease Management,
    Prescription

Type of Coverage
  Commercial, Individual, Medicare, Supplemental Medicare,
    Pet insurance

Type of Payment Plans Offered
  FFS

Geographic Areas Served
  Iowa, Kansas, Minnesota, Nebraska, North Dakota, and
  Wisconsin

Peer Review Type
  Utilization Review: Yes
  Second Surgical Opinion: Yes
  Case Management: Yes

Publishes and Distributes Report Card: Yes

Accreditation Certification
  NCQA

TJC Accreditation, Medicare Approved, Utilization Review,
  Pre-Admission Certification, State Licensure, Quality
  Assurance Program

Key Personnel
  President & CEO . . . . John Naylor
  SVP, Financial Officer . . . . Mark Baird
  VP, Human Resources . . . . Lynn Altmann
  SVP, General Counsel . . . . Jim Jacobson
  VP, Operations . . . . Kimberly Branson
  VP, General Manager . . . . Geoff Bartsh
  SVP, Government Programs. . . . . Tom Lindquist
  SVP, Marketing . . . . Rob Longendyke
  Chief Information Officer . . . . Tim Thull
  SVP, Medical Officer. . . . . John R. Mach, Jr., MD

Average Claim Compensation
  Physician's Fees Charged: 65%
  Hospital's Fees Charged: 60%

445 National Imaging Associates

7805 Hudson Road
Suite 190
St Paul, MN 55125
Toll-Free: 877-NIA-9762
www.niahealthcare.com
Subsidiary of: Magellan Healthcare
For Profit Organization: Yes
Year Founded: 1995
Number of Referral/Specialty Physicians: 4,000

Healthplan and Services Defined
  PLAN TYPE: PPO
  Model Type: Network
  Plan Specialty: Lab, Radiology
  Benefits Offered: Disease Management

Type of Coverage
  Commercial, Indemnity, Medicare, Medicaid

Type of Payment Plans Offered
  POS, DFFS, Capitated, FFS, Combination FFS & DFFS

Geographic Areas Served
  North Dakota, South Dakota, Minnesota, Wisconsin, Illinois,
  Indiana, Ohio, Michigan, Kentucky, Iowa, Missouri, Montana,
  Idaho, Nebraska, Tennessee, Kansas, Oklahoma, Utah,
  Arkansas, Arizona, Georgia, Texas, Alabama

Peer Review Type
  Utilization Review: Yes

Publishes and Distributes Report Card: Yes

Accreditation Certification
  TJC, NCQA

Key Personnel
  Chief Medical Officer. . . . . Michael J. Pentecost, MD
  SVP, Clinical Services . . . . David Hodges
  SVP, Sales . . . . Edie Jardine
  Vice President, Finance . . . . William F. Henderson

Specialty Managed Care Partners
  Enters into Contracts with Regional Business Coalitions: Yes

446   Optum Complex Medical Conditions

MN Office 102
11000 Optum Circle
Eden Prairie, MN 55344
Toll-Free: 877-801-3507
cmc_client_services@optum.com
www.myoptumhealthcomplexmedical.com
Subsidiary of: UnitedHealth Group
For Profit Organization: Yes
Year Founded: 1986

Healthplan and Services Defined
    PLAN TYPE: Multiple
    Model Type: Network
    Plan Specialty: Complex medical conditions including
        transplantation, cancer, kidney disease, congenital heart
        disease and infertility.

Type of Payment Plans Offered
    POS, Capitated, FFS

Geographic Areas Served
    Nationwide

Peer Review Type
    Utilization Review: Yes
    Case Management: Yes

Publishes and Distributes Report Card: Yes

Accreditation Certification
    URAC
    Utilization Review, Quality Assurance Program

Key Personnel
    Senior Vice President . . . . John DeSmet
    SVP, Network Solutions. . . . . Kevin O'Brien
    VP, Transplant Solutions. . . . . Heather Zick
    Chief Medical Officer . . . . Jon Friedman, MD

Specialty Managed Care Partners
    Enters into Contracts with Regional Business Coalitions: Yes

447   Spirit Dental & Vision

55 5th Street E
Suite 500
St. Paul, MN 55101
Toll-Free: 844-833-8440
www.spiritdental.com
Subsidiary of: Direct Benefits Inc.
For Profit Organization: Yes

Healthplan and Services Defined
    PLAN TYPE: Dental
    Plan Specialty: Dental, Vision
    Benefits Offered: Dental, Vision

Geographic Areas Served
    statewide

Key Personnel
    President . . . . Tom Mayer

448   UCare

500 Stinson Boulevard NE
Minneapolis, MN 55413
Phone: 612-676-6500
www.ucare.org
Secondary Address: 4310 Menard Drive, Suite 600,
    Hermantown, MN 55811, 218-336-4260
Non-Profit Organization: Yes
Year Founded: 1984
Owned by an Integrated Delivery Network (IDN): Yes
Number of Primary Care Physicians: 43,000
Total Enrollment: 147,000

Healthplan and Services Defined
    PLAN TYPE: Multiple
    Model Type: Network
    Benefits Offered: Behavioral Health, Chiropractic, Dental,
        Disease Management, Home Care, Inpatient SNF, Physical
        Therapy, Podiatry, Prescription, Psychiatric, Transplant,
        Vision, Wellness, Disability Plans available

Type of Coverage
    Medicare, Supplemental Medicare, Medicaid
    Catastrophic Illness Benefit: Unlimited

Type of Payment Plans Offered
    POS

Geographic Areas Served
    Statewide

Network Qualifications
    Pre-Admission Certification: Yes

Peer Review Type
    Utilization Review: Yes
    Second Surgical Opinion: Yes
    Case Management: Yes

Publishes and Distributes Report Card: Yes

Accreditation Certification
    NCQA
    Medicare Approved, Utilization Review, Pre-Admission
        Certification, State Licensure, Quality Assurance Program

Key Personnel
    President/CEO. . . . . Mark Traynor
    SVP/CAO . . . . Hilary Marden-Resnik
    SVP/CFO . . . . Beth Monsrud
    SVP, Public Affiars/Mkt . . . . Ghita Worcester

Specialty Managed Care Partners
    Enters into Contracts with Regional Business Coalitions: Yes

449   UnitedHealth Group

P.O. Box 1459
Minneapolis, MN 55440-1459
Toll-Free: 800-328-5979
www.unitedhealthgroup.com
For Profit Organization: Yes
Year Founded: 1974
Total Enrollment: 70,000,000

Healthplan and Services Defined
    PLAN TYPE: Medicare

Model Type: Network
Plan Specialty: Behavioral Health, Dental, Disease
 Management, PBM, Vision
Benefits Offered: Behavioral Health, Dental, Disease
 Management, Long-Term Care, Prescription, Vision,
 Wellness, Life, LTD, STD

Type of Coverage
Individual, Medicare, Supplemental Medicare, Medicaid,
 Catastrophic, Family, Military, Veterans, Group,

Geographic Areas Served
All 50 states, the District of Columbia, most U.S. territories
 & 125 countries

Key Personnel
Executive Chairman . . . . Stephen Hemsley
Chief Executive Officer . . . . David S. Wichmann
Vice-Chair . . . . Larry Renfro
Chief Financial Officer . . . . John Rex
Chief Legal Officer . . . . Marianna D. Short
Chief Marketing Officer . . . . Terry M. Clark
Chief Medical Officer . . . . Richard Migliori

450 UnitedHealthcare of Minnesota
9700 Health Care Lane
Minnetonka, MN 55343
Toll-Free: 888-545-5205
Phone: 763-797-2919
www.uhc.com
Subsidiary of: UnitedHealth Group
Year Founded: 1977

Healthplan and Services Defined
PLAN TYPE: HMO/PPO
Model Type: Network
Plan Specialty: Behavioral Health, Dental, Disease
 Management, Lab, PBM, Vision, Radiology
Benefits Offered: Behavioral Health, Chiropractic, Dental,
 Disease Management, Long-Term Care, Physical Therapy,
 Prescription, Vision, Wellness, AD&D, Life, LTD, STD

Type of Coverage
Commercial, Individual, Indemnity, Medicare, Supplemental
 Medicare, Medicaid, Catastrophic, Family, Military,
 Veterans, Group,

Geographic Areas Served
Minnesota, North Dakota, South Dakota, Hawaii, and Puerto
Rico

Network Qualifications
Pre-Admission Certification: Yes

Peer Review Type
Utilization Review: Yes
Second Surgical Opinion: Yes
Case Management: Yes

Publishes and Distributes Report Card: Yes

Accreditation Certification
TJC, NCQA

Key Personnel
CEO, MN/ND/SD . . . . Philip Kaufman

Specialty Managed Care Partners
Enters into Contracts with Regional Business Coalitions: Yes

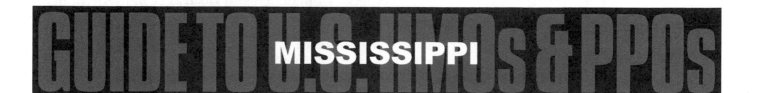

Health Insurance Coverage Status and Type of Coverage by Age

Category	All Persons		Under 18 years		Under 65 years	
	Number	%	Number	%	Number	%
Total population	2,921	-	763	-	2,469	-
Covered by some type of health insurance	2,569 *(15)*	88.0 *(0.5)*	726 *(7)*	95.2 *(0.7)*	2,119 *(15)*	85.8 *(0.6)*
Covered by private health insurance	1,763 *(25)*	60.3 *(0.8)*	367 *(11)*	48.0 *(1.4)*	1,515 *(23)*	61.4 *(1.0)*
Employer-based	1,363 *(23)*	46.7 *(0.8)*	302 *(9)*	39.6 *(1.2)*	1,261 *(21)*	51.1 *(0.9)*
Direct purchase	387 *(11)*	13.3 *(0.4)*	54 *(6)*	7.1 *(0.7)*	244 *(11)*	9.9 *(0.4)*
TRICARE	127 *(9)*	4.3 *(0.3)*	25 *(4)*	3.2 *(0.5)*	82 *(8)*	3.3 *(0.3)*
Covered by public health insurance	1,147 *(17)*	39.3 *(0.6)*	391 *(10)*	51.2 *(1.3)*	707 *(17)*	28.6 *(0.7)*
Medicaid	714 *(17)*	24.4 *(0.6)*	387 *(10)*	50.7 *(1.3)*	624 *(16)*	25.3 *(0.7)*
Medicare	561 *(7)*	19.2 *(0.3)*	4 *(1)*	0.5 *(0.2)*	121 *(7)*	4.9 *(0.3)*
VA Care	81 *(5)*	2.8 *(0.2)*	3 *(2)*	0.4 *(0.2)*	39 *(4)*	1.6 *(0.2)*
Not covered at any time during the year	352 *(15)*	12.0 *(0.5)*	37 *(5)*	4.8 *(0.7)*	350 *(15)*	14.2 *(0.6)*

Note: Numbers in thousands; Figures cover civilian noninstitutionalized population in 2017; N/A indicates that data was not available; Z represents or rounds to zero; Margin of error appears in parenthesis and is calculated using replicate weights.
Source: U.S. Census Bureau, American Community Survey, Table HIC-4_ACS. Health Insurance Coverage Status and Type of Coverage by State—All People: 2008 to 2017, Table HIC-5_ACS. Health Insurance Coverage Status and Type of Coverage by State—Children Under 18: 2008 to 2017, Table HIC-6_ACS. Health Insurance Coverage Status and Type of Coverage by State—Persons Under 65: 2008 to 2017

Mississippi

451 Allegiance Life & Health Insurance Company

2806 S Garfield Street
P.O. Box 3507
Missoula, MT 59806-3507
Toll-Free: 800-737-3137
Phone: 406-523-3122
Fax: 406-523-3124
inquire@askallegiance.com
www.allegiancelifeandhealth.com
Subsidiary of: Cigna
For Profit Organization: Yes
Year Founded: 1981

Healthplan and Services Defined
PLAN TYPE: HMO
Benefits Offered: Dental, Vision, Wellness, Pharmacy

Type of Coverage
Commercial, Individual

Geographic Areas Served
Statewide

Key Personnel
President & Owner . . . . Dirk Visser

452 Health Link PPO

808 Varsity Drive
Tupelo, MS 38801
Toll-Free: 888-855-2740
Phone: 662-377-3868
Fax: 662-377-7599
www.healthlinkppo.com
Subsidiary of: North Mississippi Medical Center
Non-Profit Organization: Yes
Year Founded: 1986
Number of Affiliated Hospitals: 30
Number of Primary Care Physicians: 1,500
Total Enrollment: 155,070

Healthplan and Services Defined
PLAN TYPE: PPO
Benefits Offered: Dental, Long-Term Care, Prescription, Transplant, Vision, Life, LTD, STD, Major Medical

Type of Coverage
Commercial, Individual

Geographic Areas Served
Mississippi and northwest Alabama

Accreditation Certification
NCQA
Medicare Approved, Utilization Review, Pre-Admission Certification, State Licensure, Quality Assurance Program

453 Humana Health Insurance of Mississippi

772 Lake Harbour Drive
Suite 3
Ridgeland, MS 39157
Toll-Free: 866-945-4376
Phone: 601-605-5130
Fax: 601-856-5222
www.humana.com
Secondary Address: 2650 Beach Boulevard, Suite 31A, Biloxi, MS 39531, 228-271-6800
For Profit Organization: Yes

Healthplan and Services Defined
PLAN TYPE: HMO/PPO
Plan Specialty: ASO
Benefits Offered: Disease Management, Prescription, Wellness

Type of Coverage
Commercial, Individual, Medicare

Geographic Areas Served
Statewide

Accreditation Certification
URAC, NCQA

Key Personnel
Market VP, LA/S. MS . . . . Rhonada Bagby

Specialty Managed Care Partners
Caremark Rx

Employer References
Tricare

454 Magnolia Health

111 E Capitol Street
Suite 500
Jackson, MS 39201
Toll-Free: 866-912-6285
www.magnoliahealthplan.com
Subsidiary of: Centene Corporation

Healthplan and Services Defined
PLAN TYPE: Multiple
Plan Specialty: Medicaid, Mississippi Children's Health Insurance Program (CHIP)
Benefits Offered: Behavioral Health, Disease Management, Prescription, Wellness, Maternity & Newborn Care; Transportation

Type of Coverage
Individual, Medicare, Medicaid

Geographic Areas Served
Statewide

Key Personnel
President & CEO . . . . Aaron Sisk

455　Molina Healthcare of Mississippi

188 E Capitol Street
Suite 700
Jackson, MS 39201
Phone: 844-826-4333
www.molinahealthcare.com
Subsidiary of: Monlina Healthcare, Inc.
For Profit Organization: Yes
Year Founded: 1980

Healthplan and Services Defined
　PLAN TYPE: Medicare
　Plan Specialty: Dental, PBM, Vision, intergrated
　　Medicare/Medicaid (Duals)
　Benefits Offered: Dental, Prescription, Vision, Wellness, Life

Geographic Areas Served
　Statewide

Key Personnel
　Plan Pres./Regional CEO . . . . Bridget Galatas
　VP, Provider Network Mgmt . . . . Bryon Grizzard
　Director, Member Services . . . . Emilio Bellizzia
　Mgr., Member Engagement. . . . . Laurie Williams, JD

456　UnitedHealthcare of Mississippi

Hattiesburg, MS 39402
Toll-Free: 888-545-5205
www.uhc.com
Subsidiary of: UnitedHealth Group
For Profit Organization: Yes
Year Founded: 1992

Healthplan and Services Defined
　PLAN TYPE: HMO/PPO
　Model Type: Network
　Plan Specialty: Behavioral Health, Dental, Disease
　　Management, PBM, Vision
　Benefits Offered: Behavioral Health, Dental, Disease
　　Management, Long-Term Care, Prescription, Vision,
　　Wellness, Life, LTD, STD

Type of Coverage
　Commercial, Individual, Indemnity, Medicare, Supplemental
　　Medicare, Medicaid, Catastrophic, Family, Military,
　　Veterans, Group,

Type of Payment Plans Offered
　FFS

Geographic Areas Served
　Statewide

Network Qualifications
　Pre-Admission Certification: Yes

Peer Review Type
　Utilization Review: Yes
　Second Surgical Opinion: Yes
　Case Management: Yes

Publishes and Distributes Report Card: Yes

Accreditation Certification
　NCQA

TJC Accreditation, Medicare Approved, Utilization Review,
　Pre-Admission Certification, State Licensure, Quality
　Assurance Program

Key Personnel
　CEO, MO . . . . Jeff Wedin

Specialty Managed Care Partners
　Enters into Contracts with Regional Business Coalitions: Yes

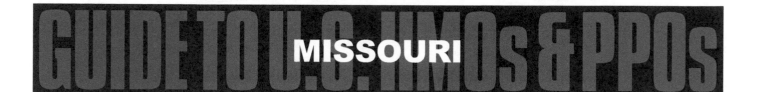
Health Insurance Coverage Status and Type of Coverage by Age

Category	All Persons		Under 18 years		Under 65 years	
	Number	%	Number	%	Number	%
Total population	6,000	-	1,465	-	5,026	-
Covered by some type of health insurance	5,452 *(17)*	90.9 *(0.3)*	1,390 *(7)*	94.9 *(0.4)*	4,483 *(17)*	89.2 *(0.3)*
Covered by private health insurance	4,236 *(30)*	70.6 *(0.5)*	940 *(16)*	64.1 *(1.1)*	3,657 *(26)*	72.8 *(0.5)*
Employer-based	3,416 *(31)*	56.9 *(0.5)*	816 *(17)*	55.7 *(1.2)*	3,142 *(28)*	62.5 *(0.6)*
Direct purchase	866 *(17)*	14.4 *(0.3)*	115 *(7)*	7.9 *(0.5)*	532 *(14)*	10.6 *(0.3)*
TRICARE	159 *(9)*	2.6 *(0.2)*	31 *(4)*	2.1 *(0.3)*	100 *(8)*	2.0 *(0.2)*
Covered by public health insurance	1,944 *(20)*	32.4 *(0.3)*	500 *(16)*	34.1 *(1.1)*	999 *(21)*	19.9 *(0.4)*
Medicaid	903 *(19)*	15.0 *(0.3)*	491 *(15)*	33.5 *(1.0)*	820 *(19)*	16.3 *(0.4)*
Medicare	1,144 *(9)*	19.1 *(0.1)*	12 *(3)*	0.8 *(0.2)*	201 *(8)*	4.0 *(0.2)*
VA Care	167 *(7)*	2.8 *(0.1)*	2 *(1)*	0.2 *(0.1)*	73 *(5)*	1.4 *(0.1)*
Not covered at any time during the year	548 *(17)*	9.1 *(0.3)*	75 *(6)*	5.1 *(0.4)*	544 *(17)*	10.8 *(0.3)*

Note: Numbers in thousands; Figures cover civilian noninstitutionalized population in 2017; N/A indicates that data was not available; Z represents or rounds to zero; Margin of error appears in parenthesis and is calculated using replicate weights.
Source: U.S. Census Bureau, American Community Survey, Table HIC-4_ACS. Health Insurance Coverage Status and Type of Coverage by State—All People: 2008 to 2017, Table HIC-5_ACS. Health Insurance Coverage Status and Type of Coverage by State—Children Under 18: 2008 to 2017, Table HIC-6_ACS. Health Insurance Coverage Status and Type of Coverage by State—Persons Under 65: 2008 to 2017

Missouri

457 American Health Care Alliance

9229 Ward Parkway
Suite 300
Kansas City, MO 64114
Toll-Free: 800-870-6252
customerservice@ahappo.com
www.americanhealthcareallianceonline.com
Mailing Address: P.O. Box 8530, Kansas City, MO
  64114-0530
Year Founded: 1990
Number of Affiliated Hospitals: 5,745
Number of Primary Care Physicians: 190,736
Number of Referral/Specialty Physicians: 285,353
Total Enrollment: 942,000
State Enrollment: 860,000

Healthplan and Services Defined
  PLAN TYPE: PPO
  Model Type: Network of PPOs
  Benefits Offered: Behavioral Health, Chiropractic,
    Complementary Medicine, Dental, Home Care, Physical
    Therapy, Podiatry, Prescription, Psychiatric, Vision,
    Wellness
  Offers Demand Management Patient Information Service:
    Yes

Geographic Areas Served
  Nationwide

Subscriber Information
  Average Annual Deductible Per Subscriber:
    Employee Only (Self): Varies
    Employee & 1 Family Member: Varies
    Employee & 2 Family Members: Varies
    Medicare: Varies
  Average Subscriber Co-Payment:
    Primary Care Physician: Varies
    Non-Network Physician: Varies
    Prescription Drugs: Varies
    Hospital ER: Varies
    Home Health Care: Varies
    Nursing Home: Varies

Publishes and Distributes Report Card: Yes

Accreditation Certification
  AAAHC, URAC, AAPI, NCQA
  TJC Accreditation, Medicare Approved, Utilization Review,
    Pre-Admission Certification, State Licensure

Key Personnel
  Executive Vice President. . . . . Phil Mehelic
    pmehelic@ahappo.com
  Director Client Service. . . . . Lisa Enslinger

458 Anthem Blue Cross & Blue Shield of Missouri

1831 Chestnut Street
St Louis, MO 63103
Phone: 719-488-7400
www.anthem.com

Subsidiary of: Anthem, Inc.
For Profit Organization: Yes

Healthplan and Services Defined
  PLAN TYPE: HMO/PPO
  Model Type: Network
  Plan Specialty: Behavioral Health, Dental, Disease
    Management, Lab, PBM, Vision, Radiology
  Benefits Offered: Behavioral Health, Dental, Disease
    Management, Inpatient SNF, Physical Therapy,
    Prescription, Psychiatric, Transplant, Vision, Wellness, Life

Type of Coverage
  Commercial, Individual, Medicare, Supplemental Medicare,
    Catastrophic

Geographic Areas Served
  All of Missouri, excluding 30 counties in the Kansas City area

Accreditation Certification
  URAC, NCQA

Key Personnel
  President. . . . . Amadou Yattassaye

459 Blue Cross Blue Shield of Kansas City

One Pershing Square
2301 Main Street
Kansas City, MO 64108
Phone: 816-395-2222
www.bluekc.com
Non-Profit Organization: Yes
Year Founded: 1982

Healthplan and Services Defined
  PLAN TYPE: PPO
  Model Type: Network
  Benefits Offered: Behavioral Health, Chiropractic, Dental,
    Physical Therapy, Podiatry, Prescription, Psychiatric

Type of Coverage
  Commercial, Individual, Medicare, Supplemental Medicare,
    Travel Insurance
  Catastrophic Illness Benefit: Maximum $2M

Type of Payment Plans Offered
  POS, FFS

Geographic Areas Served
  Serving 32 counties in greater Kansas City (including Johnson
    and Wyandotte) and northwestern Missouri

Network Qualifications
  Pre-Admission Certification: Yes

Peer Review Type
  Utilization Review: Yes

Publishes and Distributes Report Card: No

Accreditation Certification
  URAC, NCQA

Key Personnel
  President/CEO . . . . Danette Wilson
  SVP/CFO . . . . Tom Nightingale
  General Counsel/CAO . . . . Rick Kastner
  EVP, Market Innovation . . . . Erin Schneider-Stucky

SVP/Chief of Staff . . . . Kim White
SVP/CMO . . . . Greg Sweat, MD
SVP, Sales & Marketing . . . . Ron Rowe

Specialty Managed Care Partners
Enters into Contracts with Regional Business Coalitions: Yes

460 Centene Corporation

Centene Plaza
7700 Forsyth Boulevard
St. Louis, MO 63105
Phone: 314-725-4477
www.centene.com
For Profit Organization: Yes
Year Founded: 1984
Total Enrollment: 11,000,000

Healthplan and Services Defined
PLAN TYPE: HMO/PPO
Model Type: Network
Plan Specialty: Behavioral Health, Dental, PBM, Vision
Benefits Offered: Behavioral Health, Dental, Vision,
Wellness, Life, Correctional health services

Type of Coverage
Commercial, Individual, Medicare, Supplemental Medicare,
Medicaid

Geographic Areas Served
Arizona, Arkansas, California, Florida, Georgia, Indiana,
Illinois, Kansas, Louisiana, Massachusetts, Michigan,
Mississippi, Missouri, Ohio, South Carolina, Texas,
Washington, Wisconsin

Accreditation Certification
URAC, NCQA, CORE Phase III Certified

Key Personnel
VP, Sales. . . . . Wilson Gutierrez

461 Children's Mercy Pediatric Care Network

2420 Pershing Road
Suite G10
Kansas City, MO 64141
Toll-Free: 888-670-7261
Mailing Address: P.O. Box 411596, Kansas City, MO 64141
Non-Profit Organization: Yes
Year Founded: 1996
Owned by an Integrated Delivery Network (IDN): Yes
Number of Affiliated Hospitals: 31
Number of Primary Care Physicians: 200
Number of Referral/Specialty Physicians: 2,400
Total Enrollment: 49,976
State Enrollment: 49,976

Healthplan and Services Defined
PLAN TYPE: HMO
Model Type: Network, Medicaid
Benefits Offered: Behavioral Health, Dental, Disease
Management, Home Care, Inpatient SNF, Physical
Therapy, Podiatry, Prescription, Psychiatric, Vision,
Wellness

Type of Coverage
Medicaid
Catastrophic Illness Benefit: None

Geographic Areas Served
Cass, Clay, Henry, Jackson, Johnson, Lafayette, Platte, Ray,
St. Claire counties in Missouri

Subscriber Information
Average Monthly Fee Per Subscriber
(Employee + Employer Contribution):
Employee Only (Self): $0.00
Employee & 1 Family Member: $0.00
Employee & 2 Family Members: $0.00

Peer Review Type
Utilization Review: Yes
Second Surgical Opinion: Yes
Case Management: Yes

Publishes and Distributes Report Card: Yes

Key Personnel
VP/Executive Director . . . . Bob Finuf
Director, IT . . . . Bob Clark
Director, Finance . . . . Suzie Dunaway
Associate Medical Dir.. . . . . Julia Simmons, MD
Provider Relations Dir . . . . Pamela MK Johnson
Medical Director . . . . Doug Blowey, MD
Dir., Medical Economics. . . . . Kent Pack
Dir., Care Integration . . . . Candance Ramos

Average Claim Compensation
Physician's Fees Charged: 50%
Hospital's Fees Charged: 60%

Specialty Managed Care Partners
Enters into Contracts with Regional Business Coalitions: Yes

Employer References
State of Missouri, Division of Medical Services, State of
Kansas, SRS

462 Cigna Healthcare Missouri

231 S Bemiston Avenue
St. Louis, MO 63105
Phone: 314-290-7300
www.cigna.com
For Profit Organization: Yes
Year Founded: 1982

Healthplan and Services Defined
PLAN TYPE: Multiple
Benefits Offered: Behavioral Health, Dental, Disease
Management, Prescription, Vision, Wellness, AD&D, Life,
LTD, STD

Type of Coverage
Commercial, Individual, Medicare, Supplemental Medicare,
Medicaid, Part-time and hourly workers; Union

Geographic Areas Served
Coverage in only part of the state

Key Personnel
New Business Manager. . . . . Casey Beane
Regional Medical Exec. . . . . Jordan Ginsburg

Dir., Network Management . . . . Daniel Brawley
Corp. Benefits Coverage . . . . Lindsay Loftus
National Account Manager . . . . Debbie Dudley

463 Coventry Health Care of Missouri

550 Maryville Centre Drive
Suite 300
St. Louis, MO 63141
Toll-Free: 800-755-3901
www.coventryhealthcare.com
Subsidiary of: Aetna Inc.
For Profit Organization: Yes
Year Founded: 1978

Healthplan and Services Defined
  PLAN TYPE: HMO/PPO
  Other Type: POS
  Model Type: Network
  Plan Specialty: Behavioral Health, Dental, Worker's
    Compensation
  Benefits Offered: Behavioral Health, Dental, Wellness,
    Worker's Compensation

Type of Coverage
  Commercial, Individual, Medicare, Supplemental Medicare,
    Medicaid

Geographic Areas Served
  All of Eastern Missouri including St. Louis, Jefferson City,
  Columbia, Mexico, Kirksville, Hannibal, Rolla, West Plains
  and Cape Girardeau

Accreditation Certification
  URAC

Key Personnel
  Director, HR . . . . Karol Giunta
  Dir., Network Management . . . . Tim Dalbom
  Chief Financial Officer . . . . Patrick Brosnan

464 Cox Healthplans

Medical Mile Plaza
3200 S National, Building B
Springfield, MO 65807
Toll-Free: 800-205-7665
Phone: 417-269-2900
Fax: 417-269-2949
members@coxhealthplans.com
www.coxhealthplans.com
Mailing Address: P.O. Box 5750, Springfield, MO 65801-5750
Subsidiary of: CoxHealth
For Profit Organization: Yes
Number of Primary Care Physicians: 1,000
Number of Referral/Specialty Physicians: 5,000
Total Enrollment: 5,000
State Enrollment: 1,964

Healthplan and Services Defined
  PLAN TYPE: HMO/PPO
  Benefits Offered: Disease Management, Prescription,
    Wellness

Type of Coverage
  Commercial, Individual

Type of Payment Plans Offered
  POS

Geographic Areas Served
  Statewide

Key Personnel
  President. . . . . Matt Aug
  Chief Information Officer. . . . . Susan Butts
  Chief Financial Officer . . . . Lisa Odom

Specialty Managed Care Partners
  Caremark Rx

465 Delta Dental of Missouri

12399 Gravois Road
St. Louis, MO 63127
Toll-Free: 800-392-1167
Phone: 314-656-3000
service@deltadentalmo.com
www.deltadentalmo.com
Mailing Address: P.O. Box 8690, St. Louis, MO 63126-0690
Non-Profit Organization: Yes
Year Founded: 1958
Owned by an Integrated Delivery Network (IDN): Yes
State Enrollment: 1,700,000

Healthplan and Services Defined
  PLAN TYPE: Dental
  Other Type: Dental PPO
  Model Type: Group
  Plan Specialty: Dental, Vision
  Benefits Offered: Dental, Vision

Type of Coverage
  Commercial

Geographic Areas Served
  Missouri and South Carolina

Publishes and Distributes Report Card: No

Key Personnel
  President/CEO . . . . E.B. Rob Goren
  CFO/Corporate Counsel . . . . Barbara C. Bentrup
  COO/Chief Dental Officer. . . . . Ronald E. Inge, DDS
  Chief Actuary. . . . . Jonathan R. Jennings
  CIO . . . . Karl A. Mudra
  Sales/Marketing Officer . . . . Edward A. Pattarozzi

Specialty Managed Care Partners
  Enters into Contracts with Regional Business Coalitions: No

466 Dental Health Alliance

2323 Grand Boulevard
Kansas City, MO 64108
Toll-Free: 800-522-1313
ppoinforequests@sunlife.com
www.dha.com
Subsidiary of: Sunlife Financial
Year Founded: 1994
Number of Primary Care Physicians: 74,000

Total Enrollment: 1,700,000

Healthplan and Services Defined
PLAN TYPE: Dental
Other Type: Dental PPO Network
Model Type: Network, Dental PPO Network
Plan Specialty: Dental
Benefits Offered: Dental

Type of Coverage
Commercial

Type of Payment Plans Offered
POS, FFS, Combination FFS & DFFS

Geographic Areas Served
Nationwide

Network Qualifications
Pre-Admission Certification: No

Peer Review Type
Utilization Review: Yes

---

467   Essence Healthcare
13900 Riverport Drive
Maryland Heights, MO 63043
Toll-Free: 866-597-9560
Phone: 314-209-2700
Fax: 888-480-2577
customerservice@essencehealthcare.com
www.essencehealthcare.com
Secondary Address: 3330 S National Avenue, Suite 100,
Springfield, MO 65807
Year Founded: 2004
Total Enrollment: 60,000

Healthplan and Services Defined
PLAN TYPE: Medicare
Benefits Offered: Chiropractic, Dental, Disease Management,
Home Care, Inpatient SNF, Physical Therapy, Podiatry,
Prescription, Psychiatric, Vision, Wellness

Type of Coverage
Individual, Medicare

Geographic Areas Served
Missouri: Boone, Christian, Greene, Jefferson, Stone, Saint
Louis, Saint Louis City, Saint Charles, Saint Francois, and
Taney counties. Illinois: Madison, Monroe, and Saint Clair
counties

Subscriber Information
Average Monthly Fee Per Subscriber
(Employee + Employer Contribution):
Employee Only (Self): Varies
Medicare: Varies
Average Annual Deductible Per Subscriber:
Employee Only (Self): Varies
Medicare: Varies
Average Subscriber Co-Payment:
Primary Care Physician: Varies
Non-Network Physician: Varies
Prescription Drugs: Varies
Hospital ER: Varies
Home Health Care: Varies

Home Health Care Max. Days/Visits Covered: Varies
Nursing Home: Varies
Nursing Home Max. Days/Visits Covered: Varies

Key Personnel
President & CEO . . . . Richard Jones
Chief Compliance Officer . . . . Erin Venable
Chief Operating Officer . . . . Martha Butler
Chief Medical Officer . . . . Deborah Zimmerman, MD
Claims & Customer Service . . . . Dawn Walter
VP, Sales & Marketing . . . . Joel Anderson

---

**468   Government Employees Health Association
(GEHA)**
310 NE Mulberry Street
Lee's Summit, MO 64086
Toll-Free: 800-821-6136
www.geha.com
Non-Profit Organization: Yes
Year Founded: 1964

Healthplan and Services Defined
PLAN TYPE: Other
Plan Specialty: Dental, Vision, Federal employees
Benefits Offered: Dental, Disease Management, Prescription,
Vision, Wellness, Life

Type of Coverage
Commercial, Medicare
Catastrophic Illness Maximum Benefit: $5,000

Type of Payment Plans Offered
FFS

Geographic Areas Served
Nationwide

Network Qualifications
Pre-Admission Certification: Yes

Accreditation Certification
URAC

Key Personnel
President & CEO . . . . Julie Browne

Average Claim Compensation
Hospital's Fees Charged: 85%

---

469   HealthLink HMO
1831 Chestnut Street
Suite 540
St. Louis, MO 63103
Toll-Free: 800-624-2356
Phone: 314-925-6000
www.healthlink.com
For Profit Organization: Yes
Year Founded: 1985

Healthplan and Services Defined
PLAN TYPE: Multiple
Benefits Offered: Dental, Vision, Wellness, Worker's
Compensation, Life, LTD, STD, Reinsurance

Type of Coverage
Catastrophic Illness Benefit: Varies per case

Geographic Areas Served
Arkansas, Illinois, Missouri, Ohio, Kentucky, and Indiana

Network Qualifications
Pre-Admission Certification: Yes

Peer Review Type
Utilization Review: Yes
Second Surgical Opinion: No
Case Management: Yes

Accreditation Certification
URAC
Utilization Review, Pre-Admission Certification, Quality
Assurance Program

Key Personnel
President . . . . Graeme Stretch

Specialty Managed Care Partners
WellPoint Pharmacy Management, Cigna Behavioral Health,
Vision Service Plan
Enters into Contracts with Regional Business Coalitions: Yes
Gateway Purchases

Employer References
Local fifty benefits service trust, Jefferson City Public
Schools, ConAgra

---

470 Humana Health Insurance of Missouri
909 E Montclair
Suite 108
Springfield, MO 65807
Toll-Free: 800-951-0128
Phone: 417-227-5700
Fax: 417-882-2015
www.humana.com
Secondary Address: Creekwoods Commons, 215 NE
Englewood Road, Suite A, Kansas City, MO 64118,
816-459-7776
Subsidiary of: Humana
For Profit Organization: Yes

Healthplan and Services Defined
PLAN TYPE: HMO/PPO
Model Type: Network
Plan Specialty: Dental, Vision
Benefits Offered: Dental, Vision, Life, LTD, STD

Type of Coverage
Commercial, Individual

Geographic Areas Served
Statewide

Accreditation Certification
URAC, NCQA, CORE

Key Personnel
Market Manager . . . . Scott Stanton

---

471 Liberty Dental Plan of Missouri
P.O. Box 26110
Santa Ana, CA 92799-6110
Toll-Free: 877-558-6489
www.libertydentalplan.com

For Profit Organization: Yes
Year Founded: 2001
Total Enrollment: 3,000,000

Healthplan and Services Defined
PLAN TYPE: Dental
Other Type: Dental HMO
Plan Specialty: Dental
Benefits Offered: Dental

Type of Coverage
Commercial, Individual, Medicare, Medicaid, Unions

Geographic Areas Served
Statewide

Accreditation Certification
NCQA

Key Personnel
Regional Manager, MO. . . . . John McCarthy
314-489-7785
jmccarthy@libertydentalplan.com

---

472 Med-Pay
1650 Battlefield
Suite 300
Springfield, MO 65804-3706
Toll-Free: 800-777-9087
Phone: 417-886-6886
Fax: 417-886-2276
www.med-pay.com
Year Founded: 1983
State Enrollment: 26,000

Healthplan and Services Defined
PLAN TYPE: Other
Other Type: TPA, HSA, HRA
Model Type: Network
Plan Specialty: ASO, Behavioral Health, Chiropractic, Dental,
Disease Management, Lab, MSO, PBM, Vision, Radiology
Benefits Offered: Behavioral Health, Chiropractic, Dental,
Disease Management, Home Care, Inpatient SNF,
Long-Term Care, Physical Therapy, Prescription,
Transplant, Vision
Offers Demand Management Patient Information Service: Yes

Type of Coverage
Commercial, Individual

Accreditation Certification
State of MO
Utilization Review

Specialty Managed Care Partners
HCC, BCBS, Healthlink
Enters into Contracts with Regional Business Coalitions: Yes

---

473 Mercy Clinic Missouri
14528 S Outer 40 Road
Chesterfield, MO 63017
Phone: 314-432-4415
mercy.net
Subsidiary of: IBM Watson Health
Non-Profit Organization: Yes

Number of Affiliated Hospitals: 44
Number of Primary Care Physicians: 700
Number of Referral/Specialty Physicians: 2,000

Healthplan and Services Defined
PLAN TYPE: HMO
Benefits Offered: Behavioral Health, Disease Management,
Home Care, Physical Therapy, Vision, Wellness,
Non-Surgical Weight Loss, Urgent Care, Dermatology,
Rehabilitation, Breast Cancer, Orthopedics, Otosclerosis,
Pediatrics

Type of Coverage
Commercial, Individual

Geographic Areas Served
Arkansas, Kansas, Missouri, Oklahoma

Key Personnel
President & CEO. . . . . Lynn Britton
EVP, COO. . . . . Michael McCurry
EVP, Strategy & CFO . . . . Shannon Sock
EVP, Operations . . . . Donn Sorensen
SVP/CCO . . . . Tony Krawat
Chief Clinical Officer. . . . . Fred McQueary, MD
SVP/General Counsel . . . . Philip Wheeler

---

474   Sun Life Financial
2323 Grand Boulevard
Kansas City, MO 64108
Toll-Free: 816-474-2345
www.assurantemployeebenefits.com
For Profit Organization: Yes
Year Founded: 1865

Healthplan and Services Defined
PLAN TYPE: Multiple
Plan Specialty: Dental, Vision
Benefits Offered: Dental, Vision, Wellness, AD&D, Life,
LTD, STD, Subject to regulatory approvals

Type of Coverage
Commercial, Individual

Geographic Areas Served
Nationwide

Subscriber Information
Average Monthly Fee Per Subscriber
(Employee + Employer Contribution):
Employee Only (Self): Varies by plan

Accreditation Certification
NCQA

Key Personnel
President. . . . . Dan Fishbein
SVP/CFO. . . . . Neil Haynes
SVP/General Counsel . . . . Scott Davis
VP, Dental/Vision. . . . . Stacia Almquist
VP, Marketing. . . . . Ed Milano
Head of Human Resources . . . . Kathy deCastro

475   UnitedHealthcare of Missouri
13655 Riverport Drive
Maryland Heights, MO 63043
Toll-Free: 888-545-5205
Phone: 314-592-7000
www.uhc.com
Subsidiary of: UnitedHealth Group
For Profit Organization: Yes

Healthplan and Services Defined
PLAN TYPE: HMO/PPO
Model Type: Network
Plan Specialty: Behavioral Health, Dental, Disease
Management, PBM, Vision
Benefits Offered: Behavioral Health, Dental, Disease
Management, Long-Term Care, Prescription, Vision, Life,
LTD, STD

Type of Coverage
Individual, Medicare, Supplemental Medicare, Medicaid,
Catastrophic, Family, Military, Veterans, Group,

Geographic Areas Served
Statewide

Key Personnel
CEO, MO/IL . . . . Pat Quinn

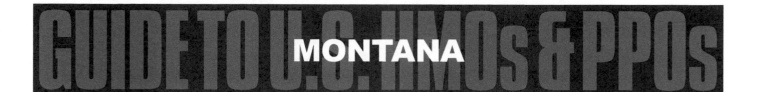

Health Insurance Coverage Status and Type of Coverage by Age

Category	All Persons		Under 18 years		Under 65 years	
	Number	%	Number	%	Number	%
Total population	1,036	-	241	-	851	-
Covered by some type of health insurance	949 (6)	91.5 (0.5)	227 (3)	94.2 (1.0)	765 (6)	89.8 (0.7)
Covered by private health insurance	697 (13)	67.2 (1.2)	137 (6)	56.7 (2.6)	581 (12)	68.3 (1.4)
Employer-based	503 (13)	48.5 (1.2)	108 (6)	44.7 (2.4)	460 (12)	54.0 (1.4)
Direct purchase	194 (8)	18.7 (0.8)	25 (4)	10.3 (1.5)	118 (7)	13.9 (0.9)
TRICARE	35 (5)	3.4 (0.4)	7 (2)	3.1 (0.8)	23 (4)	2.7 (0.5)
Covered by public health insurance	400 (11)	38.6 (1.1)	100 (6)	41.3 (2.7)	219 (11)	25.7 (1.3)
Medicaid	212 (11)	20.4 (1.1)	99 (6)	41.0 (2.7)	194 (11)	22.8 (1.3)
Medicare	203 (3)	19.6 (0.3)	1 (1)	0.4 (0.2)	23 (3)	2.6 (0.3)
VA Care	43 (3)	4.2 (0.3)	1 (1)	0.3 (0.2)	18 (2)	2.1 (0.2)
Not covered at any time during the year	88 (6)	8.5 (0.5)	14 (2)	5.8 (1.0)	87 (6)	10.2 (0.7)

Note: Numbers in thousands; Figures cover civilian noninstitutionalized population in 2017; N/A indicates that data was not available; Z represents or rounds to zero; Margin of error appears in parenthesis and is calculated using replicate weights.
Source: U.S. Census Bureau, American Community Survey, Table HIC-4_ACS. Health Insurance Coverage Status and Type of Coverage by State—All People: 2008 to 2017, Table HIC-5_ACS. Health Insurance Coverage Status and Type of Coverage by State—Children Under 18: 2008 to 2017, Table HIC-6_ACS. Health Insurance Coverage Status and Type of Coverage by State—Persons Under 65: 2008 to 2017

Montana

476   Blue Cross & Blue Shield of Montana

3645 Alice Street
P.O. Box 4309
Helena, MT 59604-4309
Toll-Free: 800-447-7828
www.bcbsmt.com
Non-Profit Organization: Yes
Year Founded: 1986
Owned by an Integrated Delivery Network (IDN): Yes
Federally Qualified: Yes
Number of Affiliated Hospitals: 58
Number of Primary Care Physicians: 1,900
Number of Referral/Specialty Physicians: 2,800
Total Enrollment: 250,000
State Enrollment: 250,000

Healthplan and Services Defined
PLAN TYPE: HMO
Model Type: Network
Plan Specialty: ASO, Behavioral Health, Chiropractic,
Dental, Disease Management, EPO, Lab, MSO, PBM,
Vision, Radiology, Worker's Compensation, UR
Benefits Offered: Behavioral Health, Chiropractic,
Complementary
Medicine, Dental, Disease Management, Home Care,
Inpatient SNF, Long-Term Care, Physical Therapy,
Podiatry, Prescription, Psychiatric, Transplant,
Vision, Wellness, Worker's Compensation, AD&D,
Life, LTD, STD
Offers Demand Management Patient Information Service:
Yes

Type of Coverage
Commercial, Individual, Indemnity, Medicare, Supplemental
Medicare, Catastrophic
Catastrophic Illness Benefit: Varies per case

Type of Payment Plans Offered
POS, DFFS, Capitated

Geographic Areas Served
Beaverhead, Big Horn, Blaine, Broadwater, Carbon, Carter,
Cascade, Choteau, Custer, Deer Lodge, Flathead, Glacier,
Hill, Jefferson, Lake, Lewis and Clark, Liberty, Lincoln,
Madison, McCone, Meagher, Mineral, Missoula,
Musselshell, Pondera, Ravalli, Sanders, Silver Bow,
Stillwater, Sweet Grass, Teton, Wheatland, Yellowstone

Subscriber Information
Average Subscriber Co-Payment:
Primary Care Physician: $15
Non-Network Physician: Deductible
Hospital ER: $75.00
Home Health Care: No deductible
Home Health Care Max. Days/Visits Covered: 180 days
Nursing Home: $300 per admit co-pay
Nursing Home Max. Days/Visits Covered: 60 days

Network Qualifications
Pre-Admission Certification: Yes

Peer Review Type
Utilization Review: Yes
Second Surgical Opinion: Yes
Case Management: Yes

Publishes and Distributes Report Card: Yes

Accreditation Certification
URAC

Key Personnel
President . . . . Monica Berner, MD
Media Contact . . . . John Doran
   406-437-6195
   John_Doran@bcbsmt.com
Media Contact . . . . Jesse Zentz
   406-437-6182
   Jesse_Zentz@bcbsmt.com

Specialty Managed Care Partners
Behavioral Health, Chiropractic, Dental, Disease
Management, Home Care, Inpatient SNF, and more
Enters into Contracts with Regional Business Coalitions: Yes

Employer References
Montana University System, Evening Post Publishing
Company, Costco Wholesale, State of Montana, Huntley
Project Schools

477   First Choice Health

1156 16th Street W
Suite 18
Billings, MT 59102-4118
Toll-Free: 888-256-6556
Fax: 406-256-9466
contact@fchn.com
www.fchn.com
For Profit Organization: Yes
Year Founded: 1996
Number of Affiliated Hospitals: 94
Number of Primary Care Physicians: 980
Number of Referral/Specialty Physicians: 1,793
Total Enrollment: 80,000
State Enrollment: 56,000

Healthplan and Services Defined
PLAN TYPE: PPO
Model Type: Open Panel & GeoExclusive
Benefits Offered: Wellness

Type of Coverage
Commercial, Individual, Private & Public Plans, Geo-specifi

Geographic Areas Served
Washington, Oregon, Alaska, Idaho, Montana, Wyoming, and
select areas of North Dakota and South Dakota

Key Personnel
Chief Executive Officer . . . . Robert L. Hunter

Specialty Managed Care Partners
Enters into Contracts with Regional Business Coalitions: Yes
First Choice Health Network (Pacific NW)

478   HCSC Insurance Services Company

560 N Park Avenue
P.O. Box 4309
Helena, MT 59604-4309
Phone: 406-437-5000
hcsc.com
Subsidiary of: Blue Cross Blue Shield Association
Non-Profit Organization: Yes
Year Founded: 1936
Number of Primary Care Physicians: 8,000

Healthplan and Services Defined
   PLAN TYPE: HMO
   Benefits Offered: Behavioral Health, Dental, Disease
      Management, Psychiatric, Wellness

Geographic Areas Served
   Statewide

Key Personnel
   Mgr., Medicaid Operations . . . . Rosemary Fowler

479   Humana Health Insurance of Montana

12600 Whitewater Dirve
Suite 150
Minnetonka, MN 55343
Toll-Free: 877-367-6990
Phone: 952-253-3540
Fax: 952-938-2787
www.humana.com
Subsidiary of: Humana
For Profit Organization: Yes

Healthplan and Services Defined
   PLAN TYPE: HMO/PPO
   Model Type: Network
   Plan Specialty: Vision
   Benefits Offered: Dental, Vision, Life, LTD, STD

Type of Coverage
   Commercial

Geographic Areas Served
   Montana is covered by the Minnesota branch

Accreditation Certification
   URAC, NCQA, CORE

Key Personnel
   Sales Manager. . . . . Dee Heinze

480   Montana Health Co-Op

5 & 6, 1005 Partridge Place
Helena, MT 59602
Toll-Free: 855-477-2900
memberservice@mhc.coop
mhc.coop
Mailing Address: P.O. Box 5358, Helena, MT 59604
Non-Profit Organization: Yes
Year Founded: 2013

Healthplan and Services Defined
   PLAN TYPE: HMO

Benefits Offered: Chiropractic, Inpatient SNF, Physical
   Therapy, Prescription, Wellness, Labs & X-Ray; Maternity;
   Occupational & Speech Therapy

Geographic Areas Served
   Statewide

Key Personnel
   Chair. . . . . Joan Miles
   Vice Chair . . . . Raymond Rogers
   Media Contact . . . . Karen Early
      208-917-1605
      kearly@mhc.coop

481   Mountain Health Co-Op

5 & 6, 1005 Patridge Place
Helena, ID 59602
Toll-Free: 855-477-2900
information@mhc.coop
mhc.coop
Non-Profit Organization: Yes
Year Founded: 2013

Healthplan and Services Defined
   PLAN TYPE: HMO
   Benefits Offered: Chiropractic, Inpatient SNF, Physical
      Therapy, Prescription, Wellness, Labs & X-Ray;
      Occupational & Speech Therapy; Maternity

Geographic Areas Served
   Statewide

Key Personnel
   Chair. . . . . Joan Miles
   Vice-Chair . . . . Raymond Rogers
   Media Contact . . . . Karen Early
      208-917-1605
      kearly@mhc.com

482   UnitedHealthcare of Montana

1212 N Washington Street
Suite 307
Spokane, WA 99201
Toll-Free: 888-545-5205
Phone: 509-324-7172
www.uhc.com
Secondary Address: 7525 SE 24th Street, Mercer Island, WA
   98040, 206-519-6472
Subsidiary of: UnitedHealth Group
For Profit Organization: Yes
Year Founded: 1986

Healthplan and Services Defined
   PLAN TYPE: HMO/PPO
   Model Type: Network
   Plan Specialty: Behavioral Health, Dental, Disease
      Management, MSO, PBM, Vision
   Benefits Offered: Behavioral Health, Chiropractic,
      Complementary Medicine, Dental, Disease Management,
      Home Care, Inpatient SNF, Long-Term Care, Physical
      Therapy, Podiatry, Prescription, Psychiatric, Transplant,
      Vision, Wellness, AD&D, Life

Type of Coverage
   Commercial, Individual, Medicare, Supplemental Medicare,
      Medicaid, Family, Military, Veterans, Group,

Type of Payment Plans Offered
   DFFS, FFS, Combination FFS & DFFS

Geographic Areas Served
   Statewide. Montana is covered by the Washington branch

Subscriber Information
   Average Monthly Fee Per Subscriber
      (Employee + Employer Contribution):
         Employee Only (Self): Varies
   Average Subscriber Co-Payment:
         Primary Care Physician: $10
         Prescription Drugs: $10/15/30
         Hospital ER: $50

Network Qualifications
   Pre-Admission Certification: Yes

Peer Review Type
   Case Management: Yes

Publishes and Distributes Report Card: Yes

Accreditation Certification
   URAC, NCQA
   State Licensure, Quality Assurance Program

Key Personnel
   Pres., West Regional Net. . . . . David Hansen

Average Claim Compensation
   Physician's Fees Charged: 70%
   Hospital's Fees Charged: 55%

Specialty Managed Care Partners
   United Behavioral Health
   Enters into Contracts with Regional Business Coalitions: No

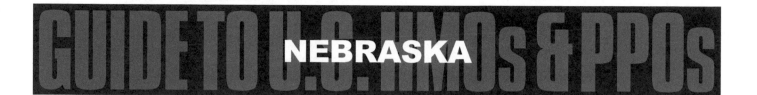
Health Insurance Coverage Status and Type of Coverage by Age

Category	All Persons		Under 18 years		Under 65 years	
	Number	%	Number	%	Number	%
Total population	1,891	-	500	-	1,609	-
Covered by some type of health insurance	1,735 (7)	91.7 (0.4)	474 (4)	94.9 (0.7)	1,454 (8)	90.4 (0.5)
Covered by private health insurance	1,435 (14)	75.9 (0.8)	348 (8)	69.6 (1.5)	1,254 (13)	77.9 (0.8)
Employer-based	1,129 (14)	59.7 (0.7)	303 (8)	60.6 (1.6)	1,062 (14)	66.0 (0.9)
Direct purchase	321 (9)	17.0 (0.5)	43 (4)	8.5 (0.8)	199 (9)	12.4 (0.5)
TRICARE	62 (5)	3.3 (0.3)	17 (3)	3.4 (0.6)	45 (5)	2.8 (0.3)
Covered by public health insurance	525 (11)	27.8 (0.6)	143 (8)	28.6 (1.6)	252 (10)	15.6 (0.7)
Medicaid	246 (11)	13.0 (0.6)	142 (8)	28.3 (1.6)	217 (11)	13.5 (0.7)
Medicare	308 (3)	16.3 (0.2)	2 (1)	0.3 (0.2)	35 (3)	2.2 (0.2)
VA Care	52 (3)	2.7 (0.2)	Z (Z)	0.1 (0.1)	20 (2)	1.3 (0.1)
Not covered at any time during the year	157 (7)	8.3 (0.4)	26 (4)	5.1 (0.7)	155 (7)	9.6 (0.5)

Note: Numbers in thousands; Figures cover civilian noninstitutionalized population in 2017; N/A indicates that data was not available; Z represents or rounds to zero; Margin of error appears in parenthesis and is calculated using replicate weights.
Source: U.S. Census Bureau, American Community Survey, Table HIC-4_ACS. Health Insurance Coverage Status and Type of Coverage by State—All People: 2008 to 2017, Table HIC-5_ACS. Health Insurance Coverage Status and Type of Coverage by State—Children Under 18: 2008 to 2017, Table HIC-6_ACS. Health Insurance Coverage Status and Type of Coverage by State—Persons Under 65: 2008 to 2017

Nebraska

483   Ameritas

5900 O Street
Lincoln, NE 68501-1889
Toll-Free: 800-311-7871
Fax: 402-325-4190
www.ameritas.com
For Profit Organization: Yes
Year Founded: 1990

Healthplan and Services Defined
  PLAN TYPE: Multiple
  Model Type: Staff
  Plan Specialty: ASO, Dental, Vision
  Benefits Offered: Dental, Vision, Life, Disability

Type of Coverage
  Commercial, Individual

Type of Payment Plans Offered
  POS, DFFS, Capitated, Combination FFS & DFFS

Geographic Areas Served
  Nationwide

Peer Review Type
  Utilization Review: Yes
  Second Surgical Opinion: Yes
  Case Management: Yes

Publishes and Distributes Report Card: Yes

Accreditation Certification
  Medicare Approved

Key Personnel
  President & CEO . . . . JoAnn M. Martin

484   Blue Cross & Blue Shield of Nebraska

1919 Aksarben Drive
P.O. Box 3248
Omaha, NE 68180
Toll-Free: 800-422-2763
Phone: 402-982-7000
sales@nebraskablue.com
www.nebraskablue.com
Secondary Address: 1233 Lincoln Mall, Lincoln, NE 68508,
  402-458-4800
Year Founded: 1939
Total Enrollment: 717,000
State Enrollment: 717,000

Healthplan and Services Defined
  PLAN TYPE: PPO
  Model Type: Network
  Benefits Offered: Behavioral Health, Chiropractic, Dental,
    Disease Management, Home Care, Inpatient SNF,
    Long-Term Care, Physical Therapy, Podiatry, Prescription,
    Psychiatric, Vision

Type of Coverage
  Commercial, Individual, Medicare, Supplemental Medicare

Geographic Areas Served
  Statewide

Publishes and Distributes Report Card: No

Key Personnel
  President/CEO . . . . Steven H. Grandfield
  EVP, Finance/Admin. Dale Mackel
  EVP, Operations . . . . Susan Courtney
  EVP, Health Delivery . . . . Dr. Joann Schaefer
  Chief Legal Officer . . . . Russell Collins
  Chief Medical Officer . . . . Debra Esser
  Chief Information Officer . . . . Rama Kolli

485   Coventry Health Care of Nebraska

15950 West Dodge Road
Omaha, NE 68118
coventryhealthcare.com
Subsidiary of: Aetna Inc.
For Profit Organization: Yes
Year Founded: 1985
Number of Affiliated Hospitals: 264
Number of Primary Care Physicians: 15,000
Total Enrollment: 5,000,000

Healthplan and Services Defined
  PLAN TYPE: HMO/PPO
  Other Type: POS
  Model Type: Network
  Plan Specialty: Behavioral Health, Dental, Worker's
    Compensation
  Benefits Offered: Behavioral Health, Dental, Wellness,
    Worker's Compensation

Type of Coverage
  Commercial, Individual, Medicare, Supplemental Medicare,
  Medicaid

Type of Payment Plans Offered
  POS

Geographic Areas Served
  Statewide

Accreditation Certification
  URAC

Key Personnel
  Health Services Manager . . . . Anne Woods

486   Delta Dental of Nebraska

1807 N 169th Plaza
Omaha, NE 68118
Toll-Free: 800-736-0710
www.deltadentalne.org
Non-Profit Organization: Yes
Year Founded: 1969

Healthplan and Services Defined
  PLAN TYPE: Dental
  Other Type: Dental PPO
  Model Type: Network
  Plan Specialty: ASO, Dental
  Benefits Offered: Dental

Type of Coverage
  Commercial, Individual
  Catastrophic Illness Benefit: None

Geographic Areas Served
Statewide

Key Personnel
President . . . . Rodney Young
Office Administrator . . . . Sally Gutowski
Sales Manager . . . . Barbara Jensen
Media Contact . . . . Clarise Tushie-Lessard
    612-224-3341
    ctushie-lessard@deltadentalmn.org

487 Humana Health Insurance of Nebraska

1415 Kimberly Road
Bettendorf, IA 52722
Toll-Free: 866-653-7275
Phone: 563-344-1242
Fax: 563-355-0730
www.humana.com
Subsidiary of: Humana
For Profit Organization: Yes

Healthplan and Services Defined
PLAN TYPE: HMO/PPO
Model Type: Network
Plan Specialty: Dental, Vision
Benefits Offered: Dental, Vision, Life, LTD, STD, Nebraska
is covered by the Iowa branch.

Geographic Areas Served
Statewide

Accreditation Certification
URAC, NCQA, CORE

488 Medica with CHI Health

331 Village Point Plaza
Suite 304
Omaha, NE 68118
Toll-Free: 800-918-6892
www.medica.com
Subsidiary of: UniNet Health Care
Number of Affiliated Hospitals: 30
Number of Primary Care Physicians: 1,400

Healthplan and Services Defined
PLAN TYPE: HMO
Benefits Offered: Behavioral Health, Chiropractic, Dental,
Disease Management, Prescription, Wellness

Geographic Areas Served
Buffalo, Burt, Butler, Cass, Colfax, Cuming, Dodge,
Douglas, Fillmore, Hall, Johnson, Lancaster, Nance, Nemaha,
Nuckolls, Otoe, Pawnee, Saline, Sarpy, Saunders, Seward,
Thayer or Washington counties

Key Personnel
President & CEO . . . . John Naylor
VP, Human Resources . . . . Lynn Altmann
SVP, Financial Officer . . . . Mark Baird
VP, General Manager . . . . Geoff Bartsh
SVP, General Counsel . . . . Jim Jacobson
SVP, Government Programs . . . . Tom Lindquist
Marketing/Communications . . . . Rob Longendyke

489 Medica: Nebraska

331 Village Point Plaza
Suite 304
Omaha, NE 68118
Toll-Free: 800-918-6892
medica.com
Year Founded: 1974
Number of Affiliated Hospitals: 170
Number of Primary Care Physicians: 7,200

Healthplan and Services Defined
PLAN TYPE: HMO
Benefits Offered: Behavioral Health, Chiropractic, Dental,
Disease Management, Prescription, Wellness, AD&D, Life

Type of Coverage
Medicare

Geographic Areas Served
Statewide

Key Personnel
President & CEO . . . . John Naylor
VP, Human Resources . . . . Lynn Altmann
SVP, Financial Officer . . . . Mark Baird
VP, General Manager . . . . Geoff Bartsh
SVP, General Counsel . . . . Jim Jacobson
SVP, Government Programs . . . . Tom Lindquist
Marketing/Communications . . . . Rob Longendyke

490 Midlands Choice

8420 W Dodge Road
Suite 210
Omaha, NE 68114
Phone: 402-390-8233
www.midlandschoice.com
For Profit Organization: Yes
Year Founded: 1993
Physician Owned Organization: Yes
Number of Affiliated Hospitals: 320
Number of Primary Care Physicians: 20,000
Total Enrollment: 615,000

Healthplan and Services Defined
PLAN TYPE: PPO
Model Type: PPO Network

Geographic Areas Served
Iowa, Nebraska, South Dakota, Colorado, and portions of
Wyoming, Kansas, Missouri, Illinois, Wisconsin and
Minnesota

Accreditation Certification
URAC

Key Personnel
President/CEO . . . . Greta Vaught
VP/Privacy Officer . . . . Daniel McCulley

Specialty Managed Care Partners
Enters into Contracts with Regional Business Coalitions: No

491 Mutual of Omaha Dental Insurance

3300 Mutual of Omaha Plaza
Omaha, NE 68175
www.mutualofomaha.com/dental
For Profit Organization: Yes
Year Founded: 1985

Healthplan and Services Defined
PLAN TYPE: Dental
Model Type: Network
Benefits Offered: Behavioral Health, Chiropractic,
    Complementary Medicine, Dental, Disease Management,
    Home Care, Inpatient SNF, Long-Term Care, Physical
    Therapy, Podiatry, Prescription, Psychiatric, Transplant,
    Vision, Wellness

Type of Coverage
Commercial, Individual

Peer Review Type
Utilization Review: Yes
Second Surgical Opinion: Yes
Case Management: Yes

Publishes and Distributes Report Card: Yes

Accreditation Certification
TJC Accreditation, Medicare Approved, Utilization Review,
    Pre-Admission Certification, State Licensure, Quality
    Assurance Program

Key Personnel
Chief Executive Officer . . . . James Blackledge
Chief Financial Officer . . . . Vibhu Sharma
General Counsel . . . . Richard Anderl
Chief Information Officer . . . . Michael Lechtenberger
Chief Marketing Officer . . . . Stephanie Pritchett

Specialty Managed Care Partners
Enters into Contracts with Regional Business Coalitions: No

492 Mutual of Omaha Health Plans

3300 Mutual of Omaha Plaza
Omaha, NE 68175
Toll-Free: 800-205-8193
www.mutualofomaha.com
For Profit Organization: Yes
Year Founded: 1909
Number of Affiliated Hospitals: 43
Number of Primary Care Physicians: 673
Number of Referral/Specialty Physicians: 1,718
Total Enrollment: 54,418
State Enrollment: 28,978

Healthplan and Services Defined
PLAN TYPE: HMO/PPO
Other Type: POS
Model Type: IPA
Plan Specialty: ASO, Behavioral Health, Chiropractic,
    Disease Management, Lab, Vision, Radiology, UR
Benefits Offered: Behavioral Health, Chiropractic, Disease
    Management, Home Care, Inpatient SNF, Long-Term Care,
    Physical Therapy, Podiatry, Prescription, Psychiatric,

Transplant, Vision, Wellness, AD&D, Life, LTD, STD,
    Critical Illness, EAP

Type of Coverage
Commercial, Individual, Indemnity, Medicare, Supplemental
    Medicare, Medicaid
Catastrophic Illness Benefit: Covered

Type of Payment Plans Offered
POS, Combination FFS & DFFS

Geographic Areas Served
Iowa: Harrison, Mills & Pottawattamie counties; Nebraska:
    Burt, Butler, Cass, Colfas, Cuming, Oakota, Dixon, Filmore,
    Johnson, Lancaster, Madison, Otoe, Salone, Saunders, Seuard,
    Stanton, Dodge, Douglas, Sampy, Washington counties

Subscriber Information
Average Monthly Fee Per Subscriber
    (Employee + Employer Contribution):
        Employee Only (Self): Varies by plan
Average Annual Deductible Per Subscriber:
        Employee Only (Self): $0.00
Average Subscriber Co-Payment:
        Primary Care Physician: $15.00
        Prescription Drugs: $15.00
        Hospital ER: $50.00
        Home Health Care: $25.00
        Home Health Care Max. Days/Visits Covered: Unlimited
        Nursing Home: $0.00
        Nursing Home Max. Days/Visits Covered: 100 days

Network Qualifications
Pre-Admission Certification: Yes

Peer Review Type
Utilization Review: Yes
Second Surgical Opinion: No
Case Management: Yes

Publishes and Distributes Report Card: Yes

Accreditation Certification
URAC, NCQA
TJC Accreditation, Utilization Review, Pre-Admission
    Certification, State Licensure, Quality Assurance Program

Key Personnel
Chairman/CEO . . . . James Blackledge
EVP/General Counsel . . . . Richard Anderl
EVP/CFO/Treasurer . . . . Vibhu Sharma
CAO . . . . Stacy Scholtz
EVP/Investment Officer . . . . Richard Hrabchak
EVP/CIO . . . . Michael Lechtenberger

Average Claim Compensation
Physician's Fees Charged: 75%
Hospital's Fees Charged: 60%

Specialty Managed Care Partners
Enters into Contracts with Regional Business Coalitions: No

Employer References
Mutual of Omaha, Forest National Bank, Nebraska Furniture
    Mart, Saint Joseph Hospital

493 UnitedHealthcare of Nebraska

2717 North 118th Street
Suite 300
Omaha, NE 68164
Toll-Free: 888-545-5205
Phone: 402-445-5000
www.uhc.com
Subsidiary of: UnitedHealth Group
For Profit Organization: Yes
Year Founded: 1984

Healthplan and Services Defined
PLAN TYPE: HMO/PPO
Model Type: Network
Plan Specialty: ASO, Behavioral Health, Chiropractic,
    Dental, Disease Management, Lab, MSO, PBM, Vision,
    Radiology
Benefits Offered: Behavioral Health, Dental, Disease
    Management, Long-Term Care, Prescription, Vision,
    Wellness, Life, LTD, STD

Type of Coverage
Commercial, Individual, Medicare, Supplemental Medicare,
    Medicaid, Catastrophic, Family, Military, Veterans, Group,

Type of Payment Plans Offered
POS, DFFS, FFS

Geographic Areas Served
Iowa: Cass, Fremont, Harrison, Mills, Mononas, Page,
Pottawattsmie, Shelby, Woodbury counties; Nebraska:
Buffalo, Burt, Butler, Dodge, Douglas, Gage, Hale, Jefferson,
Johnson, Lancaster, Madison, Nemaha, Otoe, Pierce, Platte,
Saline, Sarpy, Seward, & Washington counties

Subscriber Information
Average Subscriber Co-Payment:
    Primary Care Physician: $10.00
    Non-Network Physician: Deductible
    Prescription Drugs: $10.00
    Hospital ER: $50.00

Network Qualifications
Pre-Admission Certification: Yes

Peer Review Type
Utilization Review: Yes
Second Surgical Opinion: Yes
Case Management: Yes

Publishes and Distributes Report Card: Yes

Accreditation Certification
TJC Accreditation, Medicare Approved, Utilization Review,
    Pre-Admission Certification, State Licensure, Quality
    Assurance Program

Key Personnel
CEO, Midlands . . . . Kathy Mallatt

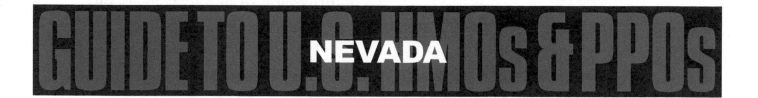
Health Insurance Coverage Status and Type of Coverage by Age

Category	All Persons		Under 18 years		Under 65 years	
	Number	%	Number	%	Number	%
Total population	2,962	-	719	-	2,508	-
Covered by some type of health insurance	2,630 *(13)*	88.8 *(0.4)*	661 *(6)*	92.0 *(0.8)*	2,181 *(13)*	87.0 *(0.5)*
Covered by private health insurance	1,921 *(19)*	64.9 *(0.7)*	435 *(10)*	60.4 *(1.3)*	1,689 *(19)*	67.4 *(0.8)*
Employer-based	1,598 *(22)*	53.9 *(0.7)*	382 *(10)*	53.2 *(1.5)*	1,472 *(21)*	58.7 *(0.8)*
Direct purchase	324 *(11)*	10.9 *(0.4)*	47 *(5)*	6.5 *(0.7)*	214 *(12)*	8.5 *(0.5)*
TRICARE	99 *(7)*	3.3 *(0.2)*	18 *(3)*	2.5 *(0.5)*	61 *(6)*	2.4 *(0.2)*
Covered by public health insurance	1,012 *(19)*	34.2 *(0.6)*	254 *(11)*	35.3 *(1.5)*	580 *(18)*	23.1 *(0.7)*
Medicaid	559 *(18)*	18.9 *(0.6)*	251 *(11)*	34.9 *(1.5)*	510 *(18)*	20.3 *(0.7)*
Medicare	495 *(6)*	16.7 *(0.2)*	4 *(1)*	0.6 *(0.2)*	64 *(5)*	2.5 *(0.2)*
VA Care	86 *(5)*	2.9 *(0.2)*	2 *(1)*	0.3 *(0.2)*	40 *(4)*	1.6 *(0.2)*
Not covered at any time during the year	333 *(13)*	11.2 *(0.4)*	58 *(6)*	8.0 *(0.8)*	327 *(13)*	13.0 *(0.5)*

Note: Numbers in thousands; Figures cover civilian noninstitutionalized population in 2017; N/A indicates that data was not available; Z represents or rounds to zero; Margin of error appears in parenthesis and is calculated using replicate weights.
Source: U.S. Census Bureau, American Community Survey, Table HIC-4_ACS. Health Insurance Coverage Status and Type of Coverage by State—All People: 2008 to 2017, Table HIC-5_ACS. Health Insurance Coverage Status and Type of Coverage by State—Children Under 18: 2008 to 2017, Table HIC-6_ACS. Health Insurance Coverage Status and Type of Coverage by State—Persons Under 65: 2008 to 2017

Nevada

494   Aetna Health of Nevada

151 Farmington Avenue
Hartford, CT 06156
Toll-Free: S 702-668-4200
Phone: N 775-687-1900
www.aetnabetterhealth.com/nevada
Subsidiary of: Aetna Inc.
For Profit Organization: Yes

Healthplan and Services Defined
PLAN TYPE: HMO/PPO
Other Type: POS
Model Type: Network
Plan Specialty: Behavioral Health, EPO, Lab, PBM,
    Radiology
Benefits Offered: Behavioral Health, Dental, Disease
    Management, Long-Term Care, Physical Therapy,
    Podiatry, Prescription, Psychiatric, Vision, Wellness, Life,
    LTD, STD

Type of Coverage
Commercial, Medicare, Supplemental Medicare, Student
    health

Geographic Areas Served
Statewide

Key Personnel
Senior Account Exec. . . . . Tim Nesbitt

495   Anthem Blue Cross & Blue Shield of Nevada

9133 W Russell Road
Las Vegas, NV 89148
Phone: 702-586-6100
www.anthem.com
Secondary Address: 5250 S Virginia Street, Reno, NV 89502,
    775-448-4000
Subsidiary of: Anthem, Inc.
For Profit Organization: Yes

Healthplan and Services Defined
PLAN TYPE: HMO/PPO
Model Type: Network
Plan Specialty: Behavioral Health, Dental, Disease
    Management, Lab, PBM, Vision, Radiology
Benefits Offered: Behavioral Health, Dental, Disease
    Management, Inpatient SNF, Physical Therapy,
    Prescription, Psychiatric, Transplant, Vision, Wellness, Life

Type of Coverage
Commercial, Individual, Medicare, Supplemental Medicare,
    Catastrophic

Geographic Areas Served
Statewide

Accreditation Certification
URAC, NCQA

Key Personnel
President . . . . Mike Murphy

496   Behavioral Healthcare Options, Inc.

2716 N Tenaya Way
Las Vegas, NV 89128
Toll-Free: 800-873-2246
www.bhoptions.com
Subsidiary of: UnitedHealthcare
Year Founded: 1991

Healthplan and Services Defined
PLAN TYPE: PPO
Model Type: Group
Plan Specialty: Behavioral Health, Mental health, addiction
    treatment, employee assistance, work-life services
Benefits Offered: Behavioral Health, Psychiatric

Accreditation Certification
URAC

497   Blue Cross Blue Shield Nevada

Desert Canyon Building 9
9133 W Russell Road
Las Vegas, NV 89148
Toll-Free: 844-396-2329
Phone: 702-586-6100
mss.anthem.com/nevada-medicaid/home.html
Subsidiary of: Anthem, Inc.
For Profit Organization: Yes
Year Founded: 2009

Healthplan and Services Defined
PLAN TYPE: HMO

Type of Coverage
Medicaid, Nevada Check Up, Taking Care of Bab

Accreditation Certification
NCQA

Key Personnel
President . . . . Mike Murphy

498   Coventry Health Care of Nevada

6720-B Rockledge Drive
Suite 800
Bethesda, MD 20817
Phone: 301-581-0600
www.coventryhealthcare.com
Subsidiary of: Aetna Inc.
For Profit Organization: Yes

Healthplan and Services Defined
PLAN TYPE: HMO/PPO
Model Type: Network
Plan Specialty: Behavioral Health, Dental, Worker's
    Compensation
Benefits Offered: Behavioral Health, Dental, Prescription,
    Wellness, Worker's Compensation

Type of Coverage
Commercial, Medicare, Medicaid

Geographic Areas Served
Statewide

Key Personnel
Director, Sales . . . . Stan Rogers
Case Manager. . . . . Joieta Ivanov

499 Health Plan of Nevada

2720 N Tenaya Way
Las Vegas, NV 89128
Toll-Free: 800-777-1840
Phone: 702-242-7300
www.healthplanofnevada.com
Subsidiary of: United HealthCare Services, Inc.
For Profit Organization: Yes
Year Founded: 1982
Total Enrollment: 418,000
State Enrollment: 25,576

Healthplan and Services Defined
PLAN TYPE: HMO
Other Type: POS, Medicare
Model Type: Network
Benefits Offered: Disease Management, Prescription,
Wellness

Type of Coverage
Commercial, Individual, Medicare, Supplemental Medicare,
Medicaid

Geographic Areas Served
Statewide

Accreditation Certification
NCQA

Key Personnel
President/CEO . . . . Jonathan W Bunker

Specialty Managed Care Partners
Express Scripts

500 Hometown Health Plan

10315 Professional Circle
Reno, NV 89521
Toll-Free: 800-336-0123
Phone: 775-982-3232
Fax: 775-982-3741
customer_service@hometownhealth.com
www.hometownhealth.com
Subsidiary of: Renown Health
Non-Profit Organization: Yes
Year Founded: 1988
Owned by an Integrated Delivery Network (IDN): Yes
Number of Affiliated Hospitals: 19
Number of Primary Care Physicians: 256
Number of Referral/Specialty Physicians: 8,917
Total Enrollment: 32,000
State Enrollment: 10,000

Healthplan and Services Defined
PLAN TYPE: Multiple
Model Type: Network
Plan Specialty: ASO, Behavioral Health, Chiropractic,
Dental, Disease Management, EPO, Lab, PBM, Vision,
Radiology, Worker's Compensation, UR

Benefits Offered: Behavioral Health, Chiropractic,
Complementary Medicine, Dental, Disease Management,
Home Care, Inpatient SNF, Physical Therapy, Podiatry,
Prescription, Psychiatric, Transplant, Vision, Wellness,
Worker's Compensation, AD&D, Life, LTD, STD,
Accupuncture
Offers Demand Management Patient Information Service: Yes

Type of Coverage
Commercial, Individual, Medicare, Supplemental Medicare

Geographic Areas Served
Statewide

Subscriber Information
Average Monthly Fee Per Subscriber
(Employee + Employer Contribution):
Employee Only (Self): Varies
Employee & 1 Family Member: Varies
Employee & 2 Family Members: Varies
Medicare: Varies
Average Annual Deductible Per Subscriber:
Employee Only (Self): Varies
Employee & 1 Family Member: Varies
Employee & 2 Family Members: Varies
Medicare: Varies
Average Subscriber Co-Payment:
Primary Care Physician: Varies
Non-Network Physician: Varies
Prescription Drugs: Varies
Hospital ER: Varies
Home Health Care: Varies
Home Health Care Max. Days/Visits Covered: Varies
Nursing Home: Varies
Nursing Home Max. Days/Visits Covered: Varies

Accreditation Certification
TJC

Key Personnel
President/CEO . . . . Ty Windfeldt

501 Humana Health Insurance of Nevada

770 E Warm Springs Road
Suite 340
Las Vegas, NV 89119
Phone: 702-837-4401
Fax: 702-562-0134
www.humana.com
Secondary Address: Pebble Marketplace Shopping Center,
1000 N Green Valley Pkwy, Suite 720, Henderson, NV 89074,
702-269-5200
Subsidiary of: Humana
For Profit Organization: Yes

Healthplan and Services Defined
PLAN TYPE: HMO/PPO
Model Type: Network
Plan Specialty: Dental, Vision
Benefits Offered: Dental, Vision, Life, LTD, STD

Type of Coverage
Commercial, Individual

Geographic Areas Served
Statewide

Accreditation Certification
URAC, NCQA, CORE

Key Personnel
Director, Sales/Marketing................. Dixon Keller

502 Liberty Dental Plan of Nevada
P.O. Box 401086
Las Vegas, NV 89140
Toll-Free: 888-401-1128
www.libertydentalplan.com
For Profit Organization: Yes
Total Enrollment: 2,000,000

Healthplan and Services Defined
PLAN TYPE: Dental
Other Type: Dental HMO
Plan Specialty: Dental
Benefits Offered: Dental

Type of Coverage
Commercial, Medicare, Medicaid, Unions

Geographic Areas Served
Statewide

Accreditation Certification
NCQA

Key Personnel
Chief Dental Officer...................... Todd Gray

503 Nevada Preferred Healthcare Providers
1050 Meadow Wood Lane
Reno, NV 89502
Toll-Free: 800-776-6959
Phone: 775-356-1159
Fax: 775-356-5746
www.universalhealthnet.com
Subsidiary of: Universal Health Services, Inc.
Non-Profit Organization: Yes
Year Founded: 1991
Number of Affiliated Hospitals: 80
Number of Primary Care Physicians: 4,483
Total Enrollment: 150,000
State Enrollment: 150,000

Healthplan and Services Defined
PLAN TYPE: PPO
Other Type: EPO
Model Type: Network
Plan Specialty: EPO, Worker's Compensation
Benefits Offered: Behavioral Health, Chiropractic, Home
    Care, Physical Therapy, Podiatry, Psychiatric, Transplant,
    Wellness, Worker's Compensation

Type of Coverage
Commercial, Individual

Type of Payment Plans Offered
POS, DFFS, FFS, Combination FFS & DFFS

Geographic Areas Served
Nevada, and limited areas in Utah

Network Qualifications
Pre-Admission Certification: Yes

Peer Review Type
Utilization Review: Yes
Second Surgical Opinion: Yes
Case Management: Yes

Publishes and Distributes Report Card: No

Specialty Managed Care Partners
Enters into Contracts with Regional Business Coalitions: Yes

Employer References
State of Nevada, CCN, PPO USA GEHA, Valley Health
    System, Pepperpill

504 Premier Access Insurance/Access Dental
P.O. Box 659010
Sacramento, CA 95865-9010
Toll-Free: 888-634-6074
Phone: 916-920-2500
Fax: 916-563-9000
info@premierlife.com
www.premierppo.com
Subsidiary of: Guardian Life Insurance Co.
For Profit Organization: Yes
Year Founded: 1989
Number of Primary Care Physicians: 1,000

Healthplan and Services Defined
PLAN TYPE: PPO
Other Type: Dental
Plan Specialty: Dental
Benefits Offered: Dental

Key Personnel
President & CEO .... Deanna M. Mulligan

505 Prominence Health Plan
1510 Meadow Wood Lane
Reno, NV 89502
Toll-Free: 800-433-3077
Phone: 775-770-9300
prominencehealthplan.com
Secondary Address: 2475 Village View Drive, Suite 100,
    Henderson, NV 89074
Subsidiary of: Universal Health Services, Inc.
For Profit Organization: Yes
Year Founded: 1993
Number of Affiliated Hospitals: 34
Number of Primary Care Physicians: 4,000
Number of Referral/Specialty Physicians: 1,500

Healthplan and Services Defined
PLAN TYPE: HMO/PPO
Other Type: POS
Model Type: Group, Network
Plan Specialty: ASO, Behavioral Health, Chiropractic, Dental,
    Disease Management, EPO, MSO, PBM, Vision, Radiology,
    Worker's Compensation

Benefits Offered: Behavioral Health, Chiropractic,
Complementary
Medicine, Dental, Disease Management, Home Care,
Inpatient SNF, Long-Term Care, Physical Therapy,
Podiatry, Prescription, Psychiatric, Transplant,
Vision, Wellness, Worker's Compensation, Routine
PE, pre and post-natal care, well baby/well child
care, mammography, GYN, prostate screenings

Type of Payment Plans Offered
POS, DFFS, FFS, Combination FFS & DFFS

Geographic Areas Served
Nevada and border communities in California and Arizona

Subscriber Information
Average Monthly Fee Per Subscriber
(Employee + Employer Contribution):
Employee Only (Self): Varies by plan
Average Subscriber Co-Payment:
Nursing Home: Varies

Network Qualifications
Pre-Admission Certification: Yes

Peer Review Type
Utilization Review: Yes
Second Surgical Opinion: Yes
Case Management: Yes

Accreditation Certification
NCQA
TJC Accreditation, Medicare Approved, Pre-Admission
Certification

Key Personnel
President/CEO . . . . David Livingston
Director of Operations . . . , , , , , , , , , , . . . Majorie Henriksen

---

506   UnitedHealthcare of Nevada
2720 N Tenaya Way
Las Vegas, NV 89128
Toll-Free: 800-701-5909
www.uhc.com
Subsidiary of: UnitedHealth Group
For Profit Organization: Yes
Year Founded: 1984

Healthplan and Services Defined
PLAN TYPE: HMO/PPO
Other Type: POS
Model Type: Network
Plan Specialty: Behavioral Health, Dental, Disease
Management, PBM, Vision
Benefits Offered: Behavioral Health, Dental, Disease
Management, Long-Term Care, Prescription, Vision,
Wellness, Life, LTD, STD

Type of Coverage
Individual, Medicare, Supplemental Medicare, Medicaid,
Catastrophic, Family, Military, Veterans, Group,

Type of Payment Plans Offered
POS, DFFS, Capitated, FFS

Geographic Areas Served
Statewide

Subscriber Information
Average Monthly Fee Per Subscriber
(Employee + Employer Contribution):
Employee Only (Self): $39.00
Average Annual Deductible Per Subscriber:
Employee Only (Self): $0
Employee & 1 Family Member: $0
Employee & 2 Family Members: $0
Medicare: $0
Average Subscriber Co-Payment:
Primary Care Physician: $0.00
Prescription Drugs: $10.00
Hospital ER: $50.00
Home Health Care: Varies
Home Health Care Max. Days/Visits Covered: Unlimited
Nursing Home: Varies
Nursing Home Max. Days/Visits Covered: 100 days

Peer Review Type
Case Management: Yes

Publishes and Distributes Report Card: Yes

Key Personnel
VP, Medicaid Nevada . . . . Kelly Simonson

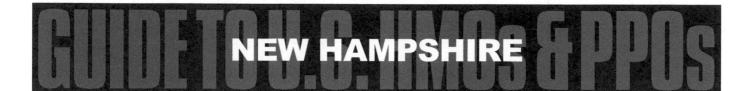

Health Insurance Coverage Status and Type of Coverage by Age

Category	All Persons		Under 18 years		Under 65 years	
	Number	%	Number	%	Number	%
Total population	1,325	-	276	-	1,098	-
Covered by some type of health insurance	1,248 (5)	94.2 (0.4)	270 (3)	97.7 (0.5)	1,022 (6)	93.1 (0.5)
Covered by private health insurance	1,016 (11)	76.7 (0.8)	194 (5)	70.2 (1.8)	857 (10)	78.1 (0.9)
Employer-based	845 (11)	63.8 (0.8)	176 (5)	63.6 (1.9)	761 (10)	69.3 (0.9)
Direct purchase	190 (8)	14.4 (0.6)	17 (3)	6.1 (0.9)	103 (7)	9.4 (0.7)
TRICARE	29 (4)	2.2 (0.3)	3 (1)	1.3 (0.4)	13 (2)	1.2 (0.2)
Covered by public health insurance	421 (9)	31.8 (0.7)	85 (6)	30.9 (2.0)	202 (9)	18.4 (0.8)
Medicaid	182 (9)	13.8 (0.7)	85 (6)	30.6 (2.0)	167 (9)	15.3 (0.8)
Medicare	254 (4)	19.2 (0.3)	1 (1)	0.5 (0.2)	36 (3)	3.3 (0.3)
VA Care	33 (3)	2.5 (0.2)	Z (Z)	0.1 (0.1)	13 (2)	1.2 (0.2)
Not covered at any time during the year	77 (5)	5.8 (0.4)	6 (1)	2.3 (0.5)	76 (5)	6.9 (0.5)

Note: Numbers in thousands; Figures cover civilian noninstitutionalized population in 2017; N/A indicates that data was not available; Z represents or rounds to zero; Margin of error appears in parenthesis and is calculated using replicate weights.
Source: U.S. Census Bureau, American Community Survey, Table HIC-4_ACS. Health Insurance Coverage Status and Type of Coverage by State—All People: 2008 to 2017, Table HIC-5_ACS. Health Insurance Coverage Status and Type of Coverage by State—Children Under 18: 2008 to 2017, Table HIC-6_ACS. Health Insurance Coverage Status and Type of Coverage by State—Persons Under 65: 2008 to 2017

New Hampshire

507   Able Insurance Agency

130 Broadway
Concord, NH 03301
Phone: 603-225-6677
able2insure.com

Healthplan and Services Defined
PLAN TYPE: HMO
Benefits Offered: Wellness, Life

Geographic Areas Served
Greater Concord Area

Key Personnel
Principal .... PJ Cistulli
   pjcj@able2insure.com
Producer .... Angela Chicoine
   angela@able2insure.com
Agent .... Kathy Coleman
   kathy@able2insure.com
Marketing Coordinator .... Samantha Sharff
   samanthaleec@gmail.com

508   Anthem Blue Cross & Blue Shield of New Hampshire

1155 Elm Street
Suite 200
Manchester, NH 03101
www.anthem.com
Subsidiary of: Anthem, Inc.
For Profit Organization: Yes

Healthplan and Services Defined
PLAN TYPE: HMO/PPO
Model Type: Network
Plan Specialty: Behavioral Health, Dental, Disease
   Management, Lab, PBM, Vision, Radiology
Benefits Offered: Behavioral Health, Dental, Disease
   Management, Inpatient SNF, Physical Therapy,
   Prescription, Psychiatric, Transplant, Vision, Wellness, Life

Type of Coverage
Commercial, Individual, Medicare, Supplemental Medicare,
   Catastrophic

Geographic Areas Served
Statewide

Accreditation Certification
URAC, NCQA

Key Personnel
President .... Lisa Guertin

509   Coventry Health Care of New Hampshire

6720-B Rockledge Drive
Suite 800
Bethesda, MD 20817
Phone: 301-581-0600
www.coventryhealthcare.com
Subsidiary of: Aetna Inc.

For Profit Organization: Yes

Healthplan and Services Defined
PLAN TYPE: HMO/PPO
Model Type: Network
Plan Specialty: Behavioral Health, Dental, Worker's
   Compensation
Benefits Offered: Behavioral Health, Dental, Prescription,
   Wellness, Worker's Compensation

Type of Coverage
Commercial, Medicare, Medicaid

Geographic Areas Served
Statewide

510   Harvard Pilgrim Health Care New Hampshire

650 Elm Street
Suite 700
Manchester, NH 03101-2596
Toll-Free: 888-888-4742
www.harvardpilgrim.org
Non-Profit Organization: Yes
Year Founded: 1977
Number of Affiliated Hospitals: 179
Number of Referral/Specialty Physicians: 53,000

Healthplan and Services Defined
PLAN TYPE: HMO/PPO
Benefits Offered: Wellness

Geographic Areas Served
Statewide

Accreditation Certification
NCQA

Key Personnel
VP, Operations NH Market .... William Brewster

511   Humana Health Insurance of New Hampshire

1 New Hampshire Avenue
Suite 125
Portsmouth, NH 03801
Toll-Free: 800-967-2370
www.humana.com
Subsidiary of: Humana
For Profit Organization: Yes

Healthplan and Services Defined
PLAN TYPE: HMO/PPO
Model Type: Network
Plan Specialty: Dental, Vision
Benefits Offered: Dental, Vision, Life, LTD, STD

Type of Coverage
Commercial

Geographic Areas Served
Statewide

Accreditation Certification
URAC, NCQA, CORE

Key Personnel
Regional President . . . . Alexander Clague

---

512 Northeast Delta Dental
One Delta Drive
P.O. Box 2002
Concord, NH 03302-2002
Toll-Free: 800-537-1715
Phone: 603-223-1000
Fax: 603-223-1199
nedelta@nedelta.com
www.nedelta.com
Non-Profit Organization: Yes
Year Founded: 1961

Healthplan and Services Defined
PLAN TYPE: Dental
Other Type: Dental PPO
Model Type: Network
Plan Specialty: ASO, Dental
Benefits Offered: Dental

Type of Coverage
Commercial, Individual
Catastrophic Illness Benefit: None

Geographic Areas Served
Maine, New Hampshire and Vermont

Key Personnel
President/CEO . . . . Thomas Raffio
Chair . . . . David B. Staples
Vice Chair . . . . Mary Ann Aldrich, RN
Treasurer . . . . Francis Boucher
Corporate Secretary . . . . Sara M. Brehm

---

513 UnitedHealthcare of New Hampshire
475 Kilvert Street
Warwick, RI 02886
Toll-Free: 888-545-5205
Phone: 401-737-6900
www.uhc.com
Subsidiary of: UnitedHealth Group
For Profit Organization: Yes
Year Founded: 1986

Healthplan and Services Defined
PLAN TYPE: HMO/PPO
Model Type: Network
Plan Specialty: Behavioral Health, Dental, Disease
  Management, MSO, PBM, Vision
Benefits Offered: Behavioral Health, Chiropractic,
  Complementary Medicine, Dental, Disease Management,
  Home Care, Inpatient SNF, Long-Term Care, Physical
  Therapy, Podiatry, Prescription, Psychiatric, Transplant,
  Vision, Wellness, AD&D, Life, LTD, STD

Type of Coverage
Commercial, Individual, Medicare, Supplemental Medicare,
  Medicaid, Catastrophic, Family, Military, Veterans, Group,

Type of Payment Plans Offered
DFFS, FFS, Combination FFS & DFFS

Geographic Areas Served
Statewide. New Hampshire is covered by the Rhode Island
branch

Subscriber Information
Average Monthly Fee Per Subscriber
  (Employee + Employer Contribution):
    Employee Only (Self): Varies
Average Subscriber Co-Payment:
  Primary Care Physician: $10
  Prescription Drugs: $10/15/30
  Hospital ER: $50

Network Qualifications
Pre-Admission Certification: Yes

Peer Review Type
Case Management: Yes

Publishes and Distributes Report Card: Yes

Accreditation Certification
URAC, NCQA
State Licensure, Quality Assurance Program

Key Personnel
CEO, CT/ME/MA/NH/RI . . . . Stephen Farrell

Average Claim Compensation
Physician's Fees Charged: 70%
Hospital's Fees Charged: 55%

Specialty Managed Care Partners
United Behavioral Health
Enters into Contracts with Regional Business Coalitions: No

---

514 Well Sense Health Plan
1155 Elm Street
Suite 600
Manchester, NH 03101
Toll-Free: 877-492-6965
NHmembers@wellsense.org
www.wellsense.org
Subsidiary of: Boston Medical Center Health Plan, Inc.
Non-Profit Organization: Yes

Healthplan and Services Defined
PLAN TYPE: Other
Other Type: Medicaid
Benefits Offered: Behavioral Health, Prescription, Vision,
  Wellness

Type of Coverage
Medicaid

Geographic Areas Served
New Hampshire

Key Personnel
Chief Medical Officer . . . . Jonathan Welch, MD
Director, Operations . . . . Carol Lacopino
Executive Director . . . . Lisa Britt

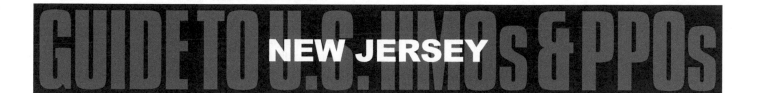
Health Insurance Coverage Status and Type of Coverage by Age

Category	All Persons		Under 18 years		Under 65 years	
	Number	%	Number	%	Number	%
Total population	8,902	-	2,094	-	7,525	-
Covered by some type of health insurance	8,214 (18)	92.3 (0.2)	2,015 (9)	96.3 (0.3)	6,851 (17)	91.0 (0.2)
Covered by private health insurance	6,413 (30)	72.0 (0.3)	1,416 (15)	67.6 (0.7)	5,574 (29)	74.1 (0.4)
Employer-based	5,523 (31)	62.0 (0.4)	1,279 (16)	61.1 (0.7)	4,979 (30)	66.2 (0.4)
Direct purchase	1,063 (22)	11.9 (0.3)	145 (8)	6.9 (0.4)	681 (19)	9.0 (0.3)
TRICARE	88 (7)	1.0 (0.1)	21 (4)	1.0 (0.2)	56 (6)	0.7 (0.1)
Covered by public health insurance	2,793 (26)	31.4 (0.3)	669 (16)	31.9 (0.8)	1,487 (25)	19.8 (0.3)
Medicaid	1,530 (26)	17.2 (0.3)	662 (16)	31.6 (0.8)	1,357 (26)	18.0 (0.3)
Medicare	1,492 (9)	16.8 (0.1)	11 (3)	0.5 (0.1)	187 (7)	2.5 (0.1)
VA Care	96 (5)	1.1 (0.1)	Z (Z)	Z (Z)	32 (3)	0.4 (Z)
Not covered at any time during the year	688 (17)	7.7 (0.2)	78 (7)	3.7 (0.3)	674 (17)	9.0 (0.2)

Note: Numbers in thousands; Figures cover civilian noninstitutionalized population in 2017; N/A indicates that data was not available; Z represents or rounds to zero; Margin of error appears in parenthesis and is calculated using replicate weights.
Source: U.S. Census Bureau, American Community Survey, Table HIC-4_ACS. Health Insurance Coverage Status and Type of Coverage by State—All People: 2008 to 2017, Table HIC-5_ACS. Health Insurance Coverage Status and Type of Coverage by State—Children Under 18: 2008 to 2017, Table HIC-6_ACS. Health Insurance Coverage Status and Type of Coverage by State—Persons Under 65: 2008 to 2017

New Jersey

515 Aetna Health of New Jersey

3 Independence Way
Suite 400
Princeton, NJ 08540-6626
Toll-Free: 855-232-3596
www.aetnabetterhealth.com/newjersey
Subsidiary of: Aetna Inc.
For Profit Organization: Yes

Healthplan and Services Defined
  PLAN TYPE: HMO/PPO
  Other Type: POS
  Model Type: Network
  Plan Specialty: Behavioral Health, EPO, Lab, PBM, Radiology
  Benefits Offered: Behavioral Health, Dental, Disease Management, Long-Term Care, Physical Therapy, Podiatry, Prescription, Psychiatric, Vision, Wellness, Life, LTD, STD

Type of Coverage
  Commercial, Medicare, Supplemental Medicare, Student health

Geographic Areas Served
  Statewide

Key Personnel
  Chief Executive Officer . . . . Glenn MacFarlane
  Chief Operating Officer . . . . Jerold Mammano
  Account Manager . . . . Michelle Rubino Knoblock
  Medical Director . . . . Cheryl Reid

516 AmeriHealth New Jersey

259 Prospect Plains Road
Building M
Cranbury, NJ 08512-3706
Toll-Free: 888-968-7241
www.amerihealthnj.com
Total Enrollment: 265,000

Healthplan and Services Defined
  PLAN TYPE: HMO/PPO
  Benefits Offered: Dental, Disease Management, Prescription, Vision, Wellness

Type of Coverage
  Commercial, Individual

Geographic Areas Served
  New Jersey

Key Personnel
  Market President . . . . Mike Munoz
  Networking Operations . . . . Ken Kobylowski
  Vice President of Sales . . . . Ryan J. Petrizzi
  Senior Medical Director . . . . Frank L. Urbano

517 Atlanticare Health Plans

2500 English Creek Avenue
Egg Harbor Township, NJ 08234
Toll-Free: 888-569-1000
Phone: 609-407-2300
webmaster@atlanticare.org
www.atlanticare.org
Subsidiary of: Geisinger Health System
Non-Profit Organization: Yes
Year Founded: 1993
Number of Affiliated Hospitals: 36
Number of Primary Care Physicians: 600
Number of Referral/Specialty Physicians: 4,000
Total Enrollment: 150,000
State Enrollment: 150,000

Healthplan and Services Defined
  PLAN TYPE: HMO/PPO
  Model Type: IPA
  Plan Specialty: ASO, Behavioral Health, Worker's Compensation, UR

Type of Payment Plans Offered
  Combination FFS & DFFS

Geographic Areas Served
  Southeastern New Jersey

Subscriber Information
  Average Subscriber Co-Payment:
    Primary Care Physician: $10.00
    Non-Network Physician: $20.00
    Prescription Drugs: $15.00
    Hospital ER: $50.00
    Home Health Care: $60
    Nursing Home: $120

Network Qualifications
  Pre-Admission Certification: Yes

Peer Review Type
  Utilization Review: Yes
  Second Surgical Opinion: Yes
  Case Management: Yes

Accreditation Certification
  TJC, URAC, NCQA

Specialty Managed Care Partners
  Horizon BC/BS of NJ

518 CHN PPO

300 American Metro Boulevard
Suite 170
Hamilton, NJ 08619
Toll-Free: 800-225-4246
Phone: 800-293-9795
www.chn.com
Subsidiary of: Consolidated Services Group
For Profit Organization: Yes
Year Founded: 1986
Number of Affiliated Hospitals: 165
Number of Primary Care Physicians: 116,000
Number of Referral/Specialty Physicians: 57,550

Total Enrollment: 975,000

Healthplan and Services Defined
PLAN TYPE: PPO
Model Type: Network
Plan Specialty: Behavioral Health, Chiropractic, EPO, Lab, Vision, Radiology, Worker's Compensation, UR
Benefits Offered: Behavioral Health, Chiropractic, Disease Management, Home Care, Inpatient SNF, Long-Term Care, Physical Therapy, Podiatry, Psychiatric, Transplant, Vision, Wellness, Worker's Compensation

Type of Coverage
Catastrophic Illness Benefit: Varies per case

Type of Payment Plans Offered
POS, DFFS, FFS

Geographic Areas Served
Connecticut, New Jersey & New York

Subscriber Information
Average Monthly Fee Per Subscriber
(Employee + Employer Contribution):
Employee Only (Self): Varies
Employee & 1 Family Member: Varies
Employee & 2 Family Members: Varies
Medicare: Varies
Average Annual Deductible Per Subscriber:
Employee Only (Self): Varies
Employee & 1 Family Member: Varies
Employee & 2 Family Members: Varies
Medicare: Varies
Average Subscriber Co-Payment:
Primary Care Physician: Varies
Non-Network Physician: Varies
Prescription Drugs: Varies
Hospital ER: Varies
Home Health Care: Varies
Home Health Care Max. Days/Visits Covered: Varies
Nursing Home: Varies
Nursing Home Max. Days/Visits Covered: Varies

Network Qualifications
Pre-Admission Certification: Yes

Peer Review Type
Utilization Review: Yes
Second Surgical Opinion: Yes
Case Management: Yes

Accreditation Certification
URAC, AAPI
TJC Accreditation, Medicare Approved, Utilization Review, Pre-Admission Certification, State Licensure, Quality Assurance Program

Key Personnel
President/CEO . . . . Craig Goldstein
SVP, Financial Operations . . . . Lee Ann Iannelli

Average Claim Compensation
Physician's Fees Charged: 33%
Hospital's Fees Charged: 40%

Specialty Managed Care Partners
Enters into Contracts with Regional Business Coalitions: Yes

---

519   **Cigna Healthcare New Jersey**
72 Princeton Highstown Road
East Windsor, NJ 08520
Phone: 609-917-2668
www.cigna.com
Secondary Address: 4 St. Michael Court, Cherry Hill, NJ 08003, 856-286-2952
For Profit Organization: Yes
Year Founded: 1982

Healthplan and Services Defined
PLAN TYPE: Multiple
Benefits Offered: Behavioral Health, Dental, Disease Management, Prescription, Vision, Wellness, AD&D, Life, LTD, STD

Type of Coverage
Commercial, Individual, Medicare, Supplemental Medicare, Medicaid

Geographic Areas Served
Statewide

Key Personnel
Cigna Pharmacy Management . . . . Craig Steel
Dir., Client Engagement . . . . Pam Lounsbury
Senior Sales Director . . . . Ann Servais

---

520   **Coventry Health Care of New Jersey**
10000 Lincoln Drive East
Suite 201
Marlton, NJ 08053
Phone: 856-988-5521
www.coventryhealthcare.com
Subsidiary of: Aetna Inc.
For Profit Organization: Yes

Healthplan and Services Defined
PLAN TYPE: HMO/PPO
Model Type: Network
Plan Specialty: Behavioral Health, Dental, Worker's Compensation
Benefits Offered: Behavioral Health, Dental, Prescription, Wellness, Worker's Compensation

Type of Coverage
Commercial, Medicare, Medicaid

Geographic Areas Served
Statewide

Key Personnel
Customer Service Rep. . . . . Pilar Capuano

---

521   **Delta Dental of New Jersey**
1639 Route 10
Parsippany, NJ 07054
Toll-Free: 800-452-9310
service@deltadentalnj.com
www.deltadentalnj.com
Mailing Address: P.O. Box 222, Parsippany, NJ 07054-0222
Non-Profit Organization: Yes
Year Founded: 1969

Healthplan and Services Defined
PLAN TYPE: Dental
Other Type: Dental HMO/PPO/POS
Model Type: Staff
Plan Specialty: Dental
Benefits Offered: Dental

Type of Coverage
Commercial

Type of Payment Plans Offered
POS, DFFS, Capitated, FFS, Combination FFS & DFFS

Geographic Areas Served
New Jersey and Connecticut

Key Personnel
President/CEO . . . . Dennis G. Wilson

522 Horizon Blue Cross Blue Shield of New Jersey
P.O. Box 820
Newark, NJ 07101
Toll-Free: 800-355-2583
www.horizonblue.com
Non-Profit Organization: Yes
Year Founded: 1932
State Enrollment: 3,800,000

Healthplan and Services Defined
PLAN TYPE: HMO/PPO
Other Type: POS
Model Type: Staff, Network
Benefits Offered: Behavioral Health, Dental, Prescription, Psychiatric, Worker's Compensation
Offers Demand Management Patient Information Service: Yes

Type of Coverage
Commercial, Individual, Indemnity, Medicare
Catastrophic Illness Benefit: None

Geographic Areas Served
Statewide

Peer Review Type
Utilization Review: Yes
Second Surgical Opinion: Yes
Case Management: Yes

Accreditation Certification
AAAHC, URAC, NCQA
TJC Accreditation, Medicare Approved, Utilization Review, Pre-Admission Certification, State Licensure, Quality Assurance Program

Key Personnel
Chairman/President/CEO . . . . Kevin P. Conlin
SVP, Operations . . . . Mark L. Barnard
SVP/CIO . . . . Douglas E. Blackwell
SVP, Human Resources . . . . Margaret M. Coons
SVP/CFO/Treasurer . . . . Dave R. Huber
General Counsel/Secretary . . . . Linda A. Willett
EVP, Commercial Business . . . . Christopher M. Lepre

Specialty Managed Care Partners
Enters into Contracts with Regional Business Coalitions: Yes

523 Horizon NJ Health
210 Silvia Street
West Trenton, NJ 08628
Toll-Free: 800-682-9090
www.horizonnjhealth.com
Subsidiary of: Horizon Blue Cross Blue Shield of NJ
Year Founded: 1993
Total Enrollment: 727,000
State Enrollment: 467,000

Healthplan and Services Defined
PLAN TYPE: PPO
Model Type: Network
Benefits Offered: Dental, Disease Management, Prescription, Vision, Wellness

Type of Coverage
Individual, Medicaid

Geographic Areas Served
Statewide

Accreditation Certification
URAC

Key Personnel
President . . . . Karen Clark
Controller/Subsidiary CFO . . . . James Dalessio
Marketing/Communications . . . . Len Kudgis
VP, Clinical Affairs/CMO . . . . Philip M Bonaparte, MD
Media Contact . . . . Carol Chernack
609-718-9290
carol_chernack@horizonnjhealth.com

524 Humana Health Insurance of New Jersey
1075 RXR Plaza
Uniondale, NY 11556
Phone: 516-247-2021
www.humana.com
Secondary Address: 5000 Ritter Road, Suite 101, Mechanicsburg, PA 17055, 866-355-5861
Subsidiary of: Humana
For Profit Organization: Yes

Healthplan and Services Defined
PLAN TYPE: HMO/PPO
Model Type: Network
Plan Specialty: Dental, Vision
Benefits Offered: Dental, Vision, Life, LTD, STD

Type of Coverage
Commercial

Geographic Areas Served
Statewide

Accreditation Certification
URAC, NCQA, CORE

Key Personnel
Reg. Dir., Contracting . . . . Michele Deverin
Regional Vice President . . . . Frank Pistone

525   Liberty Dental Plan of New Jersey

P.O. Box 26110
Santa Ana, CA 92799-6110
Toll-Free: 877-558-6489
www.libertydentalplan.com
For Profit Organization: Yes
Year Founded: 2001
Total Enrollment: 3,000,000

Healthplan and Services Defined
   PLAN TYPE: Dental
   Other Type: Dental HMO
   Plan Specialty: Dental
   Benefits Offered: Dental

Type of Coverage
   Commercial, Individual, Medicare, Medicaid, Unions

Geographic Areas Served
   Statewide

Accreditation Certification
   NCQA

526   Molina Medicaid Solutions

3705 Quakerbridge Road
Trenton, NJ 08619
Toll-Free: 800-776-6334
www.molinahealthcare.com
Subsidiary of: Molina Healthcare, Inc.
For Profit Organization: Yes

Healthplan and Services Defined
   PLAN TYPE: Medicare

Type of Coverage
   Medicaid information management sys

Geographic Areas Served
   Statewide

527   QualCare

30 Knightsbridge Road
Piscataway, NJ 08854
Toll-Free: 800-992-6613
Phone: 732-562-0833
info@qualcareinc.com
www.qualcareinc.com
Subsidiary of: QualCare Alliance Networks, Inc.
For Profit Organization: Yes
Year Founded: 1993
Federally Qualified: Yes
Number of Affiliated Hospitals: 100
Number of Primary Care Physicians: 9,000
Number of Referral/Specialty Physicians: 14,000
Total Enrollment: 750,000
State Enrollment: 750,000

Healthplan and Services Defined
   PLAN TYPE: Multiple
   Other Type: POS, TPA
   Model Type: Network

Plan Specialty: ASO, Behavioral Health, Chiropractic, Dental,
   Disease Management, EPO, Lab, MSO, PBM, Vision,
   Radiology, Worker's Compensation, UR
Benefits Offered: Behavioral Health, Chiropractic,
   Complementary
Medicine, Dental, Disease Management, Home Care,
Inpatient SNF, Long-Term Care, Physical Therapy,
Podiatry, Prescription, Psychiatric, Transplant,
Vision, Wellness, Worker's Compensation, AD&D,
Life, LTD, STD
   Offers Demand Management Patient Information Service: Yes

Type of Coverage
   Commercial

Type of Payment Plans Offered
   FFS

Geographic Areas Served
   New Jersey, Pennsylvania, New York

Peer Review Type
   Utilization Review: Yes
   Second Surgical Opinion: Yes
   Case Management: Yes

Publishes and Distributes Report Card: Yes

Accreditation Certification
   AAAHC, TJC, AAPI, NCQA
   Medicare Approved, Utilization Review, State Licensure,
   Quality Assurance Program

Key Personnel
   VP/CFO . . . . Janet Buggle
   VP, Network/Delivery. . . . . Jennifer Lagasca
   Medical Director . . . . Michael McNeil, MD

Specialty Managed Care Partners
   Multiplan

528   Trinity Health of New Jersey

Lourdes Health System
1600 Haddon Avenue
Camden, NJ 08103
Phone: 856-757-3500
www.trinity-health.org
Secondary Address: St Francis Medical Center, 601 Hamilton
   Avenue, Trenton, NJ 08629, 609-599-5000
Subsidiary of: Trinity Health
Non-Profit Organization: Yes
Year Founded: 2013
Total Enrollment: 30,000,000

Healthplan and Services Defined
   PLAN TYPE: Other
   Benefits Offered: Disease Management, Home Care,
      Long-Term Care, Psychiatric, Hospice programs, PACE
      (Program of All Inclusive Care for the Elderly)

Geographic Areas Served
   Southern New Jersey

Key Personnel
   President . . . . Reginald Blader
   Chief Nursing Officer . . . . Maria Lariccia Brennan
   Chief Information Officer. . . . . Maureen Hetu

Chief Operating Officer. . . . . Mark Nessel
VP, Medical Affairs/CMO . . . . Alan Pope

529 UnitedHealthcare of New Jersey

Iselin, NJ 08830
Toll-Free: 888-545-5205
www.uhc.com
Subsidiary of: UnitedHealth Group
For Profit Organization: Yes

Healthplan and Services Defined
  PLAN TYPE: HMO/PPO
  Model Type: Network
  Plan Specialty: Behavioral Health, Dental, Disease
    Management, PBM, Vision
  Benefits Offered: Behavioral Health, Dental, Disease
    Management, Long-Term Care, Prescription, Vision,
    Wellness, Life, LTD, STD

Type of Coverage
  Individual, Medicare, Supplemental Medicare, Medicaid,
    Catastrophic, Family, Military, Veterans, Group,

Geographic Areas Served
  Statewide

Key Personnel
  CEO, Healthplan of NJ . . . . Paul Marden

530 Zelis Healthcare

2 Crossroads Drive
Bedminster, NJ 07921
Phone: 888-311-3505
www.zelis.com
Subsidiary of: Zelis Healthcare
For Profit Organization: Yes
Year Founded: 2016
Owned by an Integrated Delivery Network (IDN): Yes

Healthplan and Services Defined
  PLAN TYPE: PPO
  Plan Specialty: Dental, Worker's Compensation
  Benefits Offered: Dental, Worker's Compensation

Type of Coverage
  Individual

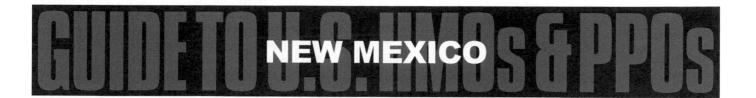

Health Insurance Coverage Status and Type of Coverage by Age

Category	All Persons		Under 18 years		Under 65 years	
	Number	%	Number	%	Number	%
Total population	2,054	-	523	-	1,709	-
Covered by some type of health insurance	1,867 *(12)*	90.9 *(0.6)*	496 *(5)*	94.9 *(0.7)*	1,526 *(12)*	89.3 *(0.7)*
Covered by private health insurance	1,119 *(22)*	54.4 *(1.1)*	232 *(9)*	44.3 *(1.7)*	935 *(21)*	54.7 *(1.2)*
Employer-based	887 *(22)*	43.2 *(1.1)*	194 *(9)*	37.1 *(1.7)*	782 *(20)*	45.7 *(1.2)*
Direct purchase	222 *(10)*	10.8 *(0.5)*	29 *(4)*	5.5 *(0.8)*	141 *(9)*	8.2 *(0.5)*
TRICARE	89 *(6)*	4.3 *(0.3)*	18 *(3)*	3.4 *(0.6)*	57 *(5)*	3.3 *(0.3)*
Covered by public health insurance	1,011 *(18)*	49.2 *(0.9)*	292 *(9)*	55.8 *(1.7)*	678 *(18)*	39.7 *(1.0)*
Medicaid	682 *(17)*	33.2 *(0.8)*	290 *(9)*	55.5 *(1.7)*	622 *(17)*	36.4 *(1.0)*
Medicare	396 *(5)*	19.3 *(0.3)*	2 *(1)*	0.5 *(0.2)*	64 *(5)*	3.8 *(0.3)*
VA Care	68 *(5)*	3.3 *(0.2)*	Z *(Z)*	0.1 *(0.1)*	32 *(3)*	1.8 *(0.2)*
Not covered at any time during the year	187 *(12)*	9.1 *(0.6)*	26 *(4)*	5.1 *(0.7)*	183 *(12)*	10.7 *(0.7)*

Note: Numbers in thousands; Figures cover civilian noninstitutionalized population in 2017; N/A indicates that data was not available; Z represents or rounds to zero; Margin of error appears in parenthesis and is calculated using replicate weights.
Source: U.S. Census Bureau, American Community Survey, Table HIC-4_ACS. Health Insurance Coverage Status and Type of Coverage by State—All People: 2008 to 2017, Table HIC-5_ACS. Health Insurance Coverage Status and Type of Coverage by State—Children Under 18: 2008 to 2017, Table HIC-6_ACS. Health Insurance Coverage Status and Type of Coverage by State—Persons Under 65: 2008 to 2017

New Mexico

---

531 Blue Cross & Blue Shield of New Mexico

5701 Balloon Fiesta Parkway NE
Albuquerque, NM 87113
Toll-Free: 800-835-8699
Phone: 505-291-3500
www.bcbsnm.com
Mailing Address: P.O. Box 27630, Albuquerque, NM
    87125-7630
Subsidiary of: Health Care Service Corporation
Non-Profit Organization: Yes
Year Founded: 1940
Owned by an Integrated Delivery Network (IDN): Yes
Number of Affiliated Hospitals: 54
Number of Primary Care Physicians: 3,322
Number of Referral/Specialty Physicians: 6,742
Total Enrollment: 367,000
State Enrollment: 367,000

Healthplan and Services Defined
  PLAN TYPE: HMO/PPO
  Other Type: EPO, CDHP
  Model Type: Network
  Plan Specialty: ASO, Behavioral Health
  Benefits Offered: Dental, Disease Management, Vision,
    Wellness, Medical, Case Management
  Offers Demand Management Patient Information Service:
    Yes
  DMPI Services Offered: Fully Insured

Type of Coverage
  Commercial, Individual, Indemnity, Supplemental Medicare

Geographic Areas Served
  Statewide

Network Qualifications
  Pre-Admission Certification: Yes

Peer Review Type
  Utilization Review: Yes
  Second Surgical Opinion: Yes

Publishes and Distributes Report Card: Yes

Accreditation Certification
  NCQA

Key Personnel
  President . . . . Kurt Shipley
  Media Contact . . . . Becky Kenny
    505-816-2012
    becky_kenny@bcbsnm.com

Specialty Managed Care Partners
  Pharmacy Manager, Prime Theraputics

---

532 Coventry Health Care of New Mexico

6720-B Rockledge Drive
Suite 800
Bethesda, MD 20817
Phone: 301-581-0600
www.coventryhealthcare.com
Subsidiary of: Aetna Inc.

For Profit Organization: Yes

Healthplan and Services Defined
  PLAN TYPE: HMO/PPO
  Model Type: Network
  Plan Specialty: Behavioral Health, Dental, Worker's
    Compensation
  Benefits Offered: Behavioral Health, Dental, Prescription,
    Wellness, Worker's Compensation

Type of Coverage
  Commercial, Medicare, Medicaid

Geographic Areas Served
  Statewide

Key Personnel
  Operations Manager . . . . Carrie Lucero

---

533 Delta Dental of New Mexico

2500 Louisiana Boulevard NE
Suite 600
Albuquerque, NM 87110
Toll-Free: 877-395-9420
Phone: 505-855-7111
Fax: 505-883-7444
www.deltadentalnm.com
Non-Profit Organization: Yes
Year Founded: 1971
Number of Primary Care Physicians: 979
State Enrollment: 390,000

Healthplan and Services Defined
  PLAN TYPE: Dental
  Other Type: Dental PPO
  Model Type: Group
  Plan Specialty: ASO, Dental, Vision
  Benefits Offered: Dental, Vision
  Offers Demand Management Patient Information Service: Yes

Type of Coverage
  Commercial

Geographic Areas Served
  Statewide

Network Qualifications
  Pre-Admission Certification: Yes

Publishes and Distributes Report Card: Yes

Key Personnel
  President/CEO . . . . Edward Lopez Jr.
  Chief Financial Officer . . . . Amy Basel
  Director, Operations . . . . Cynthia Lucero-Ali
  Director, Public Affairs. . . . . John Martinez
  Dir., Product Management. . . . . Nathalie Casado
  Sr. Admin., Corp. Service . . . . Maria Lopez
  VP, Sales/Marketing . . . . JoLou Trujillo-Ottino

Specialty Managed Care Partners
  Enters into Contracts with Regional Business Coalitions: Yes

534 HCSC Insurance Services Company

5701 Balloon Fiesta Pkywy NE
Albuquerque, NM 87113
Toll-Free: 800-835-8699
hcsc.com
Subsidiary of: Blue Cross Blue Shield Association
Non-Profit Organization: Yes
Year Founded: 1936
Number of Primary Care Physicians: 14,400

Healthplan and Services Defined
   PLAN TYPE: HMO
   Benefits Offered: Behavioral Health, Dental, Disease
      Management, Psychiatric, Wellness

Geographic Areas Served
   Statewide

535 Humana Health Insurance of New Mexico

4904 Alameda Boulevard NE
Suite A
Albuquerque, NM 87113
Toll-Free: 800-681-0680
Phone: 505-468-0500
Fax: 505-468-0554
www.humana.com
Subsidiary of: Humana
For Profit Organization: Yes

Healthplan and Services Defined
   PLAN TYPE: HMO/PPO

Type of Coverage
   Commercial, Individual

Geographic Areas Served
   Statewide

Accreditation Certification
   URAC, NCQA, CORE

Key Personnel
   Sales Representative . . . . Erica A. Gonzales

536 Molina Healthcare of New Mexico

400 Tijeras Avenue NW
Suite 200
Albuquerque, NM 87102
Toll-Free: 800-377-9594
Phone: 505-342-4660
www.molinahealthcare.com
Subsidiary of: Molina Healthcare, Inc.
For Profit Organization: Yes

Healthplan and Services Defined
   PLAN TYPE: Medicare
   Model Type: Network
   Plan Specialty: Dental, PBM, Vision, Integrated
      Medicare/Medicaid (Duals)
   Benefits Offered: Dental, Prescription, Vision, Wellness, Life

Type of Coverage
   Individual, Medicare, Supplemental Medicare, Medicaid

Geographic Areas Served
   Statewide

Key Personnel
   Vice President. . . . . Carolyn Ingram
   Chief Operating Officer . . . . Brian Martin

537 New Mexico Health Connections

2440 Louisiana Boulevard
Suite 601
Albuquerque, NM 87110
Toll-Free: 855-769-6642
Phone: 505-633-8020
Fax: 866-231-1344
mynmhc.org
Subsidiary of: Evolent Health

Healthplan and Services Defined
   PLAN TYPE: HMO
   Benefits Offered: Behavioral Health, Disease Management,
      Wellness

Geographic Areas Served
   Statewide

Key Personnel
   Chief Executive Officer . . . . Martin Hickey
   Chief Operating Officer. . . . . Anne Brennan Sapon
   Chief Medical Officer . . . . Mark Epstein, MD
   Chief Compliance Officer. . . . . Angela Vigil
   Chief Information Officer . . . . Richard Hilliard
   Chief Financial Officer . . . . Nathan Johns

538 Presbyterian Health Plan

9521 San Mateo Boulevard NE
Albuquerque, NM 87113
Toll-Free: 800-356-2219
Phone: 505-923-5700
info@phs.org
www.phs.org
Non-Profit Organization: Yes
Year Founded: 1908
Number of Affiliated Hospitals: 28
Number of Primary Care Physicians: 18,843
Number of Referral/Specialty Physicians: 4,850
Total Enrollment: 400,000
State Enrollment: 400,000

Healthplan and Services Defined
   PLAN TYPE: HMO
   Other Type: POS
   Model Type: Contracted Network
   Benefits Offered: Disease Management, Inpatient SNF,
      Prescription

Type of Coverage
   Commercial, Medicare, Medicaid

Type of Payment Plans Offered
   POS, DFFS, Capitated, FFS

Geographic Areas Served
   Statewide

Subscriber Information
Average Monthly Fee Per Subscriber
(Employee + Employer Contribution):
Employee Only (Self): Varies by plan
Average Subscriber Co-Payment:
Primary Care Physician: $10.00
Prescription Drugs: $0
Hospital ER: $50.00

Accreditation Certification
NCQA

Key Personnel
Chair/President/CEO. . . . . Dale Maxwell
Vice Chair . . . . Teresa Kline

Employer References
State of New Mexico, Albuquerque Public Schools, Intel
Corporation

---

539 Presbyterian Medicare Advantage Plans

The Cooper Center
9521 San Mateo Boulevard NE
Albuquerque, NM 87113
Toll-Free: 800-979-5343
Phone: 505-923-6060
info@phs.org
www.phs.org

Healthplan and Services Defined
PLAN TYPE: Medicare
Benefits Offered: Chiropractic, Dental, Disease Management,
Home Care, Inpatient SNF, Physical Therapy, Podiatry,
Prescription, Psychiatric, Vision, Wellness, Hearing;
Rehabilitation; Durable Medical Equipment;
Transportation

Type of Coverage
Individual, Medicare

Geographic Areas Served
Bernalillo, Cibola, Rio Arriba, Sandoval, Santa Fe, Socorro,
Torrance and Valencia

Key Personnel
Chair . . . . Katharine Winograd
Vice Chair . . . . Brian Burnett

---

540 United Concordia of New Mexico

4401 Deer Path Road
Harrisburg, PA 17110
Phone: 717-260-6800
www.unitedconcordia.com
For Profit Organization: Yes
Year Founded: 1971
Total Enrollment: 7,800,000

Healthplan and Services Defined
PLAN TYPE: Dental
Plan Specialty: Dental
Benefits Offered: Dental

Type of Coverage
Commercial, Individual, Military personnel & families

Geographic Areas Served
Nationwide

Accreditation Certification
URAC

Key Personnel
Contact. . . . . Beth Rutherford
717-260-7659
beth.rutherford@ucci.com

---

541 UnitedHealthcare of New Mexico

8801 Horizon Blvd NE
Albuquerque, NM 87113
Toll-Free: 877-236-0826
www.uhc.com
Subsidiary of: UnitedHealth Group
For Profit Organization: Yes

Healthplan and Services Defined
PLAN TYPE: HMO/PPO
Model Type: Network
Plan Specialty: Behavioral Health, Dental, Disease
Management, PBM, Vision
Benefits Offered: Behavioral Health, Dental, Disease
Management, Long-Term Care, Prescription, Vision,
Wellness, Life, LTD, STD

Type of Coverage
Individual, Medicare, Supplemental Medicare, Medicaid,
Catastrophic, Family, Military, Veterans, Group,

Geographic Areas Served
Statewide

Key Personnel
VP, Health Services. . . . . Tracy Townsend

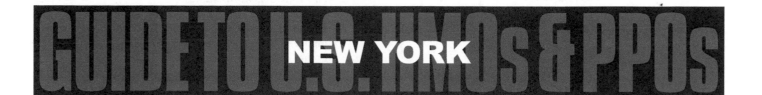
Health Insurance Coverage Status and Type of Coverage by Age

Category	All Persons		Under 18 years		Under 65 years	
	Number	%	Number	%	Number	%
Total population	19,608	-	4,403	-	16,542	-
Covered by some type of health insurance	18,495 *(27)*	94.3 *(0.1)*	4,286 *(12)*	97.3 *(0.2)*	15,450 *(27)*	93.4 *(0.2)*
Covered by private health insurance	13,124 *(59)*	66.9 *(0.3)*	2,718 *(26)*	61.7 *(0.6)*	11,340 *(58)*	68.6 *(0.4)*
Employer-based	10,965 *(56)*	55.9 *(0.3)*	2,278 *(24)*	51.7 *(0.5)*	9,758 *(55)*	59.0 *(0.3)*
Direct purchase	2,587 *(38)*	13.2 *(0.2)*	480 *(19)*	10.9 *(0.4)*	1,833 *(34)*	11.1 *(0.2)*
TRICARE	166 *(9)*	0.8 *(Z)*	37 *(4)*	0.8 *(0.1)*	109 *(7)*	0.7 *(Z)*
Covered by public health insurance	7,766 *(49)*	39.6 *(0.2)*	1,837 *(25)*	41.7 *(0.5)*	4,844 *(49)*	29.3 *(0.3)*
Medicaid	5,157 *(49)*	26.3 *(0.3)*	1,826 *(25)*	41.5 *(0.5)*	4,560 *(48)*	27.6 *(0.3)*
Medicare	3,381 *(15)*	17.2 *(0.1)*	25 *(4)*	0.6 *(0.1)*	461 *(13)*	2.8 *(0.1)*
VA Care	265 *(8)*	1.3 *(Z)*	4 *(2)*	0.1 *(Z)*	104 *(6)*	0.6 *(Z)*
Not covered at any time during the year	1,113 *(27)*	5.7 *(0.1)*	118 *(9)*	2.7 *(0.2)*	1,091 *(27)*	6.6 *(0.2)*

Note: Numbers in thousands; Figures cover civilian noninstitutionalized population in 2017; N/A indicates that data was not available; Z represents or rounds to zero; Margin of error appears in parenthesis and is calculated using replicate weights.
Source: U.S. Census Bureau, American Community Survey, Table HIC-4_ACS. Health Insurance Coverage Status and Type of Coverage by State—All People: 2008 to 2017, Table HIC-5_ACS. Health Insurance Coverage Status and Type of Coverage by State—Children Under 18: 2008 to 2017, Table HIC-6_ACS. Health Insurance Coverage Status and Type of Coverage by State—Persons Under 65: 2008 to 2017

New York

542 Aetna Health of New York
151 Farmington Avenue
Hartford, CT 06156
Toll-Free: 800-872-3862
www.aetna.com
Subsidiary of: Aetna Inc.
For Profit Organization: Yes
Year Founded: 1986
Number of Affiliated Hospitals: 61
Number of Primary Care Physicians: 2,691
Total Enrollment: 154,162
State Enrollment: 154,162

Healthplan and Services Defined
PLAN TYPE: HMO/PPO
Model Type: Network
Plan Specialty: Behavioral Health, Dental, EPO, Lab, PBM, Vision, Radiology
Benefits Offered: Behavioral Health, Dental, Disease Management, Long-Term Care, Physical Therapy, Podiatry, Prescription, Psychiatric, Vision, Wellness, Life, LTD, STD

Type of Coverage
Commercial, Supplemental Medicare, Medicaid, Student health
Catastrophic Illness Benefit: Varies per case

Type of Payment Plans Offered
POS, Capitated

Geographic Areas Served
Statewide

Network Qualifications
Pre-Admission Certification: Yes

Peer Review Type
Utilization Review: Yes
Second Surgical Opinion: No
Case Management: Yes

Publishes and Distributes Report Card: Yes

Accreditation Certification
NCQA
TJC Accreditation, Medicare Approved, Utilization Review, Pre-Admission Certification, State Licensure, Quality Assurance Program

Key Personnel
Sr. Dir., Care Management . . . . Matt Tang

Specialty Managed Care Partners
Enters into Contracts with Regional Business Coalitions: Yes

543 Affinity Health Plan
1776 Eastchester Road
Bronx, NY 10461
Toll-Free: 866-247-5678
Fax: 718-794-7804
mainoffice@affinityplan.org
www.affinityplan.org

Non-Profit Organization: Yes
Year Founded: 1986
Number of Affiliated Hospitals: 60
Number of Primary Care Physicians: 1,400
Number of Referral/Specialty Physicians: 5,000
Total Enrollment: 134,837
State Enrollment: 134,837

Healthplan and Services Defined
PLAN TYPE: HMO
Model Type: Staff

Type of Coverage
Medicaid

Geographic Areas Served
NY Metropolitan Area

Accreditation Certification
TJC Accreditation, Medicare Approved, Utilization Review, State Licensure

Key Personnel
President/CEO . . . . Michael G. Murphy
Chief Compliance Officer . . . . Lisa Mingione
Chief Marketing Officer . . . . Denise J. Pesich
Director, Medicaid . . . . Adrian Robert
Chief Financial Officer . . . . Steve Giasi

544 AlphaCare
335 Adams Street
Suite 2600
Brooklyn, NY 11201
Toll-Free: 855-363-6110
www.alphacare.com
Subsidiary of: Magellan Health
For Profit Organization: Yes

Healthplan and Services Defined
PLAN TYPE: Multiple
Plan Specialty: Chronic illness and long-term care.
Benefits Offered: Long-Term Care

Type of Coverage
Medicare, Medicaid

Geographic Areas Served
Bronx, Brooklyn, Manhattan, Queens and Westchester counties

Key Personnel
CEO . . . . Daniel M. Parietti

545 BlueCross BlueShield of Western New York
257 W Genesee Street
Buffalo, NY 14202-2657
Toll-Free: 800-544-2583
Phone: 716-884-2800
www.bcbswny.com
Mailing Address: P.O. Box 80, Buffalo, NY 14240-0080
Non-Profit Organization: Yes
Year Founded: 1936
Total Enrollment: 555,405
State Enrollment: 197,194

Healthplan and Services Defined
    PLAN TYPE: HMO/PPO
    Other Type: POS, EPO
    Plan Specialty: Dental, Lab, Vision
    Benefits Offered: Dental, Disease Management, Prescription, Vision, Wellness

Type of Coverage
    Commercial, Medicare, Supplemental Medicare, Medicaid

Geographic Areas Served
    Statewide

Key Personnel
    President/CEO . . . . David W. Anderson
    EVP/CFO . . . . Stephen T. Swift
    Senior VP, Operations. . . . . Christopher M. Leardini
    SVP, Chief Sales Officer. . . . . David Busch
    SVP, Network Officer . . . . Ronald Mornelli
    SVP, Human Resources . . . . Douglas Parks
    SVP, Medical Officer . . . . Thomas E. Schenk, MD

Specialty Managed Care Partners
    Wellpoint Pharmacy Management

---

546   BlueShield of Northeastern New York

40 Century Hill Drive
Latham, NY 12110
Toll-Free: 800-888-1238
Phone: 518-220-4600
customerservice@bsneny.com
www.bsneny.com
Mailing Address: P.O. Box 15013, Albany, NY 12212
Non-Profit Organization: Yes
Year Founded: 1946
Total Enrollment: 193,498
State Enrollment: 72,563

Healthplan and Services Defined
    PLAN TYPE: HMO/PPO
    Other Type: POS, EPO
    Plan Specialty: Dental
    Benefits Offered: Dental, Disease Management, Prescription, Wellness

Type of Coverage
    Commercial, Medicare, Supplemental Medicare, Medicaid

Type of Payment Plans Offered
    POS, FFS

Geographic Areas Served
    Albany, Clinton, Columbia, Essex, Fulton, Green, Montgomery, Schoharie, Schenectedy, Warren and Washington counties

Accreditation Certification
    NCQA

Key Personnel
    President/CEO . . . . David W. Anderson
    Chief Financial Officer . . . . Stephen T. Swift
    SVP/General Counsel . . . . Kenneth J. Sodaro, Esq.
    SVP, Chief Sales Officer. . . . . David Busch
    SVP, Operations . . . . Christopher Leardini
    SVP, Network Officer . . . . Ronald Mornelli

Chief Medical Officer . . . . Thomas E. Schenk, MD

Specialty Managed Care Partners
    Wellpoint Pharmacy Management

---

547   CareCentrix: New York

3 Huntington Quadrangle
Suite 200S
Melville, NY 11747
Toll-Free: 800-808-1902
carecentrix.com
Year Founded: 1996
Number of Primary Care Physicians: 8,000

Healthplan and Services Defined
    PLAN TYPE: HMO
    Benefits Offered: Home Care, Physical Therapy, Durable Medical Equipment; Occupational & Respiratory Theraoy; Orthotics; Prosthetics

Key Personnel
    SVP, Business Development . . . . Judy Platkin

---

548   CDPHP Medicare Plan

500 Patroon Creek Boulevard
Albany, NY 12206-1057
Toll-Free: 888-248-6522
Phone: 518-641-3950
www.cdphp.com
Year Founded: 1984
Total Enrollment: 400,000

Healthplan and Services Defined
    PLAN TYPE: Medicare
    Benefits Offered: Chiropractic, Dental, Disease Management, Home Care, Inpatient SNF, Physical Therapy, Podiatry, Prescription, Psychiatric, Vision, Wellness

Type of Coverage
    Individual, Medicare

Geographic Areas Served
    Statewide

Subscriber Information
    Average Monthly Fee Per Subscriber
      (Employee + Employer Contribution):
        Employee Only (Self): Varies
        Medicare: Varies
    Average Annual Deductible Per Subscriber:
        Employee Only (Self): Varies
        Medicare: Varies
    Average Subscriber Co-Payment:
        Primary Care Physician: Varies
        Non-Network Physician: Varies
        Prescription Drugs: Varies
        Hospital ER: Varies
        Home Health Care: Varies
        Home Health Care Max. Days/Visits Covered: Varies
        Nursing Home: Varies
        Nursing Home Max. Days/Visits Covered: Varies

549 CDPHP: Capital District Physicians' Health Plan

500 Patroon Creek Boulevard
Albany, NY 12206-1057
Toll-Free: 800-777-2273
Phone: 518-641-3700
www.cdphp.com
Non-Profit Organization: Yes
Year Founded: 1984
Number of Primary Care Physicians: 5,000
Total Enrollment: 350,000
State Enrollment: 350,000

Healthplan and Services Defined
 PLAN TYPE: HMO/PPO
 Other Type: POS, ASO
 Model Type: IPA
 Benefits Offered: Dental, Disease Management, Prescription, Wellness

Type of Coverage
 Commercial, Individual, Medicare, Medicaid

Geographic Areas Served
 Albany, Broome, Chenango, Columbia, Delaware, Dutchess, Essex, Fulton, Greene, Hamilton, Herkimer, Madison, Montgomery, Oneida, Orange, Ostego, Rensselaer, Saratoga, Schenectady, Schoharie, Tioga, Ulster, Warren, and Washington counties

Subscriber Information
 Average Monthly Fee Per Subscriber
  (Employee + Employer Contribution):
   Employee Only (Self): $64.41
   Employee & 2 Family Members: $175.47
 Average Subscriber Co-Payment:
  Primary Care Physician: $10
  Prescription Drugs: $5-20

Accreditation Certification
 NCQA

Key Personnel
 President/CEO . . . . John D. Bennett, MD
 Chief Operating Officer . . . . Barbara A. Downs
 SVP, General Counsel . . . . Frederick B. Galt
 SVP, Strategy Officer . . . . Robert R. Hinckley
 SVP, Financial Officer. . . . . Bethany R. Smith
 Chief Medical Officer . . . . . . Richard H. Dal Col, MD, MPH
 SVP, Marketing . . . . Brian J. Morrissey

550 Coventry Health Care of New York

6720-B Rockledge Drive
Suite 800
Bethesda, MD 20817
Phone: 301-581-0600
www.coventryhealthcare.com
Subsidiary of: Aetna Inc.
For Profit Organization: Yes

Healthplan and Services Defined
 PLAN TYPE: HMO/PPO
 Model Type: Network

 Plan Specialty: Behavioral Health, Dental, Worker's Compensation
 Benefits Offered: Behavioral Health, Dental, Prescription, Wellness, Worker's Compensation

Type of Coverage
 Commercial, Medicare, Medicaid

Geographic Areas Served
 Statewide

Key Personnel
 Vice President . . . . Tom Downey

551 Davis Vision

Capital Region Health Park, Suite 301
711 Troy-Schenectady Road
Latham, NY 12110
Toll-Free: 800-773-2847
www.davisvision.com
Secondary Address: Davis Vision Corporate Headquarters, 175 E Houston Street, San Antonio, TX 78205, 800-328-4728
Subsidiary of: Versant Health
For Profit Organization: Yes
Year Founded: 1964
Number of Primary Care Physicians: 30,000
Total Enrollment: 55,000,000

Healthplan and Services Defined
 PLAN TYPE: Vision
 Model Type: Network
 Plan Specialty: Vision
 Benefits Offered: Vision
 Offers Demand Management Patient Information Service: Yes

Type of Payment Plans Offered
 DFFS, Capitated, FFS

Geographic Areas Served
 National & Puerto Rico, Guam, Saipan, Dominican Republic

Subscriber Information
 Average Monthly Fee Per Subscriber
  (Employee + Employer Contribution):
   Employee Only (Self): Varies by plan
   Medicare: Varies

Network Qualifications
 Pre-Admission Certification: No

Peer Review Type
 Utilization Review: Yes
 Second Surgical Opinion: Yes
 Case Management: Yes

Publishes and Distributes Report Card: Yes

Accreditation Certification
 NCQA, COLTS Certification
 TJC Accreditation

Key Personnel
 President . . . . Danny Bentley
 EVP, Strategy/Manufacture. . . . . Scott Hamey
 Chief Information Officer . . . . Walt Meffert
 Chief Medical Officer . . . . Jeff Smith

Average Claim Compensation
Physician's Fees Charged: 75%

Specialty Managed Care Partners
Enters into Contracts with Regional Business Coalitions: Yes

---

552   Delta Dental of New York

One Delta Drive
Mechanicsburg, PA 17055-6999
Toll-Free: 800-932-0783
www.deltadentalins.com
Mailing Address: P.O. Box 1803, Alpharetta, GA 30023
Non-Profit Organization: Yes

Healthplan and Services Defined
PLAN TYPE: Dental
Other Type: Dental PPO
Plan Specialty: Dental
Benefits Offered: Dental

Type of Coverage
Commercial, Individual

Geographic Areas Served
Statewide

Key Personnel
President & CEO . . . . Tony Barth
Chief Financial Officer . . . . Michael Castro
Chief Legal Officer . . . . Michael Hankinson
EVP, Sales & Marketing . . . . Belinda Martinez
Chief Operating Officer . . . . Nilesh Patel

---

553   Dentcare Delivery Systems

333 Earle Ovington Boulevard
Uniondale, NY 11553-3608
Toll-Free: 800-468-0608
Phone: 516-542-2200
Fax: 516-794-3186
www.dentcaredeliverysystems.org
Subsidiary of: Healthplex
Non-Profit Organization: Yes
Year Founded: 1978

Healthplan and Services Defined
PLAN TYPE: Dental
Model Type: IPA
Plan Specialty: Dental
Benefits Offered: Dental

Type of Coverage
Commercial, Individual
Catastrophic Illness Benefit: None

Type of Payment Plans Offered
FFS

Geographic Areas Served
Statewide

Accreditation Certification
NCQA
Utilization Review, Quality Assurance Program

Key Personnel
Treasurer . . . . Deborah Wissing

---

554   Elderplan

6323 Seventh Avenue
Brooklyn, NY 11220
Toll-Free: 866-360-1934
www.elderplan.org
Subsidiary of: MJHS
Non-Profit Organization: Yes
Year Founded: 1985
Number of Affiliated Hospitals: 35
Number of Primary Care Physicians: 1,200
Number of Referral/Specialty Physicians: 3,800
Total Enrollment: 16,000
State Enrollment: 15,000

Healthplan and Services Defined
PLAN TYPE: Medicare
Other Type: Medicare Advantage
Model Type: Network
Plan Specialty: ASO, Behavioral Health, Chiropractic, Dental, Disease Management, EPO, Lab, Vision, Radiology
Benefits Offered: Behavioral Health, Chiropractic, Complementary
Medicine, Dental, Disease Management, Home Care, Inpatient SNF, Long-Term Care, Physical Therapy, Podiatry, Prescription, Psychiatric, Transplant, Vision, Hearing; Durable Medical Equipment; Speech Therapy; Transportation

Type of Coverage
Medicare

Type of Payment Plans Offered
FFS

Geographic Areas Served
Brooklyn, Bronx, Manhattan, Queens and Staten Island

Subscriber Information
Average Monthly Fee Per Subscriber
(Employee + Employer Contribution):
Medicare: No premium
Average Annual Deductible Per Subscriber:
Medicare: $0.00
Average Subscriber Co-Payment:
Primary Care Physician: $0.00 co-pay
Prescription Drugs: $5.00/9.00
Hospital ER: $50.00
Home Health Care: $0.00
Home Health Care Max. Days/Visits Covered: 365 days
Nursing Home Max. Days/Visits Covered: 200 days

Network Qualifications
Pre-Admission Certification: Yes

Peer Review Type
Utilization Review: Yes
Second Surgical Opinion: Yes
Case Management: Yes

Publishes and Distributes Report Card: No

Accreditation Certification
TJC Accreditation, Medicare Approved, Utilization Review, State Licensure, Quality Assurance Program

Specialty Managed Care Partners
    HomeFirst, Maxore
    Enters into Contracts with Regional Business Coalitions: Yes

555   EmblemHealth

55 Water Street
New York, NY 10041-8190
Toll-Free: 877-411-3625
www.emblemhealth.com
Non-Profit Organization: Yes
Year Founded: 1985

Healthplan and Services Defined
    PLAN TYPE: Other
    Model Type: IPA
    Plan Specialty: ASO, Chiropractic, Dental, Disease
        Management, EPO, Vision, Radiology
    Benefits Offered: Behavioral Health, Chiropractic,
        Complementary Medicine, Dental, Disease Management,
        Home Care, Inpatient SNF, Physical Therapy, Podiatry,
        Prescription, Psychiatric, Transplant, Vision, Wellness

Type of Payment Plans Offered
    Capitated

Geographic Areas Served
    City employees and retirees under 65: Queens, Nassau,
    Suffolk

Accreditation Certification
    URAC, NCQA
    TJC Accreditation, Medicare Approved, Utilization Review,
        Pre-Admission Certification, State Licensure, Quality
        Assurance Program

Key Personnel
    President & CEO . . . . Karen M. Ignagni
    Administrative Officer . . . . Michael Palmateer
    Chief Legal Officer . . . . Jeffrey D. Chansler
    Human Resources . . . . Mariann E. Drohan
    Chief Marketing Officer . . . . Beth A. Leonard
    Chief Compliance Officer . . . . Debra M. Lightner
    Chief Medical Officer . . . . Navarra Rodriguez, MD

556   EmblemHealth Enhanced Care Plus (HARP)

55 Water Street
New York, NY 10041-8190
Toll-Free: 855-283-2146
www.emblemhealth.com
Subsidiary of: EmblemHealth
Non-Profit Organization: Yes

Healthplan and Services Defined
    PLAN TYPE: Other
    Benefits Offered: Behavioral Health, Dental, Home Care,
        Inpatient SNF, Prescription, Psychiatric, Vision, Wellness,
        Maternity care; Therapy for TB; Hospice; Labs & X-Ray;
        Substance Abuse services; Durable Medical Equipment;
        HIV testing

Geographic Areas Served
    Bronx, Queens, Brooklyn, Manhattan, Staten Island, Nassau,
    Suffolk and Westchester

Key Personnel
    President & CEO . . . . Karen M. Ignagni
    Administrative Officer . . . . Michael Palmateer
    Chief Legal Officer . . . . Jeffrey D. Chansler
    Human Resources . . . . Mariann E. Drohan
    Chief Marketing Officer . . . . Beth A. Leonard
    Chief Compliance Officer . . . . Debra M. Lightner
    Chief Medical Officer . . . . Navarra Rodriguez, MD

557   Empire BlueCross BlueShield

15 MetroTech Center
Brooklyn, NY 11201
Toll-Free: 800-331-1476
www.empireblue.com
Subsidiary of: Anthem, Inc.

Healthplan and Services Defined
    PLAN TYPE: HMO/PPO
    Model Type: Network
    Plan Specialty: Behavioral Health, Dental, Disease
        Management, Lab, PBM, Vision, Radiology
    Benefits Offered: Behavioral Health, Dental, Disease
        Management, Inpatient SNF, Physical Therapy,
        Prescription, Psychiatric, Transplant, Vision, Wellness, Life

Type of Coverage
    Commercial, Individual, Medicare, Supplemental Medicare,
    Catastrophic

Geographic Areas Served
    Serving the 28 eastern and southeastern counties of New York
    State

Accreditation Certification
    URAC

Key Personnel
    Provider Network Manager . . . . Paula Kynalis
    VP/COO . . . . Errol L. Pierre
    Regional Vice President . . . . Dominic DePiano

558   Excellus BlueCross BlueShield

165 Court Street
Rochester, NY 14647
Toll-Free: 877-883-9577
www.excellusbcbs.com
Non-Profit Organization: Yes
Year Founded: 1985
Total Enrollment: 1,500,000

Healthplan and Services Defined
    PLAN TYPE: HMO
    Model Type: IPA
    Benefits Offered: Disease Management, Prescription,
        Wellness

Type of Payment Plans Offered
    POS, Combination FFS & DFFS

Geographic Areas Served
    Central New York, the Rochester area and Utica-Watertown

Publishes and Distributes Report Card: Yes

Accreditation Certification
NCQA
TJC Accreditation, Medicare Approved, Utilization Review, State Licensure, Quality Assurance Program

Key Personnel
Chief Executive Officer. . . . . Christopher C. Booth

---

559   **Fidelis Care**
95-25 Queens Boulevard
Rego Park, NY 11374
Toll-Free: 888-FIDELIS
www.fideliscare.org
For Profit Organization: Yes
Year Founded: 1993
Number of Primary Care Physicians: 42,000
Total Enrollment: 625,000
State Enrollment: 625,000

Healthplan and Services Defined
PLAN TYPE: Multiple
Model Type: Network
Benefits Offered: Behavioral Health, Chiropractic, Dental, Disease Management, Home Care, Inpatient SNF, Physical Therapy, Podiatry, Prescription, Psychiatric, Vision, Wellness

Type of Coverage
Individual, Medicare, Medicaid

Geographic Areas Served
53 counties in New York State

Subscriber Information
Average Monthly Fee Per Subscriber
(Employee + Employer Contribution):
Employee Only (Self): Varies
Medicare: Varies
Average Annual Deductible Per Subscriber:
Employee Only (Self): Varies
Medicare: Varies
Average Subscriber Co-Payment:
Primary Care Physician: Varies
Non-Network Physician: Varies
Prescription Drugs: Varies
Hospital ER: Varies
Home Health Care: Varies
Home Health Care Max. Days/Visits Covered: Varies
Nursing Home: Varies
Nursing Home Max. Days/Visits Covered: Varies

Key Personnel
CEO . . . . Patrick Frawley
President/COO. . . . . David Thomas
Director, IT . . . . Gary Crane
Chief Medical Officer . . . . Sanjiv Shah, MD
VP, Communications. . . . . Darla Skiermont

560   **GHI Medicare Plan**
55 Water Street Lobby
New York, NY 10041-8190
Toll-Free: 877-411-3625
www.emblemhealth.com
Subsidiary of: EmblemHealth
Year Founded: 1931
Total Enrollment: 53,000

Healthplan and Services Defined
PLAN TYPE: Medicare
Benefits Offered: Chiropractic, Dental, Disease Management, Home Care, Inpatient SNF, Physical Therapy, Podiatry, Prescription, Psychiatric, Vision, Wellness

Type of Coverage
Individual, Medicare

Geographic Areas Served
Statewide

Subscriber Information
Average Monthly Fee Per Subscriber
(Employee + Employer Contribution):
Employee Only (Self): Varies
Medicare: Varies
Average Annual Deductible Per Subscriber:
Employee Only (Self): Varies
Medicare: Varies
Average Subscriber Co-Payment:
Primary Care Physician: Varies
Non-Network Physician: Varies
Prescription Drugs: Varies
Hospital ER: Varies
Home Health Care: Varies
Home Health Care Max. Days/Visits Covered: Varies
Nursing Home: Varies
Nursing Home Max. Days/Visits Covered: Varies

Key Personnel
President/CEO. . . . . Karen M. Ignagni
EVP/Chief Admin Officer . . . . Michael . Palmateer
Chief Legal Officer. . . . . Jeffrey D. Chansler
Chief, Human Resources . . . . Mariann E. Drohan
Chief Marketing Officer . . . . Beth A. Leonard
Chief Compliance Officer . . . . Debra M. Lightner

---

561   **Guardian Life Insurance Company of America**
7 Hanover Square
H-6-D
New York, NY 10004
Toll-Free: 888-482-7342
www.guardianlife.com
Subsidiary of: Guardian
For Profit Organization: Yes
Year Founded: 1860
Owned by an Integrated Delivery Network (IDN): Yes
Number of Affiliated Hospitals: 2,966
Number of Primary Care Physicians: 121,815
Number of Referral/Specialty Physicians: 193,137
Total Enrollment: 205,677

Healthplan and Services Defined
PLAN TYPE: HMO/PPO
Model Type: Network
Plan Specialty: Chiropractic, Dental, Disease Management,
   Lab, PBM, Vision, Radiology, UR
Benefits Offered: Behavioral Health, Chiropractic,
   Complementary Medicine, Dental, Disease Management,
   Home Care, Physical Therapy, Podiatry, Prescription,
   Psychiatric, Vision, Wellness, AD&D, Life, LTD, STD

Type of Coverage
Commercial, Individual, Indemnity

Type of Payment Plans Offered
Combination FFS & DFFS

Geographic Areas Served
Nationwide

Subscriber Information
Average Monthly Fee Per Subscriber
   (Employee + Employer Contribution):
      Employee Only (Self): Varies by plan

Peer Review Type
Utilization Review: Yes
Second Surgical Opinion: Yes
Case Management: Yes

Publishes and Distributes Report Card: Yes

Accreditation Certification
URAC, NCQA

Key Personnel
President/CEO . . . . Deanna M. Mulligan
EVP/CIO . . . . Dean A. Del Vecchio
EVP/General Counsel . . . . Eric R. Dinallo
EVP/CFO . . . . Michael Ferik
EVP/Human Resources . . . . Diana L. Scott
Chief Investment Officer . . . . Thomas G. Sorell, CFA

Specialty Managed Care Partners
Health Net
Enters into Contracts with Regional Business Coalitions: Yes

562 Healthfirst
100 Church Street
New York, NY 10007
Toll-Free: 888-260-1010
healthfirst.org
Non-Profit Organization: Yes
Number of Affiliated Hospitals: 6

Healthplan and Services Defined
PLAN TYPE: Multiple
Benefits Offered: Dental, Inpatient SNF, Physical Therapy,
   Vision, Wellness

Type of Coverage
Medicare, Medicaid, Child Health Plus; Managed Long Ter

Key Personnel
President & CEO . . . . Pat Wang
Chief Operating Officer . . . . Steve Black
Chief Financial Officer . . . . John J. Bermel
Chief Clinical Officer . . . . Jay Schechtman, MD

Chief Legal Officer . . . . Linda Tiano
Human Resources . . . . Sean Kane
Chief Information Officer . . . . G.T. Sweeney

563 Healthplex
333 Earle Ovington Boulevard
Suite 300
Uniondale, NY 11553
Toll-Free: 800-468-0608
info@healthplex.com
www.healthplex.com
For Profit Organization: Yes
Year Founded: 1977
Number of Primary Care Physicians: 2,855
Number of Referral/Specialty Physicians: 448
Total Enrollment: 3,500,000

Healthplan and Services Defined
PLAN TYPE: Dental
Other Type: Dental HMO/PPO
Model Type: IPA
Plan Specialty: Dental
Benefits Offered: Dental

Type of Coverage
Commercial, Individual, Indemnity

Type of Payment Plans Offered
POS, DFFS, Capitated, FFS, Combination FFS & DFFS

Geographic Areas Served
New Jersey & New York

Subscriber Information
Average Monthly Fee Per Subscriber
   (Employee + Employer Contribution):
      Employee Only (Self): $159.00
      Employee & 1 Family Member: $264.00
      Employee & 2 Family Members: $350.00
Average Annual Deductible Per Subscriber:
      Employee Only (Self): $0
      Employee & 1 Family Member: $0
      Employee & 2 Family Members: $0

Network Qualifications
Pre-Admission Certification: No

Peer Review Type
Utilization Review: Yes
Second Surgical Opinion: Yes
Case Management: Yes

Accreditation Certification
NCQA
Utilization Review, Quality Assurance Program

Key Personnel
President/CEO . . . . Christopher Schmidt
Controller . . . . Mary Jean Kelly
Human Resources . . . . Eileen Scaturro

Specialty Managed Care Partners
Enters into Contracts with Regional Business Coalitions: Yes

564 Humana Health Insurance of New York

125 Wolf Road
Suite 501
Albany, NY 12205
Toll-Free: 800-967-2370
Fax: 518-435-0412
www.humana.com
Secondary Address: 290 Elwood Davis Road, Suite 225,
Liverpool, NY 13088
Subsidiary of: Humana
For Profit Organization: Yes

Healthplan and Services Defined
PLAN TYPE: HMO/PPO
Model Type: Network
Plan Specialty: Dental, Vision
Benefits Offered: Dental, Vision, Life, LTD, STD

Type of Coverage
Commercial

Geographic Areas Served
Statewide

Accreditation Certification
URAC, NCQA, CORE

Key Personnel
Market Manager...................... Andre Dowdie

565 Independent Health

511 Farber Lakes Drive
Buffalo, NY 14221
Toll-Free: 800-501-3439
Phone: 716-631-3001
www.lndependenthealth.com
Non-Profit Organization: Yes
Year Founded: 1980
Number of Affiliated Hospitals: 35
Number of Primary Care Physicians: 1,125
Number of Referral/Specialty Physicians: 1,626
Total Enrollment: 365,000
State Enrollment: 365,000

Healthplan and Services Defined
PLAN TYPE: HMO/PPO
Model Type: IPA
Plan Specialty: EPO
Benefits Offered: Behavioral Health, Chiropractic, Dental,
Disease Management, Home Care, Inpatient SNF, Physical
Therapy, Podiatry, Prescription, Psychiatric, Transplant,
Vision, Wellness

Type of Coverage
Commercial, Individual, Indemnity, Medicare, Medicaid,
Choice
Catastrophic Illness Benefit: Varies per case

Type of Payment Plans Offered
POS, Combination FFS & DFFS

Geographic Areas Served
Allegany, Cattaraugus, Chautauqua, Erie, Genesee, Niagara,
Orleans & Wyoming counties of western New York

Subscriber Information
Average Monthly Fee Per Subscriber
(Employee + Employer Contribution):
Employee Only (Self): Varies by plan

Network Qualifications
Pre-Admission Certification: Yes

Peer Review Type
Utilization Review: Yes
Second Surgical Opinion: Yes
Case Management: Yes

Publishes and Distributes Report Card: No

Accreditation Certification
TJC, NCQA
Utilization Review, Pre-Admission Certification, State
Licensure, Quality Assurance Program

Key Personnel
President/CEO .... Michael W. Cropp, MD
EVP/COO .... John Rodgers
EVP/CFO........................... Mike Hudson
EVP, General Counsel .... John Mineo
Chief Medical Officer........ Thomas J. Foels, MD, MMM
EVP, Human Resources............... Patricia Clabeaux

Specialty Managed Care Partners
Enters into Contracts with Regional Business Coalitions: No

566 Independent Health Medicare Plan

511 Farber Lakes Drive
Buffalo, NY 14221
Toll-Free: 800-501-3439
Phone: 716-631-3001
www.independenthealth.com
Non-Profit Organization: Yes
Year Founded: 1980

Healthplan and Services Defined
PLAN TYPE: Medicare
Benefits Offered: Chiropractic, Dental, Disease Management,
Home Care, Inpatient SNF, Physical Therapy, Podiatry,
Prescription, Psychiatric, Vision, Wellness

Type of Coverage
Individual, Medicare

Geographic Areas Served
Statewide

Subscriber Information
Average Monthly Fee Per Subscriber
(Employee + Employer Contribution):
Employee Only (Self): Varies
Medicare: Varies
Average Annual Deductible Per Subscriber:
Employee Only (Self): Varies
Medicare: Varies
Average Subscriber Co-Payment:
Primary Care Physician: Varies
Non-Network Physician: Varies
Prescription Drugs: Varies
Hospital ER: Varies
Home Health Care: Varies

Home Health Care Max. Days/Visits Covered: Varies
Nursing Home: Varies
Nursing Home Max. Days/Visits Covered: Varies

Key Personnel
President and CEO . . . . Michael W Cropp, MD
EVP/COO . . . . John Rodgers
EVP/CFO . . . . Mark Johnson
EVP, General Counsel . . . . John Mineo
Chief Medical Officer . . . . Thomas J. Foels, MD
EVP, Human Resources. . . . . Patricia Clabeaux

567 Island Group Administration, Inc.
3 Toilsome Lane
East Hampton, NY 11937
Toll-Free: 800-926-2306
Phone: 631-324-2306
Fax: 631-324-7021
www.islandgroupadmin.com
For Profit Organization: Yes
Year Founded: 1990
Federally Qualified: No
Number of Affiliated Hospitals: 9,055
Number of Primary Care Physicians: 21,010
Total Enrollment: 52,000

Healthplan and Services Defined
PLAN TYPE: PPO
Model Type: TPA
Plan Specialty: Dental, Vision, Radiology, Worker's
Compensation, UR, Medical
Benefits Offered: Chiropractic, Dental, Disease Management,
Home Care, Podiatry, Prescription, Psychiatric, Transplant,
Vision, Wellness, Worker's Compensation, Medical,
Hospital

Type of Coverage
Commercial, Individual, Varies

Geographic Areas Served
Nationwide

Subscriber Information
Average Monthly Fee Per Subscriber
(Employee + Employer Contribution):
Employee Only (Self): Varies by plan

Peer Review Type
Utilization Review: Yes
Second Surgical Opinion: Yes
Case Management: Yes

Accreditation Certification
Utilization Review, Pre-Admission Certification, State
Licensure

Key Personnel
President . . . . Alan Kaplan
VP, Operations . . . . Rosemarie Nuzzi
EVP, Provider Relations . . . . Lynn Kaplan
Supervisor, Plan Mngmnt. . . . . Cindy Bacon
Case Review . . . . Lucille Dunn, RN

Specialty Managed Care Partners
Standard Security; CareMark PBM

568 Liberty Dental Plan of New York
One Rockefeller Plaza
11th Floor
New York, NY 10020
Toll-Free: 888-700-1246
www.libertydentalplan.com
For Profit Organization: Yes
Total Enrollment: 2,000,000

Healthplan and Services Defined
PLAN TYPE: Dental
Other Type: Dental HMO
Plan Specialty: Dental
Benefits Offered: Dental

Type of Coverage
Commercial, Medicare, Medicaid, Unions

Geographic Areas Served
Statewide

Accreditation Certification
NCQA

Key Personnel
President & CEO. . . . . Amir Neshat
EVP, Compliance Officer. . . . . John Carvelli
Chief Financial Officer . . . . Maja Kapic
General Counsel . . . . Lisa Wright
Chief Operating Officer . . . . Rohan Reid
Chief Dental Officer. . . . . Todd Gray

569 Liberty Health Advantage HMO
1 Huntington Quadrangle
Suite 3N01
Melville, NY 11747
Toll-Free: 866-542-4269
Fax: 631-227-3484
www.lhany.com

Healthplan and Services Defined
PLAN TYPE: HMO
Plan Specialty: Integrated Medicare/Medicaid (Duals)
Benefits Offered: Chiropractic, Dental, Disease Management,
Home Care, Inpatient SNF, Physical Therapy, Podiatry,
Prescription, Psychiatric, Vision, Wellness

Type of Coverage
Individual, Medicare, Supplemental Medicare, Medicaid

Geographic Areas Served
New York City and Nassau County

Subscriber Information
Average Monthly Fee Per Subscriber
(Employee + Employer Contribution):
Employee Only (Self): Varies
Medicare: Varies
Average Annual Deductible Per Subscriber:
Employee Only (Self): Varies
Medicare: Varies
Average Subscriber Co-Payment:
Primary Care Physician: Varies
Non-Network Physician: Varies
Prescription Drugs: Varies

Hospital ER: Varies
Home Health Care: Varies
Home Health Care Max. Days/Visits Covered: Varies
Nursing Home: Varies
Nursing Home Max. Days/Visits Covered: Varies

Key Personnel
VP of Operations . . . . Lucy Oliva

570 MagnaCare

One Penn Plaza
53rd Floor
New York, NY 10119
Toll-Free: 800-235-7267
Phone: 516-282-8000
www.magnacare.com
Secondary Address: 1600 Stewart Avenue, Suite 700,
    Westbury, NY 11590
For Profit Organization: Yes
Year Founded: 1990
Number of Affiliated Hospitals: 260
Number of Primary Care Physicians: 70,000
Number of Referral/Specialty Physicians: 58,000
Total Enrollment: 1,326,000
State Enrollment: 928,200

Healthplan and Services Defined
PLAN TYPE: PPO
Model Type: Network
Plan Specialty: ASO, Behavioral Health, Chiropractic,
    Dental, Lab, Radiology, Worker's Compensation, UR
Benefits Offered: Behavioral Health, Chiropractic, Dental,
    Home Care, Inpatient SNF, Physical Therapy, Podiatry,
    Prescription, Psychiatric, Worker's Compensation,
    Correctional health services

Type of Coverage
Commercial, Individual, Leased Network Arrangement

Type of Payment Plans Offered
DFFS

Geographic Areas Served
New Jersey and New York

Subscriber Information
Average Monthly Fee Per Subscriber
    (Employee + Employer Contribution):
        Employee Only (Self): Varies
Average Subscriber Co-Payment:
        Home Health Care: Varies
        Home Health Care Max. Days/Visits Covered: Varies
        Nursing Home: Varies
        Nursing Home Max. Days/Visits Covered: Varies

Network Qualifications
Pre-Admission Certification: Yes

Peer Review Type
Utilization Review: Yes
Second Surgical Opinion: No
Case Management: Yes

Accreditation Certification
TJC Accreditation, Utilization Review, Pre-Admission
    Certification, State Licensure, Quality Assurance Program

Key Personnel
President & CEO . . . . Simeon Schindelman
VP of Finance . . . . Vanessa Hargrave
Chairman . . . . Joseph Berardo, Jr
Chief Legal Officer. . . . . Adam Young
Chief Compliance Officer . . . . Joseph Brennan
SVP, Human Resources . . . . Julie Bank

Average Claim Compensation
Physician's Fees Charged: 50%
Hospital's Fees Charged: 60%

Specialty Managed Care Partners
American Psych Systems, Intra State Choice Management
    Chiropractic

Employer References
Local 947, District Council of Painters #9

571 Meritain Health

300 Corporate Parkway
Amherst, NY 14226
Toll-Free: 888-324-5789
service@meritain.com
www.meritain.com
Subsidiary of: Aetna
For Profit Organization: Yes

Healthplan and Services Defined
PLAN TYPE: Multiple
Model Type: Network
Plan Specialty: Dental, Disease Management, Vision,
    Radiology, UR
Benefits Offered: Dental, Prescription, Vision
Offers Demand Management Patient Information Service: Yes

Type of Coverage
Commercial

Geographic Areas Served
Nationwide

Accreditation Certification
URAC
TJC Accreditation, Medicare Approved, Utilization Review,
    Pre-Admission Certification, State Licensure, Quality
    Assurance Program

Key Personnel
Cheief Executive Officer . . . . Mark T. Bertolini
President . . . . Karen S. Lynch

Average Claim Compensation
Physician's Fees Charged: 78%
Hospital's Fees Charged: 90%

572 MetroPlus Health Plan

160 Water Street
3rd Floor
New York, NY 10038
Toll-Free: 800-303-9626
Fax: 212-908-8601
www.metroplus.org
Subsidiary of: New York City Health Hospitals Corporation
Non-Profit Organization: Yes
Year Founded: 1985
Owned by an Integrated Delivery Network (IDN): Yes
Number of Affiliated Hospitals: 11
Number of Primary Care Physicians: 12,000
Total Enrollment: 332,128
State Enrollment: 332,128

Healthplan and Services Defined
  PLAN TYPE: Medicare
  Model Type: Network
  Benefits Offered: Dental, Disease Management, Prescription, Vision, Wellness, Nurse management line, TeleHealth

Type of Coverage
  Medicare, Medicaid, Child Health Plus, Family Health Pl

Geographic Areas Served
  Brooklyn, Bronx, Manhattan and Queens

Accreditation Certification
  TJC Accreditation

Key Personnel
  President/CEO . . . . Arnold Saperstein
  Chief Customer Officer . . . . Gail L. Smith
  Chief Financial Officer. John Cuba
  Chief Operating Officer . . . . Seth Diamond
  Chief HR Officer . . . . Ryan Harris
  Chief Information Officer . . . . Susan Sun

Specialty Managed Care Partners
  Enters into Contracts with Regional Business Coalitions: Yes

573 Molina Healthcare of New York

5232 Witz Drive
North Syracuse, NY 13212
Toll-Free: 800-223-7242
molinahealthcare.com
For Profit Organization: Yes
Year Founded: 1980

Healthplan and Services Defined
  PLAN TYPE: Medicare
  Plan Specialty: Dental, PBM, Vision, Integrated Medicare/Medicaid (Duals)
  Benefits Offered: Dental, Prescription, Vision, Wellness, Life

Geographic Areas Served
  Statewide

Key Personnel
  Chief Executive Officer . . . . Colleen Schmidt
  Chief Operating Officer . . . . Gary Billy

574 MVP Health Care

625 State Street
P.O. Box 2207
Schenectady, NY 12301-2207
Toll-Free: 800-777-4793
Phone: 518-370-4793
Fax: 518-370-0830
mvphealthcare.com
Secondary Address: 62 Merchants Row, Williston, VT 05495, 802-264-6500
Non-Profit Organization: Yes
Total Enrollment: 700,000

Healthplan and Services Defined
  PLAN TYPE: Multiple
  Benefits Offered: Chiropractic, Dental, Disease Management, Home Care, Inpatient SNF, Physical Therapy, Podiatry, Prescription, Psychiatric, Vision, Wellness

Type of Coverage
  Commercial, Individual, Medicare

Geographic Areas Served
  New York, Vermont

Accreditation Certification
  NCQA

Key Personnel
  CEO/Director . . . . Denise Gonick, Esq.
  President/COO . . . . Christopher Del Vecchio
  EVP/CFO. . . . . Karla A. Austen
  EVP, General Counsel . . . . Monice Barbero
  VP, Human Resources . . . . Lynn Manning
  Chief Information Officer . . . . Michael Della Villa
  VP/Chief Actuary . . . . Kathleen Fish
  VP, Marketing/Comm. Ted Herman
  VP, Pharmacy . . . . Jim Hopsicker
  VP, Client Engagement. . . . . Augusta Martin
  VP, Sales . . . . Kelly Smith

575 Nova Healthcare Administrators

6400 Main Street
Suite 210
Williamsville, NY 14221
Toll-Free: 800-999-5703
Phone: 716-773-2122
sales@novahealthcare.com
www.novahealthcare.com
Subsidiary of: Independent Health Association, Inc.
For Profit Organization: Yes
Year Founded: 1982
Total Enrollment: 210,000

Healthplan and Services Defined
  PLAN TYPE: Multiple
  Plan Specialty: ASO, Dental
  Benefits Offered: Dental, Disease Management, Prescription, Wellness

Type of Coverage
  Commercial, Indemnity

Geographic Areas Served
Nationwide

Network Qualifications
Pre-Admission Certification: Yes

Peer Review Type
Utilization Review: Yes
Second Surgical Opinion: Yes
Case Management: Yes

Key Personnel
President............................. Laura Hirsch

Specialty Managed Care Partners
Express Scripts

576 Oscar Health
295 Lafayette Street
New York, NY 10012
Toll-Free: 855-672-2788
guides@hioscar.com
www.hioscar.com
Subsidiary of: Mulberry Health, Inc.
For Profit Organization: Yes
Year Founded: 2012

Healthplan and Services Defined
PLAN TYPE: PPO
Benefits Offered: Inpatient SNF, Physical Therapy,
Prescription, Psychiatric, Wellness, Labs & Imaging;
Occupational & Speech Therapy

Geographic Areas Served
New York, California, and Texas

Key Personnel
Co-Founder .... Joshua Kushner
Co-Founder .... Mario Schlosser
Co-Founder.......................... Kevin Nazemi

577 Quality Health Plans of New York
2805 Veterans Memorial Highway
Suite 17
Ronkonkoma, NY 11779
Toll-Free: 877-233-7058
www.qhpny.com
Secondary Address: Quality Health Plans of New York
Claims, P.O. Box 340397, Tampa, FL 33694-0397
Year Founded: 2003
Physician Owned Organization: Yes
Total Enrollment: 19,000

Healthplan and Services Defined
PLAN TYPE: Medicare
Other Type: Medicare HMO

Type of Coverage
Supplemental Medicare

Geographic Areas Served
13 counties in Florida

Key Personnel
Chief Executive Officer.................. Frank Olsen
Compliance Officer.................... Monique Slater

578 Trinity Health of New York
Saint Joseph's Health
301 Prospect Avenue
Syracuse, NY 13203
Phone: 315-448-5111
www.trinity-health.org
Secondary Address: St. Peter's Health Partners, 315 S Manning
Boulevard, Albany, NY 12208, 518-525-1111
Subsidiary of: Trinity Health
Non-Profit Organization: Yes
Year Founded: 2013
Total Enrollment: 30,000,000

Healthplan and Services Defined
PLAN TYPE: Other
Benefits Offered: Disease Management, Home Care,
Long-Term Care, Psychiatric, Hospice programs, PACE
(Program of All Inclusive Care for the Elderly)

Geographic Areas Served
Western New York and Albany

Key Personnel
President/CEO .... Leslie Paul Luke
VP, Integrity/Compliance......... Jennifer Reschke Bolster
COO/CNO .... AnneMarie W. Czyz
VP, Human Resources.................... Erika Duncan
Chief Information Officer.............. Charles J. Fennell
VP, Development .... Vincent J. Kuss
Chief Strategy Officer................. Mark E. Murphy
Chief Financial Officer .... Meredith Price
General Counsel .... Lowell A. Seifter, Esq.
Chief Medical Officer................ Joseph W. Spinale

579 United Concordia of New York
4401 Deer Path Road
Harrisburg, PA 17110
Toll-Free: 800-232-0366
www.unitedconcordia.com
For Profit Organization: Yes
Year Founded: 1971
Total Enrollment: 7,800,000

Healthplan and Services Defined
PLAN TYPE: Dental
Plan Specialty: Dental
Benefits Offered: Dental

Type of Coverage
Commercial, Individual, Military personnel & families

Geographic Areas Served
Nationwide

Accreditation Certification
URAC

Key Personnel
Contact.......................... Beth Rutherford
717-260-7659
beth.rutherford@ucci.com

580   UnitedHealthcare of New York

1 Pennsylvania Plaza
Suite 8
New York, NY 10119
Toll-Free: 866-633-2446
www.uhc.com
Subsidiary of: UnitedHealth Group
For Profit Organization: Yes
Year Founded: 1987
Federally Qualified: Yes

Healthplan and Services Defined
  PLAN TYPE: HMO/PPO
  Model Type: Network
  Plan Specialty: Behavioral Health, Dental, Disease
    Management, PBM, Vision
  Benefits Offered: Behavioral Health, Dental, Disease
    Management, Long-Term Care, Prescription, Vision,
    Wellness, Life, LTD, STD

Type of Coverage
  Individual, Medicare, Supplemental Medicare, Medicaid,
    Catastrophic, Family, Military, Veterans, Group,

Type of Payment Plans Offered
  DFFS, Capitated

Geographic Areas Served
  Statewide

Network Qualifications
  Pre-Admission Certification: Yes

Peer Review Type
  Utilization Review: Yes
  Second Surgical Opinion: Yes
  Case Management: Yes

Publishes and Distributes Report Card: Yes

Accreditation Certification
  TJC Accreditation, Medicare Approved, Utilization Review,
    Pre-Admission Certification, State Licensure, Quality
    Assurance Program

Key Personnel
  VP, Sales & Marketing . . . . David Willhoft

Specialty Managed Care Partners
  Enters into Contracts with Regional Business Coalitions: Yes

581   Univera Healthcare

205 Park Club Lane
Buffalo, NY 14221
Toll-Free: 800-499-1275
www.univerahealthcare.com
Mailing Address: P.O. Box 211256, Eagan, MN 55121
Subsidiary of: The Lifetime Healthcare Companies
Non-Profit Organization: Yes
Number of Affiliated Hospitals: 35
Number of Primary Care Physicians: 5,700
Total Enrollment: 1,500,000
State Enrollment: 1,500,000

Healthplan and Services Defined
  PLAN TYPE: HMO

Model Type: Network
Plan Specialty: ASO, Behavioral Health, Chiropractic, Dental,
  Disease Management, EPO, Lab, MSO, PBM, Vision,
  Radiology, Worker's Compensation, UR
Benefits Offered: Behavioral Health, Chiropractic,
  Complementary Medicine, Dental, Disease Management,
  Home Care, Inpatient SNF, Long-Term Care, Physical
  Therapy, Podiatry, Prescription, Psychiatric, Transplant,
  Vision, Wellness, Worker's Compensation, Life

Type of Coverage
  Commercial, Individual, Medicare

Geographic Areas Served
  Allegany, Cattaraugus, Chautauqua, Erie, Genesee, Niagara,
  Orleans and Wyoming counties

Subscriber Information
  Average Monthly Fee Per Subscriber
    (Employee + Employer Contribution):
      Employee Only (Self): Varies by plan
  Average Subscriber Co-Payment:
    Primary Care Physician: Varies
    Prescription Drugs: Varies

Publishes and Distributes Report Card: Yes

Accreditation Certification
  NCQA

Key Personnel
  President . . . . Arthur G. Wingerter
  Chief Executive Officer. . . . . Christopher C. Booth
  Chief Financial Officer . . . . Dorothy Coleman
  Chief Medical Officer . . . . Richard P. Vienne
  VP, Sales . . . . Pamela J. Pawenski
  VP, Communications . . . . Peter B Kates
    716-857-4495
    peter.kates@univerahealthcare.com

582   Universal American Medicare Plans

44 South Broadway
Suite 1200
White Plains, NY 10601-4411
Phone: 914-934-5200
Fax: 914-934-0700
www.universalamerican.com
Subsidiary of: Wellcare Health Plans
Number of Primary Care Physicians: 4,200
Total Enrollment: 2,000,000

Healthplan and Services Defined
  PLAN TYPE: Medicare
  Other Type: HMO-POS, PPO, PFFS
  Benefits Offered: Prescription

Type of Coverage
  Individual, Medicare

Geographic Areas Served
  Texas, New York, Maine

Subscriber Information
  Average Monthly Fee Per Subscriber
    (Employee + Employer Contribution):
      Employee Only (Self): Varies

Medicare: Varies
Average Annual Deductible Per Subscriber:
    Employee Only (Self): Varies
    Medicare: Varies
Average Subscriber Co-Payment:
    Primary Care Physician: Varies
    Non-Network Physician: Varies
    Prescription Drugs: Varies
    Hospital ER: Varies

Key Personnel

Chairman & CEO . . . . Richard A Barasch
Chief Financial Officer . . . . Steven H. Black
SVP, Market Operations. . . . . Erin Page
EVP, Health Care Services . . . . . . Theodore M. Carpenter Jr.
EVP, General Counsel . . . . Anthony L. Wolk

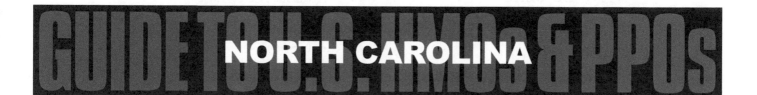

NORTH CAROLINA

Health Insurance Coverage Status and Type of Coverage by Age

Category	All Persons		Under 18 years		Under 65 years	
	Number	%	Number	%	Number	%
Total population	10,071	-	2,451	-	8,482	-
Covered by some type of health insurance	8,995 *(24)*	89.3 *(0.2)*	2,332 *(11)*	95.2 *(0.3)*	7,413 *(25)*	87.4 *(0.3)*
Covered by private health insurance	6,752 *(43)*	67.0 *(0.4)*	1,380 *(20)*	56.3 *(0.8)*	5,780 *(41)*	68.1 *(0.5)*
Employer-based	5,213 *(44)*	51.8 *(0.4)*	1,127 *(19)*	46.0 *(0.8)*	4,734 *(43)*	55.8 *(0.5)*
Direct purchase	1,519 *(26)*	15.1 *(0.3)*	183 *(9)*	7.5 *(0.4)*	959 *(24)*	11.3 *(0.3)*
TRICARE	446 *(15)*	4.4 *(0.2)*	120 *(7)*	4.9 *(0.3)*	321 *(14)*	3.8 *(0.2)*
Covered by public health insurance	3,491 *(33)*	34.7 *(0.3)*	1,029 *(21)*	42.0 *(0.8)*	1,942 *(32)*	22.9 *(0.4)*
Medicaid	1,863 *(33)*	18.5 *(0.3)*	1,021 *(22)*	41.7 *(0.9)*	1,671 *(32)*	19.7 *(0.4)*
Medicare	1,833 *(11)*	18.2 *(0.1)*	8 *(2)*	0.3 *(0.1)*	286 *(9)*	3.4 *(0.1)*
VA Care	286 *(9)*	2.8 *(0.1)*	5 *(2)*	0.2 *(0.1)*	142 *(7)*	1.7 *(0.1)*
Not covered at any time during the year	1,076 *(24)*	10.7 *(0.2)*	119 *(8)*	4.8 *(0.3)*	1,069 *(24)*	12.6 *(0.3)*

Note: Numbers in thousands; Figures cover civilian noninstitutionalized population in 2017; N/A indicates that data was not available; Z represents or rounds to zero; Margin of error appears in parenthesis and is calculated using replicate weights.
Source: U.S. Census Bureau, American Community Survey, Table HIC-4_ACS. Health Insurance Coverage Status and Type of Coverage by State—All People: 2008 to 2017, Table HIC-5_ACS. Health Insurance Coverage Status and Type of Coverage by State—Children Under 18: 2008 to 2017, Table HIC-6_ACS. Health Insurance Coverage Status and Type of Coverage by State—Persons Under 65: 2008 to 2017

North Carolina

583 Aetna Health of North Carolina
151 Farmington Avenue
Hartford, CT 06156
Toll-Free: 800-872-3862
Phone: 860-273-0123
www.aetna.com
Subsidiary of: Aetna Inc.
For Profit Organization: Yes

Healthplan and Services Defined
PLAN TYPE: HMO/PPO
Other Type: POS
Model Type: Network
Plan Specialty: Behavioral Health, EPO, Lab, PBM, Radiology
Benefits Offered: Behavioral Health, Dental, Disease Management, Long-Term Care, Physical Therapy, Podiatry, Prescription, Psychiatric, Vision, Wellness, Life, LTD, STD

Type of Coverage
Commercial, Student health

Geographic Areas Served
Statewide

584 Blue Cross Blue Shield of North Carolina
4615 Univerisity Drive
Durham, NC 27707
Toll-Free: 800-228-6216
Phone: 919-765-4600
www.bluecrossnc.com
Mailing Address: P.O. Box 2291, DurhamNC 27702-2291
Non-Profit Organization: Yes
Year Founded: 1933
Total Enrollment: 3,890,000

Healthplan and Services Defined
PLAN TYPE: HMO/PPO
Model Type: Network
Plan Specialty: ASO, Behavioral Health, Chiropractic, Dental, Disease Management, Lab, PBM, Vision, Radiology, UR
Benefits Offered: Behavioral Health, Chiropractic, Complementary Medicine, Dental, Disease Management, Home Care, Inpatient SNF, Long-Term Care, Physical Therapy, Podiatry, Prescription, Psychiatric, Transplant, Vision, Wellness, AD&D, Life, LTD, STD

Type of Coverage
Commercial, Individual, Supplemental Medicare

Type of Payment Plans Offered
POS, DFFS, FFS, Combination FFS & DFFS

Geographic Areas Served
Statewide

Peer Review Type
Utilization Review: Yes
Second Surgical Opinion: Yes
Case Management: Yes

Accreditation Certification
NCQA
State Licensure

Key Personnel
President & CEO . . . . Patrick Conway
SVP, Operating Officer . . . . Gerald Petkau
SVP, Financial Officer . . . . Mitch Perry
Chief Information. . . . . Jo Abernathy
Service Operations. . . . . Lisa Cade
Chief Medical Officer . . . . Rahul Rajkumar

Average Claim Compensation
Physician's Fees Charged: 43%
Hospital's Fees Charged: 35%

585 Cigna Healthcare North Carolina
900 Cottage Grove Road
Bloomfield, CT 06002
Toll-Free: 800-244-6224
www.cigna.com
For Profit Organization: Yes

Healthplan and Services Defined
PLAN TYPE: Multiple
Benefits Offered: Behavioral Health, Dental, Disease Management, Prescription, Vision, Wellness, AD&D, Life, LTD, STD

Type of Coverage
Commercial, Individual, Medicare, Supplemental Medicare, Medicaid, Part-time and hourly workers; Union

Geographic Areas Served
Statewide

Key Personnel
President/General Manager . . . . Charles Pitts
Dir., Network Contracting. . . . . Jennifer Ketner
VP, Sales, Mid-Atlantic . . . . William Vogelpohl
New Business Manager . . . . Cameron Starnes
Sr. Dir., Clinical IT . . . . Robert Wayne Barker
IT Manager . . . . Tammy Champion

586 Coventry Health Care of the Carolinas
1720 South Sykes Drive
Bismark, ND 58504
Toll-Free: SC 888-935-7284
Phone: NC 800-935-7284
coventryhealthcare.com
Subsidiary of: Aetna Inc.
For Profit Organization: Yes
Total Enrollment: 5,000,000
State Enrollment: 187,000

Healthplan and Services Defined
PLAN TYPE: HMO/PPO
Model Type: Network
Plan Specialty: Behavioral Health, Dental, Worker's Compensation
Benefits Offered: Behavioral Health, Dental, Prescription, Wellness, Worker's Compensation

Type of Coverage
Commercial, Individual, Medicare, Medicaid

Geographic Areas Served
North and South Carolina

Key Personnel
Mgr., Network Development . . . . Colleen Andrews
CFO . . . . Dewey Brown

---

587 Crescent Health Solutions

1200 Ridgefield Boulevard
Suite 215
Asheville, NC 28806
Toll-Free: 800-707-7726
Phone: 828-670-9145
Fax: 828-670-9155
www.crescenths.com
Year Founded: 1999
Physician Owned Organization: Yes
Number of Affiliated Hospitals: 4,000
Number of Primary Care Physicians: 1,900
Number of Referral/Specialty Physicians: 2,400
Total Enrollment: 40,000
State Enrollment: 40,000

Healthplan and Services Defined
PLAN TYPE: PPO
Benefits Offered: Disease Management, Prescription,
Wellness, Case Management, UR, TPA Services

Type of Coverage
Commercial, Individual

Geographic Areas Served
North Carolina, South Carolina, Georgia, and Oklahoma

Peer Review Type
Utilization Review: Yes
Case Management: Yes

Key Personnel
CEO . . . . Andrew L. Wilson
VP, Operations/Business . . . . Desiree Greene
CFO . . . . Stephanie Weil
TPA Claims Manager . . . . Cindy Beaver
Provider Relations Mgr . . . . Delane Stiles
Chief Medical Officer . . . . W. Virgil Thrash, MD
Director of Sales . . . . Blake Spell

---

588 Delta Dental of North Carolina

4242 Six Forks Road
Suite 970
Raleigh, NC 27609
Toll-Free: 800-587-9514
www.deltadentalnc.org
Secondary Address: Customer Service, P.O. Box 1596,
Indianapolis, IN 46206-1596
Non-Profit Organization: Yes

Healthplan and Services Defined
PLAN TYPE: Dental
Other Type: Dental PPO
Plan Specialty: Dental

Benefits Offered: Dental

Type of Coverage
Commercial, Individual

Type of Payment Plans Offered
POS, DFFS, FFS

Geographic Areas Served
Statewide

Key Personnel
President/CEO . . . . Curtis Ladig

---

589 Envolve Vision

112 Zebulon Court
P.O. Box 7548
Rocky Mount, NC 27804
Toll-Free: 800-334-3937
Fax: 877-940-9243
visionbenefits.envolvehealth.com
For Profit Organization: Yes
Number of Primary Care Physicians: 20,000

Healthplan and Services Defined
PLAN TYPE: Vision
Model Type: Network
Plan Specialty: Vision
Benefits Offered: Vision

Type of Coverage
Commercial, Medicare, Supplemental Medicare, Medicaid

Type of Payment Plans Offered
POS, DFFS, Capitated, FFS, Combination FFS & DFFS

Geographic Areas Served
Nationwide

Peer Review Type
Utilization Review: Yes
Case Management: Yes

Accreditation Certification
AAAHC, NCQA, State Licensure

Key Personnel
President/CEO . . . . David Lavely
SVP, Information Systems . . . . Juan Marrero
SVP, Regulatory Affairs . . . . Larry Keeley
SVP, Finance . . . . George Verrastro
Chief Operating Officer . . . . Michael Grover

Employer References
Wilmer-Hutchins Independent School D+strict

---

590 FirstCarolinaCare

42 Memorial Drive
Pinehurst, NC 28374
Phone: 910-715-8100
www.firstcarolinacare.com
Subsidiary of: FirstHealth of the Carolinas
Non-Profit Organization: Yes
Total Enrollment: 13,000
State Enrollment: 13,000

Healthplan and Services Defined
   PLAN TYPE: HMO
   Offers Demand Management Patient Information Service:
      Yes
   DMPI Services Offered: Nurse Helpline

Type of Coverage
   Individual

Key Personnel
   President . . . . Craig Humphrey

---

591   Humana Health Insurance of North Carolina
5955 Carnegie Boulevard
Suite 100
Charlotte, NC 28209
Toll-Free: 800-211-2389
Phone: 704-643-1009
www.humana.com
Secondary Address: Westover Gallery of Shoppes, 1420
   Westover Terr., Suite C, Greensboro, NC 27408,
   336-547-2701
For Profit Organization: Yes

Healthplan and Services Defined
   PLAN TYPE: HMO/PPO
   Plan Specialty: ASO
   Benefits Offered: Disease Management, Prescription,
      Wellness

Type of Coverage
   Commercial, Individual

Geographic Areas Served
   Statewide

Accreditation Certification
   URAC, NCQA, CORE

Specialty Managed Care Partners
   Caremark Rx

Employer References
   Tricare

---

592   MedCost
165 Kimel Park Drive
Winston Salem, NC 27103
Toll-Free: 800-217-5097
www.medcost.com
Secondary Address: 1915 Rexford Road, Suite 430, Charlotte,
   NC 28211, 704-525-1473
Subsidiary of: Carolinas HealthCare System
For Profit Organization: Yes
Year Founded: 1983
Number of Affiliated Hospitals: 191
Number of Primary Care Physicians: 12,349
Number of Referral/Specialty Physicians: 21,295
Total Enrollment: 670,000
State Enrollment: 670,000

Healthplan and Services Defined
   PLAN TYPE: PPO
   Model Type: Network

Plan Specialty: UR, PPO Network, Maternity Management,
   Case Management, Nurse Coaching
Benefits Offered: Behavioral Health, Dental, Home Care,
   Inpatient SNF, Long-Term Care, Physical Therapy,
   Podiatry, Psychiatric, Transplant, Vision, Wellness,
   Medical, Hospice, Durable Medical Equipment

Type of Coverage
   Commercial

Type of Payment Plans Offered
   FFS

Geographic Areas Served
   North Carolina, South Carolina, and Virginia

Subscriber Information
   Average Subscriber Co-Payment:
      Primary Care Physician: Varies
      Non-Network Physician: Varies
      Prescription Drugs: Varies
      Hospital ER: Varies
      Home Health Care: Varies
      Home Health Care Max. Days/Visits Covered: Varies
      Nursing Home: Varies
      Nursing Home Max. Days/Visits Covered: Varies

Peer Review Type
   Utilization Review: Yes
   Second Surgical Opinion: Yes
   Case Management: Yes

Publishes and Distributes Report Card: Yes

Accreditation Certification
   URAC

Key Personnel
   Senior Vice President . . . . Kathryn Showalter
   Chief Financial Officer . . . . Greg Bray

---

593   United Concordia of North Carolina
10700 Sikes Place
Suite 331
Charlotte, NC 28277
Phone: 704-845-8224
www.unitedconcordia.com
For Profit Organization: Yes
Year Founded: 1971
Total Enrollment: 7,800,000

Healthplan and Services Defined
   PLAN TYPE: Dental
   Plan Specialty: Dental
   Benefits Offered: Dental

Type of Coverage
   Commercial, Individual, Military personnel & families

Geographic Areas Served
   Nationwide

Accreditation Certification
   URAC

Key Personnel

Contact. . . . . Beth Rutherford
717-260-7659
beth.rutherford@ucci.com

---

594   UnitedHealthcare of North Carolina

8601 Six Forks Road
Raleigh, NC 27615
Toll-Free: 888-835-9637
www.uhc.com
Subsidiary of: UnitedHealth Group
For Profit Organization: Yes
Year Founded: 1985

Healthplan and Services Defined
PLAN TYPE: HMO/PPO
Model Type: Network
Plan Specialty: Behavioral Health, Dental, Disease
     Management, PBM, Vision
Benefits Offered: Behavioral Health, Dental, Disease
     Management, Long-Term Care, Prescription, Vision,
     Wellness, Life, LTD, STD

Type of Coverage
Individual, Medicare, Supplemental Medicare, Medicaid,
     Catastrophic, Family, Military, Veterans, Group,
Catastrophic Illness Benefit: Maximum $2M

Type of Payment Plans Offered
POS, DFFS, FFS, Combination FFS & DFFS

Geographic Areas Served
Statewide

Subscriber Information
Average Subscriber Co-Payment:
     Primary Care Physician: $10.00
     Non-Network Physician: 20%
     Prescription Drugs: $10.00
     Hospital ER: $35.00
     Home Health Care: $0
     Home Health Care Max. Days/Visits Covered: 30 days
     Nursing Home: 20%
     Nursing Home Max. Days/Visits Covered: 30 days

Network Qualifications
Pre-Admission Certification: Yes

Peer Review Type
Utilization Review: Yes
Second Surgical Opinion: No
Case Management: Yes

Publishes and Distributes Report Card: Yes

Accreditation Certification
TJC Accreditation, Utilization Review, Pre-Admission
     Certification, State Licensure, Quality Assurance Program

Key Personnel
CEO, Community Plan NC. . . . . Anita Bachmann

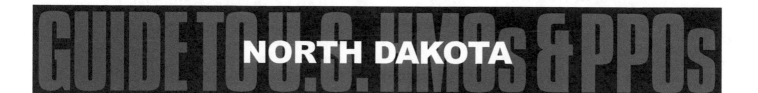

Health Insurance Coverage Status and Type of Coverage by Age

Category	All Persons		Under 18 years		Under 65 years	
	Number	%	Number	%	Number	%
Total population	738	-	184	-	632	-
Covered by some type of health insurance	683 (5)	92.5 (0.6)	170 (3)	92.5 (1.4)	576 (5)	91.2 (0.8)
Covered by private health insurance	589 (9)	79.8 (1.2)	138 (5)	75.0 (2.7)	511 (9)	80.9 (1.4)
Employer-based	454 (9)	61.5 (1.2)	117 (5)	63.7 (2.7)	426 (9)	67.4 (1.4)
Direct purchase	140 (5)	19.0 (0.6)	19 (3)	10.1 (1.4)	87 (4)	13.7 (0.7)
TRICARE	28 (4)	3.9 (0.5)	7 (2)	3.7 (0.9)	21 (3)	3.3 (0.5)
Covered by public health insurance	190 (7)	25.8 (1.0)	40 (5)	21.8 (2.5)	88 (7)	13.9 (1.1)
Medicaid	82 (7)	11.2 (0.9)	39 (5)	21.4 (2.5)	73 (7)	11.6 (1.1)
Medicare	114 (2)	15.4 (0.3)	1 (Z)	0.4 (0.2)	12 (1)	1.8 (0.2)
VA Care	20 (2)	2.7 (0.3)	Z (Z)	0.1 (0.1)	9 (2)	1.4 (0.2)
Not covered at any time during the year	56 (5)	7.5 (0.6)	14 (3)	7.5 (1.4)	55 (5)	8.8 (0.8)

Note: Numbers in thousands; Figures cover civilian noninstitutionalized population in 2017; N/A indicates that data was not available; Z represents or rounds to zero; Margin of error appears in parenthesis and is calculated using replicate weights.
Source: U.S. Census Bureau, American Community Survey, Table HIC-4_ACS. Health Insurance Coverage Status and Type of Coverage by State—All People: 2008 to 2017, Table HIC-5_ACS. Health Insurance Coverage Status and Type of Coverage by State—Children Under 18: 2008 to 2017, Table HIC-6_ACS. Health Insurance Coverage Status and Type of Coverage by State—Persons Under 65: 2008 to 2017

North Dakota

595 Aetna Health of North Dakota

151 Farmington Avenue
Hartford, CT 06156
Toll-Free: 800-872-3862
Phone: 860-273-0123
www.aetna.com
Subsidiary of: Aetna Inc.
For Profit Organization: Yes

Healthplan and Services Defined
PLAN TYPE: PPO
Other Type: POS
Model Type: Network
Plan Specialty: Behavioral Health, EPO, Lab, PBM,
   Radiology
Benefits Offered: Behavioral Health, Disease Management,
   Long-Term Care, Physical Therapy, Podiatry, Prescription,
   Psychiatric, Wellness, Life, LTD, STD

Type of Coverage
Commercial, Student health

Type of Payment Plans Offered
POS, FFS

Geographic Areas Served
Statewide

Key Personnel
Vice President .... Joe Harris
Operations Manager .... Sandy Bauer

596 Coventry Health Care of North Dakota

4810 16th Avenue South
Fargo, ND 58103
Phone: 701-248-0457
www.coventryhealthcare.com
Subsidiary of: Aetna Inc.
For Profit Organization: Yes

Healthplan and Services Defined
PLAN TYPE: HMO/PPO
Model Type: Network
Plan Specialty: Behavioral Health, Dental, Worker's
   Compensation
Benefits Offered: Behavioral Health, Dental, Prescription,
   Wellness, Worker's Compensation

Type of Coverage
Commercial, Medicare, Medicaid

Geographic Areas Served
Statewide

Key Personnel
Operations Manager .... Leah Loerch
Chief Strategy Officer .... Ener Hawks
Service Operations Mgr. .... Sandra Bauer

597 Heart of America Health Plan

P.O. Box 1999
Fargo, ND 58107
Toll-Free: 877-652-1845
Phone: 701-776-5848
Fax: 605-328-6811
www.sanfordhealthplan.org/heart-of-america
Subsidiary of: Sanford Health Plan
Non-Profit Organization: Yes
Year Founded: 1982
Number of Affiliated Hospitals: 1
Number of Primary Care Physicians: 15
Number of Referral/Specialty Physicians: 500
Total Enrollment: 1,000
State Enrollment: 2,049

Healthplan and Services Defined
PLAN TYPE: HMO
Model Type: Group
Benefits Offered: Behavioral Health, Disease Management,
   Podiatry, Psychiatric, Wellness, LTD, Substance Abuse,
   Maternity

Type of Coverage
Medicare, Supplemental Medicare

Type of Payment Plans Offered
POS, DFFS

Geographic Areas Served
North Central North Dakota: Pierce, Rolette, Bottineau,
   McHenry, Towner, Ward and Renville counties in North
   Dakota and portions of Benson, Wells, Sheridan, McLean,
   Mountrail and Burke counties

Subscriber Information
Average Annual Deductible Per Subscriber:
   Employee Only (Self): $600
   Employee & 1 Family Member: $0
   Employee & 2 Family Members: $0
   Medicare: $0
Average Subscriber Co-Payment:
   Primary Care Physician: $10.00
   Non-Network Physician: 20%
   Prescription Drugs: $0.00
   Hospital ER: $30.00

Accreditation Certification
TJC Accreditation

Average Claim Compensation
Physician's Fees Charged: 1%
Hospital's Fees Charged: 1%

Employer References
Federal Employee Plan

598   Humana Health Insurance of North Dakota

12600 Whitewater Drive
Suite 150
Minnetonka, MN 55343
Toll-Free: 877-367-6990
Phone: 952-253-3540
Fax: 952-938-2787
www.humana.com
Subsidiary of: Humana
For Profit Organization: Yes

Healthplan and Services Defined
  PLAN TYPE: HMO/PPO
  Model Type: Network
  Plan Specialty: Dental, Vision
  Benefits Offered: Dental, Vision, Life, LTD, STD

Type of Coverage
  Commercial

Geographic Areas Served
  North Dakota is covered by the Minnesota branch

Accreditation Certification
  URAC, NCQA, CORE

Key Personnel
  Sales Representative . . . . Jim Simmers

599   Medica: North Dakota

1711 Gold Drive South
Suite 210
Fargo, ND 58103
Phone: 701-293-4700
www.medica.com
Non-Profit Organization: Yes
Year Founded: 1974
Number of Affiliated Hospitals: 158
Number of Primary Care Physicians: 24,000
Total Enrollment: 1,600,000

Healthplan and Services Defined
  PLAN TYPE: HMO
  Model Type: IPA
  Benefits Offered: Behavioral Health, Chiropractic, Dental,
    Disease Management, Prescription, Wellness, AD&D, Life,
    LTD, STD
  Offers Demand Management Patient Information Service:
    Yes

Type of Coverage
  Medicare
  Catastrophic Illness Benefit: Covered

Type of Payment Plans Offered
  Capitated, FFS, Combination FFS & DFFS

Geographic Areas Served
  Aitkin, Anoka, Becker, Beltrami, Benton, Big Stone, Blue
  Earth, Brown, Carlton, Carver, Cass, Chisago, Clay,
  Clearwater, Cottonwood, Crow Wing, Dakota, Dodge,
  Douglas, Fillmore, Goodhue, Grant, Hennepin, Hubbard,
  Isanti, Itaska, Kanabec, Kandiyohi, Koochiching, Jackson,
  Lac Qui Parle, Lake, Le Sueur, Lincoln, Lyon, Mahnomen,
  McLeod, Meeker, Mille Lacs, Morrison, Murray, Nicollet,

Norman, Olnsted, Otter Tail, Pine, Polk, Pope, Ramsey,
Renville, Rice, Rock, Scott

Subscriber Information
  Average Monthly Fee Per Subscriber
    (Employee + Employer Contribution):
      Employee Only (Self): Varies by plan
  Average Subscriber Co-Payment:
    Primary Care Physician: $15.00
    Non-Network Physician: Deductible + 20%
    Prescription Drugs: $11.00
    Hospital ER: $60.00
    Home Health Care: 20%
    Nursing Home: 20%

Network Qualifications
  Pre-Admission Certification: Yes

Peer Review Type
  Utilization Review: Yes
  Second Surgical Opinion: Yes
  Case Management: Yes

Publishes and Distributes Report Card: Yes

Accreditation Certification
  NCQA
  TJC Accreditation, Medicare Approved, Utilization Review,
    Pre-Admission Certification, State Licensure, Quality
    Assurance Program

Average Claim Compensation
  Physician's Fees Charged: 65%
  Hospital's Fees Charged: 60%

Specialty Managed Care Partners
  Express Scrips, Vision Service Plan, National Healthcare
    Resources, Cigna Behavioral Resources
  Enters into Contracts with Regional Business Coalitions: Yes

Employer References
  Construction Industry Laborers Welfare Fund-Jefferson City,
    District 9 Machinists (Missouri/Welfare Plan), Government
    Employees Hospital Association/GEHA, Missouri Highway
    & Transportation Department/Highway Patrol

600   Noridian Insurance Services Inc.

4510 13th Avenue S
Fargo, ND 58121
Toll-Free: 800-575-9643
www.mynisi.com
For Profit Organization: Yes

Healthplan and Services Defined
  PLAN TYPE: PPO
  Plan Specialty: Dental, Vision
  Benefits Offered: Dental, Long-Term Care, Vision, AD&D,
    Life, LTD, STD

Type of Coverage
  Commercial, Individual, Indemnity

Geographic Areas Served
  North Dakota and Northwest Minnesota

601 UnitedHealthcare of North Dakota

9700 Health Care Lane
Minnetonka, MN 55343
Toll-Free: 888-545-5205
Phone: 763-797-2919
www.uhc.com
Subsidiary of: UnitedHealth Group
For Profit Organization: Yes
Year Founded: 1977

Healthplan and Services Defined
  PLAN TYPE: HMO/PPO
  Model Type: Network
  Plan Specialty: Behavioral Health, Dental, Disease
    Management, Lab, PBM, Vision, Radiology
  Benefits Offered: Behavioral Health, Dental, Disease
    Management, Home Care, Long-Term Care, Physical
    Therapy, Prescription, Psychiatric, Vision, Wellness,
    AD&D, Life, LTD, STD
  Offers Demand Management Patient Information Service:
    Yes

Type of Coverage
  Commercial, Individual, Indemnity, Medicare, Supplemental
    Medicare, Medicaid, Catastrophic, Family, Military,
    Veterans, Group,
  Catastrophic Illness Benefit: Varies per case

Geographic Areas Served
  Statewide. North Dakota is covered by the Minnesota branch

Publishes and Distributes Report Card: Yes

Accreditation Certification
  TJC Accreditation, Medicare Approved

Key Personnel
  CEO, MN/ND/SD . . . . Philip Kaufman

Specialty Managed Care Partners
  Enters into Contracts with Regional Business Coalitions: Yes

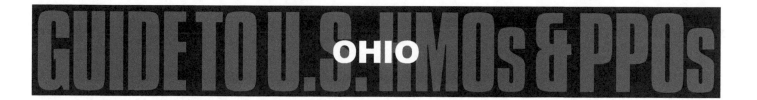

Health Insurance Coverage Status and Type of Coverage by Age

Category	All Persons		Under 18 years		Under 65 years	
	Number	%	Number	%	Number	%
Total population	11,485	-	2,759	-	9,615	-
Covered by some type of health insurance	10,799 (22)	94.0 (0.2)	2,634 (11)	95.5 (0.4)	8,938 (23)	93.0 (0.2)
Covered by private health insurance	7,934 (43)	69.1 (0.4)	1,731 (21)	62.8 (0.8)	6,775 (39)	70.5 (0.4)
Employer-based	6,763 (44)	58.9 (0.4)	1,581 (21)	57.3 (0.7)	6,095 (41)	63.4 (0.4)
Direct purchase	1,387 (23)	12.1 (0.2)	152 (7)	5.5 (0.3)	768 (19)	8.0 (0.2)
TRICARE	191 (10)	1.7 (0.1)	40 (5)	1.4 (0.2)	121 (9)	1.3 (0.1)
Covered by public health insurance	4,316 (38)	37.6 (0.3)	1,023 (22)	37.1 (0.8)	2,508 (36)	26.1 (0.4)
Medicaid	2,415 (38)	21.0 (0.3)	1,014 (22)	36.8 (0.8)	2,239 (36)	23.3 (0.4)
Medicare	2,127 (12)	18.5 (0.1)	16 (3)	0.6 (0.1)	322 (10)	3.3 (0.1)
VA Care	269 (8)	2.3 (0.1)	3 (1)	0.1 (0.1)	111 (6)	1.2 (0.1)
Not covered at any time during the year	686 (22)	6.0 (0.2)	125 (10)	4.5 (0.4)	677 (22)	7.0 (0.2)

Note: Numbers in thousands; Figures cover civilian noninstitutionalized population in 2017; N/A indicates that data was not available; Z represents or rounds to zero; Margin of error appears in parenthesis and is calculated using replicate weights.
Source: U.S. Census Bureau, American Community Survey, Table HIC-4_ACS. Health Insurance Coverage Status and Type of Coverage by State—All People: 2008 to 2017, Table HIC-5_ACS. Health Insurance Coverage Status and Type of Coverage by State—Children Under 18: 2008 to 2017, Table HIC-6_ACS. Health Insurance Coverage Status and Type of Coverage by State—Persons Under 65: 2008 to 2017

Ohio

602 Aetna Health of Ohio

7400 W Campus Road
New Albany, OH 43054
Toll-Free: 855-364-0974
www.aetnabetterhealth.com/ohio
Subsidiary of: Aetna Inc.
For Profit Organization: Yes

Healthplan and Services Defined
PLAN TYPE: HMO/PPO
Other Type: POS
Model Type: Network
Plan Specialty: Behavioral Health, Dental, EPO, Lab, PBM,
   Vision, Radiology
Benefits Offered: Behavioral Health, Dental, Disease
   Management, Long-Term Care, Physical Therapy,
   Podiatry, Prescription, Psychiatric, Vision, Wellness, Life,
   LTD, STD

Type of Coverage
Commercial, Medicare, Medicaid, Student health

Type of Payment Plans Offered
POS

Geographic Areas Served
Statewide

Subscriber Information
Average Subscriber Co-Payment:
   Prescription Drugs: $5.00
   Home Health Care Max. Days/Visits Covered: Unlimited

Network Qualifications
Pre-Admission Certification: No

Peer Review Type
Utilization Review: Yes
Second Surgical Opinion: Yes
Case Management: Yes

Publishes and Distributes Report Card: Yes

Accreditation Certification
NCQA
TJC Accreditation, Utilization Review, Pre-Admission
   Certification, State Licensure, Quality Assurance Program

Key Personnel
CEO, Medicaid Ohio . . . . Tony Solem

Specialty Managed Care Partners
Enters into Contracts with Regional Business Coalitions: Yes

603 Anthem Blue Cross & Blue Shield of Ohio

4361 Irwin Simpson Road
Mason, OH 45040
Toll-Free: 800-483-2311
www.anthem.com
Secondary Address: 6740 N High Street, Worthington, OH
   43085, 614-528-4581
Subsidiary of: Anthem, Inc.
For Profit Organization: Yes
Year Founded: 1944

Owned by an Integrated Delivery Network (IDN): Yes
Number of Affiliated Hospitals: 568
Number of Primary Care Physicians: 25,000
Number of Referral/Specialty Physicians: 61,728

Healthplan and Services Defined
PLAN TYPE: PPO
Plan Specialty: ASO, Behavioral Health, Chiropractic, Dental,
   Disease Management, Lab, PBM, Vision, Radiology,
   Worker's Compensation, UR
Benefits Offered: Behavioral Health, Chiropractic, Dental,
   Disease Management, Home Care, Inpatient SNF, Physical
   Therapy, Podiatry, Prescription, Psychiatric, Transplant,
   Vision, Wellness, Worker's Compensation
Offers Demand Management Patient Information Service: Yes
DMPI Services Offered: Iris Program, Care Wise (24/7 Nurse
   Line), Dental, Vision

Type of Coverage
Commercial, Individual, Indemnity, Medicare, Catastrophic

Type of Payment Plans Offered
POS, DFFS, Capitated, FFS

Geographic Areas Served
Statewide

Subscriber Information
Average Monthly Fee Per Subscriber
   (Employee + Employer Contribution):
      Employee Only (Self): Proprietary
      Employee & 1 Family Member: Proprietary
      Employee & 2 Family Members: Proprierary
      Medicare: Proprietary
Average Annual Deductible Per Subscriber:
      Employee Only (Self): Proprietary
      Employee & 1 Family Member: Proprietary
      Employee & 2 Family Members: Proprietary
      Medicare: Proprietary

Network Qualifications
Pre-Admission Certification: Yes

Peer Review Type
Utilization Review: Yes
Second Surgical Opinion: Yes
Case Management: Yes

Accreditation Certification
URAC, NCQA
TJC Accreditation, Medicare Approved, Utilization Review,
   Pre-Admission Certification, State Licensure, Quality
   Assurance Program

Key Personnel
President . . . . Steve Martenet

Specialty Managed Care Partners
Anthem Dental, Anthem Prescription Management LLC,
   Anthem Vision, Anthem Life

604 Aultcare Corporation

2600 Sixth Street SW
Canton, OH 44710
Toll-Free: 800-344-8858
Phone: 330-363-6360
www.aultcare.com
Non-Profit Organization: Yes
Year Founded: 1985
Number of Affiliated Hospitals: 14
Number of Primary Care Physicians: 3,500
Number of Referral/Specialty Physicians: 6,800
Total Enrollment: 500,000
State Enrollment: 5,151

Healthplan and Services Defined
 PLAN TYPE: HMO/PPO
 Model Type: Network
 Benefits Offered: Chiropractic, Dental, Disease Management,
 Inpatient SNF, Podiatry, Vision, Wellness, Worker's
 Compensation, STD, Flexible Spending Accounts

Type of Coverage
 Commercial, Individual

Geographic Areas Served
 Carroll, Holmes, Stark, Summit, Tuscarawas and Wayne
 counties

Network Qualifications
 Pre-Admission Certification: Yes

Peer Review Type
 Utilization Review: Yes
 Second Surgical Opinion: Yes
 Case Management: Yes

Accreditation Certification
 NCQA

Key Personnel
 CEO/President . . . . Rick Haines

Employer References
 Maytag, Timken Company

605 CareSource Ohio

230 N Main Street
Dayton, OH 45402
Toll-Free: 844-607-2830
Phone: 937-224-3300
www.caresource.com
Secondary Address: 5900 Landerbrook Drive, Suite 300,
 Mayfield Heights, OH 44124, 216-839-1001
Non-Profit Organization: Yes
Total Enrollment: 1,000,000

Healthplan and Services Defined
 PLAN TYPE: Medicare
 Other Type: Medicaid

Type of Coverage
 Medicare, Medicaid

Geographic Areas Served
 Statewide

Key Personnel
 President & CEO . . . . Erhardt Preitauer
 COO . . . . L. Tarlton Thomas III
 CFO . . . . David Goltz
 CIO. . . . . Pauk Stoddard
 CAO . . . . Dan McCabe

606 Delta Dental of Ohio

4100 Okemos Road
Okemos, MI 48864
Toll-Free: 800-524-0149
www.deltadentaloh.com
Mailing Address: P.O. Box 9085, Farmington Hills, MI
 48333-9085
Non-Profit Organization: Yes
Year Founded: 1960

Healthplan and Services Defined
 PLAN TYPE: Dental
 Other Type: Dental PPO
 Plan Specialty: Dental
 Benefits Offered: Dental

Type of Coverage
 Commercial

Type of Payment Plans Offered
 POS

Geographic Areas Served
 Statewide

Peer Review Type
 Second Surgical Opinion: Yes
 Case Management: No

Publishes and Distributes Report Card: Yes

Accreditation Certification
 Utilization Review

Key Personnel
 Controller . . . . Jennifer Needham, CPA
 Exec. Dir., Sales/Account. . . . . Bryan Leddy
 Senior Account Manager. . . . . Cathy Dorocak
 Account Executive. Daniel Parker

Specialty Managed Care Partners
 Enters into Contracts with Regional Business Coalitions: Yes

607 EyeMed Vision Care

4000 Luxottica Place
Mason, OH 45040
Toll-Free: 866-939-3633
portal.eyemedvisioncare.com
Subsidiary of: Luxxotica
For Profit Organization: Yes
Year Founded: 1988
Total Enrollment: 43,000,000

Healthplan and Services Defined
 PLAN TYPE: Vision
 Plan Specialty: Vision
 Benefits Offered: Vision

Type of Coverage
Commercial

Key Personnel
President .... Lukas Ruecker
SVP, Operations .... Matt MacDonald

608 Humana Health Insurance of Ohio

4555 Lake Forest Drive
Suite 650
Cincinnati, OH 45242
Phone: 513-563-3042
Fax: 513-442-7668
www.humana.com
Secondary Address: 6050 Oaktree Boulevard, Suite 100,
Independence, OH 44131, 614-210-8001
For Profit Organization: Yes
Year Founded: 1979
Owned by an Integrated Delivery Network (IDN): Yes

Healthplan and Services Defined
PLAN TYPE: HMO/PPO
Model Type: Group
Plan Specialty: ASO, Dental, Vision, Radiology, Worker's
Compensation
Benefits Offered: Behavioral Health, Chiropractic, Disease
Management, Inpatient SNF, Physical Therapy, Podiatry,
Prescription, Psychiatric, Transplant, Vision, Wellness
Offers Demand Management Patient Information Service:
Yes

Type of Coverage
Commercial, Individual, Medicare, Medicaid

Type of Payment Plans Offered
POS, DFFS, Capitated, FFS, Combination FFS & DFFS

Geographic Areas Served
Statewide

Subscriber Information
Average Subscriber Co-Payment:
Home Health Care: $0
Nursing Home: $0

Peer Review Type
Utilization Review: Yes
Case Management: Yes

Publishes and Distributes Report Card: No

Accreditation Certification
URAC, NCQA, CORE
Utilization Review, Pre-Admission Certification, State
Licensure, Quality Assurance Program

Key Personnel
Sales Manager .... Susan Schoen

Specialty Managed Care Partners
Enters into Contracts with Regional Business Coalitions: No

609 Medical Mutual

2060 E 9th Street
Cleveland, OH 44115
Toll-Free: 800-382-5729
www.medmutual.com
Year Founded: 1934

Healthplan and Services Defined
PLAN TYPE: HMO
Model Type: Staff
Benefits Offered: Prescription

Type of Coverage
Commercial, Individual, Medicare

Type of Payment Plans Offered
DFFS, Capitated, FFS, Combination FFS & DFFS

Geographic Areas Served
Statewide

Publishes and Distributes Report Card: Yes

Accreditation Certification
NCQA

Key Personnel
Chairman, President & CEO............. Rick Chiricosta
EVP, Chief Health Officer................ Kathy Golovan
EVP, Financial Officer.................... Ray Mueller
Chief Information Officer .... John Kish
Chief Medical Officer .... Tere Koenig
Chief Marketing Officer .... Steffany Larkins

Specialty Managed Care Partners
Enters into Contracts with Regional Business Coalitions: Yes

610 Medical Mutual Services

1602, 3636 Copley Road
Copley, OH 44321
Toll-Free: 800-762-8130
Phone: 330-666-0337
www.supermednetwork.com
Subsidiary of: SuperMed Network
Number of Primary Care Physicians: 24,000
Total Enrollment: 144,000

Healthplan and Services Defined
PLAN TYPE: PPO
Benefits Offered: Chiropractic, Physical Therapy, Podiatry,
Psychiatric

Type of Coverage
Commercial, Self Funded, Insurance Companies

Geographic Areas Served
South Carolina, Georgia, Ohio

Accreditation Certification
TJC, NCQA

611 MediGold

6150 East Broad Street
Suite EE320
Columbus, OH 43213-1574
Toll-Free: 800-964-4525
Fax: 614-546-3108
www.medigold.com
Subsidiary of: Mount Carmel Health Plan
Non-Profit Organization: Yes
Year Founded: 1997
Federally Qualified: Yes
Number of Affiliated Hospitals: 23
Number of Primary Care Physicians: 1,050
Number of Referral/Specialty Physicians: 1,850
Total Enrollment: 55,000
State Enrollment: 55,000

Healthplan and Services Defined
  PLAN TYPE: Medicare
  Model Type: Network, Medicare
  Benefits Offered: Behavioral Health, Chiropractic, Dental,
    Disease Management, Home Care, Inpatient SNF, Physical
    Therapy, Podiatry, Prescription, Psychiatric, Vision,
    Wellness, Medical, OP Services, Drug Coverage

Type of Coverage
  Individual, Medicare
  Catastrophic Illness Benefit: Unlimited

Type of Payment Plans Offered
  Combination FFS & DFFS

Geographic Areas Served
  31 counties in Ohio

Subscriber Information
  Average Monthly Fee Per Subscriber
    (Employee + Employer Contribution):
      Employee Only (Self): Varies
      Medicare: Varies
  Average Annual Deductible Per Subscriber:
      Employee Only (Self): Varies
      Medicare: Varies
  Average Subscriber Co-Payment:
      Primary Care Physician: Varies
      Non-Network Physician: Varies
      Prescription Drugs: Varies
      Hospital ER: Varies
      Home Health Care: Varies
      Home Health Care Max. Days/Visits Covered: Varies
      Nursing Home: Varies
      Nursing Home Max. Days/Visits Covered: Varies

Network Qualifications
  Pre-Admission Certification: Yes

Peer Review Type
  Utilization Review: Yes
  Case Management: Yes

Publishes and Distributes Report Card: Yes

Accreditation Certification
  TJC Accreditation, Medicare Approved, Utilization Review,
    Pre-Admission Certification, State Licensure, Quality
    Assurance Program

Key Personnel
  President/CEO . . . . Mike Demand, PhD
  Chief Admin Officer . . . . Chuck Alvarado
  VP, Network Management . . . . Matt Barrett
  VP, Finance . . . . Juan Fraiz
  VP, Health Services . . . . Karen Phillippi
  VP, Compliance/Governance . . . . Larry Pliskin, JD
  CMO/Medical Director . . . . Greg Wise, MD

Specialty Managed Care Partners
  PBM-CAREMARK

Employer References
  Timken, Mount Carmel Trinity

612 Molina Healthcare of Ohio

3000 Corporate Exchange Drive
Columbus, OH 43231
Toll-Free: 800-642-4168
www.molinahealthcare.com
Subsidiary of: Molina Healthcare, Inc.
For Profit Organization: Yes
Year Founded: 1980
Physician Owned Organization: Yes

Healthplan and Services Defined
  PLAN TYPE: Medicare
  Model Type: Network
  Plan Specialty: Integrated Medicare/Medicaid (Duals)
  Benefits Offered: Chiropractic, Dental, Home Care, Inpatient
    SNF, Long-Term Care, Podiatry, Vision

Type of Coverage
  Commercial, Medicare, Supplemental Medicare, Medicaid

Accreditation Certification
  URAC, NCQA

Key Personnel
  Plan President . . . . Ami Cole
  Vice President . . . . Holly Saelens
  Dir., Finance/Analytics . . . . Sara Huffman
  VP, Network Management . . . . Amy Conn

613 Ohio Health Choice

P.O. Box 2090
Akron, OH 44309-2090
Toll-Free: 800-554-0027
www.ohiohealthchoice.com
Mailing Address: P.O. Box 3619, Akron, OH 44309-3619
For Profit Organization: Yes
Year Founded: 1982
Number of Affiliated Hospitals: 199
Number of Primary Care Physicians: 28,000
Total Enrollment: 370,000
State Enrollment: 370,000

Healthplan and Services Defined
  PLAN TYPE: PPO
  Model Type: Network
  Plan Specialty: Chiropractic, Disease Management, EPO, UR
  Benefits Offered: Behavioral Health, Chiropractic, Disease
    Management, Home Care, Inpatient SNF, Long-Term Care,

Physical Therapy, Podiatry, Psychiatric, Transplant, Wellness, Audiology, durable medical equipment, sleep disorder services, speech therapy

Type of Coverage
Commercial, Individual, Indemnity, Medicare

Type of Payment Plans Offered
POS, FFS

Geographic Areas Served
Throughout Ohio as well as the contiguous counties of Boone, Boyd, Campbell, Grant and Kenton in Kentucky; Dearborn in Indiana; Mercer and Erie in Pennsylvania; and Wood, Hancock and Ohio in West Virginia

Peer Review Type
Utilization Review: Yes
Second Surgical Opinion: Yes
Case Management: Yes

---

614 Ohio State University Health Plan Inc.

700 Ackerman Road
Suite 1007
Columbus, OH 43202
Toll-Free: 800-678-6269
Phone: 614-292-4700
OSUHealthPlanCS@osumc.edu
www.osuhealthplan.com
Non-Profit Organization: Yes
Year Founded: 1991
Number of Affiliated Hospitals: 95
Number of Primary Care Physicians: 3,250
Number of Referral/Specialty Physicians: 7,950
Total Enrollment: 52,000
State Enrollment: 52,000

Healthplan and Services Defined
PLAN TYPE: Multiple
Model Type: IPA
Plan Specialty: ASO, Behavioral Health, Disease Management, EPO
Benefits Offered: Behavioral Health, Chiropractic, Complementary Medicine, Dental, Disease Management, Home Care, Inpatient SNF, Physical Therapy, Podiatry, Prescription, Psychiatric, Transplant, Vision, Wellness
Offers Demand Management Patient Information Service: Yes
DMPI Services Offered: Faculty and Staff Assistance Program, University Health Connection

Type of Payment Plans Offered
DFFS, Capitated, Combination FFS & DFFS

Geographic Areas Served
Ohio State University employees and their dependents

Subscriber Information
Average Annual Deductible Per Subscriber:
Employee Only (Self): $0
Employee & 1 Family Member: $0
Employee & 2 Family Members: $0
Medicare: $0
Average Subscriber Co-Payment:
Primary Care Physician: $15.00

Non-Network Physician: 30%
Prescription Drugs: 20% (generic)
Hospital ER: $75.00
Home Health Care: 20%
Home Health Care Max. Days/Visits Covered: Unlimited
Nursing Home: $0
Nursing Home Max. Days/Visits Covered: 60 days

Network Qualifications
Pre-Admission Certification: Yes

Peer Review Type
Utilization Review: Yes
Second Surgical Opinion: No
Case Management: Yes

Publishes and Distributes Report Card: No

Accreditation Certification
NCQA
TJC Accreditation, Medicare Approved, Utilization Review, Pre-Admission Certification, State Licensure, Quality Assurance Program

Key Personnel
CFO/CAO. . . . . Kelly Hamilton
Medical Director . . . . Rob Cooper, MD
Dir, Pharmacy Benefits . . . . Greg Wilson
Chief Information Officer . . . . Tom Gessells
Dir, Mkting/Communication. . . . . Susan Meyer

Specialty Managed Care Partners
Enters into Contracts with Regional Business Coalitions: No

Employer References
Ohio State University

---

615 OhioHealth Group

155 East Broad Street
Suite 1700
Columbus, OH 43215
Toll-Free: 800-455-4460
Phone: 614-566-0056
www.ohiohealthgroup.com
For Profit Organization: Yes
Year Founded: 1985
Physician Owned Organization: Yes
Number of Affiliated Hospitals: 75
Number of Primary Care Physicians: 6,900
Total Enrollment: 100,000
State Enrollment: 100,000

Healthplan and Services Defined
PLAN TYPE: PPO
Model Type: TPA
Benefits Offered: Disease Management, Prescription, Wellness

Type of Coverage
Commercial, Individual

Geographic Areas Served
Statewide

Peer Review Type
Utilization Review: Yes
Case Management: Yes

616 Paramount Elite Medicare Plan

1901 Indian Wood Circle
Maumee, OH 43537
Toll-Free: 800-462-3589
Phone: 419-887-2525
Fax: 419-887-2039
paramount.memberservices@promedica.org
www.paramounthealthcare.com
Mailing Address: P.O. Box 928, Toledo, OH 43697-0928
Subsidiary of: ProMedica Health System
Year Founded: 1988
Number of Affiliated Hospitals: 34
Number of Primary Care Physicians: 1,900
Total Enrollment: 187,000

Healthplan and Services Defined
PLAN TYPE: Medicare
Other Type: HMO
Benefits Offered: Chiropractic, Dental, Disease Management,
Home Care, Inpatient SNF, Physical Therapy, Podiatry,
Prescription, Psychiatric, Vision

Type of Coverage
Individual, Medicare

Geographic Areas Served
Ohio: Lucas and Wood counties; Michigan: Monroe County

Subscriber Information
Average Monthly Fee Per Subscriber
(Employee + Employer Contribution):
Employee Only (Self): Varies
Medicare: Varies
Average Annual Deductible Per Subscriber:
Employee Only (Self): Varies
Medicare: Varies
Average Subscriber Co-Payment:
Primary Care Physician: Varies
Non-Network Physician: Varies
Prescription Drugs: Varies
Hospital ER: Varies
Home Health Care: Varies
Home Health Care Max. Days/Visits Covered: Varies
Nursing Home: Varies
Nursing Home Max. Days/Visits Covered: Varies

Key Personnel
President . . . . Lori Johnston
VP, Finance . . . . Stacey Bock
Dir., Care Management. Deb Woody
VP, Health Services . . . . John Meier

617 Paramount Health Care

1901 Indian Wood Circle
Maumee, OH 43537
Toll-Free: 800-462-3589
Phone: 419-887-2500
paramount.marketing@promedica.org
www.paramounthealthcare.com
Secondary Address: 106 Park Place, Dundee, MI 48131,
734-529-7800
Subsidiary of: ProMedica Health System

For Profit Organization: Yes
Year Founded: 1988
Number of Affiliated Hospitals: 34
Number of Primary Care Physicians: 1,900
Number of Referral/Specialty Physicians: 900
Total Enrollment: 187,000

Healthplan and Services Defined
PLAN TYPE: HMO/PPO
Model Type: Network
Benefits Offered: Prescription

Geographic Areas Served
Northwest Ohio and Southeast Michigan

Subscriber Information
Average Monthly Fee Per Subscriber
(Employee + Employer Contribution):
Employee Only (Self): Varies by plan
Average Annual Deductible Per Subscriber:
Employee Only (Self): Varies
Employee & 1 Family Member: Varies
Employee & 2 Family Members: Varies
Average Subscriber Co-Payment:
Primary Care Physician: Varies
Prescription Drugs: Varies
Hospital ER: $25.00
Home Health Care: $0
Home Health Care Max. Days/Visits Covered: Unlimited
Nursing Home: $0
Nursing Home Max. Days/Visits Covered: 100 days

Network Qualifications
Pre-Admission Certification: Yes

Peer Review Type
Second Surgical Opinion: Yes

Publishes and Distributes Report Card: Yes

Accreditation Certification
URAC, NCQA

Key Personnel
President . . . . Lori Johnston
VP, Finance . . . . Stacey Bock
Dir., Care Management. Deb Woody
VP, Health Services . . . . John Meier

618 Prime Time Health Medicare Plan

214 Dartmouth Avenue SW
Canton, OH 44710
Toll-Free: 800-577-5084
Phone: 330-363-7407
www.primetimehealthplan.com
Mailing Address: P.O. Box 6905, Canton, OH 44706
Subsidiary of: Aultcare
Year Founded: 1997
Total Enrollment: 20,000
State Enrollment: 20,000

Healthplan and Services Defined
PLAN TYPE: Medicare

Benefits Offered: Chiropractic, Dental, Disease Management, Home Care, Inpatient SNF, Physical Therapy, Podiatry, Prescription, Psychiatric, Vision, Wellness

Type of Coverage
Individual, Medicare, Medicaid

Geographic Areas Served
Portage, Medina, Summit, Stark, Carroll, Columbiana, Holmes, Harrison, Trumbull, Mahoning, Tuscarawas and Wayne counties

Subscriber Information
Average Monthly Fee Per Subscriber
(Employee + Employer Contribution):
Employee Only (Self): Varies
Medicare: Varies
Average Annual Deductible Per Subscriber:
Employee Only (Self): Varies
Medicare: Varies
Average Subscriber Co-Payment:
Primary Care Physician: Varies
Non-Network Physician: Varies
Prescription Drugs: Varies
Hospital ER: Varies
Home Health Care: Varies
Home Health Care Max. Days/Visits Covered: Varies
Nursing Home: Varies
Nursing Home Max. Days/Visits Covered: Varies

Key Personnel
President/CEO . . . . Rick Haines

---

619   S&S HealthCare Strategies

1385 Kemper Meadow Drive
Cincinnati, OH 45240
Toll-Free: 800-717-2872
Fax: 513-772-9174
servicedesk@ss-healthcare.com
www.ss-healthcare.com
Subsidiary of: International Managed Care Strategies
Year Founded: 1994

Healthplan and Services Defined
PLAN TYPE: Other
Plan Specialty: Third Party Administrator
Benefits Offered: Dental, Prescription, Vision

Type of Payment Plans Offered
POS, DFFS, FFS

Peer Review Type
Second Surgical Opinion: No
Case Management: No

Publishes and Distributes Report Card: Yes

Specialty Managed Care Partners
Enters into Contracts with Regional Business Coalitions: Yes

---

620   SummaCare Medicare Advantage Plan

1200 East Market Street
Akron, OH 44308-4018
Toll-Free: 800-996-8411
www.summacare.com

Subsidiary of: Summa Health System
For Profit Organization: Yes
Year Founded: 1993
Physician Owned Organization: Yes
Number of Affiliated Hospitals: 60
Number of Primary Care Physicians: 10,000
Total Enrollment: 26,000
State Enrollment: 73,724

Healthplan and Services Defined
PLAN TYPE: Medicare
Model Type: IPA, PPO, POS
Benefits Offered: Behavioral Health, Chiropractic, Complementary Medicine, Dental, Disease Management, Home Care, Inpatient SNF, Physical Therapy, Podiatry, Prescription, Psychiatric, Transplant, Vision, Wellness, AD&D, Life
Offers Demand Management Patient Information Service: Yes
DMPI Services Offered: Nurses Line

Type of Coverage
Medicare
Catastrophic Illness Benefit: Covered

Type of Payment Plans Offered
POS, DFFS, FFS

Geographic Areas Served
Northeast Ohio: Cuyahoga, Geauga, Medina, Portage, Stark, Summit, Wayne, Tuscarawas, Ashtabula, Caroll, Mahoning, Trumbull & Lorain counties

Subscriber Information
Average Monthly Fee Per Subscriber
(Employee + Employer Contribution):
Employee Only (Self): Proprietary
Average Annual Deductible Per Subscriber:
Employee Only (Self): $0
Employee & 1 Family Member: $0
Employee & 2 Family Members: $0
Medicare: $45.00
Average Subscriber Co-Payment:
Primary Care Physician: $5.00/10.00
Prescription Drugs: $5.00/10.00
Hospital ER: $50.00
Home Health Care: $0 if in-network
Home Health Care Max. Days/Visits Covered: 30 days
Nursing Home: $0 if in-network
Nursing Home Max. Days/Visits Covered: 100 days

Network Qualifications
Pre-Admission Certification: Yes

Peer Review Type
Utilization Review: Yes
Second Surgical Opinion: Yes
Case Management: Yes

Accreditation Certification
NCQA
TJC Accreditation, Medicare Approved, Utilization Review, Pre-Admission Certification, State Licensure, Quality Assurance Program

Specialty Managed Care Partners
Enters into Contracts with Regional Business Coalitions: Yes

Akron Regional Development Board, Canton Regional
Chamber of Commerce, Home Builders Association

Employer References
Goodyear, Summa Health System, Cuyahoga County,
University of Akron, Akron Public Schools

621 Superior Dental Care

6683 Centerville Business Parkway
Centerville, OH 45459
Toll-Free: 800-762-3159
Phone: 937-438-0283
www.superiordental.com
Year Founded: 1986
Physician Owned Organization: Yes

Healthplan and Services Defined
  PLAN TYPE: Dental
  Model Type: Network, POS
  Plan Specialty: Dental
  Benefits Offered: Dental, Vision

Type of Payment Plans Offered
  FFS

Geographic Areas Served
  Ohio, Kentucky and Indiana

Publishes and Distributes Report Card: Yes

Key Personnel
  Chairman . . . . Richard W. Portune
  President . . . . L. Don Shumaker

622 The Dental Care Plus Group

100 Crowne Point Place
Cincinnati, OH 45241
Toll-Free: 800-367-9466
Phone: 513-554-1100
Fax: 513-554-3187
www.dentalcareplus.com
For Profit Organization: Yes
Year Founded: 1986
Physician Owned Organization: Yes
Number of Primary Care Physicians: 246,000
Total Enrollment: 300,000

Healthplan and Services Defined
  PLAN TYPE: Multiple
  Model Type: IPA
  Plan Specialty: Dental, Vision
  Benefits Offered: Dental, Vision

Type of Payment Plans Offered
  POS

Geographic Areas Served
  Ohio, Kentucky and Indiana

Peer Review Type
  Utilization Review: Yes

Key Personnel
  President and CEO . . . . Anthony A. Cook
  VP, Financial Officer . . . . Robert C. Hodgkins, Jr.
  Chief Operating Officer . . . . Jodi Fronczek

Chief Information Officer . . . . Tom Koch
Marketing/Communications . . . . Julie Lange
Director of Sales . . . . Jodi Duncan

623 The Health Plan of the Ohio Valley/Mountaineer Region

Toll-Free: 800-624-6961
www.healthplan.org
Non-Profit Organization: Yes
Year Founded: 1979
Federally Qualified: Yes
Number of Affiliated Hospitals: 63
Number of Primary Care Physicians: 4,000
Number of Referral/Specialty Physicians: 1,000
Total Enrollment: 380,000
State Enrollment: 380,000

Healthplan and Services Defined
  PLAN TYPE: HMO/PPO
  Other Type: POS
  Model Type: IPA
  Plan Specialty: ASO, Disease Management, Worker's
    Compensation, UR, TPA
  Benefits Offered: Behavioral Health, Chiropractic, Disease
    Management, Home Care, Inpatient SNF, Physical Therapy,
    Podiatry, Prescription, Psychiatric, Transplant, Vision,
    Worker's Compensation, AD&D, Life, LTD, STD
  Offers Demand Management Patient Information Service: No

Type of Coverage
  Individual, Medicare, Medicaid
  Catastrophic Illness Benefit: Unlimited

Type of Payment Plans Offered
  POS, DFFS

Geographic Areas Served
  Ohio & Central West Virginia

Subscriber Information
  Average Monthly Fee Per Subscriber
    (Employee + Employer Contribution):
      Employee Only (Self): Varies
      Medicare: Varies
  Average Annual Deductible Per Subscriber:
      Employee Only (Self): Varies
      Medicare: Varies
  Average Subscriber Co-Payment:
      Primary Care Physician: Varies
      Non-Network Physician: Varies
      Prescription Drugs: Varies
      Hospital ER: Varies
      Home Health Care: Varies
      Home Health Care Max. Days/Visits Covered: Varies
      Nursing Home: Varies
      Nursing Home Max. Days/Visits Covered: Varies

Network Qualifications
  Pre-Admission Certification: Yes

Peer Review Type
  Utilization Review: Yes
  Second Surgical Opinion: Yes
  Case Management: Yes

Publishes and Distributes Report Card: Yes

Accreditation Certification
NCQA
TJC Accreditation, Medicare Approved, Utilization Review,
Pre-Admission Certification, State Licensure, Quality
Assurance Program

Key Personnel
President/CEO................... James M. Pennington
Chief Financial Officer .... Jeffrey M. Knight
VP, Network Services .... Jason Landers
VP of Clinical Services .... John Fischer
Chief Information Officer.................. Bob Roset
Human Resources .... Carla Bell

---

624 **Trinity Health of Ohio**
Mount Carmel Health System
6150 E Broad Street
Columbus, OH 43213
Phone: 614-234-6000
www.trinity-health.org
Subsidiary of: Trinity Health
Non-Profit Organization: Yes
Year Founded: 2013
Total Enrollment: 30,000,000

Healthplan and Services Defined
PLAN TYPE: Other
Benefits Offered: Disease Management, Home Care,
Long-Term Care, Psychiatric, Hospice programs, PACE
(Program of All Inclusive Care for the Elderly)

Geographic Areas Served
Greater Central Ohio

Key Personnel
President .... Daniel Wendorff
Medical Director .... Loren Ledheiser
Chief Operating Officer............... Michael Ceballos

---

625 **UnitedHealthcare of Ohio**
2800 Corporate Exchange Drive
Suite 200
Columbus, OH 43231
Toll-Free: 888-545-5205
Phone: 614-890-6852
www.uhc.com
Subsidiary of: UnitedHealth Group
For Profit Organization: Yes
Year Founded: 1980

Healthplan and Services Defined
PLAN TYPE: HMO/PPO
Model Type: Network
Plan Specialty: Behavioral Health, Dental, Disease
Management, PBM, Vision
Benefits Offered: Behavioral Health, Dental, Disease
Management, Long-Term Care, Prescription, Vision,
Wellness, Life, LTD, STD

Type of Coverage
Individual, Medicare, Supplemental Medicare, Medicaid,
Catastrophic, Family, Military, Veterans, Group,

Geographic Areas Served
Statewide

Subscriber Information
Average Subscriber Co-Payment:
Primary Care Physician: $15.00
Prescription Drugs: $15.00

Accreditation Certification
NCQA

Key Personnel
CEO, Ohio.............................. Kurt Lewis

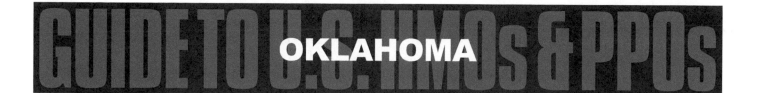
Health Insurance Coverage Status and Type of Coverage by Age

Category	All Persons		Under 18 years		Under 65 years	
	Number	%	Number	%	Number	%
Total population	3,851	-	1,019	-	3,267	-
Covered by some type of health insurance	3,306 *(11)*	85.8 *(0.3)*	936 *(6)*	91.9 *(0.5)*	2,726 *(11)*	83.4 *(0.3)*
Covered by private health insurance	2,465 *(18)*	64.0 *(0.5)*	536 *(11)*	52.6 *(1.1)*	2,098 *(18)*	64.2 *(0.5)*
Employer-based	1,950 *(18)*	50.6 *(0.5)*	453 *(10)*	44.4 *(1.0)*	1,770 *(17)*	54.2 *(0.5)*
Direct purchase	516 *(10)*	13.4 *(0.3)*	68 *(5)*	6.7 *(0.5)*	316 *(10)*	9.7 *(0.3)*
TRICARE	151 *(8)*	3.9 *(0.2)*	35 *(4)*	3.5 *(0.4)*	103 *(7)*	3.1 *(0.2)*
Covered by public health insurance	1,333 *(14)*	34.6 *(0.4)*	453 *(10)*	44.4 *(0.9)*	765 *(13)*	23.4 *(0.4)*
Medicaid	697 *(13)*	18.1 *(0.3)*	440 *(9)*	43.2 *(0.9)*	633 *(13)*	19.4 *(0.4)*
Medicare	694 *(6)*	18.0 *(0.2)*	16 *(3)*	1.6 *(0.3)*	127 *(6)*	3.9 *(0.2)*
VA Care	125 *(5)*	3.2 *(0.1)*	2 *(1)*	0.2 *(0.1)*	60 *(5)*	1.9 *(0.1)*
Not covered at any time during the year	545 *(12)*	14.2 *(0.3)*	82 *(5)*	8.1 *(0.5)*	541 *(12)*	16.6 *(0.3)*

Note: Numbers in thousands; Figures cover civilian noninstitutionalized population in 2017; N/A indicates that data was not available; Z represents or rounds to zero; Margin of error appears in parenthesis and is calculated using replicate weights.
Source: U.S. Census Bureau, American Community Survey, Table HIC-4_ACS. Health Insurance Coverage Status and Type of Coverage by State—All People: 2008 to 2017, Table HIC-5_ACS. Health Insurance Coverage Status and Type of Coverage by State—Children Under 18: 2008 to 2017, Table HIC-6_ACS. Health Insurance Coverage Status and Type of Coverage by State—Persons Under 65: 2008 to 2017

Oklahoma

626 Aetna Health of Oklahoma
151 Farmington Avenue
Hartford, CT 06156
Toll-Free: 800-872-3862
www.stateofok.aetna.com
Subsidiary of: Aetna Inc.
For Profit Organization: Yes

Healthplan and Services Defined
PLAN TYPE: HMO/PPO
Other Type: POS
Model Type: Network
Plan Specialty: Behavioral Health, EPO, Lab, PBM,
Radiology
Benefits Offered: Behavioral Health, Dental, Disease
Management, Long-Term Care, Physical Therapy,
Podiatry, Prescription, Psychiatric, Vision, Wellness, Life,
LTD, STD

Type of Coverage
Commercial, Student health

Geographic Areas Served
Statewide

Key Personnel
Sales Executive . . . . Mike Knox

627 Ascension At Home
Jane Phillips Regional Home Care
219 N Virginia
Bartlesville, OK 74003
Phone: 918-907-3010
Fax: 844-721-8184
ascensionathome.com
Subsidiary of: Ascension
Non-Profit Organization: Yes

Healthplan and Services Defined
PLAN TYPE: Other
Plan Specialty: Disease Management
Benefits Offered: Dental, Disease Management, Home Care,
Wellness, Ambulance & Transportation; Nursing Service;
Short-and-long-term care management planning; Hospice

Geographic Areas Served
Texas, Alabama, Indiana, Kansas, Michigan, Mississippi,
Oklahoma, Wisconsin

Key Personnel
President . . . . Kirk Allen
Dir., Home Health Service . . . . Darcy Burthay

628 Blue Cross & Blue Shield of Oklahoma
1400 S Boston
Tulsa, OK 74119
Toll-Free: 800-942-5837
Phone: 918-551-3500
www.bcbsok.com
Mailing Address: P.O. Box 3283, Tulsa, OK 74102-3283
Non-Profit Organization: Yes

Year Founded: 1940
Number of Affiliated Hospitals: 88
Number of Primary Care Physicians: 1,551
Number of Referral/Specialty Physicians: 6,000
Total Enrollment: 600,000
State Enrollment: 600,000

Healthplan and Services Defined
PLAN TYPE: HMO/PPO
Model Type: IPA
Plan Specialty: ASO, Behavioral Health, Chiropractic, Dental,
Disease Management, Lab, MSO, PBM, Vision, Radiology,
UR
Benefits Offered: Behavioral Health, Chiropractic, Dental,
Disease Management, Home Care, Inpatient SNF,
Long-Term Care, Physical Therapy, Podiatry, Prescription,
Psychiatric, Transplant, Vision, Worker's Compensation,
Life, LTD, STD

Type of Coverage
Commercial, Individual, Indemnity, Medicare, Supplemental
Medicare, Student health, Short-term

Type of Payment Plans Offered
POS, FFS

Geographic Areas Served
Statewide

Subscriber Information
Average Annual Deductible Per Subscriber:
Employee Only (Self): $500.00
Average Subscriber Co-Payment:
Primary Care Physician: $10.00
Prescription Drugs: 10/20/30%

Network Qualifications
Pre-Admission Certification: Yes

Peer Review Type
Utilization Review: Yes
Second Surgical Opinion: Yes
Case Management: Yes

Accreditation Certification
URAC

Key Personnel
President . . . . Ted Haynes
VP of Sales & Marketing . . . . Stephania Grober
Communications/Pub Rel. . . . . Lauren Cusick
918-551-2002
lauren_cusick@bcbsok.com

Specialty Managed Care Partners
Enters into Contracts with Regional Business Coalitions: Yes

Employer References
Federal Employee Program, The Williams Companies,
OneOK, Helmerich & Payne, Bank of Oklahoma

629 Cigna HealthCare of Tennessee
900 Cottage Grove Road
Bloomfield, CT 06002
Toll-Free: 800-244-6224
www.cigna.com
For Profit Organization: Yes

Healthplan and Services Defined
   PLAN TYPE: HMO/PPO
   Plan Specialty: Behavioral Health, Dental, Vision
   Benefits Offered: Behavioral Health, Dental, Disease
      Management, Prescription, Vision, AD&D, Life, LTD,
      STD

Type of Coverage
   Commercial, Individual

Type of Payment Plans Offered
   POS

Key Personnel
   President, TN . . . . Greg Allen

---

630   CommunityCare
Williams Center Tower II
2 West 2nd Street, Suite 100
Tulsa, OK 74103
Toll-Free: 800-278-7563
Phone: 918-594-5200
ccare@ccok.com
www.ccok.com
For Profit Organization: Yes
Total Enrollment: 500,000

Healthplan and Services Defined
   PLAN TYPE: Multiple
   Benefits Offered: Disease Management, Prescription, Vision,
      Wellness

Type of Coverage
   Commercial, Medicare, Supplemental Medicare

Type of Payment Plans Offered
   POS

Geographic Areas Served
   Oklahoma

---

631   Delta Dental of Oklahoma
16 NW 63rd Street
Oklahoma City, OK 73116
Toll-Free: 800-522-0188
Phone: 405-607-2100
customerservice@deltadentalok.org
www.deltadentalok.org
Secondary Address: Customer Service Department, P.O. Box
   54709, Oklahoma City, OK 73154-1709
Non-Profit Organization: Yes
Year Founded: 1973
Number of Primary Care Physicians: 1,500
Total Enrollment: 1,000,000

Healthplan and Services Defined
   PLAN TYPE: Dental
   Other Type: Dental PPO
   Model Type: Network
   Plan Specialty: ASO, Dental
   Benefits Offered: Dental

Type of Coverage
   Commercial, Individual, Group
   Catastrophic Illness Benefit: None

Geographic Areas Served
   Statewide

Subscriber Information
   Average Subscriber Co-Payment:
      Prescription Drugs: $0
      Home Health Care: $0
      Nursing Home: $0

Key Personnel
   President & CEO . . . . John Gladden
   Chief Financial Officer . . . . Frank Turbeville
   Chief Operating Officer . . . . Tania Graham
   Chief Information Officer . . . . David Jones
   Vice President of Sales . . . . Lan Miller

---

632   HCSC Insurance Services Company
1400 S Boston Avenue
Tulsa, OK 74119
Phone: 918-560-3500
hcsc.com
Subsidiary of: Blue Cross Blue Shield Association
Non-Profit Organization: Yes
Year Founded: 1936
Number of Primary Care Physicians: 15,600

Healthplan and Services Defined
   PLAN TYPE: HMO
   Benefits Offered: Behavioral Health, Dental, Disease
      Management, Psychiatric, Wellness

Geographic Areas Served
   Statewide

---

633   Humana Health Insurance of Oklahoma
6808 S Memorial Drive
Suite 202
Tulsa, OK 74133
Toll-Free: 800-681-0637
Phone: 918-237-4707
Fax: 918-499-2297
www.humana.com
Subsidiary of: Humana
For Profit Organization: Yes

Healthplan and Services Defined
   PLAN TYPE: HMO/PPO
   Model Type: Network
   Plan Specialty: Dental, Vision
   Benefits Offered: Dental, Vision, Life, LTD, STD

Type of Coverage
   Commercial, Individual

Geographic Areas Served
   Statewide

Accreditation Certification
   URAC, NCQA, CORE

Key Personnel
   Sales Representative . . . . Linda Bell

634 Mercy Clinic Oklahoma

5201 W Memorial Road
Oklahoma City, OK 73142
Phone: 405-755-4050
mercy.net
Subsidiary of: IBM Watson Health
Non-Profit Organization: Yes
Number of Affiliated Hospitals: 44
Number of Primary Care Physicians: 700
Number of Referral/Specialty Physicians: 2,000

Healthplan and Services Defined
 PLAN TYPE: HMO
  Benefits Offered: Behavioral Health, Disease Management,
    Home Care, Inpatient SNF, Physical Therapy, Podiatry,
    Vision, Wellness, Non-Surgical Weight Loss; Urgent Care;
    Dermatology; Rehabilitation; Breast Cancer; Orthopedics;
    Ostoclerosis; Pediatrics

Geographic Areas Served
 Arkansas, Kansas, Missouri, and Oklahoma

635 UnitedHealthcare of Oklahoma

5800 Granite Parkway
Suite 900
Plano, TX 75024
Toll-Free: 888-545-5205
Phone: 469-633-9200
www.uhc.com
Subsidiary of: UnitedHealth Group
For Profit Organization: Yes
Year Founded: 1986

Healthplan and Services Defined
 PLAN TYPE: HMO/PPO
 Model Type: Network
 Plan Specialty: Behavioral Health, Dental, Disease
   Management, PBM, Vision
 Benefits Offered: Behavioral Health, Dental, Disease
   Management, Long-Term Care, Prescription, Vision,
   Wellness, AD&D, Life, LTD, STD

Type of Coverage
 Commercial, Individual, Medicare, Supplemental Medicare,
   Medicaid, Catastrophic, Family, Military, Veterans, Group,

Geographic Areas Served
 Statewide. Oklahoma is covered by the Texas branch

Network Qualifications
 Pre-Admission Certification: Yes

Publishes and Distributes Report Card: Yes

Accreditation Certification
 AAPI, NCQA

Key Personnel
 CEO, TX/OK . . . . David Milich

Specialty Managed Care Partners
 Enters into Contracts with Regional Business Coalitions: Yes

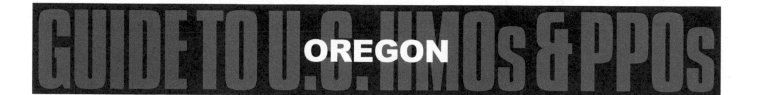

Health Insurance Coverage Status and Type of Coverage by Age

Category	All Persons		Under 18 years		Under 65 years	
	Number	%	Number	%	Number	%
Total population	4,103	-	928	-	3,405	-
Covered by some type of health insurance	3,822 (12)	93.2 (0.3)	895 (6)	96.4 (0.5)	3,127 (12)	91.8 (0.4)
Covered by private health insurance	2,770 (22)	67.5 (0.5)	562 (12)	60.6 (1.3)	2,333 (21)	68.5 (0.6)
Employer-based	2,174 (23)	53.0 (0.6)	492 (11)	53.0 (1.2)	1,987 (23)	58.3 (0.7)
Direct purchase	639 (14)	15.6 (0.3)	70 (5)	7.5 (0.6)	370 (12)	10.9 (0.3)
TRICARE	84 (7)	2.0 (0.2)	12 (3)	1.3 (0.3)	41 (5)	1.2 (0.2)
Covered by public health insurance	1,629 (20)	39.7 (0.5)	377 (11)	40.6 (1.2)	949 (19)	27.9 (0.6)
Medicaid	944 (20)	23.0 (0.5)	375 (11)	40.4 (1.1)	858 (20)	25.2 (0.6)
Medicare	776 (7)	18.9 (0.2)	3 (1)	0.4 (0.1)	97 (6)	2.8 (0.2)
VA Care	124 (5)	3.0 (0.1)	1 (1)	0.1 (0.1)	54 (3)	1.6 (0.1)
Not covered at any time during the year	281 (12)	6.8 (0.3)	33 (4)	3.6 (0.5)	278 (12)	8.2 (0.4)

Note: Numbers in thousands; Figures cover civilian noninstitutionalized population in 2017; N/A indicates that data was not available; Z represents or rounds to zero; Margin of error appears in parenthesis and is calculated using replicate weights.
Source: U.S. Census Bureau, American Community Survey, Table HIC-4_ACS. Health Insurance Coverage Status and Type of Coverage by State—All People: 2008 to 2017, Table HIC-5_ACS. Health Insurance Coverage Status and Type of Coverage by State—Children Under 18: 2008 to 2017, Table HIC-6_ACS. Health Insurance Coverage Status and Type of Coverage by State—Persons Under 65: 2008 to 2017

Oregon

636 Aetna Health of Oregon

151 Farmington Avenue
Hartford, CT 06156
Toll-Free: 800-872-3862
Phone: 860-273-0123
www.aetna.com
Subsidiary of: Aetna Inc.
For Profit Organization: Yes

Healthplan and Services Defined
PLAN TYPE: PPO
Other Type: POS
Model Type: Network
Plan Specialty: Behavioral Health, EPO, Lab, PBM,
Radiology
Benefits Offered: Behavioral Health, Disease Management,
Long-Term Care, Physical Therapy, Podiatry, Prescription,
Psychiatric, Wellness, Life, LTD, STD

Type of Coverage
Commercial, Student health

Type of Payment Plans Offered
POS, FFS

Geographic Areas Served
Statewide

Key Personnel
Senior Product Manager.................. Jordan Fields

637 AllCare Health

1701 NE 7th Street
Grants Pass, OR 97526
Toll-Free: 888-460-0185
Phone: 541-471-4106
Fax: 541-471-3784
info@allcarehealth.com
www.allcarehealth.com
Secondary Address: 3629 Aviation Way, Medford, OR 97504,
541-734-5520
Year Founded: 1995
Number of Primary Care Physicians: 1,500
Total Enrollment: 54,000
State Enrollment: 54,000

Healthplan and Services Defined
PLAN TYPE: Medicare
Plan Specialty: Medicaid
Benefits Offered: Chiropractic, Dental, Disease Management,
Home Care, Inpatient SNF, Physical Therapy, Podiatry,
Prescription, Psychiatric, Vision, Wellness

Type of Coverage
Individual, Medicare, Medicaid

Geographic Areas Served
Southern Oregon (Josephine, Jackson, Curry counties and
Glendale and Azalea in Douglas County)

Subscriber Information
Average Monthly Fee Per Subscriber
(Employee + Employer Contribution):

Employee Only (Self): Varies
Medicare: Varies
Average Annual Deductible Per Subscriber:
Employee Only (Self): Varies
Medicare: Varies
Average Subscriber Co-Payment:
Primary Care Physician: Varies
Non-Network Physician: Varies
Prescription Drugs: Varies
Hospital ER: Varies
Home Health Care: Varies
Home Health Care Max. Days/Visits Covered: Varies
Nursing Home: Varies
Nursing Home Max. Days/Visits Covered: Varies

Key Personnel
Chair .... Thomas Eagan
Vice Chair........................ Katherine Johnston
Secretary/Treasurer................... Susan Seereiter

638 Atrio Health Plans

2270 NW Aviation Drive
Suite 3
Roseburg, OR 97470
Toll-Free: 877-672-8620
Fax: 541-672-8670
www.atriohp.com
Secondary Address: 3025 Ryan Drive SE, Salem, OR 97701

Healthplan and Services Defined
PLAN TYPE: Medicare
Other Type: HMO, PPO
Benefits Offered: Chiropractic, Dental, Disease Management,
Home Care, Inpatient SNF, Physical Therapy, Podiatry,
Prescription, Psychiatric, Vision, Wellness

Type of Coverage
Individual, Medicare

Geographic Areas Served
Douglas, Klamath, Josephine, Jackson, Marion, Polk, and
Deschutes counties

Subscriber Information
Average Monthly Fee Per Subscriber
(Employee + Employer Contribution):
Employee Only (Self): Varies
Medicare: Varies
Average Annual Deductible Per Subscriber:
Employee Only (Self): Varies
Medicare: Varies
Average Subscriber Co-Payment:
Primary Care Physician: Varies
Non-Network Physician: Varies
Prescription Drugs: Varies
Hospital ER: Varies
Home Health Care: Varies
Home Health Care Max. Days/Visits Covered: Varies
Nursing Home: Varies
Nursing Home Max. Days/Visits Covered: Varies

Accreditation Certification
URAC

639 CareOregon Health Plan

315 SW Fifth Avenue
Portland, OR 97204
Toll-Free: 800-224-4840
Phone: 503-416-4100
www.careoregon.org
Non-Profit Organization: Yes
Year Founded: 1993
Number of Affiliated Hospitals: 33
Number of Primary Care Physicians: 950
Number of Referral/Specialty Physicians: 3,000
Total Enrollment: 250,000
State Enrollment: 250,000

Healthplan and Services Defined
PLAN TYPE: Medicare
Plan Specialty: Dental
Benefits Offered: Dental, Prescription, Vision, Wellness,
    Maternity and Family Planning

Type of Coverage
Medicare

Geographic Areas Served
20 counties in Oregon. careOregon Advantage is available
for residents of Clackamas, Clatsop, Columbia, Jackson,
Josephine, Marion, Multnomah, Polk and Washington
counties

Key Personnel
President/CEO . . . . Eric C. Hunter
Chief Financial Officer . . . . Teresa Learn
Chief Operating Officer . . . . Greg Morgan
Chief Medical Officer . . . . Amit Shah, MD
Chief Legal Officer . . . . Erin Fair Taylor

640 Dental Health Services of Oregon

205 SE Spokane Street
Suite 334
Portland, OR 97202
Toll-Free: 800-637-6453
Phone: 503-281-1771
Fax: 503-968-0187
www.dentalhealthservices.com
For Profit Organization: Yes
Year Founded: 1974

Healthplan and Services Defined
PLAN TYPE: Dental
Plan Specialty: Dental
Benefits Offered: Dental

Geographic Areas Served
California, Oregon, and Washington State

Accreditation Certification
URAC, NCQA

Key Personnel
Founder . . . . Godfrey Pernell

641 First Choice Health

10260 SW Greenburg Road
Suite 400
Portland, OR 97223
Phone: 877-287-2922
Fax: 503-652-8087
contact@fchn.com
www.fchn.com
For Profit Organization: Yes
Year Founded: 1996
Number of Affiliated Hospitals: 94
Number of Primary Care Physicians: 980
Number of Referral/Specialty Physicians: 1,793

Healthplan and Services Defined
PLAN TYPE: PPO
Benefits Offered: Wellness

Type of Coverage
Commercial, Individual, Private & Public Plans, Geo-specifi

Geographic Areas Served
Washington, Oregon, Alaska, Idaho, Montana, Wyoming, and
select areas of North Dakota and South Dakota

Key Personnel
Director of Sales, Oregon . . . . James Cassel

642 Humana Health Insurance of Oregon

1498 SE Tech Center Pl
Suite 300
Vancouver, WA 98683
Toll-Free: 800-781-4203
Phone: 360-253-7523
Fax: 360-253-7524
www.humana.com
Subsidiary of: Humana
For Profit Organization: Yes

Healthplan and Services Defined
PLAN TYPE: HMO/PPO
Model Type: Network
Plan Specialty: Dental, Vision
Benefits Offered: Dental, Disease Management, Prescription,
    Vision, Wellness, Life, LTD, STD

Type of Coverage
Commercial

Geographic Areas Served
Statewide

Accreditation Certification
URAC, NCQA, CORE

Key Personnel
Market President . . . . Catherine Field

643 Kaiser Permanente Northwest

500 NE Multnomah Street
Suite 100
Portland, OR 97232
Phone: 503-813-3860
thrive.kaiserpermanente.org/care-near-oregon-washington

Subsidiary of: Kaiser Permanente
Non-Profit Organization: Yes
Year Founded: 1977
Number of Primary Care Physicians: 880
State Enrollment: 523,967

Healthplan and Services Defined
 PLAN TYPE: HMO
 Model Type: Network
 Plan Specialty: Dental, Lab, Radiology
 Benefits Offered: Behavioral Health, Dental, Disease
  Management, Prescription, Vision, Wellness, Worker's
  Compensation

Type of Coverage
 Individual, Medicare, Supplemental Medicare, Medicaid

Geographic Areas Served
 Oregon & Washington

Accreditation Certification
 NCQA

Key Personnel
 President . . . . Ruth Williams-Brinkley

---

644 LifeMap

P.O. Box 1271, MS E8L
Portland, OR 97207-1271
Toll-Free: 800-794-5390
Fax: 855-854-4570
lifemapco.com
Subsidiary of: Cambia Health Solutions
Year Founded: 1984

Healthplan and Services Defined
 PLAN TYPE: Other
 Plan Specialty: Short-term Medical
 Benefits Offered: Dental, Vision, AD&D, Life

Geographic Areas Served
 Alaska, Idaho, Montana, Oregon, Utah, Washington, and
 Wyoming

Key Personnel
 President & CEO. . . . . Chris Blanton
 Director of Finance . . . . Randy Lowell
 VP, Sales & Marketing. . . . . Peter Mueller
 Operations & Technology . . . . Scott Wilkinson
 VP, Rick Management . . . . Jim Clark

---

645 Managed HealthCare Northwest

422 East Burnside Street, Suite 215
P.O. Box 4629
Portland, OR 97208-4629
Phone: 503-413-5800
Fax: 503-413-5801
www.mhninc.com
Subsidiary of: Legacy Health & Adventist Medical Center
For Profit Organization: Yes
Year Founded: 1988
Number of Affiliated Hospitals: 21
Number of Primary Care Physicians: 1,228
Number of Referral/Specialty Physicians: 4,757

Total Enrollment: 125,000

Healthplan and Services Defined
 PLAN TYPE: PPO
 Model Type: Network
 Plan Specialty: Worker's Compensation, MCO,
  Precertification, Utilization Review
 Benefits Offered: Disease Management, Wellness, Worker's
  Compensation, MCO, Precertification, Utilization Review,
  Case Management

Type of Coverage
 Commercial, Individual

Geographic Areas Served
 Oregon: Clackamas, Clatsop, Columbia, Coos, Hood River,
 Lane, Marion, Multnomah, Polk, Wasco, Washington &
 Yamhill; Washington: Clark, Cowlitz, Klickitat & Skamania
 counties

Peer Review Type
 Utilization Review: Yes
 Second Surgical Opinion: Yes
 Case Management: Yes

Publishes and Distributes Report Card: No

Key Personnel
 President/CEO . . . . Dolores Russell
 Director, Info/Finance . . . . David Pyle
 Provider Relations. . . . . Nita Patterson
 Claims Coordinator . . . . Robyn Fischer

Specialty Managed Care Partners
 Enters into Contracts with Regional Business Coalitions: Yes

---

646 Moda Health Oregon

601 SW Second Avenue
Portland, OR 97204
Phone: 855-718-1767
individualplans@modahealth.com
modahealth.com
Mailing Address: P.O. Box 40384, Portland, OR 97240-0384
Year Founded: 1955

Healthplan and Services Defined
 PLAN TYPE: Multiple
 Plan Specialty: Dental, Disease Management, Health Coaches
 Benefits Offered: Dental, Disease Management, Prescription,
  Wellness

Geographic Areas Served
 Statewide, Alaska, and Washington

Key Personnel
 Chief Executive Officer . . . . Robert Gootee
 President. . . . . William Johnson, MD
 Executive Vice President . . . . Steve Wynne
 Strategic Communications . . . . Jonathan Nicholas
  503-219-3673
  jonathan.nicholas@modahealth.com

647   PacificSource Health Plans

110 International Way
Springfield, OR 97477
Toll-Free: 800-624-6052
Phone: 541-686-1242
www.pacificsource.com
Mailing Address: P.O. Box 7068, Springfield, OR 97475-0068
Non-Profit Organization: Yes
Year Founded: 1933
Number of Referral/Specialty Physicians: 46,300
Total Enrollment: 275,000

Healthplan and Services Defined
  PLAN TYPE: Multiple
  Plan Specialty: Dental, PBM, Vision
  Benefits Offered: Dental, Disease Management, Prescription,
    Vision, Wellness

Type of Coverage
  Commercial, Individual, Medicare

Type of Payment Plans Offered
  POS, Combination FFS & DFFS

Geographic Areas Served
  Oregon, Montana & Idaho

Key Personnel
  President/CEO . . . . Ken Provencher
  EVP, Operating Officer . . . . Erick Doolen
  EVP, Financial Officer . . . . Peter Davidson
  EVP, Medical Officer. . . . . Dan Roth, MD
  EVP/Strategy & Marketing . . . . Sharon Thomson

648   PacificSource Health Plans

110 International Way
Springfield, OR 97477
Toll-Free: 800-624-6052
Phone: 541-686-1242
www.pacificsource.com
Mailing Address: P.O. Box 7068, Springfield, OR 97475-0068
Non-Profit Organization: Yes
Year Founded: 1933
Number of Referral/Specialty Physicians: 46,300
Total Enrollment: 275,000

Healthplan and Services Defined
  PLAN TYPE: HMO/PPO
  Benefits Offered: Dental, Disease Management, Prescription,
    Vision, Wellness

Type of Coverage
  Commercial, Individual

Type of Payment Plans Offered
  POS, Combination FFS & DFFS

Geographic Areas Served
  Oregon, Idaho & Montana

649   Providence Health Plan

P.O. Box 4327
Portland, OR 97208-4327
Toll-Free: 800-878-4445
Phone: 503-574-7500
healthplans.providence.org
Non-Profit Organization: Yes
Year Founded: 1985

Healthplan and Services Defined
  PLAN TYPE: Multiple
  Model Type: IPA, Group, PHO
  Plan Specialty: Disease Management, EPO, Vision, UR
  Benefits Offered: Behavioral Health, Chiropractic,
    Complementary Medicine, Disease Management, Home
    Care, Inpatient SNF, Physical Therapy, Podiatry,
    Prescription, Psychiatric, Transplant, Vision, Wellness

Type of Coverage
  Commercial, Individual, Medicare, Medicaid

Type of Payment Plans Offered
  POS, FFS

Geographic Areas Served
  Oregon: Clackamas, Clark, Columbia, Crook, Deschutes,
    Hood River, Jefferson, Lane, Marion, Multnomah,
    Washington, Wheeler; Washington: Clark

Peer Review Type
  Utilization Review: Yes
  Second Surgical Opinion: Yes
  Case Management: Yes

Publishes and Distributes Report Card: Yes

Accreditation Certification
  NCQA
  Medicare Approved, Utilization Review, Pre-Admission
    Certification, State Licensure, Quality Assurance Program

Key Personnel
  Chief Executive Officer . . . . Michael Cotton
  Chief Financial Officer . . . . Michael White
  Chief Medical Officer . . . . Robert Gluckman
  Adminstrative Officer. . . . . Alison Schrupp
  Chief Compliance Officer . . . . Carrie Smith
  Chief Marketing Officer . . . . Brad Garrigues

Average Claim Compensation
  Physician's Fees Charged: 55%
  Hospital's Fees Charged: 48%

Specialty Managed Care Partners
  PBH Behavioral Health, ARGUS (PBM), Complementary
    Health Care, Well Partner
  Enters into Contracts with Regional Business Coalitions: No

Employer References
  Providence Health System, PeaceHealth, Portland Public
    School District, Oregon PERS, Tektonix

650　Regence BlueCross BlueShield of Oregon

P.O. Box 1071
Portland, OR 97207
Toll-Free: 888-367-2117
www.regence.com
Subsidiary of: Regence
Non-Profit Organization: Yes
Total Enrollment: 2,400,000
State Enrollment: 730,000

Healthplan and Services Defined
PLAN TYPE: Multiple
Model Type: Network
Benefits Offered: Dental, Prescription, Vision, Wellness,
　Life, Preventive Care

Type of Coverage
Commercial, Individual, Supplemental Medicare

Key Personnel
President/Revenue Officer . . . . Angela Dowling
Chief Medical Officer . . . . Richard Popiel

651　Samaritan Health Plan Operations

2300 NW Walnut Boulevard
Corvallis, OR 97330
Toll-Free: 800-832-4580
Phone: 541-768-4550
www.samhealthplans.org
Subsidiary of: Samaritan Health Services
Year Founded: 1993

Healthplan and Services Defined
PLAN TYPE: Multiple
Benefits Offered: Chiropractic, Dental, Disease Management,
　Home Care, Inpatient SNF, Physical Therapy, Podiatry,
　Prescription, Psychiatric, Vision, Wellness

Type of Coverage
Individual, Medicare

Geographic Areas Served
Statewide

Key Personnel
Chief Executive Officer . . . . Kelley C. Kaiser
Chief Operating Officer . . . . Kim R. Whitley
Chief Medical Officer . . . . Kevin Ewanchyna, MD
Chief Financial Officer . . . . Daniel B. Smith

652　Trillium Community Health Plan

UO Riverfront Research Park
1800 Milrace Drive
Eugene, OR 97403
Toll-Free: 877-600-5472
Phone: 541-485-2155
Fax: 866-703-0958
trilliumchp.com
Mailing Address: P.O. Box 11740, Eugene, OR 97440-3940

Healthplan and Services Defined
PLAN TYPE: Multiple
Benefits Offered: Chiropractic, Dental, Disease Management,
　Home Care, Inpatient SNF, Physical Therapy, Podiatry,
　Prescription, Psychiatric, Vision, Wellness, Durable
　Medical Equipment; Hearing Aids

Type of Coverage
Individual, Medicare

Geographic Areas Served
Serving Eugene, Springfield and the following counties:
Benton, Clackamas, Clatsop, Deschutes, Douglas, Hood
River, Jackson, Josephine, Klamath, Lane, Lincoln, Linn,
Malheur, Marion, Polk, Umatilla, Wasco, Washington and
Yamhill

Accreditation Certification
NCQA

Key Personnel
Chief Executive Officer . . . . Chris Ellertson
Vice President, Finance . . . . Justin Lyman
Chief Operating Officer . . . . Amy Williams
Chief Medical Officer . . . . Thomas K. Wuest, MD

653　United Concordia of Oregon

4401 Deer Path Road
Harrisburg, PA 17110
Phone: 717-260-6800
www.unitedconcordia.com
For Profit Organization: Yes
Year Founded: 1971
Total Enrollment: 7,800,000

Healthplan and Services Defined
PLAN TYPE: Dental
Plan Specialty: Dental
Benefits Offered: Dental

Type of Coverage
Commercial, Individual, Military personnel & families

Geographic Areas Served
Nationwide

Accreditation Certification
URAC

Key Personnel
Contact. . . . . Beth Rutherford
　717-260-7659
　beth.rutherford@ucci.com

654　UnitedHealthcare of Oregon

5 Centerpointe Drive
Suite 600
Lake Oswego, OR 97035
Toll-Free: 888-545-5205
Phone: 503-603-7355
www.uhc.com
Subsidiary of: UnitedHealth Group
For Profit Organization: Yes

Healthplan and Services Defined
PLAN TYPE: HMO/PPO
Model Type: Network
Plan Specialty: Behavioral Health, Dental, Disease
　Management, PBM, Vision

Benefits Offered: Behavioral Health, Dental, Disease
Management, Long-Term Care, Prescription, Vision,
Wellness, Life, LTD, STD

Type of Coverage
Individual, Medicare, Supplemental Medicare, Medicaid,
Catastrophic, Family, Military, Veterans, Group,

Geographic Areas Served
Statewide

Key Personnel
Regional Growth Officer . . . . Gary Daniels

---

655   Willamette Dental Group

6950 NE Campus Way
Hillsboro, OR 97124
Toll-Free: 855-433-6825
Fax: 503-952-2200
info@willamettedental.com
www.willamettedental.com
For Profit Organization: Yes
Year Founded: 1970

Healthplan and Services Defined
PLAN TYPE: Dental
Model Type: Staff
Plan Specialty: Dental
Benefits Offered: Dental

Type of Payment Plans Offered
POS, FFS

Geographic Areas Served
Oregon, Washington and Idaho

Peer Review Type
Case Management: Yes

Publishes and Distributes Report Card: No

Key Personnel
President & CEO . . . . Dr. Eugene Skourtes, DMD

Specialty Managed Care Partners
Enters into Contracts with Regional Business Coalitions: No

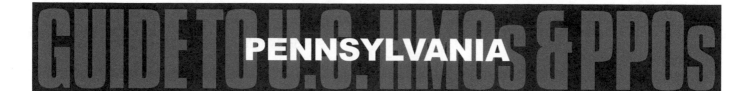
Health Insurance Coverage Status and Type of Coverage by Age

Category	All Persons		Under 18 years		Under 65 years	
	Number	%	Number	%	Number	%
Total population	12,602	-	2,835	-	10,405	-
Covered by some type of health insurance	11,910 *(21)*	94.5 *(0.2)*	2,710 *(10)*	95.6 *(0.3)*	9,723 *(20)*	93.4 *(0.2)*
Covered by private health insurance	9,143 *(34)*	72.5 *(0.3)*	1,837 *(18)*	64.8 *(0.6)*	7,663 *(33)*	73.6 *(0.3)*
Employer-based	7,470 *(37)*	59.3 *(0.3)*	1,660 *(18)*	58.5 *(0.6)*	6,758 *(35)*	64.9 *(0.3)*
Direct purchase	1,916 *(23)*	15.2 *(0.2)*	189 *(9)*	6.7 *(0.3)*	1,020 *(19)*	9.8 *(0.2)*
TRICARE	183 *(8)*	1.5 *(0.1)*	26 *(4)*	0.9 *(0.1)*	104 *(7)*	1.0 *(0.1)*
Covered by public health insurance	4,641 *(31)*	36.8 *(0.2)*	1,037 *(17)*	36.6 *(0.6)*	2,514 *(30)*	24.2 *(0.3)*
Medicaid	2,484 *(29)*	19.7 *(0.2)*	1,026 *(17)*	36.2 *(0.6)*	2,225 *(30)*	21.4 *(0.3)*
Medicare	2,506 *(13)*	19.9 *(0.1)*	19 *(4)*	0.7 *(0.1)*	381 *(11)*	3.7 *(0.1)*
VA Care	264 *(7)*	2.1 *(0.1)*	2 *(1)*	0.1 *(Z)*	98 *(5)*	0.9 *(Z)*
Not covered at any time during the year	692 *(21)*	5.5 *(0.2)*	125 *(9)*	4.4 *(0.3)*	682 *(21)*	6.6 *(0.2)*

Note: Numbers in thousands; Figures cover civilian noninstitutionalized population in 2017; N/A indicates that data was not available; Z represents or rounds to zero; Margin of error appears in parenthesis and is calculated using replicate weights.
Source: U.S. Census Bureau, American Community Survey, Table HIC-4_ACS. Health Insurance Coverage Status and Type of Coverage by State—All People: 2008 to 2017, Table HIC-5_ACS. Health Insurance Coverage Status and Type of Coverage by State—Children Under 18: 2008 to 2017, Table HIC-6_ACS. Health Insurance Coverage Status and Type of Coverage by State—Persons Under 65: 2008 to 2017

Pennsylvania

656 Aetna Health of Pennsylvania

2000 Market Street
Philadelphia, PA 19103
Toll-Free: 866-638-1232
www.aetnabetterhealth.com/pennsylvania
Subsidiary of: Aetna Inc.
For Profit Organization: Yes

Healthplan and Services Defined
PLAN TYPE: HMO/PPO
Other Type: POS
Model Type: Network
Plan Specialty: Behavioral Health, EPO, Lab, PBM,
Radiology
Benefits Offered: Behavioral Health, Dental, Disease
Management, Long-Term Care, Physical Therapy,
Podiatry, Prescription, Psychiatric, Vision, Wellness, Life,
LTD, STD

Type of Coverage
Commercial, Medicaid, Student health

Geographic Areas Served
Statewide

Key Personnel
Director, Operations..................... Leander Monk

657 American HealthCare Group

1910 Cochran Road
Manor Oak One, Suite 405
Pittsburgh, PA 15220
Phone: 412-563-8800
Fax: 412-563-8319
american-healthcare.net
For Profit Organization: Yes
Year Founded: 1996

Healthplan and Services Defined
PLAN TYPE: Other
Model Type: Network
Plan Specialty: ASO, Chiropractic, Dental, MSO, Worker's
Compensation
Benefits Offered: Behavioral Health, Chiropractic,
Complementary
Medicine, Dental, Disease Management, Home Care,
Inpatient SNF, Long-Term Care, Physical Therapy,
Podiatry, Prescription, Psychiatric, Transplant,
Vision, Wellness, Worker's Compensation, School
wellness programs, on-site immunizations, support
services for public housing

Type of Payment Plans Offered
FFS

Geographic Areas Served
Pennsylvania, Eastern Ohio, Northwestern Virginia

Peer Review Type
Utilization Review: Yes
Second Surgical Opinion: Yes
Case Management: Yes

Accreditation Certification
State Licensure

Key Personnel
President & CEO.................. Robert E. Hagan, Jr.
412-563-7804
bhagan@american-healthcare.net
Accounts Recievable .... Lynn Hagan
412-563-7805
lhagan@american-healthcare.net
Dir., Health Benefits........................ Erin Hart
412-563-7807
ehart@american-healthcare.net
Dir., Wellness Services .... Liz Hagan Kanche
412-563-7854
lhkanche@american-healthcare.net
Marketing Manager .... Sarah Kelly
skelly@american-healthcare.net

658 AmeriHealth Pennsylvania

1901 Market Street
Philadelphia, PA 19103-1480
Toll-Free: 866-681-7373
www.amerihealth.com
Year Founded: 1995
Total Enrollment: 265,000

Healthplan and Services Defined
PLAN TYPE: HMO/PPO
Benefits Offered: Dental, Disease Management, Prescription,
Vision, Wellness

Type of Coverage
Commercial, Individual

Geographic Areas Served
Pennsylvania

659 Berkshire Health Partners

P.O. Box 14744
Reading, PA 19612-4744
Toll-Free: 866-257-0445
Phone: 610-372-8044
bhp.org
Non-Profit Organization: Yes
Year Founded: 1986
Physician Owned Organization: Yes

Healthplan and Services Defined
PLAN TYPE: PPO

Type of Coverage
Commercial, Individual, Indemnity, Catastrophic
Catastrophic Illness Benefit: Varies per case

Geographic Areas Served
Berks, Upper Bucks, Carbon, Northern Lancaster, Lehigh,
Montgomery, Northampton and Schuylkill counties

Peer Review Type
Utilization Review: Yes
Second Surgical Opinion: Yes
Case Management: Yes

Accreditation Certification
  URAC, NCQA

---

660   Capital BlueCross

2500 Elmerton Avenue
Harrisburg, PA 17177
Phone: 717-541-7000
www.capbluecross.com
Non-Profit Organization: Yes
Year Founded: 1938

Healthplan and Services Defined
  PLAN TYPE: HMO/PPO
  Plan Specialty: Dental, Vision
  Benefits Offered: Dental, Home Care, Inpatient SNF,
    Physical Therapy, Prescription, Psychiatric, Transplant,
    Vision, Wellness

Type of Coverage
  Commercial

Type of Payment Plans Offered
  FFS

Geographic Areas Served
  21 counties in central Pennsylvania and the Lehigh Valley

Peer Review Type
  Second Surgical Opinion: Yes
  Case Management: Yes

Accreditation Certification
  TJC Accreditation, Medicare Approved, Utilization Review,
    Pre-Admission Certification, State Licensure, Quality
    Assurance Program

Key Personnel
  President & CEO . . . . Gary D. St. Hilaire
  SVP/CFO/Treasurer . . . . Harvey Littman
  SVP/CMO . . . . Jennifer Chambers, MD
  CCO/SVP, Risk Management . . . . William B. Reineberg
  SVP, Human Resources . . . . Steven J. Krupinski
  Commercial Group Sales . . . . Jack Jaroh
  SVP/Marketing Officer . . . . Donna K. Lencki

---

661   Delta Dental of Pennsylvania

One Delta Drive
Mechanicsburg, PA 17055-6999
Toll-Free: 800-932-0783
www.deltadentalins.com
Mailing Address: P.O. Box 1803, Alpharetta, GA 30023
Non-Profit Organization: Yes

Healthplan and Services Defined
  PLAN TYPE: Dental
  Other Type: Dental PPO
  Plan Specialty: Dental
  Benefits Offered: Dental

Type of Coverage
  Commercial, Individual

Geographic Areas Served
  Statewide

Key Personnel
  President & CEO . . . . Tony Barth
  Chief Financial Officer . . . . Michael Castro
  Chief Legal Officer . . . . Michael Hankinson
  EVP, Sales & Marketing . . . . Belinda Martinez
  Chief Operating Officer . . . . Nilesh Patel

---

662   Devon Health Services

1100 First Avenue
King of Prussia, PA 19406
Toll-Free: 800-431-2273
Fax: 800-221-0002
customerservice@devonhealth.com
www.devonhealth.com
For Profit Organization: Yes
Year Founded: 1991
Physician Owned Organization: Yes

Healthplan and Services Defined
  PLAN TYPE: PPO
  Model Type: Network
  Plan Specialty: Chiropractic, Dental, Lab, Vision, Radiology,
    Worker's Compensation, Group Health & Pharmacy Plans;
    Acupuncture
  Benefits Offered: Chiropractic, Dental, Inpatient SNF,
    Physical Therapy, Vision, Worker's Compensation, Group
    Health & Pharmacy Plans

Type of Coverage
  Commercial

Type of Payment Plans Offered
  DFFS, FFS, Combination FFS & DFFS

Geographic Areas Served
  Pennsylvania, New Jersey, and Delaware

Publishes and Distributes Report Card: No

Key Personnel
  President. . . . . Dean Vaden
  Chief Operating Officer . . . . Marie McDaniel
  Regional VP of Sales . . . . David Williams

Average Claim Compensation
  Physician's Fees Charged: 55%
  Hospital's Fees Charged: 58%

Specialty Managed Care Partners
  Medimpact
  Enters into Contracts with Regional Business Coalitions: Yes

Employer References
  Mid-Jersey trucking Industry & Local 701 Welfare Fund,
    Pennsylvania Public School Health Care Trust, International
    Brotherhood of Teamsters

---

663   Gateway Health

Four Gateway Center
444 Liberty Ave, Suite 2100
Pittsburgh, PA 15222-1222
Toll-Free: 800-392-1147
www.gatewayhealthplan.com
For Profit Organization: Yes
Year Founded: 1992

State Enrollment: 300,000

Healthplan and Services Defined
PLAN TYPE: HMO
Other Type: Medicaid
Model Type: Network
Plan Specialty: Dental, Disease Management, Vision, UR, Prospective Care Managment; Dual Eligibility; Chronic Special Needs
Benefits Offered: Chiropractic, Dental, Disease Management, Home Care, Inpatient SNF, Physical Therapy, Podiatry, Prescription, Transplant, Vision, Wellness

Type of Coverage
Medicare, Medicaid

Type of Payment Plans Offered
DFFS, Capitated, FFS

Geographic Areas Served
Allegheny, Armstrong, Beaver, Berks, Blair, Butler, Cambria, Clarion, Cumberland, Dauphin, Erie, Fayette, Greene, Indiana, Jefferson, Lawrence, Lehigh, Mercer, Montour, Northumberland, Schulkill, Somerset, Washington and Westmoreland counties

Peer Review Type
Utilization Review: Yes
Second Surgical Opinion: Yes
Case Management: Yes

Accreditation Certification
NCQA
Utilization Review, State Licensure, Quality Assurance Program

Key Personnel
President & CEO . . . . Patricia J. Darnley
Chief Financial Officer . . . . Sharon Kelley
Chief Medical Officer . . . . Steven Szebenyi, MD

Specialty Managed Care Partners
Clarity Vision, Dental Benefit Providers, National Imaging Association, Merck-Medco

664   Geisinger Health Plan
100 North Academy Avenue
Danville, PA 17822
Toll-Free: 800-275-6401
www.geisinger.org/health-plan
Non-Profit Organization: Yes
Year Founded: 1985
Number of Affiliated Hospitals: 110
Number of Primary Care Physicians: 3,500
Number of Referral/Specialty Physicians: 27,000
Total Enrollment: 540,000

Healthplan and Services Defined
PLAN TYPE: HMO/PPO
Model Type: Network
Benefits Offered: Chiropractic, Dental, Disease Management, Home Care, Inpatient SNF, Physical Therapy, Podiatry, Prescription, Psychiatric, Vision, Wellness

Type of Coverage
Commercial, Individual, Medicare, Supplemental Medicare, CHIP

Geographic Areas Served
42 counties in Pennsylvania

Accreditation Certification
NCQA

Key Personnel
President/CEO . . . . David T. Feinberg, MD

665   Health Partners Plans
901 Market Street
Suite 500
Philadelphia, PA 19107
Phone: 215-849-9606
contact@hpplans.com
www.healthpartnersplans.com
Non-Profit Organization: Yes
Year Founded: 1984
Physician Owned Organization: Yes
Number of Affiliated Hospitals: 43
Number of Primary Care Physicians: 6,400
Total Enrollment: 263,200

Healthplan and Services Defined
PLAN TYPE: Medicare
Other Type: Medicaid
Benefits Offered: Chiropractic, Dental, Disease Management, Home Care, Inpatient SNF, Physical Therapy, Podiatry, Prescription, Psychiatric, Vision, Wellness

Type of Coverage
Medicare, Medicaid, CHIP

Geographic Areas Served
Bucks, Chester, Delaware, Lancaster, Lehigh, Montgomery, Northampton, and Philadelphia counties

Key Personnel
President/CEO . . . . William S. George
SVP/CIO . . . . Joe Brand
EVP, Finance/Admin/CFO . . . . Eric Huss
SVP, Communications/Mkt . . . . Michelle Davidson
SVP, Medicare/Operations . . . . Jenny Fong

666   HealthAmerica
3721 TecPort Drive
P.O. Box 67103
Harrisburg, PA 17106-7103
Toll-Free: 800-788-6445
healthamerica.coventryhealthcare.com
Secondary Address: 11 Stanwix Street, Suite 2300, Pittsburgh, PA 15222, 800-735-4404
Subsidiary of: Coventry Health Care
For Profit Organization: Yes
Year Founded: 1974
Owned by an Integrated Delivery Network (IDN): Yes

Healthplan and Services Defined
PLAN TYPE: Multiple
Model Type: Network

Plan Specialty: ASO, Behavioral Health, Chiropractic, Dental, Disease Management, Lab, Vision, Radiology
Benefits Offered: Behavioral Health, Chiropractic, Complementary Medicine, Dental, Disease Management, Home Care, Inpatient SNF, Physical Therapy, Podiatry, Prescription, Psychiatric, Transplant, Vision, Wellness

Type of Coverage
Commercial, Individual, Medicare

Type of Payment Plans Offered
POS, Capitated, FFS

Geographic Areas Served
Statewide

Peer Review Type
Utilization Review: Yes
Case Management: Yes

Accreditation Certification
TJC, NCQA
Medicare Approved, Utilization Review, Pre-Admission Certification, State Licensure, Quality Assurance Program

Key Personnel
Chief Executive Officer . . . . Mark T. Bertolini

Specialty Managed Care Partners
ValueOptions, CareMark, Dominion Dental (WPA) Delta Dental (EPA), Quest Diagnostics (EPA) LabCorp (WPA), National Vision Administrators (NVA)

Employer References
Federal Government, Penn State University, US Airways, City of Pittsburgh, General Motors

667   Highmark Blue Cross Blue Shield

501 Penn Avenue Place
Pittsburgh, PA 15222
Toll-Free: 800-816-5527
www.highmarkbcbs.com
Mailing Address: P.O. Box 226, Pittsburgh, PA 15222
For Profit Organization: Yes
Year Founded: 1996
Owned by an Integrated Delivery Network (IDN): Yes

Healthplan and Services Defined
PLAN TYPE: HMO/PPO
Model Type: IPA
Benefits Offered: Dental, Disease Management, Prescription, Vision, Wellness
Offers Demand Management Patient Information Service: Yes

Type of Coverage
Commercial, Individual
Catastrophic Illness Benefit: Unlimited

Type of Payment Plans Offered
POS, DFFS, Capitated, FFS, Combination FFS & DFFS

Geographic Areas Served
Western and Northeastern Pennsylvania

Peer Review Type
Utilization Review: Yes
Second Surgical Opinion: No

Case Management: Yes

Publishes and Distributes Report Card: No

Accreditation Certification
URAC, NCQA
Medicare Approved, Pre-Admission Certification, State Licensure

Key Personnel
President . . . . Deborah L. Rice-Johnson
Chief Medical Officer . . . . Charles Deshazer, MD
EVP, Healthcare Services . . . . Thomas Pellathy
EVP/COO/CFO/Treasurer. . . . . Karen Hanlon
Secretary . . . . Thomas L. Vankirk, Esq.

Average Claim Compensation
Physician's Fees Charged: 50%
Hospital's Fees Charged: 61%

Specialty Managed Care Partners
Enters into Contracts with Regional Business Coalitions: No

668   Highmark Blue Shield

Camp Hill Service Center
1800 Center Street
Camp Hill, PA 17011
Phone: 717-302-5000
www.highmarkblueshield.com
Non-Profit Organization: Yes
Year Founded: 1932
Total Enrollment: 5,300,000

Healthplan and Services Defined
PLAN TYPE: PPO
Model Type: Network
Benefits Offered: Disease Management, Prescription, Wellness

Type of Payment Plans Offered
POS, DFFS, Combination FFS & DFFS

Geographic Areas Served
Central Pennsylvania

Peer Review Type
Second Surgical Opinion: Yes

Publishes and Distributes Report Card: Yes

Accreditation Certification
URAC, NCQA

Key Personnel
President . . . . Deborah L. Rice-Johnson

Specialty Managed Care Partners
Enters into Contracts with Regional Business Coalitions: Yes

669   Humana Health Insurance of Pennsylvania

5000 Ritter Road
Suite 101
Mechanicsburg, PA 17055
Toll-Free: 866-355-5861
Phone: 717-766-6040
Fax: 717-795-1951
www.humana.com

Secondary Address: 325 Sentry Parkway, Suite 200, Philadelphia, PA 19422
Subsidiary of: Humana
For Profit Organization: Yes

Healthplan and Services Defined
PLAN TYPE: HMO/PPO
Model Type: Network
Plan Specialty: Dental, Vision
Benefits Offered: Dental, Vision, Life, LTD, STD

Type of Coverage
Commercial

Geographic Areas Served
Statewide

Accreditation Certification
URAC, NCQA, CORE

Key Personnel
Provider Exec. Consultant . . . . Holli Masci

---

670 Independence Blue Cross

1901 Market Street
2nd Floor
Philadelphia, PA 19103
Toll-Free: 800-275-2583
www.ibx.com
Non-Profit Organization: Yes
Year Founded: 1986
Total Enrollment: 9,500,000
State Enrollment: 2,500,000

Healthplan and Services Defined
PLAN TYPE: HMO/PPO
Benefits Offered: Dental, Prescription, Vision, Worker's Compensation, AD&D, Life, LTD, STD

Type of Coverage
Individual, Indemnity, Medicaid

Type of Payment Plans Offered
DFFS, FFS, Combination FFS & DFFS

Geographic Areas Served
24 states and the District of Columbia

Network Qualifications
Pre-Admission Certification: Yes

Peer Review Type
Utilization Review: Yes
Second Surgical Opinion: No
Case Management: Yes

Publishes and Distributes Report Card: Yes

Accreditation Certification
NCQA
TJC Accreditation, Medicare Approved, Utilization Review, Pre-Admission Certification, State Licensure, Quality Assurance Program

Key Personnel
President & CEO . . . . Daniel J. Hilferty
Chief Operating Officer . . . . Yvette Bright
Chief Financial Officer . . . . Gregory Deavens

General Counsel/Secretary . . . . Thomas A. Hutton, Esq.

Specialty Managed Care Partners
Magellan Behavioral Health, United Concorida, Medco Health Solutions
Enters into Contracts with Regional Business Coalitions: Yes

---

671 InterGroup Services

401 Shady Avenue
Suite B108
Pittsburgh, PA 15206
Phone: 412-363-0600
Fax: 412-363-0900
www.igs-ppo.com
Secondary Address: 1 S Bacton Hill Road], 2nd Floor, Malvern, PA 19355, 800-537-9389
For Profit Organization: Yes
Year Founded: 1985

Healthplan and Services Defined
PLAN TYPE: PPO
Model Type: Network
Plan Specialty: ASO, Behavioral Health, Chiropractic, EPO, Lab, MSO, PBM, Vision, Radiology, Worker's Compensation
Benefits Offered: Behavioral Health, Disease Management, Prescription, Wellness, Worker's Compensation

Type of Coverage
Commercial

Geographic Areas Served
Pennsylvania, New Jersey, Delaware and West Virginia

Network Qualifications
Pre-Admission Certification: Yes

Specialty Managed Care Partners
Chiropractic Network

---

672 Penn Highlands Healthcare

204 Hospital Avenue
DuBois, PA 15801
Phone: 814-371-2200
www.phhealthcare.org
Non-Profit Organization: Yes
Year Founded: 2011
Number of Affiliated Hospitals: 4
Number of Primary Care Physicians: 363

Healthplan and Services Defined
PLAN TYPE: PPO
Model Type: IPA
Plan Specialty: ASO, Behavioral Health, Disease Management, EPO, Lab, MSO, Radiology, Worker's Compensation, UR
Benefits Offered: Behavioral Health, Chiropractic, Disease Management, Home Care, Inpatient SNF, Long-Term Care, Physical Therapy, Podiatry, Psychiatric, Transplant, Wellness, Worker's Compensation
Offers Demand Management Patient Information Service: Yes

Type of Coverage
Commercial

Type of Payment Plans Offered
POS, DFFS, Combination FFS & DFFS

Geographic Areas Served
Cameron, Centre, Clarion, Clearfield, Elk, Forest, Jefferson and McKean counties

Network Qualifications
Pre-Admission Certification: Yes

Peer Review Type
Utilization Review: Yes
Second Surgical Opinion: No
Case Management: Yes

Publishes and Distributes Report Card: Yes

Accreditation Certification
AAAHC, URAC
TJC Accreditation, Medicare Approved, Pre-Admission Certification, State Licensure

Key Personnel
Chief Executive Officer . . . . Steven M. Fontaine

Average Claim Compensation
Physician's Fees Charged: 1%
Hospital's Fees Charged: 1%

Specialty Managed Care Partners
Enters into Contracts with Regional Business Coalitions: No

673   Preferred Health Care

Urban Place
480 New Holland Ave, Suite 7203
Lancaster, PA 17602
Phone: 717-560-9290
Fax: 717-560-2312
info@phcunity.com
www.phcunity.com
Non-Profit Organization: Yes
Year Founded: 1984
Number of Affiliated Hospitals: 19
Number of Primary Care Physicians: 1,900

Healthplan and Services Defined
PLAN TYPE: PPO
Model Type: Network
Offers Demand Management Patient Information Service: Yes

Type of Payment Plans Offered
FFS

Geographic Areas Served
Statewide

Peer Review Type
Utilization Review: Yes
Case Management: Yes

Accreditation Certification
TJC Accreditation, Medicare Approved, Utilization Review, Pre-Admission Certification, State Licensure, Quality Assurance Program

Key Personnel
President & CEO. . . . . Eric E. Buck

VP, Operations. . . . . Sherry Wolgemuth
Financial Services . . . . Kathy Roth
Provider Relations . . . . Lynne Ostrowski

674   Preferred Healthcare System

P.O. Box 1015
Duncansville, PA 16635
Toll-Free: 800-238-9900
Phone: 814-317-5063
Fax: 814-317-5139
www.phsppo.com
For Profit Organization: Yes
Year Founded: 1985
Physician Owned Organization: Yes

Healthplan and Services Defined
PLAN TYPE: PPO
Model Type: Network
Plan Specialty: ASO, Behavioral Health, Chiropractic, Dental, Disease Management, EPO, PBM, Vision, Worker's Compensation, Health
Benefits Offered: Behavioral Health, Chiropractic, Complementary Medicine, Dental, Disease Management, Home Care, Inpatient SNF, Long-Term Care, Physical Therapy, Podiatry, Prescription, Psychiatric, Transplant, Vision, Wellness, AD&D, Life, STD, Durable Medical Equipment

Type of Coverage
Commercial, Individual, Indemnity
Catastrophic Illness Benefit: Maximum $1M

Type of Payment Plans Offered
Combination FFS & DFFS

Geographic Areas Served
South Central Pennsylvania

Peer Review Type
Utilization Review: Yes
Second Surgical Opinion: Yes

Publishes and Distributes Report Card: No

Accreditation Certification
TJC Accreditation, Utilization Review, Pre-Admission Certification, State Licensure, Quality Assurance Program

Key Personnel
President . . . . Maureen Frucella
Chief Executive Officer . . . . Brian Brumbaugh

Average Claim Compensation
Physician's Fees Charged: 70%
Hospital's Fees Charged: 70%

Specialty Managed Care Partners
Enters into Contracts with Regional Business Coalitions: Yes

675   South Central Preferred Health Network

3421 Concord Road
York, PA 17402
Toll-Free: 800-842-1768
Phone: 717-851-6800
www.scp-ppo.com

Non-Profit Organization: Yes
Year Founded: 1992
Number of Affiliated Hospitals: 16
Number of Primary Care Physicians: 6,150
Number of Referral/Specialty Physicians: 1,275
Total Enrollment: 33,000
State Enrollment: 33,000

Healthplan and Services Defined
PLAN TYPE: PPO
Model Type: PHO
Plan Specialty: Behavioral Health, Chiropractic, Radiology
Benefits Offered: Behavioral Health, Chiropractic, Home
    Care, Inpatient SNF, Long-Term Care, Physical Therapy,
    Podiatry, Psychiatric, Transplant

Type of Coverage
Catastrophic Illness Benefit: None

Type of Payment Plans Offered
Capitated

Geographic Areas Served
Cumberland, Dauphin, Lebanon, Perry and Northern York
counties

Subscriber Information
Average Monthly Fee Per Subscriber
    (Employee + Employer Contribution):
        Employee Only (Self): $6.75 per employee

Network Qualifications
Pre-Admission Certification: No

Peer Review Type
Utilization Review: Yes

Average Claim Compensation
Physician's Fees Charged: 64%
Hospital's Fees Charged: 70%

676 Trinity Health of Pennsylvania

Mercy Health System
One W Elm St, Suite 100
Conshohocken, PA 19428
Phone: 610-567-6000
www.trinity-health.org
Secondary Address: St Mary Medical Center, 1201
    Langhorne-Newtown Road, Langhorne, PA 19047,
    215-710-2000
Subsidiary of: Trinity Health
Non-Profit Organization: Yes
Year Founded: 2013
Total Enrollment: 30,000,000

Healthplan and Services Defined
PLAN TYPE: Other
Benefits Offered: Disease Management, Home Care,
    Long-Term Care, Psychiatric, Hospice programs, PACE
    (Program of All Inclusive Care for the Elderly)

Geographic Areas Served
Statewide

Key Personnel
President/CEO . . . . Susan Croushore

677 United Concordia Dental

4401 Deer Path Road
Harrisburg, PA 17110
Phone: 717-260-6800
www.unitedconcordia.com
Subsidiary of: Highmark, Inc.
For Profit Organization: Yes
Year Founded: 1971
Total Enrollment: 7,800,000

Healthplan and Services Defined
PLAN TYPE: Dental
Plan Specialty: Dental
Benefits Offered: Dental

Type of Coverage
Commercial, Individual

Geographic Areas Served
Nationwide

Accreditation Certification
URAC

Key Personnel
President & COO . . . . Timothy J. Constantine
Contact. . . . . Beth Rutherford
    717-260-7659
    beth.rutherford@ucci.com

678 United Concordia of Pennsylvania

4401 Deer Path Road
Harrisburg, PA 17110
Phone: 717-260-6800
www.unitedconcordia.com
For Profit Organization: Yes
Year Founded: 1971
Total Enrollment: 7,800,000

Healthplan and Services Defined
PLAN TYPE: Dental
Plan Specialty: Dental
Benefits Offered: Dental

Type of Coverage
Commercial, Individual, Military personnel & families

Geographic Areas Served
Nationwide

Accreditation Certification
URAC

Key Personnel
Contact. . . . . Beth Rutherford
    717-260-7659
    beth.rutherford@ucci.com

679 UnitedHealthcare of Pennsylvania

1001 Brinton Road
Pittsburgh, PA 15221
Toll-Free: 888-545-5205
Phone: 412-858-4000
www.uhc.com
Subsidiary of: UnitedHealth Group

For Profit Organization: Yes

Healthplan and Services Defined
PLAN TYPE: HMO/PPO
Model Type: Network
Plan Specialty: Behavioral Health, Dental, Disease
   Management, PBM, Vision
Benefits Offered: Behavioral Health, Dental, Disease
   Management, Long-Term Care, Prescription, Vision,
   Wellness, Life, LTD, STD

Type of Coverage
Individual, Medicare, Supplemental Medicare, Medicaid,
   Catastrophic, Family, Military, Veterans, Group,

Type of Payment Plans Offered
DFFS

Geographic Areas Served
Statewide

Publishes and Distributes Report Card: Yes

Accreditation Certification
AAPI, NCQA

Key Personnel
CEO, PA/DE . . . . Dan Tropeano

---

680 UPMC Health Plan

600 Grant Street
Pittsburgh, PA 15219
Toll-Free: 888-876-2756
www.upmchealthplan.com
Subsidiary of: University of Pittsburgh Medical Center
For Profit Organization: Yes
Year Founded: 1996
Physician Owned Organization: Yes
Number of Affiliated Hospitals: 125
Number of Primary Care Physicians: 23,300
Total Enrollment: 101,000
State Enrollment: 209,211

Healthplan and Services Defined
PLAN TYPE: Multiple
Benefits Offered: Behavioral Health, Chiropractic,
   Complementary Medicine, Dental, Disease Management,
   Home Care, Inpatient SNF, Physical Therapy, Podiatry,
   Prescription, Psychiatric, Transplant, Vision, Wellness

Type of Coverage
Commercial, Individual, Medicare, Medicaid

Type of Payment Plans Offered
POS

Geographic Areas Served
26 counties in western Pennsylvania

Subscriber Information
Average Monthly Fee Per Subscriber
   (Employee + Employer Contribution):
      Employee Only (Self): Varies
      Employee & 1 Family Member: Varies
      Employee & 2 Family Members: Varies
      Medicare: Varies
Average Annual Deductible Per Subscriber:

Employee Only (Self): Varies
Employee & 1 Family Member: Varies
Employee & 2 Family Members: Varies
Medicare: Varies
Average Subscriber Co-Payment:
   Primary Care Physician: Varies
   Non-Network Physician: Varies
   Prescription Drugs: Varies
   Hospital ER: Varies
   Home Health Care: Varies
   Home Health Care Max. Days/Visits Covered: Varies
   Nursing Home: Varies
   Nursing Home Max. Days/Visits Covered: Varies

Accreditation Certification
NCQA

Key Personnel
President/CEO . . . . Diane Holder
VP, Business Development . . . . Kim Jacobs
CAO/COO . . . . Mary Beth Jenkins
VP, Government Relations . . . . Sheryl Kashuba
Marketing/Communications . . . . Sheri Manning
Chief Pharmacy Officer . . . . Chronis Manolis, RPh
Chief Medical Officer . . . . Stephen Perkins, MD
VP, Medicare . . . . Helene Weinraub

---

681 UPMC Susquehanna

700 High Street
Williamsport, PA 17701
Phone: 570-321-1000
www.susquehannahealth.org
For Profit Organization: Yes
Year Founded: 1994
Physician Owned Organization: Yes
Number of Affiliated Hospitals: 24
Number of Primary Care Physicians: 1,090

Healthplan and Services Defined
PLAN TYPE: PPO
Model Type: Network
Plan Specialty: Disease Management, Lab, Cancer,
   orthopedics, heart & vascular, maternty care
Benefits Offered: Disease Management, Home Care,
   Long-Term Care, Prescription, Wellness

Type of Coverage
Catastrophic Illness Benefit: Maximum $2M

Geographic Areas Served
Central & Northeastern Pennsylvania

Subscriber Information
Average Monthly Fee Per Subscriber
   (Employee + Employer Contribution):
      Employee Only (Self): $140
      Employee & 1 Family Member: $275
      Employee & 2 Family Members: $410
Average Annual Deductible Per Subscriber:
   Employee Only (Self): $500
Average Subscriber Co-Payment:
   Primary Care Physician: $30.00
   Non-Network Physician: $52.00

Hospital ER: $75.00
Home Health Care: 15%
Home Health Care Max. Days/Visits Covered: 100 days
Nursing Home Max. Days/Visits Covered:
  30/confinement

Network Qualifications
Pre-Admission Certification: Yes

Peer Review Type
Utilization Review: Yes
Second Surgical Opinion: Yes

Publishes and Distributes Report Card: No

Accreditation Certification
Medicare Approved, Utilization Review, Pre-Admission
  Certification, State Licensure, Quality Assurance Program

Key Personnel
President/CEO .... Steven P. Johnson, Jr

Specialty Managed Care Partners
Enters into Contracts with Regional Business Coalitions: Yes

---

682 Vale-U-Health

800 Plaza Drive
Suite 230
Belle Vernon, PA 15012
Phone: 724-379-4011
Fax: 724-379-4354
www.valeuhealth.com
Non-Profit Organization: Yes
Year Founded: 1995
Number of Affiliated Hospitals: 1
Number of Primary Care Physicians: 156
Total Enrollment: 2,375

Healthplan and Services Defined
PLAN TYPE: PPO
Model Type: PHO
Plan Specialty: Radiology
Benefits Offered: Disease Management, Podiatry,
  Psychiatric, Wellness, 40 specialties including allergy &
  immunology, cardiology, dermatology & geriatrics.

Type of Coverage
Commercial, Individual
Catastrophic Illness Benefit: Covered

Geographic Areas Served
Monongahela Valley

Subscriber Information
Average Annual Deductible Per Subscriber:
  Employee Only (Self): $200.00
  Employee & 1 Family Member: $400.00
  Employee & 2 Family Members: $400.00

Peer Review Type
Case Management: Yes

Accreditation Certification
TJC, CARF, COA and AOA

Key Personnel
Chief Executive Officer.................... Susan Flynn
  smf@vuhealth.com

Director of Operations .... Jois J. Weaver
  ljw@vuhealth.com
Care & Quality Management .... Trina L. Curcio
  tlc@vuhealth.com
Claims Adjudicator .... Hillary Rodenz
  hrodenz@vuhealth.com

---

683 Valley Preferred

1605 N Cedar Crest Boulevard
Suite 411
Allentown, PA 18104-2351
Toll-Free: 800-955-6620
Phone: 610-969-0485
Fax: 610-969-0439
info@valleypreferred.com
www.valleypreferred.com
Non-Profit Organization: Yes
Year Founded: 1994
Physician Owned Organization: Yes
Federally Qualified: Yes
Number of Affiliated Hospitals: 18
Number of Primary Care Physicians: 778
Number of Referral/Specialty Physicians: 2,977
Total Enrollment: 174,309
State Enrollment: 174,209

Healthplan and Services Defined
PLAN TYPE: Multiple
Model Type: PHO

Geographic Areas Served
Lehigh, Northampton, Berks, Bucks, Montgomery, Dauphin,
  Schuylkill, Columbia, Luzerne, Carbon and Lackawanna
  counties

Accreditation Certification
TJC, NCQA

Key Personnel
Chair .... Gregory G. Kile
Executive Director .... Mark Wendling, MD
Associate Executive Dir. .... Laura J. Mertz, CBC
Medical Director .... Jonathan Burke, MD
Associate Medical Dir................. Nicole Sully, DO

Specialty Managed Care Partners
Enters into Contracts with Regional Business Coalitions: No
NPRHCC

---

684 Value Behavioral Health of Pennsylvania

PO Box 1840
Cranberry Township, PA 16066
Toll-Free: 877-615-8503
pawebmaster@beaconhealthoptions.com
www.vbh-pa.com
Subsidiary of: A Beacon Health Options Company
For Profit Organization: Yes
Year Founded: 1999
Physician Owned Organization: Yes
Number of Referral/Specialty Physicians: 6,000
Total Enrollment: 22,000,000

Healthplan and Services Defined
PLAN TYPE: PPO
Model Type: Network
Plan Specialty: ASO, Behavioral Health, UR
Benefits Offered: Behavioral Health, Psychiatric, EAP

Type of Coverage
Commercial, Indemnity, Medicaid

Type of Payment Plans Offered
POS, DFFS, Combination FFS & DFFS

Geographic Areas Served
Armstrong, Beaver, Butler, Crawford, Fayette, Greene, Indiana, Lawrence, Mercer, Venango, Washington and Westmoreland counties

Peer Review Type
Case Management: Yes

Publishes and Distributes Report Card: Yes

Accreditation Certification
TJC, URAC, NCQA, CARF, COA and AOA

Key Personnel
Chief Executive Officer . . . . Laverne Cichon
Chief Financial Officer. . . . . Diane Werksman

Health Insurance Coverage Status and Type of Coverage by Age

Category	All Persons		Under 18 years		Under 65 years	
	Number	%	Number	%	Number	%
Total population	N/A	-	N/A	-	N/A	-
Covered by some type of health insurance	N/A	N/A	N/A	N/A	N/A	N/A
Covered by private health insurance	N/A	N/A	N/A	N/A	N/A	N/A
Employer-based	N/A	N/A	N/A	N/A	N/A	N/A
Direct purchase	N/A	N/A	N/A	N/A	N/A	N/A
TRICARE	N/A	N/A	N/A	N/A	N/A	N/A
Covered by public health insurance	N/A	N/A	N/A	N/A	N/A	N/A
Medicaid	N/A	N/A	N/A	N/A	N/A	N/A
Medicare	N/A	N/A	N/A	N/A	N/A	N/A
VA Care	N/A	N/A	N/A	N/A	N/A	N/A
Not covered at any time during the year	N/A	N/A	N/A	N/A	N/A	N/A

Note: Figures cover civilian noninstitutionalized population in 2017; N/A indicates that data was not available.
Source: U.S. Census Bureau, American Community Survey, Table HIC-4_ACS. Health Insurance Coverage Status and Type of Coverage by State—All People: 2008 to 2017, Table HIC-5_ACS. Health Insurance Coverage Status and Type of Coverage by State—Children Under 18: 2008 to 2017, Table HIC-6_ACS. Health Insurance Coverage Status and Type of Coverage by State—Persons Under 65: 2008 to 2017

Puerto Rico

685 BlueCross BlueShield of Puerto Rico

P.O. Box 363628
San Juan, PR 00936-3628
Toll-Free: 800-981-4860
Phone: 787-277-6544
Fax: 855-887-8275
Year Founded: 1959

Healthplan and Services Defined
PLAN TYPE: Multiple
Benefits Offered: Chiropractic, Dental, Disease Management,
Home Care, Inpatient SNF, Physical Therapy, Podiatry,
Prescription, Psychiatric, Vision, Wellness

Type of Coverage
Individual, Medicare, Supplemental Medicare

Geographic Areas Served
Puerto Rico

Accreditation Certification
TJC, URAC, NCQA

686 First Medical Health Plan

Lote #510 00966, Frontage Road
Guaynabo, PR 00966
Toll-Free: 888-318-0274
Phone: 787-474-3999
www.firstmedicalpr.com
For Profit Organization: Yes
Year Founded: 1977
Number of Affiliated Hospitals: 12
Total Enrollment: 180,000
State Enrollment: 180,000

Healthplan and Services Defined
PLAN TYPE: Multiple
Plan Specialty: Dental
Benefits Offered: Dental, Disease Management, Wellness

Key Personnel
President . . . . Francisco Javier Artau Feliciano

687 Humana Health Insurance of Puerto Rico

383 Franklin Delano Roosevelt Avenue
San Juan, PR 00918
Toll-Free: 800-314-3121
Fax: 888-899-6762
www.humana.com
Subsidiary of: Humana
For Profit Organization: Yes

Healthplan and Services Defined
PLAN TYPE: HMO/PPO
Model Type: Network
Plan Specialty: Dental, Vision
Benefits Offered: Dental, Vision, Life, LTD, STD

Type of Coverage
Commercial

Accreditation Certification
URAC, NCQA, CORE

Key Personnel
President, Puerto Rico . . . . Luis A. Torres Olivera
Finance Director, PR . . . . Jose Mercado

688 InnovaCare Health

173 Bridge Plaza N
Fort Lee, NJ 07024
Phone: 201-969-2300
info@innovacarehealth.com
innovacarehealth.com

Healthplan and Services Defined
PLAN TYPE: Medicare

Type of Coverage
Medicare

Geographic Areas Served
Puerto Rico

Key Personnel
President & CEO . . . . Richard Shinto
Chief Financial Officer . . . . Douglas Malton
General Counsel . . . . Christopher Joyce
Administrative Officer . . . . Penelope Kokkinides
Chief Accounting Officer . . . . Michael J. Sortino
Chief Actuary Officer . . . . Jonathan A. Meyers
Chief Information Officer . . . . S Bhasker

689 Medical Card System (MCS)

MCS Plaza, 1st Fl, Suite 105, 255
Ave. Ponce de León
San Juan, PR 00916-1919
Toll-Free: 888-758-1616
Phone: 787-281-2800
www.mcs.com.pr
For Profit Organization: Yes
Year Founded: 1983
Number of Affiliated Hospitals: 57
Number of Primary Care Physicians: 11
Total Enrollment: 300,000

Healthplan and Services Defined
PLAN TYPE: Multiple
Model Type: Group, Network
Plan Specialty: ASO, Behavioral Health, Chiropractic, Dental,
Disease Management, EPO, Lab, MSO, PBM, Vision,
Radiology
Benefits Offered: Behavioral Health, Chiropractic,
Complementary Medicine, Dental, Disease Management,
Home Care, Inpatient SNF, Physical Therapy, Podiatry,
Prescription, Psychiatric, Transplant, Vision, Wellness, Life,
LTD

Type of Coverage
Commercial, Individual, Indemnity, Medicare, Supplemental
Medicare, Medicaid, Catastrophic

Type of Payment Plans Offered
POS, Capitated

Geographic Areas Served
Statewide

Subscriber Information
Average Monthly Fee Per Subscriber
(Employee + Employer Contribution):
Employee Only (Self): Varies
Employee & 1 Family Member: Varies
Employee & 2 Family Members: Varies
Medicare: Varies
Average Annual Deductible Per Subscriber:
Employee Only (Self): Varies
Employee & 1 Family Member: Varies
Employee & 2 Family Members: Varies
Medicare: Varies
Average Subscriber Co-Payment:
Primary Care Physician: Varies
Non-Network Physician: Varies
Prescription Drugs: Varies
Hospital ER: Varies
Home Health Care: Varies
Home Health Care Max. Days/Visits Covered: Varies
Nursing Home: Varies
Nursing Home Max. Days/Visits Covered: Varies

Network Qualifications
Pre-Admission Certification: Yes

Peer Review Type
Utilization Review: Yes
Second Surgical Opinion: Yes
Case Management: Yes

Accreditation Certification
Medicare Approved, Pre-Admission Certification, State
Licensure

Key Personnel
President . . . . Roberto Pando
Chief Financial Officer . . . . Jos, Aponte Amador
Chief Compliance Officer . . . . Mait, Morales Mart¡nez
VP of Clinical Operations . . . . Ixel Rivera
Chief Revenue Officer. . . . . Richard Luna
SVP, Human Resources . . . . Gretchen Muiz
Chief Medical Officer . . . . In,s Hern ndez, MD

Employer References
Sensormatic, El Nuevo Dia, Pan Pepin, Nypro Puerto Rico,
Cardinal Health

690 MMM Holdings
350 Carlos E Chardon Avenue
Suite 500
San Juan, PR 00918
Phone: 787-622-3000
www.mmm-pr.com
Subsidiary of: InnovaCare, Inc.
For Profit Organization: Yes
Year Founded: 2001
Total Enrollment: 126,000

Healthplan and Services Defined
  PLAN TYPE: Multiple

Type of Coverage
Individual, Medicare, Medicaid

Geographic Areas Served
Puerto Rico

Accreditation Certification
NCQA

Key Personnel
President. . . . . Orlando Gonzalez
CEO. . . . . Richard Shinto
Chief Operating Officer . . . . Manuel Sanchez Sierra
Chief Financial Officer. . . . . Carlos Vivaldi
Chief Medical Officer . . . . Diego Rosso Flores

691 PMC Medicare Choice
350 Chardon Avenue
Suite 500, Torre Chardon
San Juan, PR 00926-2709
Toll-Free: 866-516-7700
Phone: 787-625-2126
www.pmcpr.org
Mailing Address: P.O. Box 366292, San Juan, PR 00936-6292
Subsidiary of: MMM Holdings, Inc.
For Profit Organization: Yes
Year Founded: 2000
Number of Primary Care Physicians: 7
Total Enrollment: 53,000

Healthplan and Services Defined
  PLAN TYPE: Medicare
  Model Type: Network
  Benefits Offered: Behavioral Health, Chiropractic, Home
    Care, Inpatient SNF, Podiatry, Prescription, Vision,
    Wellness

Type of Coverage
Medicare

Geographic Areas Served
Puerto Rico

Accreditation Certification
NCQA

Key Personnel
President . . . . Orlando Gonzalez, Esq.
Chief Executive Officer. . . . . Richard Shinto, MD

692 UnitedHealthcare of Puerto Rico
9700 Health Care Lane
Minnetonka, MN 55343
Toll-Free: 888-545-5205
Phone: 763-797-2919
www.uhc.com
Subsidiary of: UnitedHealth Group
Year Founded: 1977

Healthplan and Services Defined
  PLAN TYPE: HMO/PPO
  Model Type: Network
  Plan Specialty: Behavioral Health, Dental, Disease
    Management, Lab, PBM, Vision, Radiology

Benefits Offered: Behavioral Health, Chiropractic, Dental,
Disease Management, Long-Term Care, Physical Therapy,
Prescription, Vision, Wellness, AD&D, Life, LTD, STD

Type of Coverage

Commercial, Individual, Indemnity, Medicare, Supplemental
Medicare, Medicaid, Catastrophic, Family, Military,
Veterans, Group,

Geographic Areas Served

Statewide. Puerto Rico is covered by the Minnesota branch

Network Qualifications

Pre-Admission Certification: Yes

Peer Review Type

Utilization Review: Yes
Second Surgical Opinion: Yes
Case Management: Yes

Publishes and Distributes Report Card: Yes

Accreditation Certification

TJC, NCQA

Key Personnel

CEO, MN/ND/SD/PR . . . . Philip Kaufman

Specialty Managed Care Partners

Enters into Contracts with Regional Business Coalitions: Yes

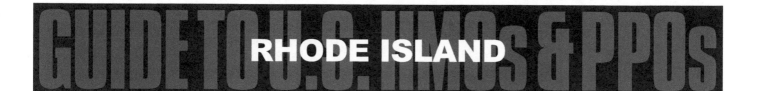

Health Insurance Coverage Status and Type of Coverage by Age

Category	All Persons		Under 18 years		Under 65 years	
	Number	%	Number	%	Number	%
Total population	1,044	-	224	-	874	-
Covered by some type of health insurance	996 (4)	95.4 (0.4)	219 (2)	97.9 (0.6)	826 (5)	94.5 (0.5)
Covered by private health insurance	727 (13)	69.6 (1.2)	144 (6)	64.4 (2.3)	626 (11)	71.6 (1.3)
Employer-based	594 (12)	56.9 (1.2)	127 (6)	56.6 (2.3)	541 (11)	61.9 (1.3)
Direct purchase	151 (9)	14.4 (0.9)	17 (3)	7.6 (1.4)	94 (8)	10.7 (0.9)
TRICARE	23 (3)	2.2 (0.3)	6 (2)	2.6 (0.9)	13 (3)	1.5 (0.3)
Covered by public health insurance	397 (11)	38.0 (1.1)	85 (5)	38.1 (2.3)	235 (11)	26.9 (1.3)
Medicaid	242 (11)	23.2 (1.1)	85 (5)	38.0 (2.3)	217 (11)	24.8 (1.3)
Medicare	189 (4)	18.1 (0.4)	2 (1)	0.8 (0.4)	27 (3)	3.1 (0.3)
VA Care	22 (2)	2.1 (0.2)	Z (Z)	Z (Z)	8 (2)	0.9 (0.2)
Not covered at any time during the year	48 (4)	4.6 (0.4)	5 (1)	2.1 (0.6)	48 (5)	5.5 (0.5)

Note: Numbers in thousands; Figures cover civilian noninstitutionalized population in 2017; N/A indicates that data was not available; Z represents or rounds to zero; Margin of error appears in parenthesis and is calculated using replicate weights.
Source: U.S. Census Bureau, American Community Survey, Table HIC-4_ACS. Health Insurance Coverage Status and Type of Coverage by State—All People: 2008 to 2017, Table HIC-5_ACS. Health Insurance Coverage Status and Type of Coverage by State—Children Under 18: 2008 to 2017, Table HIC-6_ACS. Health Insurance Coverage Status and Type of Coverage by State—Persons Under 65: 2008 to 2017

Rhode Island

693   Aetna Health of Rhode Island

151 Farmington Avenue
Hartford, CT 06156
Toll-Free: 800-872-3862
Phone: 860-273-0123
www.aetna.com
Subsidiary of: Aetna Inc.
For Profit Organization: Yes

Healthplan and Services Defined
  PLAN TYPE: PPO
  Other Type: POS
  Model Type: Network
  Plan Specialty: Behavioral Health, EPO, Lab, PBM,
    Radiology
  Benefits Offered: Behavioral Health, Disease Management,
    Long-Term Care, Physical Therapy, Podiatry, Prescription,
    Psychiatric, Wellness, Life, LTD, STD

Type of Coverage
  Commercial, Student health

Type of Payment Plans Offered
  POS, FFS

Geographic Areas Served
  Statewide

Key Personnel
  Dir., Enterprise Comm. . . . . Stephanie Crowley

694   Blue Cross & Blue Shield of Rhode Island

500 Exchange Street
Providence, RI 02903
Toll-Free: 800-637-3718
Phone: 401-459-1000
www.bcbsri.com
Subsidiary of: Health and Wellness Institute
Non-Profit Organization: Yes
Year Founded: 1939
Number of Primary Care Physicians: 100,000
Total Enrollment: 600,000

Healthplan and Services Defined
  PLAN TYPE: HMO
  Model Type: Staff
  Plan Specialty: Dental, Vision
  Benefits Offered: Dental, Disease Management, Home Care,
    Inpatient SNF, Prescription, Vision, Wellness

Type of Coverage
  Commercial, Individual, Medicare

Type of Payment Plans Offered
  DFFS

Geographic Areas Served
  Statewide

Subscriber Information
  Average Monthly Fee Per Subscriber
    (Employee + Employer Contribution):
      Employee Only (Self): Varies

      Employee & 1 Family Member: Varies
      Employee & 2 Family Members: Varies
      Medicare: Varies
  Average Annual Deductible Per Subscriber:
    Employee Only (Self): Varies
    Employee & 1 Family Member: Varies
    Employee & 2 Family Members: Varies

Peer Review Type
  Case Management: Yes

Publishes and Distributes Report Card: Yes

Accreditation Certification
  URAC, NCQA

Key Personnel
  President & CEO . . . . Kim A. Keck
  EVP/CFO . . . . Mark Stewart
  EVP/CAO/General Counsel . . . . Michele Lederberg
  EVP/Care Integration . . . . Kevin Splaine
  SVP/Chief Medical Officer . . . . Gus Manocchia, MD
  EVP/Customer Services . . . . Melissa Cummings

695   Coventry Health Care of Rhode Island

6720-B Rockledge Drive
Suite 800
Bethesda, MD 20817
Phone: 301-581-0600
www.coventryhealthcare.com
Subsidiary of: Aetna Inc.
For Profit Organization: Yes

Healthplan and Services Defined
  PLAN TYPE: HMO/PPO
  Model Type: Network
  Plan Specialty: Behavioral Health, Dental, Worker's
    Compensation
  Benefits Offered: Behavioral Health, Dental, Prescription,
    Wellness, Worker's Compensation

Type of Coverage
  Commercial, Medicare, Medicaid

Geographic Areas Served
  Statewide

696   CVS CareMark

One CVS Drive
Woonsocket, MO 02895
Toll-Free: 800-746-7287
cvshealth.com
For Profit Organization: Yes
Year Founded: 1963
Owned by an Integrated Delivery Network (IDN): Yes
Number of Affiliated Hospitals: 650
Number of Primary Care Physicians: 60,000
Total Enrollment: 70,000,000

Healthplan and Services Defined
  PLAN TYPE: Other
  Other Type: PBM
  Model Type: Staff
  Plan Specialty: Disease Management, PBM

Benefits Offered: Disease Management, Prescription

Type of Payment Plans Offered
POS, DFFS, FFS

Geographic Areas Served
Nationwide

Peer Review Type
Second Surgical Opinion: Yes
Case Management: Yes

Publishes and Distributes Report Card: Yes

Accreditation Certification
TJC, URAC

Key Personnel
President & CEO........................ Larry J Merlo
EVP/COO .... Jonathan C. Roberts
EVP, Chief Financial Offc .... David M Denton
Executive Vice President............. Thomas M Moriarty
Executive Vice President.............. Helena B Foulkes
EVP & Chief Medical Off......... Troyen A. Brennan, MD
SVP, Chief Human Resource .... Lisa Bisaccia
SVP, Chief Info Officer................. Stephen J Gold
Executive Vice President................ J David Joyner

Specialty Managed Care Partners
Enters into Contracts with Regional Business Coalitions: Yes

---

697   Humana Health Insurance of Rhode Island
125 Wolf Road
Suite 501
Albany, NY 12205
Toll-Free: 800-967-2370
Fax: 518-435-0412
www.humana.com
Subsidiary of: Humana
For Profit Organization: Yes

Healthplan and Services Defined
PLAN TYPE: HMO/PPO
Model Type: Network
Plan Specialty: Dental, Vision
Benefits Offered: Dental, Vision, Life, LTD, STD

Type of Coverage
Commercial

Geographic Areas Served
Rhode Island is covered by the New York branch

Accreditation Certification
URAC, NCQA, CORE

Key Personnel
President & CEO..................... Bruce Broussard
Chief Medical Officer................. Roy A. Beveridge
Chief Consumer Officer.................. Jody L. Bilney
Human Resources........................ Tim Huval
Chief Financial Officer .... Brian Kane
Chief Information Officer .... Brian LeClaire
General Counsel............... Christopher M. Todoroff

---

698   Neighborhood Health Plan of Rhode Island
910 Douglas Pike
Smithfield, RI 02917
Toll-Free: 800-963-1001
Phone: 401-459-6000
Fax: 401-459-6175
www.nhpri.org
Non-Profit Organization: Yes
Year Founded: 1994
Number of Primary Care Physicians: 900
Number of Referral/Specialty Physicians: 2,700
Total Enrollment: 190,000
State Enrollment: 190,000

Healthplan and Services Defined
PLAN TYPE: HMO
Model Type: Network
Benefits Offered: Behavioral Health, Disease Management,
Inpatient SNF, Prescription, Wellness

Type of Coverage
Commercial, Individual, Medicare, Medicaid

Peer Review Type
Case Management: Yes

Publishes and Distributes Report Card: Yes

Accreditation Certification
NCQA

Key Personnel
President/CEO...................... Peter M. Marino
Chief Financial Officer.................. Frank Meaney
Chief of Staff........................ David Burnett
Chief Marketing Officer .... Brenda Whittle
Chief Medical Officer .... Francisco Trilla, MD
Chief Information Officer .... Jeffrey Meyer

---

699   Tufts Health Plan: Rhode Island
75 Fountain Street
Providence, RI 02902
www.tuftshealthplan.com
Secondary Address: 705 Mt Auburn Street, Watertown, MA
02742, 617-972-9400
Non-Profit Organization: Yes
Year Founded: 1979
Number of Affiliated Hospitals: 90
Number of Primary Care Physicians: 25,000
Number of Referral/Specialty Physicians: 12,500
Total Enrollment: 1,018,589

Healthplan and Services Defined
PLAN TYPE: Multiple
Model Type: IPA
Plan Specialty: ASO, Behavioral Health, Chiropractic,
Disease Management, EPO, Lab, PBM, Vision, Radiology,
UR, Pharmacy
Benefits Offered: Behavioral Health, Chiropractic,
Complementary Medicine, Disease Management, Home
Care, Inpatient SNF, Physical Therapy, Podiatry,
Prescription, Psychiatric, Transplant, Vision, Wellness

Type of Coverage
Commercial, Individual, Medicare, Supplemental Medicare, Medicaid

Type of Payment Plans Offered
POS, DFFS, FFS, Combination FFS & DFFS

Geographic Areas Served
Massachusetts, New Hampshire and Rhode Island

Subscriber Information
Average Monthly Fee Per Subscriber
(Employee + Employer Contribution):
Employee Only (Self): $190.00-220.00
Employee & 2 Family Members: $800.00-950.00
Medicare: $150.00
Average Annual Deductible Per Subscriber:
Employee Only (Self): $1000.00
Employee & 1 Family Member: $500.00
Employee & 2 Family Members: $3000.00
Average Subscriber Co-Payment:
Primary Care Physician: $10.00
Non-Network Physician: 20%
Prescription Drugs: $10/20/35
Hospital ER: $50.00
Home Health Care: $0
Home Health Care Max. Days/Visits Covered: 120 days
Nursing Home: $0
Nursing Home Max. Days/Visits Covered: 120 days

Network Qualifications
Pre-Admission Certification: No

Peer Review Type
Utilization Review: Yes
Case Management: Yes

Publishes and Distributes Report Card: Yes

Accreditation Certification
TJC, AAPI, NCQA

Key Personnel
Chief Executive Officer. . . . . Thomas Croswell

Average Claim Compensation
Physician's Fees Charged: 75%
Hospital's Fees Charged: 70%

Specialty Managed Care Partners
Advance PCS, Private Healthe Care Systems

Employer References
Commonwealth of Massachuestts, Fleet Boston, Roman Catholic Archdiocese of Boston, City of Boston, State Street Corporation

---

700   UnitedHealthcare of Rhode Island
475 Kilvert Street
Warwick, RI 02886
Toll-Free: 888-545-5205
Phone: 401-737-6900
www.uhc.com
Subsidiary of: UnitedHealth Group
For Profit Organization: Yes
Year Founded: 1983
Owned by an Integrated Delivery Network (IDN): Yes

Healthplan and Services Defined
PLAN TYPE: HMO/PPO
Model Type: Network
Plan Specialty: Behavioral Health, Chiropractic, Dental, Disease Management, Lab, PBM, Vision, Radiology
Benefits Offered: Behavioral Health, Dental, Disease Management, Long-Term Care, Prescription, Vision, Wellness, Life, LTD, STD

Type of Coverage
Commercial, Individual, Medicare, Supplemental Medicare, Medicaid, Catastrophic, Family, Military, Veterans, Group,

Type of Payment Plans Offered
Combination FFS & DFFS

Geographic Areas Served
Rhode Island, Massachusetts, Maine, New Hampshire, Vermont

Publishes and Distributes Report Card: Yes

Accreditation Certification
AAPI, NCQA

Key Personnel
CEO, CT/ME/MA/NH/RI . . . . Stephen Farrell

Specialty Managed Care Partners
G Tec, State of RI

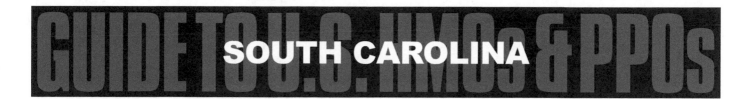

Health Insurance Coverage Status and Type of Coverage by Age

Category	All Persons		Under 18 years		Under 65 years	
	Number	%	Number	%	Number	%
Total population	4,928	-	1,169	-	4,080	-
Covered by some type of health insurance	4,387 *(17)*	89.0 *(0.3)*	1,109 *(8)*	94.9 *(0.5)*	3,542 *(17)*	86.8 *(0.4)*
Covered by private health insurance	3,225 *(25)*	65.4 *(0.5)*	645 *(14)*	55.1 *(1.1)*	2,705 *(26)*	66.3 *(0.6)*
Employer-based	2,528 *(28)*	51.3 *(0.6)*	549 *(14)*	47.0 *(1.1)*	2,265 *(26)*	55.5 *(0.6)*
Direct purchase	681 *(16)*	13.8 *(0.3)*	70 *(6)*	6.0 *(0.5)*	410 *(12)*	10.1 *(0.3)*
TRICARE	239 *(12)*	4.8 *(0.2)*	46 *(5)*	3.9 *(0.5)*	146 *(10)*	3.6 *(0.2)*
Covered by public health insurance	1,833 *(19)*	37.2 *(0.4)*	505 *(12)*	43.2 *(1.1)*	1,007 *(18)*	24.7 *(0.4)*
Medicaid	957 *(19)*	19.4 *(0.4)*	499 *(12)*	42.7 *(1.1)*	854 *(18)*	20.9 *(0.5)*
Medicare	987 *(9)*	20.0 *(0.2)*	6 *(2)*	0.6 *(0.2)*	162 *(8)*	4.0 *(0.2)*
VA Care	157 *(6)*	3.2 *(0.1)*	1 *(1)*	0.1 *(0.1)*	72 *(4)*	1.8 *(0.1)*
Not covered at any time during the year	542 *(17)*	11.0 *(0.3)*	60 *(6)*	5.1 *(0.5)*	538 *(17)*	13.2 *(0.4)*

Note: Numbers in thousands; Figures cover civilian noninstitutionalized population in 2017; N/A indicates that data was not available; Z represents or rounds to zero; Margin of error appears in parenthesis and is calculated using replicate weights.

Source: U.S. Census Bureau, American Community Survey, Table HIC-4_ACS. Health Insurance Coverage Status and Type of Coverage by State—All People: 2008 to 2017, Table HIC-5_ACS. Health Insurance Coverage Status and Type of Coverage by State—Children Under 18: 2008 to 2017, Table HIC-6_ACS. Health Insurance Coverage Status and Type of Coverage by State—Persons Under 65: 2008 to 2017

South Carolina

701 Aetna Health of South Carolina

151 Farmington Avenue
Hartford, CT 06156
Toll-Free: 800-872-3862
Phone: 860-273-0123
www.aetna.com
Subsidiary of: Aetna Inc.
For Profit Organization: Yes

Healthplan and Services Defined
PLAN TYPE: PPO
Other Type: POS
Model Type: Network
Plan Specialty: Behavioral Health, EPO, Lab, PBM,
  Radiology
Benefits Offered: Behavioral Health, Dental, Disease
  Management, Long-Term Care, Physical Therapy,
  Podiatry, Prescription, Psychiatric, Vision, Wellness, Life,
  LTD, STD

Type of Coverage
Commercial, Supplemental Medicare, Student health

Geographic Areas Served
29 counties

702 Blue Cross & Blue Shield of South Carolina

P.O. Box 100300
Columbia, SC 29202-3300
Toll-Free: 888-410-2227
www.southcarolinablues.com
For Profit Organization: Yes
Year Founded: 1946
Number of Affiliated Hospitals: 64
Number of Primary Care Physicians: 3,434
Number of Referral/Specialty Physicians: 5,473
Total Enrollment: 950,000
State Enrollment: 950,000

Healthplan and Services Defined
PLAN TYPE: HMO/PPO
Model Type: Network
Plan Specialty: ASO, Behavioral Health, Chiropractic,
  Dental, Disease Management, EPO, Lab, PBM, Vision,
  Radiology, UR
Benefits Offered: Behavioral Health, Chiropractic,
  Complementary Medicine, Dental, Disease Management,
  Physical Therapy, Podiatry, Prescription, Psychiatric,
  Transplant, Vision, Wellness
Offers Demand Management Patient Information Service:
  Yes

Type of Coverage
Commercial, Individual, Medicare

Type of Payment Plans Offered
POS, DFFS, Capitated, FFS, Combination FFS & DFFS

Geographic Areas Served
Statewide

Network Qualifications
Pre-Admission Certification: Yes

Peer Review Type
Utilization Review: Yes
Second Surgical Opinion: Yes

Publishes and Distributes Report Card: Yes

Accreditation Certification
URAC, NCQA
TJC Accreditation, Utilization Review, Pre-Admission
  Certification, State Licensure, Quality Assurance Program

Key Personnel
President . . . . Scott Graves

Specialty Managed Care Partners
Enters into Contracts with Regional Business Coalitions: Yes

703 BlueChoice Health Plan of South Carolina

P.O. Box 6170
Columbia, SC 29260-6170
Toll-Free: 800-868-2528
www.bluechoicesc.com
For Profit Organization: Yes
Year Founded: 1984
Owned by an Integrated Delivery Network (IDN): Yes
Federally Qualified: Yes
Number of Affiliated Hospitals: 68
Number of Primary Care Physicians: 7,700
Number of Referral/Specialty Physicians: 4,199
Total Enrollment: 205,000
State Enrollment: 205,000

Healthplan and Services Defined
PLAN TYPE: Multiple
Model Type: IPA
Plan Specialty: ASO, Disease Management, EPO, PBM,
  Vision, UR
Benefits Offered: Behavioral Health, Chiropractic,
  Complementary Medicine, Dental, Disease Management,
  Home Care, Inpatient SNF, Physical Therapy, Podiatry,
  Prescription, Psychiatric, Transplant, Vision, Wellness,
  AD&D, Life, LTD, STD, EAP
Offers Demand Management Patient Information Service: Yes

Type of Coverage
Commercial, Individual, Medicare, Medicaid, Medicare
  Advantage
Catastrophic Illness Benefit: Maximum $2M

Type of Payment Plans Offered
POS, DFFS, Combination FFS & DFFS

Geographic Areas Served
Statewide

Subscriber Information
Average Annual Deductible Per Subscriber:
  Employee Only (Self): $0
  Employee & 1 Family Member: $0
  Employee & 2 Family Members: $0
Average Subscriber Co-Payment:
  Primary Care Physician: $15.00
  Non-Network Physician: $25.00

Prescription Drugs: $3 tier
Hospital ER: 10%
Home Health Care: 10%
Home Health Care Max. Days/Visits Covered: Unlimited
Nursing Home Max. Days/Visits Covered: 120 days

Network Qualifications
Pre-Admission Certification: Yes

Peer Review Type
Utilization Review: Yes
Second Surgical Opinion: Yes
Case Management: Yes

Publishes and Distributes Report Card: Yes

Accreditation Certification
NCQA
Quality Assurance Program

Key Personnel
President .... Scott Graves

Average Claim Compensation
Physician's Fees Charged: 65%
Hospital's Fees Charged: 65%

Specialty Managed Care Partners
Companion Benefit Alternatives (CBA)

Employer References
Alltel Corporation, Bank of America, Kimberley Clark,
BellSouth, United Parcel Service

704 Cigna Healthcare South Carolina

900 Cottage Grove Road
Bloomfield, CT 06002
Toll-Free: 800-244-6224
www.cigna.com
For Profit Organization: Yes
Year Founded: 1982

Healthplan and Services Defined
PLAN TYPE: Multiple
Benefits Offered: Behavioral Health, Dental, Disease
Management, Prescription, Vision, Wellness, AD&D, Life,
LTD, STD

Type of Coverage
Commercial, Individual, Medicare, Supplemental Medicare,
Medicaid, Part-time and hourly workers; Union

Geographic Areas Served
Statewide

Key Personnel
President/General Manager .... Charles Pitts
Operations Director .... Deborah Rodriguez
VP, Sales, Mid-Atlantic .... William Vogelpohl
Provider Contracting .... Karen Wood

705 Delta Dental of South Carolina

1320 Main Street
Suite 650
Columbia, SC 29201
Toll-Free: 800-529-3268
Phone: 803-731-2495
service@deltadentalmo.com
www.deltadentalsc.com
Mailing Address: P.O. Box 8690, St. Louis, MO 63126-0690
Non-Profit Organization: Yes
Year Founded: 1969

Healthplan and Services Defined
PLAN TYPE: Dental
Other Type: Dental PPO
Model Type: Network
Plan Specialty: ASO, Dental
Benefits Offered: Dental

Type of Coverage
Commercial, Individual
Catastrophic Illness Benefit: None

Geographic Areas Served
South Carolina and Missouri

Key Personnel
President/CEO .... E.B. Rob Goren
CFO/Corporate Counsel .... Barbara C. Bentrup
COO/Chief Dental Officer. .... Ronald E. Inge
Chief Actuary. .... Jonathan R. Jennings
Chief Information Officer .... Karl A. Mudra
Sales/Marketing Officer .... Edward A. Pattarozzi

706 Humana Health Insurance of South Carolina

240 Harbison Boulevard
Suite H
Columbia, SC 29212
Toll-Free: 877-486-2622
Phone: 803-865-7663
Fax: 803-865-1760
www.humana.com
Secondary Address: 1025 Woodruff Road, Suite J108,
Greenville, SC 29607, 864-968-2307
Subsidiary of: Humana
For Profit Organization: Yes

Healthplan and Services Defined
PLAN TYPE: HMO/PPO
Model Type: Network
Plan Specialty: Dental, Vision
Benefits Offered: Dental, Vision, Life, LTD, STD

Type of Coverage
Commercial

Geographic Areas Served
Statewide

Accreditation Certification
URAC, NCQA, CORE

Key Personnel
Market Vice President .... Al Hernandez

707 InStil Health

P.O. Box 100294
Mail Code AG-795
Columbia, SC 29202-3294
Toll-Free: 800-444-5445
Phone: 803-763-6620
sandy.collins@myinstil.com
www.myinstil.com
Subsidiary of: Celerian Group
For Profit Organization: Yes
Total Enrollment: 30,000

Healthplan and Services Defined
  PLAN TYPE: Medicare
  Plan Specialty: ASO
  Benefits Offered: Behavioral Health, Disease Management,
    Home Care, Physical Therapy, Psychiatric, Wellness

Type of Coverage
  Medicare, Supplemental Medicare

Accreditation Certification
  URAC

Key Personnel
  Network Manager . . . . Sandy Collins
  Provider Relations . . . . Carlotta Rose
    803-666-3705
    carlotta.rose@myinstil.com
  Service Consultant . . . . Julie Drew
    843-525-9416
    theresa.curtis-barnes@myinstil.com
  Assistant VP . . . . Jennifer N. Mashura
    803-763-6623
    jennifer.mashura@myinstil.com

708 Molina Healthcare of South Carolina

4105 Faber Place Drive
Suite 120
North Charleston, SC 29405
Toll-Free: 855-882-3901
www.molinahealthcare.com
Subsidiary of: Molina Healthcare, Inc.
For Profit Organization: Yes

Healthplan and Services Defined
  PLAN TYPE: Medicare
  Model Type: Network
  Plan Specialty: Dental, PBM, Vision, Integrated
    Medicare/Medicaid (Duals)
  Benefits Offered: Dental, Prescription, Vision, Wellness, Life

Type of Coverage
  Individual, Medicare, Supplemental Medicare, Medicaid

Geographic Areas Served
  Statewide

Key Personnel
  Plan President . . . . Dora Wilson
  Chief Medical Officer. . . . . Cheryl R. Shafer, MD
  Chief Compliance Officer . . . . Niurka Adorno, Esq.
  Health Plan Operations. . . . . John Segars
  Dir., Provider Services. . . . . Jennifer Marze

709 Select Health of South Carolina

P.O. Box 40849
Charleston, SC 29423
Toll-Free: 800-741-6605
Phone: 843-569-1759
Fax: 800-575-0419
www.selecthealthofsc.com
Subsidiary of: AmeriHealth Mercy
For Profit Organization: Yes
Total Enrollment: 330,000
State Enrollment: 330,000

Healthplan and Services Defined
  PLAN TYPE: HMO
  Model Type: Medicaid
  Plan Specialty: Medicaid
  Benefits Offered: Chiropractic, Disease Management, Home
    Care, Inpatient SNF, Physical Therapy, Prescription,
    Psychiatric, Transplant, Vision, Wellness, Transportation;
    Hearing; Durable Medical Equipment; Family Planning;
    Labs & X-rays; Speech Therapy

Type of Coverage
  Medicaid

Geographic Areas Served
  Statewide

Peer Review Type
  Case Management: Yes

Publishes and Distributes Report Card: Yes

Accreditation Certification
  TJC, URAC, NCQA

Key Personnel
  Regional President . . . . Rebecca Engelman
  Market President. . . . . Courtnay Thompson
  Market CMO . . . . Kirt Caton, MD
  Director, Member Services . . . . Kevin Vaughan
  Dir., Provider Network. . . . . Peggy Vickery

710 UnitedHealthcare of South Carolina

107 Westpark Boulevard
Suite 110
Columbia, SC 29210
Toll-Free: 888-545-5205
Phone: 803-274-2819
www.uhc.com
Subsidiary of: UnitedHealth Group
For Profit Organization: Yes

Healthplan and Services Defined
  PLAN TYPE: HMO/PPO
  Model Type: Network
  Plan Specialty: Behavioral Health, Dental, Disease
    Management, PBM, Vision
  Benefits Offered: Behavioral Health, Dental, Disease
    Management, Long-Term Care, Prescription, Vision,
    Wellness, Life, LTD, STD

Type of Coverage
  Individual, Medicare, Supplemental Medicare, Medicaid,
    Catastrophic, Family, Military, Veterans, Group,

Geographic Areas Served
Statewide

Accreditation Certification
AAPI, NCQA

Key Personnel
VP, Network Management . . . . Stephen Daniels

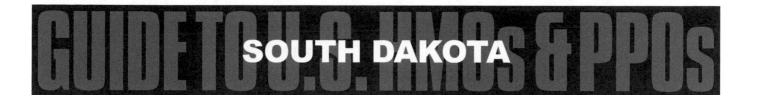

Health Insurance Coverage Status and Type of Coverage by Age

Category	All Persons		Under 18 years		Under 65 years	
	Number	%	Number	%	Number	%
Total population	852	-	224	-	716	-
Covered by some type of health insurance	774 (5)	90.9 (0.6)	211 (3)	93.8 (1.0)	639 (5)	89.3 (0.7)
Covered by private health insurance	624 (8)	73.2 (1.0)	148 (4)	66.2 (1.9)	538 (8)	75.1 (1.1)
Employer-based	473 (9)	55.6 (1.1)	123 (5)	55.0 (2.1)	444 (10)	62.0 (1.3)
Direct purchase	152 (7)	17.8 (0.8)	21 (2)	9.2 (1.1)	92 (6)	12.8 (0.9)
TRICARE	33 (5)	3.9 (0.6)	9 (2)	4.1 (0.9)	23 (4)	3.3 (0.5)
Covered by public health insurance	263 (7)	30.9 (0.8)	73 (5)	32.7 (2.0)	131 (7)	18.3 (1.0)
Medicaid	123 (6)	14.5 (0.7)	73 (5)	32.5 (2.0)	110 (6)	15.4 (0.9)
Medicare	150 (2)	17.6 (0.3)	1 (Z)	0.4 (0.2)	18 (2)	2.5 (0.3)
VA Care	33 (3)	3.9 (0.3)	Z (Z)	Z (Z)	13 (2)	1.9 (0.3)
Not covered at any time during the year	77 (5)	9.1 (0.6)	14 (2)	6.2 (1.0)	77 (5)	10.7 (0.7)

Note: Numbers in thousands; Figures cover civilian noninstitutionalized population in 2017; N/A indicates that data was not available; Z represents or rounds to zero; Margin of error appears in parenthesis and is calculated using replicate weights.
Source: U.S. Census Bureau, American Community Survey, Table HIC-4_ACS. Health Insurance Coverage Status and Type of Coverage by State—All People: 2008 to 2017, Table HIC-5_ACS. Health Insurance Coverage Status and Type of Coverage by State—Children Under 18: 2008 to 2017, Table HIC-6_ACS. Health Insurance Coverage Status and Type of Coverage by State—Persons Under 65: 2008 to 2017

South Dakota

711 Avera Health Plans

3816 S Elmwood Avenue
Sioux Falls, SD 57105-6583
Phone: 605-322-4500
sales@averahealthplans.com
www.averahealthplans.com
Secondary Address: Archway Plaza, 522 S Arch Street,
   Aberdeen, SD 57401, 605-262-4500
Total Enrollment: 63,000
State Enrollment: 63,000

Healthplan and Services Defined
   PLAN TYPE: HMO
   Benefits Offered: Disease Management, Prescription,
      Wellness, Health Education, EAP

Type of Coverage
   Commercial, Individual

Type of Payment Plans Offered
   POS

Geographic Areas Served
   Statewide

Accreditation Certification
   URAC

Key Personnel
   Chief Executive Officer . . . . Debra Muller
   SVP, Financial Services . . . . Jim Breckenridge
   Chief Operations Officer . . . . Fred Slunecka

712 DakotaCare

2600 W 49th Street
Sioux Falls, SD 57117-7406
Toll-Free: 800-325-5598
Phone: 605-334-4000
customer-service@dakotacare.com
www.dakotacare.com
Subsidiary of: Avera Health
For Profit Organization: Yes
Year Founded: 1986
Physician Owned Organization: Yes
Number of Affiliated Hospitals: 74
Number of Primary Care Physicians: 825
Number of Referral/Specialty Physicians: 950
Total Enrollment: 118,600
State Enrollment: 24,310

Healthplan and Services Defined
   PLAN TYPE: HMO
   Model Type: IPA
   Plan Specialty: ASO, Behavioral Health, Chiropractic,
      Dental, Disease Management, Lab, PBM, Vision,
      Radiology, UR
   Benefits Offered: Behavioral Health, Chiropractic,
      Complementary Medicine, Dental, Disease Management,
      Home Care, Inpatient SNF, Physical Therapy, Podiatry,
      Prescription, Psychiatric, Transplant, Vision, Wellness,
      AD&D, Life, LTD, STD

Offers Demand Management Patient Information Service: No

Type of Payment Plans Offered
   POS, FFS

Geographic Areas Served
   HMO: all counties in South Dakota; TPA: Nationwide

Subscriber Information
   Average Monthly Fee Per Subscriber
      (Employee + Employer Contribution):
         Employee Only (Self): Varies by plan
   Average Annual Deductible Per Subscriber:
      Employee & 1 Family Member: $1500
   Average Subscriber Co-Payment:
      Primary Care Physician: $25.00
      Non-Network Physician: $25.00
      Hospital ER: $150.00

Network Qualifications
   Pre-Admission Certification: Yes

Peer Review Type
   Utilization Review: Yes
   Case Management: Yes

Publishes and Distributes Report Card: No

Accreditation Certification
   URAC
   Utilization Review, Pre-Admission Certification, State
      Licensure, Quality Assurance Program

Key Personnel
   Chief Operating Officer . . . . Rhonda K. Mack
      dkrogman@dakotacare.com
   Business Development . . . . Greg Jasmer
   VP, Medical Management . . . . Rich Jones

Specialty Managed Care Partners
   Prescription benefits - CVS Caremark, Chiropractic - CASD,
      Transplant - Optum, Dental Benefits - Companion Life, Life
      Insurance Benefits - Companion Life, Sun Life Standard,
      STD/LTD - Companion Life
   Enters into Contracts with Regional Business Coalitions: No

713 Delta Dental of South Dakota

P.O. Box 1157
Pierre, SD 57501
Toll-Free: 877-841-1478
Fax: 605-494-2566
benefit@deltadentalsd.com
www.deltadentalsd.com
Non-Profit Organization: Yes
Year Founded: 1963
Total Enrollment: 60,000,000
State Enrollment: 340,000

Healthplan and Services Defined
   PLAN TYPE: Dental
   Other Type: Dental PPO
   Model Type: Network
   Plan Specialty: ASO, Dental
   Benefits Offered: Dental

Type of Coverage
   Commercial, Individual

Catastrophic Illness Benefit: None

Geographic Areas Served
Statewide

Key Personnel
President & CEO . . . . Scott Jones
VP, Operations. Mick Heckenlaible
VP, Finance . . . . Kirby Scott
VP, Underwriting . . . . Jeff Miller
VP, Information Tech . . . . Gene Tetzlaff

714   First Choice of the Midwest

100 S Spring Avenue
Suite 220
Sioux Falls, SD 57104-3660
Toll-Free: 888-246-9949
Phone: 605-332-5955
Fax: 605-332-5953
info@1choicem.com
www.1choicem.com
Mailing Address: P.O. Box 5078, Sioux Falls, SD 57117-5078
For Profit Organization: Yes
Year Founded: 1997
Owned by an Integrated Delivery Network (IDN): Yes
Number of Referral/Specialty Physicians: 6,924
Total Enrollment: 87,000
State Enrollment: 25,000

Healthplan and Services Defined
  PLAN TYPE: PPO
  Model Type: Network, Open Staff
  Plan Specialty: ASO, Behavioral Health, Chiropractic,
    Disease Management, EPO, Lab, Radiology, Worker's
    Compensation
  Benefits Offered: Behavioral Health, Chiropractic,
    Complementary Medicine, Home Care, Inpatient SNF,
    Long-Term Care, Physical Therapy, Podiatry, Prescription,
    Psychiatric, Transplant, Vision, Wellness, Worker's
    Compensation, Durable Medical Equipment

Type of Payment Plans Offered
  DFFS

Geographic Areas Served
  Colorado, Idaho, Iowa, Minnesota, Montana, Nebraska,
  North Dakota, South Dakota, Utah, and Wyoming

Network Qualifications
  Pre-Admission Certification: No

Accreditation Certification
  TJC, NCQA

Average Claim Compensation
  Physician's Fees Charged: 85%
  Hospital's Fees Charged: 90%

Specialty Managed Care Partners
  Enters into Contracts with Regional Business Coalitions: Yes

715   Humana Health Insurance of South Dakota

1415 Kimberly Road
Bettendorf, IA 52722
Toll-Free: 800-653-7275
Phone: 563-344-1242
Fax: 563-355-0730
www.humana.com
Subsidiary of: Humana
For Profit Organization: Yes

Healthplan and Services Defined
  PLAN TYPE: HMO/PPO
  Model Type: Network
  Plan Specialty: Dental, Vision
  Benefits Offered: Dental, Vision, Life, LTD, STD

Type of Coverage
  Commercial, Medicare

Geographic Areas Served
  Statewide. South Dakota is covered by the Iowa branch

Accreditation Certification
  URAC, NCQA, CORE

Key Personnel
  N Central Reg. President . . . . Chuck Dow

716   UnitedHealthcare of South Dakota

9700 Health Care Lane
Minnetonka, MN 55343
Toll-Free: 888-545-5205
Phone: 763-797-2919
www.uhc.com
Subsidiary of: UnitedHealth Group
Year Founded: 1977

Healthplan and Services Defined
  PLAN TYPE: HMO/PPO
  Model Type: Network
  Plan Specialty: Behavioral Health, Dental, Disease
    Management, Lab, PBM, Vision, Radiology
  Benefits Offered: Behavioral Health, Chiropractic, Dental,
    Disease Management, Long-Term Care, Physical Therapy,
    Prescription, Vision, Wellness, AD&D, Life, LTD, STD

Type of Coverage
  Commercial, Individual, Indemnity, Medicare, Supplemental
    Medicare, Medicaid, Catastrophic, Family, Military,
    Veterans, Group,

Geographic Areas Served
  Statewide. South Dakota is covered by the Minnesota branch

Network Qualifications
  Pre-Admission Certification: Yes

Peer Review Type
  Utilization Review: Yes
  Second Surgical Opinion: Yes
  Case Management: Yes

Publishes and Distributes Report Card: Yes

Accreditation Certification
  TJC, NCQA

Key Personnel

CEO, MN/ND/SD/PR . . . . Philip Kaufman

Specialty Managed Care Partners

Enters into Contracts with Regional Business Coalitions: Yes

---

717 Wellmark Blue Cross & Blue Shield of South Dakota

1601 W Madison Street
Sioux Falls, SD 57104
Toll-Free: 800-524-9242
Phone: 605-373-7200
www.wellmark.com
Secondary Address: 1331 Grand Avenue, Des Moines, IA
50309, 515-376-4500
For Profit Organization: Yes
Owned by an Integrated Delivery Network (IDN): Yes
Number of Affiliated Hospitals: 6,000
Number of Primary Care Physicians: 600,000
Total Enrollment: 1,800,000
State Enrollment: 300,000

Healthplan and Services Defined
  PLAN TYPE: Multiple
  Model Type: Network
  Plan Specialty: ASO, Behavioral Health, Chiropractic,
     Dental, Disease Management, EPO, Lab, PBM, Vision,
     Radiology, UR
  Benefits Offered: Behavioral Health, Chiropractic,
     Complementary Medicine, Dental, Disease Management,
     Home Care, Inpatient SNF, Physical Therapy, Podiatry,
     Prescription, Psychiatric, Transplant, Vision, Wellness,
     AD&D, Life, LTD, STD

Type of Coverage
  Commercial, Individual, Indemnity, Medicare, Supplemental
     Medicare, Medicaid, Catastrophic
  Catastrophic Illness Benefit: Maximum $1M

Geographic Areas Served
  South Dakota and Iowa

Publishes and Distributes Report Card: Yes

Accreditation Certification
  AAAHC, TJC, URAC, NCQA

Key Personnel
  Chairman/CEO . . . . John D. Forsyth
  Chief Financial Officer . . . . David Brown
  Chief Information Officer . . . . Paul Eddy
  Administrative & Legal . . . . Cory R. Harris
  Business Development . . . . Laura Jackson
  Executive VP, Operations . . . . Vicki Signor

Specialty Managed Care Partners
  American Health Ways

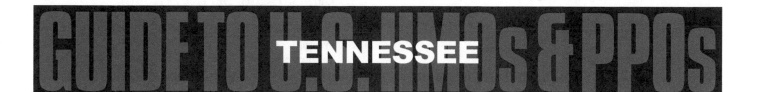

Health Insurance Coverage Status and Type of Coverage by Age

Category	All Persons		Under 18 years		Under 65 years	
	Number	%	Number	%	Number	%
Total population	6,613	-	1,600	-	5,571	-
Covered by some type of health insurance	5,983 *(19)*	90.5 *(0.3)*	1,530 *(8)*	95.6 *(0.5)*	4,946 *(19)*	88.8 *(0.3)*
Covered by private health insurance	4,381 *(34)*	66.3 *(0.5)*	928 *(16)*	58.0 *(1.0)*	3,773 *(33)*	67.7 *(0.6)*
Employer-based	3,506 *(35)*	53.0 *(0.5)*	807 *(17)*	50.4 *(1.1)*	3,227 *(33)*	57.9 *(0.6)*
Direct purchase	895 *(17)*	13.5 *(0.3)*	102 *(7)*	6.4 *(0.4)*	538 *(14)*	9.7 *(0.3)*
TRICARE	225 *(12)*	3.4 *(0.2)*	44 *(4)*	2.7 *(0.3)*	148 *(9)*	2.7 *(0.2)*
Covered by public health insurance	2,433 *(27)*	36.8 *(0.4)*	673 *(16)*	42.1 *(1.0)*	1,420 *(27)*	25.5 *(0.5)*
Medicaid	1,362 *(27)*	20.6 *(0.4)*	659 *(16)*	41.2 *(0.9)*	1,223 *(26)*	21.9 *(0.5)*
Medicare	1,232 *(10)*	18.6 *(0.1)*	15 *(3)*	1.0 *(0.2)*	219 *(9)*	3.9 *(0.2)*
VA Care	181 *(7)*	2.7 *(0.1)*	5 *(2)*	0.3 *(0.1)*	94 *(6)*	1.7 *(0.1)*
Not covered at any time during the year	629 *(19)*	9.5 *(0.3)*	71 *(7)*	4.4 *(0.5)*	625 *(19)*	11.2 *(0.3)*

Note: Numbers in thousands; Figures cover civilian noninstitutionalized population in 2017; N/A indicates that data was not available; Z represents or rounds to zero; Margin of error appears in parenthesis and is calculated using replicate weights.
Source: U.S. Census Bureau, American Community Survey, Table HIC-4_ACS. Health Insurance Coverage Status and Type of Coverage by State—All People: 2008 to 2017, Table HIC-5_ACS. Health Insurance Coverage Status and Type of Coverage by State—Children Under 18: 2008 to 2017, Table HIC-6_ACS. Health Insurance Coverage Status and Type of Coverage by State—Persons Under 65: 2008 to 2017

Tennessee

718   Aetna Health of Tennessee
151 Farmington Avenue
Hartford, CT 06156
Toll-Free: 800-872-3862
Phone: 860-273-0123
www.aetna.com
Subsidiary of: Aetna Inc.
For Profit Organization: Yes

Healthplan and Services Defined
PLAN TYPE: HMO/PPO
Other Type: POS
Model Type: Network
Plan Specialty: Behavioral Health, EPO, Lab, PBM,
    Radiology
Benefits Offered: Behavioral Health, Dental, Disease
    Management, Long-Term Care, Physical Therapy,
    Podiatry, Prescription, Psychiatric, Vision, Wellness, Life,
    LTD, STD

Type of Coverage
Commercial, Student health

Geographic Areas Served
Statewide

Key Personnel
Senior Medical Director . . . . Steve Serra

719   Amerigroup Tennessee
22 Century Boulevard
Suite 310
Nashville, TN 37214
Toll-Free: 800-600-4441
Phone: 615-316-2400
www.myamerigroup.com/tn
Subsidiary of: Anthem, Inc.
For Profit Organization: Yes
Year Founded: 2007

Healthplan and Services Defined
PLAN TYPE: HMO

Type of Coverage
Taking Care of Baby and Me

Geographic Areas Served
Statewide

Accreditation Certification
NCQA

Key Personnel
Chief Operating Officer . . . . Robert Garnett
Manager I, Child Programs . . . . JoAnne Hunnicutt
Mgr., Provider Relations . . . . Baretta Johnson

720   Baptist Health Services Group
350 N Humphreys Boulevard
4th Floor
Memphis, TN 38120
Toll-Free: 800-522-2474
Phone: 901-227-2474
bhsginfo@bmhcc.org
www.bhsgonline.org
Subsidiary of: Baptist Memorial Health Care Corporation
Non-Profit Organization: Yes
Year Founded: 1984
Number of Affiliated Hospitals: 50
Number of Primary Care Physicians: 4,000
Number of Referral/Specialty Physicians: 2,073
Total Enrollment: 423,244

Healthplan and Services Defined
PLAN TYPE: Other
Model Type: Network, Provider Spons. Network
Plan Specialty: Disease Management, Lab, Worker's
    Compensation
Benefits Offered: Disease Management, Home Care,
    Long-Term Care, Physical Therapy, Podiatry, Transplant,
    Wellness, Orthopedics; Diabeties; Dialysis; Durable
    Medical Equipment; Occupational Therapy; Prosthetics
Offers Demand Management Patient Information Service: No

Geographic Areas Served
E Arkansas, SW Kentucky, N Mississipi, SE Missouri, and W
Tennessee

Subscriber Information
Average Monthly Fee Per Subscriber
    (Employee + Employer Contribution):
        Employee Only (Self): n/a
Average Annual Deductible Per Subscriber:
        Employee Only (Self): n/a
Average Subscriber Co-Payment:
        Primary Care Physician: n/a

Publishes and Distributes Report Card: No

Key Personnel
Chief Executive Officer . . . . David Elliott

Average Claim Compensation
Physician's Fees Charged: 1%
Hospital's Fees Charged: 1%

Specialty Managed Care Partners
Enters into Contracts with Regional Business Coalitions: Yes

721   Blue Cross & Blue Shield of Tennessee
1 Cameron Hill Circle
Chattanooga, TN 37402
Toll-Free: 800-565-9140
Phone: 423-535-5600
www.bcbst.com
Secondary Address: 85 North Danny Thomas Boulevard,
    Memphis, TN 38103-2398, 901-544-2111
Non-Profit Organization: Yes
Year Founded: 1945
Number of Affiliated Hospitals: 130
Number of Primary Care Physicians: 2,490

Number of Referral/Specialty Physicians: 15,000
Total Enrollment: 3,000,000
State Enrollment: 3,000,000

Healthplan and Services Defined
  PLAN TYPE: Multiple
  Plan Specialty: Dental, Disease Management, Vision
  Benefits Offered: Dental, Disease Management, Prescription,
    Vision, Wellness

Type of Coverage
  Medicaid

Key Personnel
  President & CEO . . . . JD Hickey
  EVP, CFO . . . . John Giblin
  EVP, COO . . . . Scott Pierce
  SVP, CMO . . . . Andrea D. Willis
  SVP, Senior Products . . . . Todd Ray
  SVP, Marketing . . . . Henry Smith
  SVP, Government Relations . . . . Dakasha Winton
  SVP, Human Resources . . . . Karen Ward
  SVP, General Counsel . . . . Anne Hance
  SVP, Communications . . . . Roy Vaughn

Specialty Managed Care Partners
  Magellen Health Services

Employer References
  State, local and government employees

722 Cigna-HealthSpring

500 Great Circle Road
Nashville, TN 37228
Toll-Free: 888-705-2933
www.cigna.com/medicare/cigna-healthspring
For Profit Organization: Yes
Year Founded: 1995
Number of Affiliated Hospitals: 42
Number of Primary Care Physicians: 4,300
Total Enrollment: 345,000
State Enrollment: 17,844

Healthplan and Services Defined
  PLAN TYPE: Medicare
  Model Type: Network
  Plan Specialty: ASO, EPO
  Benefits Offered: Behavioral Health, Chiropractic, Disease
    Management, Home Care, Inpatient SNF, Physical
    Therapy, Podiatry, Prescription, Psychiatric, Transplant,
    Vision

Type of Coverage
  Commercial, Medicare, Supplemental Medicare,
    Catastrophic, Medicare PPO
  Catastrophic Illness Benefit: Covered

Type of Payment Plans Offered
  POS, DFFS, Capitated, Combination FFS & DFFS

Geographic Areas Served
  Tennessee, Northern Mississippi, Northern Georgia

Subscriber Information
  Average Monthly Fee Per Subscriber
    (Employee + Employer Contribution):

Employee Only (Self): Varies by plan
  Medicare: $0
Average Subscriber Co-Payment:
  Primary Care Physician: Varies by plan

Network Qualifications
  Minimum Years of Practice: 3
  Pre-Admission Certification: Yes

Peer Review Type
  Utilization Review: Yes
  Case Management: Yes

Accreditation Certification
  AAAHC, URAC

Key Personnel
  COO/Market Manager . . . . Casey McKeon

Average Claim Compensation
  Physician's Fees Charged: 65%
  Hospital's Fees Charged: 80%

Specialty Managed Care Partners
  Magellaw, Black Vision, MedImpact

Employer References
  Lifeway, Ingram Industries, AmSouth Banks

723 Coventry Health & Life Ins. Co. of Tennessee

5350 Poplar Avenue
Suite 310
Memphis, TN 38119
Phone: 901-763-0141
www.coventryhealthcare.com
Subsidiary of: Aetna Inc.
For Profit Organization: Yes

Healthplan and Services Defined
  PLAN TYPE: HMO/PPO
  Model Type: Network
  Plan Specialty: Behavioral Health, Dental, Worker's
    Compensation
  Benefits Offered: Behavioral Health, Dental, Prescription,
    Wellness, Worker's Compensation, Life

Type of Coverage
  Commercial, Individual, Medicare, Medicaid

Geographic Areas Served
  Tennessee, Mississippi and Arkansas

Key Personnel
  Product Manager . . . . Kiersten Claeys
  Product Implementation . . . . Allen Shannon

724 Delta Dental of Tennessee

240 Venture Circle
Nashville, TN 37228
Toll-Free: 800-223-3104
Fax: 615-244-8108
www.deltadentaltn.com
Non-Profit Organization: Yes
Year Founded: 1965
State Enrollment: 1,500,000

Healthplan and Services Defined
PLAN TYPE: Dental
Other Type: Dental PPO
Model Type: Network
Plan Specialty: ASO, Dental
Benefits Offered: Dental

Type of Coverage
Commercial, Individual
Catastrophic Illness Benefit: None

Geographic Areas Served
Statewide

Key Personnel
President/CEO . . . . Philip A. Wenk
Senior VP, Operations . . . . Kaye Martin
Chief Financial Officer . . . . Jeff Ballard
VP, Sales/Account Manager . . . . Jay Reavis

725 Health Choice LLC

1661 International Place
Suite 150
Memphis, TN 38120
Phone: 901-821-6700
contactus@myhealthchoice.com
www.myhealthchoice.com
Year Founded: 1985
Number of Affiliated Hospitals: 24
Number of Primary Care Physicians: 1,400
Total Enrollment: 518,000
State Enrollment: 518,000

Healthplan and Services Defined
PLAN TYPE: PPO
Model Type: PHO
Plan Specialty: ASO, Behavioral Health, Chiropractic,
Disease Management, EPO, Lab, MSO, PBM, Radiology,
Worker's Compensation, UR

Type of Payment Plans Offered
DFFS, FFS, Combination FFS & DFFS

Geographic Areas Served
Tennessee: Shelby, Tipton, Fayette; Arkansas: Crittenden,
Cross; Mississippi: Tunica, Desoto; Missouri: Pemiscott

Network Qualifications
Pre-Admission Certification: Yes

Peer Review Type
Utilization Review: Yes
Second Surgical Opinion: Yes
Case Management: Yes

Accreditation Certification
AAAHC
TJC Accreditation, Medicare Approved, Utilization Review,
Pre-Admission Certification, State Licensure, Quality
Assurance Program

Key Personnel
President/CEO . . . . Mitch Graves

Specialty Managed Care Partners
Lakeside Behavioral Health, Med Impact PEM
Memphis Business Group On Health

Employer References
City of Memphis Employees, Shelby County Government,
Memphis Light Gas and Water, Methodist HealthCare
Associates, St. Jude Children's Hospital

726 Humana Health Insurance of Tennessee

6515 Poplar Avenue
Suite 108
Memphis, TN 38119
Toll-Free: 866-254-1218
Fax: 901-685-0194
www.humana.com
Secondary Address: 320 Seven Springs Way, Suite 200,
Brentwood, TN 37027, 877-365-1197
For Profit Organization: Yes

Healthplan and Services Defined
PLAN TYPE: HMO/PPO
Plan Specialty: ASO
Benefits Offered: Disease Management, Prescription,
Wellness

Type of Coverage
Commercial, Individual

Geographic Areas Served
Statewide

Accreditation Certification
URAC, NCQA, CORE

Key Personnel
S Region Media Relations . . . . Mitch Lubitz

Specialty Managed Care Partners
Caremark Rx

Employer References
Tricare

727 Initial Group

6556 Jocelyn Hollow Road
Nashville, TN 37205
Toll-Free: 866-295-6586
Phone: 865-546-1893
Fax: 615-352-8782
information@initialgroup.com
www.initialgroup.com
Mailing Address: P.O. Box 58735, Nashville, TN 37205-8735
Subsidiary of: Baptist Health System of East Tennessee
For Profit Organization: Yes
Year Founded: 1994
Number of Affiliated Hospitals: 190
Number of Primary Care Physicians: 12,000
Number of Referral/Specialty Physicians: 4,000
Total Enrollment: 200,000
State Enrollment: 106,364

Healthplan and Services Defined
PLAN TYPE: PPO
Model Type: Network
Plan Specialty: Behavioral Health, Lab, Radiology, Worker's
Compensation

Benefits Offered: Behavioral Health, Home Care, Inpatient
SNF, Physical Therapy, Podiatry, Psychiatric, Transplant,
Wellness, Worker's Compensation, Life, LTD

Type of Coverage
Commercial, Medicare
Catastrophic Illness Benefit: Covered

Type of Payment Plans Offered
POS

Geographic Areas Served
East Tennessee region (i.e., KY, NC, VA, TN, GA and AL)

Subscriber Information
Average Monthly Fee Per Subscriber
(Employee + Employer Contribution):
Employee Only (Self): Varies by plan
Average Annual Deductible Per Subscriber:
Employee Only (Self): $250.00
Employee & 2 Family Members: $500.00
Average Subscriber Co-Payment:
Primary Care Physician: $15.00
Prescription Drugs: $5.00/10.00
Hospital ER: $30.00
Home Health Care: $30.00

Network Qualifications
Pre-Admission Certification: Yes

Peer Review Type
Utilization Review: Yes
Second Surgical Opinion: Yes
Case Management: Yes

Accreditation Certification
URAC
TJC Accreditation, Medicare Approved, Utilization Review,
Pre-Admission Certification, State Licensure, Quality
Assurance Program

Specialty Managed Care Partners
Health System

---

728   UnitedHealthcare of Tennessee
8 Cadillac Drive
Suite 100
Brentwood, TN 37027
Toll-Free: 800-695-1273
www.uhc.com
Subsidiary of: UnitedHealth Group
For Profit Organization: Yes
Year Founded: 1992

Healthplan and Services Defined
PLAN TYPE: HMO/PPO
Model Type: Network
Plan Specialty: ASO, Behavioral Health, Chiropractic,
Dental, Disease Management, EPO, Lab, MSO, PBM,
Vision, Radiology, UR
Benefits Offered: Behavioral Health, Dental, Disease
Management, Long-Term Care, Prescription, Vision,
Wellness, AD&D, Life, LTD, STD

Type of Coverage
Commercial, Individual, Indemnity, Medicare, Supplemental
Medicare, Medicaid, Catastrophic, Family, Military,
Veterans, Group,
Catastrophic Illness Benefit: Covered

Geographic Areas Served
Statewide

Network Qualifications
Pre-Admission Certification: Yes

Accreditation Certification
AAPI, NCQA

Key Personnel
President & CEO . . . . Rita Johnson-Mills

Specialty Managed Care Partners
United Health Group, Spectra, United Behavioral Health
Enters into Contracts with Regional Business Coalitions: Yes

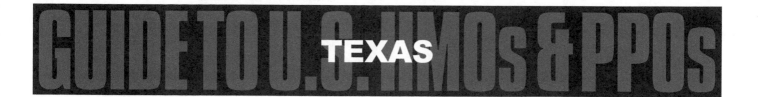

Health Insurance Coverage Status and Type of Coverage by Age

Category	All Persons		Under 18 years		Under 65 years	
	Number	%	Number	%	Number	%
Total population	27,837	-	7,782	-	24,467	-
Covered by some type of health insurance	23,020 *(48)*	82.7 *(0.2)*	6,947 *(28)*	89.3 *(0.3)*	19,713 *(46)*	80.6 *(0.2)*
Covered by private health insurance	17,326 *(70)*	62.2 *(0.3)*	4,103 *(39)*	52.7 *(0.5)*	15,523 *(66)*	63.4 *(0.3)*
Employer-based	14,324 *(74)*	51.5 *(0.3)*	3,556 *(39)*	45.7 *(0.5)*	13,317 *(71)*	54.4 *(0.3)*
Direct purchase	3,098 *(45)*	11.1 *(0.2)*	487 *(20)*	6.3 *(0.3)*	2,234 *(41)*	9.1 *(0.2)*
TRICARE	822 *(22)*	3.0 *(0.1)*	185 *(10)*	2.4 *(0.1)*	560 *(19)*	2.3 *(0.1)*
Covered by public health insurance	8,053 *(52)*	28.9 *(0.2)*	3,037 *(39)*	39.0 *(0.5)*	4,871 *(51)*	19.9 *(0.2)*
Medicaid	4,767 *(50)*	17.1 *(0.2)*	3,009 *(39)*	38.7 *(0.5)*	4,296 *(50)*	17.6 *(0.2)*
Medicare	3,730 *(17)*	13.4 *(0.1)*	39 *(4)*	0.5 *(0.1)*	553 *(12)*	2.3 *(0.1)*
VA Care	591 *(14)*	2.1 *(Z)*	12 *(3)*	0.2 *(Z)*	322 *(10)*	1.3 *(Z)*
Not covered at any time during the year	4,817 *(48)*	17.3 *(0.2)*	835 *(27)*	10.7 *(0.3)*	4,755 *(47)*	19.4 *(0.2)*

Note: Numbers in thousands; Figures cover civilian noninstitutionalized population in 2017; N/A indicates that data was not available; Z represents or rounds to zero; Margin of error appears in parenthesis and is calculated using replicate weights.
Source: U.S. Census Bureau, American Community Survey, Table HIC-4_ACS. Health Insurance Coverage Status and Type of Coverage by State—All People: 2008 to 2017, Table HIC-5_ACS. Health Insurance Coverage Status and Type of Coverage by State—Children Under 18: 2008 to 2017, Table HIC-6_ACS. Health Insurance Coverage Status and Type of Coverage by State—Persons Under 65: 2008 to 2017

329

Texas

729 Aetna Health of Texas

P.O. Box 569150
Dallas, TX 75356-9150
Toll-Free: 800-306-8612
www.aetnabetterhealth.com/texas
Subsidiary of: Aetna Inc.
For Profit Organization: Yes

Healthplan and Services Defined
PLAN TYPE: HMO/PPO
Other Type: POS
Model Type: Network
Plan Specialty: Behavioral Health, EPO, Lab, PBM,
Radiology
Benefits Offered: Behavioral Health, Dental, Disease
Management, Long-Term Care, Physical Therapy,
Podiatry, Prescription, Psychiatric, Vision, Wellness, Life,
LTD, STD

Type of Coverage
Commercial, Medicaid, Student health

Geographic Areas Served
Statewide

Key Personnel
CEO . . . . Patrina Fowler
COO . . . . Eleanor Rivera
CMO . . . . Dr. Angela Moemeka, MD
Dir., Network Management . . . . Mary Downey
Dir., Medical Management . . . . Laqueda Bell

730 Alliance Regional Health Network

1501 S Coulter Street
Amarillo, TX 79106
Phone: 806-354-1000
Fax: 806-354-1122
www.nwtexashealthcare.com
Subsidiary of: Northwest Texas Healthcare System
For Profit Organization: Yes
Year Founded: 1986
Number of Affiliated Hospitals: 25
Number of Primary Care Physicians: 550
Total Enrollment: 80,000
State Enrollment: 79,500

Healthplan and Services Defined
PLAN TYPE: PPO
Model Type: Network
Plan Specialty: Behavioral Health, Radiology, Blood
Management Program; Diabetes; Sleep Disorders; Surgery
Benefits Offered: Behavioral Health, Disease Management,
Prescription, Wellness, Worker's Compensation,
Occupational therapy

Geographic Areas Served
Northwest Texas

Network Qualifications
Pre-Admission Certification: Yes

Accreditation Certification
Medicare Approved, Utilization Review, State Licensure,
Quality Assurance Program

Key Personnel
Chief Executive Officer . . . . Ryan Chandler
Chief Operating Officer . . . . Randall Castillo
Chief Medical Officer . . . . Brian Weis
Chief Nursing Officer . . . . Douglas Coffey
Assistant Administrator . . . . Jason Madsen
Chair . . . . Sonja Clark

Employer References
City of Amarillo, Affilate Foods, Potter County,
TPMHMR/State Center, Boys Ranch

731 American National Insurance Company

One Moody Plaza
1 Moody Avenue
Galveston, TX 77550
Toll-Free: 800-899-6503
www.americannational.com
Total Enrollment: 5,000,000

Healthplan and Services Defined
PLAN TYPE: PPO
Benefits Offered: AD&D, Life

Type of Coverage
Supplemental Medicare, Supplemental health, credit disabil

Geographic Areas Served
Nationwide and Puerto Rico

Key Personnel
President & CEO . . . . Robert L. Moody

732 American PPO

391 East Las Colinas Boulevard
Suite 130
Irving, TX 75039
Phone: 972-533-0081
Fax: 972-871-2005
www.americanppo.com
For Profit Organization: Yes
Year Founded: 2000
Number of Affiliated Hospitals: 305
Number of Primary Care Physicians: 10,000
Number of Referral/Specialty Physicians: 13,000

Healthplan and Services Defined
PLAN TYPE: PPO
Model Type: Network
Benefits Offered: Behavioral Health, Chiropractic, Dental,
Disease Management, Home Care, Inpatient SNF,
Long-Term Care, Physical Therapy, Prescription, Vision
Offers Demand Management Patient Information Service: Yes

Type of Coverage
Commercial

Type of Payment Plans Offered
Combination FFS & DFFS

Geographic Areas Served
Arkansas, Louisiana, Mississippi, Missouri, Oklahoma, Tennessee and Texas

Specialty Managed Care Partners
Enters into Contracts with Regional Business Coalitions: Yes

---

733   Amerigroup Texas
2505 N Highway 360 Service Road E
Suite 300
Grand Prairie, TX 75050
Toll-Free: 800-600-4441
www.myamerigroup.com/tx
Subsidiary of: Anthem, Inc.
For Profit Organization: Yes
Year Founded: 1996

Healthplan and Services Defined
PLAN TYPE: HMO

Type of Coverage
Medicaid

Accreditation Certification
URAC, NCQA

Key Personnel
Chief Financial Officer.................. Debbie Hefley
Provider Account Manager .... Christopher Harris

---

734   Ascension At Home
13737 Noel Road
Suite 1400
Dallas, TX 75240
Phone: 314-733-8000
ascensionathome.com
Secondary Address: Providence Home Care, 301 Owen Lane, Waco, TX 76710, 254-523-6970
Subsidiary of: Ascension

Healthplan and Services Defined
PLAN TYPE: Other
Plan Specialty: Disease Management
Benefits Offered: Dental, Disease Management, Home Care, Vision, Wellness, Ambulance & Transportation; Nursing Service; Short-and-long-term care management planning; Hospice

Geographic Areas Served
Texas, Alabama, Indiana, Kansas, Michigan, Mississippi, Oklahoma, Wisconsin

Key Personnel
President................................. Kirk Allen
Dir., Home Health Service............... Darcy Burthay

---

735   Avesis: Texas
Toll-Free: 866-884-4986
www.avesis.com
Subsidiary of: Guardian Life Insurance Co.
Year Founded: 1978
Number of Primary Care Physicians: 25,000
Total Enrollment: 3,500,000

Healthplan and Services Defined
PLAN TYPE: PPO
Other Type: Vision, Dental
Model Type: Network
Plan Specialty: Dental, Vision, Hearing
Benefits Offered: Dental, Vision

Type of Coverage
Commercial

Type of Payment Plans Offered
POS, Capitated, Combination FFS & DFFS

Geographic Areas Served
Nationwide and Puerto Rico

Publishes and Distributes Report Card: Yes

Accreditation Certification
AAAHC, NCQA
TJC Accreditation

Key Personnel
Regional VP, Center/Mid W .... Melissa Jones

---

736   Blue Cross & Blue Shield of Texas
1001 E Lookout Drive
Richardson, TX 75082
Phone: 972-766-6900
media@bcbstx.com
www.bcbstx.com
Year Founded: 1984
Number of Affiliated Hospitals: 451
Number of Primary Care Physicians: 3,800
State Enrollment: 4,700,000

Healthplan and Services Defined
PLAN TYPE: HMO/PPO
Model Type: Network
Plan Specialty: Behavioral Health, Disease Management, Lab
Benefits Offered: Behavioral Health, Disease Management, Physical Therapy, Prescription, Psychiatric, Wellness

Type of Coverage
Commercial, Individual, Medicare, Supplemental Medicare
Catastrophic Illness Benefit: Unlimited

Type of Payment Plans Offered
POS, DFFS, Capitated, FFS, Combination FFS & DFFS

Geographic Areas Served
Statewide

Subscriber Information
Average Monthly Fee Per Subscriber
(Employee + Employer Contribution):
Employee Only (Self): Varies by plan
Average Subscriber Co-Payment:
Home Health Care Max. Days/Visits Covered: 60 days
Nursing Home Max. Days/Visits Covered: 60 days

Network Qualifications
Pre-Admission Certification: Yes

Peer Review Type
Utilization Review: Yes
Second Surgical Opinion: Yes
Case Management: Yes

Publishes and Distributes Report Card: Yes

Accreditation Certification
NCQA
TJC Accreditation, Medicare Approved, Utilization Review, Pre-Admission Certification, State Licensure, Quality Assurance Program

Key Personnel
President .... Dan McCoy
Chief Medical Officer .... Esteban Lopez, MD
DSVP, Sales & Marketing.............. Darrell Beckett
VP, Government Relations .... Lee Spangler, JD
VP, Business Performance .... Erin Barney

Average Claim Compensation
Physician's Fees Charged: 1%
Hospital's Fees Charged: 1%

Specialty Managed Care Partners
Magellen Behavioral Health
Enters into Contracts with Regional Business Coalitions: Yes

Employer References
American Airlines, Halliburton, Texas Instruments, Texas A&M System, JBS

737   Care N' Care
1701 River Run
Suite 402
Fort Worth, TX 76107
Toll-Free: 800-994-1076
cnchealthplan.com
Year Founded: 2008

Healthplan and Services Defined
PLAN TYPE: Medicare
Other Type: HMO & PPO
Benefits Offered: Dental, Home Care, Physical Therapy, Podiatry, Prescription, Durable Medical Equipment; Labs & X-rays; Ocupational & Speech Therapy; Outpatient Surgery; Therapeutic Radiology

Geographic Areas Served
Tarrant, Johnson, Dallas, Collin, Denton, Rockwall and parts of Parker County

Key Personnel
Chief Executive Officer .... Wendy Karsten
Medical Director................... S. David Lloyd, MD
SVP, Sales & Operations .... Scott Hancock
Compliance Director .... Nakia Smith

738   Care1st Medicare Advantage Plan Texas
601 Potrero Grande Drive
Monterey Park, CA 91755
Toll-Free: 800-544-0088
www.care1st.com
Subsidiary of: Care1st Health Plan

Healthplan and Services Defined
PLAN TYPE: Medicare
Benefits Offered: Behavioral Health, Long-Term Care, Prescription

Type of Coverage
Medicare

739   Careington Solutions
7400 Gaylord Parkway
Frisco, TX 75034
Toll-Free: 800-400-8789
www1.careington.com
Year Founded: 1979

Healthplan and Services Defined
PLAN TYPE: Other
Other Type: DHMO
Plan Specialty: Dental
Benefits Offered: Dental

Type of Coverage
Commercial, Individual

Geographic Areas Served
Statewide

Key Personnel
Chief Executive Officer.................. Barbara Fasola
Chief Financial Officer .... Melissa Baumann
Sales & Marketing .... Stewart Sweda
General Counsel................. Amanda Rinker Horton
SVP, Sales & Marketing .... Chuck Misasi
SVP, Client Relations .... Wendy Sideris
SVP, Information Systems .... Rashmi Jain

740   Christus Health Plan
919 Hidden Ridge Drive
Irving, TX 75038
Toll-Free: 844-282-3025
Fax: 469-282-2013
CHRISTUS.HP.MemberService.Inquiry@christushealth.org
www.christushealthplan.org

Healthplan and Services Defined
PLAN TYPE: Multiple
Benefits Offered: Dental, Disease Management, Inpatient SNF, Vision, Wellness

Type of Coverage
Individual, Medicare

Geographic Areas Served
Texas and New Mexico

Key Personnel
Chief Executive Officer .... Nancy Horstmann
Director, Health Plans.................... Ron Hirasaki
Dir., Health Plan Sales .... Matt Miles

741   Cigna HealthCare of Texas
900 Cottage Grove Road
Bloomfield, CT 06002
Toll-Free: 800-244-6224
www.cigna.com
For Profit Organization: Yes

Healthplan and Services Defined
PLAN TYPE: HMO

Plan Specialty: Behavioral Health, Dental, Vision
Benefits Offered: Behavioral Health, Dental, Disease
Management, Prescription, Vision, AD&D, Life, LTD,
STD

Type of Coverage
Commercial, Individual

Type of Payment Plans Offered
POS, DFFS, Capitated, FFS, Combination FFS & DFFS

Peer Review Type
Utilization Review: Yes
Second Surgical Opinion: Yes
Case Management: Yes

Publishes and Distributes Report Card: Yes

Accreditation Certification
URAC, NCQA
Utilization Review, Pre-Admission Certification, State
Licensure, Quality Assurance Program

Key Personnel
President/GM, TX/OK . . . . Thomas LaMonte

Average Claim Compensation
Physician's Fees Charged: 1%
Hospital's Fees Charged: 1%

Specialty Managed Care Partners
Quest
Enters into Contracts with Regional Business Coalitions: Yes

742 Community First Health Plans

12238 Silicon Drive
Suite 100
San Antonio, TX 78249
Toll-Free: 800-434-2347
Phone: 210-227-2347
www.cfhp.com
Secondary Address: Avenida Guadalupe, 1410 Guadalupe
Street, Suite 222, San Antonio, TX 78207
Subsidiary of: University Health System
Non-Profit Organization: Yes
Year Founded: 1995
Total Enrollment: 110,000
State Enrollment: 110,000

Healthplan and Services Defined
PLAN TYPE: HMO/PPO
Benefits Offered: Disease Management, Wellness

Type of Coverage
Commercial, Medicaid, CHIP

Geographic Areas Served
Bexar and surrounding seven counties

Key Personnel
Chair . . . . Rene Escobedo
Vice Chair . . . . Paul Nguyen
President/CEO . . . . Greg Gieseman
VP/CFO . . . . Barbara Holmes
VP/CMO . . . . Priti Mody-Bailey
VP, Operations . . . . Brian Wheeler

743 Concentra

5080 Spectrum Drive
Suite 1200W
Addison, TX 75001
Toll-Free: 866-944-6046
www.concentra.com
For Profit Organization: Yes

Healthplan and Services Defined
PLAN TYPE: Other
Plan Specialty: Worker's Compensation, Workers'
compensation and occupational health (wellness,
ergonomics, drug screening and occupational therapy)
Benefits Offered: Wellness, Worker's Compensation

Type of Coverage
Commercial

Key Personnel
President & CEO . . . . Keith Newton
Chief Financial Officer . . . . Su Zan Nelson
SVP, Human Resources . . . . Dani Kendall
SVP, Medical Officer . . . . John Anderson
EVP, Marketing & Sales . . . . John deLorimier

744 Consumers Direct Insurance Services (CDIS)

14785 Preston Road
Suite 550
Dallas, TX 75254
Toll-Free: 855-788-2583
texasmedicarehealth.com
Subsidiary of: Blue Cross Blue Shield of Texas
Year Founded: 1997

Healthplan and Services Defined
PLAN TYPE: Multiple
Benefits Offered: Dental, Wellness

Type of Coverage
Individual, Medicare, Supplemental Medicare, Medicaid,
Short-term Insurance

Geographic Areas Served
Statewide

Key Personnel
President . . . . Scott Loochtan
Executive Vice President . . . . Jenn Hemann

745 Coventry Health Care of Texas

3220 Keller Springs Road
Suite 106
Carrolton, TX 75006
Phone: 972-416-6323
www.coventryhealthcare.com
Subsidiary of: Aetna Inc.
For Profit Organization: Yes

Healthplan and Services Defined
PLAN TYPE: HMO/PPO
Model Type: Network
Plan Specialty: Behavioral Health, Dental, Worker's
Compensation

Benefits Offered: Behavioral Health, Dental, Prescription, Wellness, Worker's Compensation

Type of Coverage
Commercial, Medicare, Medicaid

Geographic Areas Served
Statewide

Key Personnel
Vice President . . . . William Baker
Customer Service Rep. . . . . Carrie Ramirez

746 Dental Source: Dental Health Care Plans

101 Parklane Boulevard
Suite 301
Sugar Land, TX 77478
Toll-Free: 877-493-6282
Phone: 866-481-9473
Fax: 281-313-7155
www.densource.com
For Profit Organization: Yes
Number of Primary Care Physicians: 149
State Enrollment: 1,500

Healthplan and Services Defined
PLAN TYPE: Dental
Model Type: Network
Plan Specialty: Dental
Benefits Offered: Dental

Type of Coverage
Commercial, Individual, Indemnity

Geographic Areas Served
Kansas and Missouri

747 FCL Dental

101 Parklane Boulevard
Suite 301
Sugar Land, TX 77478
Toll-Free: 877-493-6282
Phone: 281-313-7150
www.fcldental.com
For Profit Organization: Yes
Year Founded: 1986

Healthplan and Services Defined
PLAN TYPE: Dental
Other Type: PPO
Plan Specialty: Dental, Vision
Benefits Offered: Dental, Vision

Subscriber Information
Average Annual Deductible Per Subscriber:
Employee Only (Self): $0
Employee & 1 Family Member: $0
Employee & 2 Family Members: $0
Medicare: $0
Average Subscriber Co-Payment:
Primary Care Physician: $9.00

748 FirstCare Health Plans

12940 N Highway 183
Austin, TX 78750
Toll-Free: 800-431-7737
www.firstcare.com
Secondary Address: Customer Service, 1901 W Loop 289, Suite 9, Lubbock, TX 79407
Subsidiary of: Covenant Health
For Profit Organization: Yes
Year Founded: 1985
Number of Affiliated Hospitals: 210
Number of Primary Care Physicians: 18,900

Healthplan and Services Defined
PLAN TYPE: Multiple

Type of Coverage
Commercial, Individual, Medicaid, CHIP

Geographic Areas Served
143 counties in Texas

Key Personnel
President . . . . Darnell Dent
Product/Project Manager . . . . Jim Locke

749 Galaxy Health Network

2261 Brookhollow Plaza Drive
Suite 106
Arlington, TX 76011
Toll-Free: 800-975-3322
Phone: 817-633-5822
Fax: 817-633-5729
contracting@ghn-mci.com
www.galaxyhealth.net
Mailing Address: P.O. Box 201425, Arlington, TX 76006
For Profit Organization: Yes
Year Founded: 1993
Number of Affiliated Hospitals: 2,700
Number of Primary Care Physicians: 400,000
Number of Referral/Specialty Physicians: 47,000
Total Enrollment: 3,500,000
State Enrollment: 3,200,000

Healthplan and Services Defined
PLAN TYPE: PPO
Model Type: Network
Benefits Offered: Disease Management, Prescription, Wellness
Offers Demand Management Patient Information Service: Yes

Type of Coverage
Catastrophic Illness Benefit: Varies per case

Type of Payment Plans Offered
POS, DFFS, FFS, Combination FFS & DFFS

Geographic Areas Served
Nationwide

Subscriber Information
Average Monthly Fee Per Subscriber
(Employee + Employer Contribution):
Employee Only (Self): Varies by plan
Average Annual Deductible Per Subscriber:

Employee Only (Self): $500.00
Employee & 1 Family Member: $1000.00
Employee & 2 Family Members: $1000.00
Average Subscriber Co-Payment:
Primary Care Physician: $10.00

Network Qualifications
Pre-Admission Certification: Yes

Peer Review Type
Utilization Review: Yes
Second Surgical Opinion: Yes
Case Management: Yes

Publishes and Distributes Report Card: Yes

Accreditation Certification
URAC
Utilization Review, Pre-Admission Certification, State
Licensure, Quality Assurance Program

Key Personnel
President.............................. P.J. Shane, Jr
pjshanejr@ghn-mci.com
Director, Managed Care................. Bridget Shadle
Administrative Manager .... Venus Warner
vmatthews@ghn-mci.com

Specialty Managed Care Partners
Enters into Contracts with Regional Business Coalitions: Yes

---

750 HCSC Insurance Services Company
1001 E Lookout Drive
Richardson, TX 75082
Phone: 912-766-6900
hcsc.com
Subsidiary of: Blue Cross Blue Shield Association
Non-Profit Organization: Yes
Year Founded: 1936
Number of Primary Care Physicians: 111,500

Healthplan and Services Defined
PLAN TYPE: HMO
Benefits Offered: Behavioral Health, Dental, Disease
Management, Psychiatric, Wellness

Geographic Areas Served
Statewide

Key Personnel
Dir., Medicaid Programs .... Walter Goodnight

---

751 HealthSmart
222 West Las Colinas Boulevard
Suite 500N
Irving, TX 75039
Toll-Free: 800-687-0500
Phone: 214-574-3546
www.healthsmart.com
For Profit Organization: Yes
Year Founded: 1983
Total Enrollment: 1,000,000

Healthplan and Services Defined
PLAN TYPE: PPO

Model Type: Network
Plan Specialty: MSO, PBM
Benefits Offered: Disease Management, Wellness, Business
intelligence; web-based reporting; employer clinics

Type of Coverage
Catastrophic Illness Benefit: Varies per case

Type of Payment Plans Offered
POS, DFFS, FFS, Combination FFS & DFFS

Subscriber Information
Average Monthly Fee Per Subscriber
(Employee + Employer Contribution):
Employee Only (Self): Varies
Employee & 1 Family Member: Varies
Employee & 2 Family Members: Varies
Medicare: Varies
Average Annual Deductible Per Subscriber:
Employee Only (Self): Varies
Employee & 1 Family Member: Varies
Employee & 2 Family Members: Varies
Medicare: Varies
Average Subscriber Co-Payment:
Primary Care Physician: Varies
Non-Network Physician: Varies
Hospital ER: Varies
Home Health Care: Varies
Home Health Care Max. Days/Visits Covered: Varies
Nursing Home: Varies
Nursing Home Max. Days/Visits Covered: Varies

Network Qualifications
Minimum Years of Practice: 1
Pre-Admission Certification: Yes

Peer Review Type
Utilization Review: Yes
Second Surgical Opinion: Yes
Case Management: Yes

Publishes and Distributes Report Card: Yes

Accreditation Certification
URAC
Medicare Approved, Utilization Review, Pre-Admission
Certification, State Licensure, Quality Assurance Program

Key Personnel
Chief Executive Officer .... Phil Christianson
Chief Client Officer .... Les McPhearson
Government Affairs .... Loren Claypool
VP, Client Services.................... Marc Zech
Chief Clinical Officer .... Pamela Coffey
General Counsel....................... Sarah Bittner
Chief Financial Officer .... Matthew Thompson
Chief Sales Officer..................... Tom Mafale
Chief Information Officer................ Donald Couch

Specialty Managed Care Partners
Enters into Contracts with Regional Business Coalitions: Yes

Employer References
Garland ISD, Richardson ISD, Nokia, Tenet Health System,
Gulf Stream Aerospace

752 Horizon Health Corporation

1965 Lakepointe Drive
Suite 100
Lewisville, TX 75057
Toll-Free: 800-931-4646
bhs@horizonhealth.com
www.horizonhealth.com
Subsidiary of: Universal Health Solutions, Inc.
For Profit Organization: Yes
Year Founded: 1981
Number of Affiliated Hospitals: 2,000
Number of Primary Care Physicians: 17,000
Number of Referral/Specialty Physicians: 18,531
Total Enrollment: 120,000

Healthplan and Services Defined
   PLAN TYPE: PPO
   Model Type: Staff
   Plan Specialty: Behavioral Health, UR
   Benefits Offered: Behavioral Health, Psychiatric,
      Rehabilitation Services

Type of Coverage
   Commercial, Indemnity

Type of Payment Plans Offered
   POS, DFFS, Capitated, FFS, Combination FFS & DFFS

Geographic Areas Served
   All 50 United States, Canada, Puerto Rico, Mexico, England,
   and the Virgin Islands

Subscriber Information
   Average Monthly Fee Per Subscriber
      (Employee + Employer Contribution):
         Employee & 2 Family Members: Varies by plan

Network Qualifications
   Pre-Admission Certification: Yes

Peer Review Type
   Utilization Review: Yes
   Case Management: Yes

Publishes and Distributes Report Card: Yes

Accreditation Certification
   URAC, NCQA

Key Personnel
   President . . . . Jack DeVaney

Specialty Managed Care Partners
   Enters into Contracts with Regional Business Coalitions: Yes
   Employer Health Coalition

Employer References
   American Greetings, Saint Gobain Corporation, Broodwing,
   Jeld-Wen, The Pep Boys

753 Humana Health Insurance of Texas

8119 Datapoint Drive
San Antonio, TX 78229
Toll-Free: 800-611-1456
Phone: 210-615-5100
Fax: 210-617-1251
www.humana.com

Secondary Address: 1221 S MoPac Expressway, Suite 300,
   Austin, TX 78746, 800-967-2971
For Profit Organization: Yes
Year Founded: 1983

Healthplan and Services Defined
   PLAN TYPE: HMO/PPO
   Model Type: Network
   Benefits Offered: Disease Management, Prescription,
      Wellness
   Offers Demand Management Patient Information Service: Yes

Type of Coverage
   Commercial, Individual
   Catastrophic Illness Benefit: Covered

Geographic Areas Served
   Statewide

Peer Review Type
   Utilization Review: Yes
   Second Surgical Opinion: Yes
   Case Management: Yes

Publishes and Distributes Report Card: Yes

Accreditation Certification
   URAC, NCQA, CORE
   TJC Accreditation, Medicare Approved, Utilization Review,
      Pre-Admission Certification, State Licensure, Quality
      Assurance Program

Key Personnel
   Reginal VP, Operations . . . . Charles Majdalani
   Regional President. . . . . William C. White

Average Claim Compensation
   Physician's Fees Charged: 80%
   Hospital's Fees Charged: 80%

Specialty Managed Care Partners
   Enters into Contracts with Regional Business Coalitions: Yes

754 KelseyCare Advantage

11511 Shadow Creek Parkway
Pearland, TX 77584
Toll-Free: 866-302-9336
Phone: 713-442-5646
www.kelseycareadvantage.com

Healthplan and Services Defined
   PLAN TYPE: Multiple
   Other Type: HMO/POS
   Benefits Offered: Behavioral Health, Chiropractic, Dental,
      Disease Management, Home Care, Podiatry, Prescription,
      Vision, Wellness, Hearing; Outpatient Rehabilitation;
      Prosthetic

Type of Coverage
   Medicare, Medicare Advantage

Key Personnel
   President . . . . Marnie Matheny
   VP, Operations . . . . Theresa Devivar
   Medical Director . . . . Dr. Donald Aga

755   Liberty Dental Plan of Texas

P.O. Box 26110
Santa Ana, CA 92799-6110
Toll-Free: 877-558-6489
www.libertydentalplan.com
For Profit Organization: Yes
Year Founded: 2008
Total Enrollment: 3,000,000

Healthplan and Services Defined
  PLAN TYPE: Dental
  Other Type: Dental HMO
  Plan Specialty: Dental
  Benefits Offered: Dental

Type of Coverage
  Commercial, Individual, Medicare, Medicaid, Unions

Geographic Areas Served
  Statewide

Accreditation Certification
  NCQA

Key Personnel
  Senior Vice President . . . . Bill Henderson
    bhenderson@libertydentalplan.com
  Network Manager, Texas . . . . Deborah Kinder
    dkinder@libertydentalplan.com
  Operations Manager, Texas . . . . Margaret Stark
    mstark@libertydentalplan.com

756   MHNet Behavioral Health

9606 N. Mopac Expressway
Stonebridge Plaza 1, Suite 600
Austin, TX 78759
Toll-Free: 888-646-6889
Fax: 724-741-4552
www.mhnet.com
Mailing Address: PO Box 209010, Austin, TX 78720-9010
For Profit Organization: Yes
Year Founded: 1985
Number of Affiliated Hospitals: 134
Number of Referral/Specialty Physicians: 2,000
Total Enrollment: 2,000,000

Healthplan and Services Defined
  PLAN TYPE: Multiple
  Model Type: IPA
  Plan Specialty: Behavioral Health, Employee Assistance
    Programs and Managed Behavioral Health Care
  Benefits Offered: Behavioral Health, Psychiatric
  Offers Demand Management Patient Information Service:
    Yes
  DMPI Services Offered: Psychiatric Illness

Type of Payment Plans Offered
  POS, DFFS, Capitated, FFS, Combination FFS & DFFS

Geographic Areas Served
  Nationwide

Network Qualifications
  Minimum Years of Practice: 1
  Pre-Admission Certification: Yes

Peer Review Type
  Utilization Review: Yes
  Second Surgical Opinion: Yes
  Case Management: Yes

Publishes and Distributes Report Card: Yes

Accreditation Certification
  URAC, NCQA

Key Personnel
  Chairman & CEO . . . . Mark T. Bertolini

Average Claim Compensation
  Physician's Fees Charged: 30%
  Hospital's Fees Charged: 30%

Specialty Managed Care Partners
  Enters into Contracts with Regional Business Coalitions: Yes

757   Molina Healthcare of Texas

5605 N MacArthur Boulevard
Suite 400
Irving, TX 75038
Toll-Free: 877-665-4622
www.molinahealthcare.com
Subsidiary of: Molina Healthcare, Inc.
For Profit Organization: Yes
Year Founded: 1980
Physician Owned Organization: Yes

Healthplan and Services Defined
  PLAN TYPE: Medicare
  Model Type: Network
  Plan Specialty: Integrated Medicare/Medicaid (Duals)
  Benefits Offered: Chiropractic, Dental, Home Care, Inpatient
    SNF, Long-Term Care, Podiatry, Vision

Type of Coverage
  Commercial, Medicare, Supplemental Medicare, Medicaid

Accreditation Certification
  URAC, NCQA

Key Personnel
  Dir., Finance/Analytics . . . . Harvey Birch
  Chief Financial Officer . . . . Susan Carmack

758   Ora Quest Dental Plans

101 Parklane Boulevard
Suite 301
Sugar Land, TX 77478
Toll-Free: 800-660-6064
Phone: 281-313-7170
Fax: 281-313-7155
info@oraquest.com
www.oraquest.com
For Profit Organization: Yes

Healthplan and Services Defined
  PLAN TYPE: Dental
  Other Type: Dental HMO
  Model Type: Network
  Plan Specialty: Dental
  Benefits Offered: Dental

Type of Coverage
Commercial, Individual, Medicare, Medicaid

Subscriber Information
Average Annual Deductible Per Subscriber:
Employee Only (Self): $0

759 Parkland Community Health Plan

P.O. Box 569005
Dallas, TX 75356-9005
Toll-Free: 888-672-2277
www.parklandhmo.com
Non-Profit Organization: Yes
Year Founded: 1999
Number of Affiliated Hospitals: 25
Number of Primary Care Physicians: 3,000

Healthplan and Services Defined
PLAN TYPE: HMO
Model Type: Network
Benefits Offered: Behavioral Health, Chiropractic, Home
Care, Inpatient SNF, Physical Therapy, Podiatry,
Prescription, Psychiatric, Transplant, Vision

Type of Coverage
Medicaid, Medicaid STAR, CHIP

Type of Payment Plans Offered
POS, FFS

Geographic Areas Served
Dallas, Collin, Ellis, Hunt, Kaufman, Navarro and Rockwall
counties

Network Qualifications
Pre-Admission Certification: Yes

Peer Review Type
Utilization Review: Yes
Second Surgical Opinion: Yes
Case Management: Yes

Accreditation Certification
Utilization Review, Pre-Admission Certification, State
Licensure, Quality Assurance Program

Key Personnel
President & CEO. . . . . Frederick P. Cerise, MD
EVP, Financial Officer . . . . Richard Humphrey
Chief Operating Officer . . . . David Lopez
EVP, Medical Officer . . . . Roberto de la Cruz, MD

Specialty Managed Care Partners
Comprehensive Behavioral Care, Block Vision

760 Scott & White Health Plan

1206 West Campus Drive
Temple, TX 76502
Toll-Free: 800-321-7947
www.swhp.org
Secondary Address: 204 I-35, Suite 100, Georgetown, TX
78628, 512-930-6040
Non-Profit Organization: Yes
Year Founded: 1982
Owned by an Integrated Delivery Network (IDN): Yes

Number of Affiliated Hospitals: 18
Number of Primary Care Physicians: 1,000
Total Enrollment: 200,000
State Enrollment: 200,000

Healthplan and Services Defined
PLAN TYPE: Multiple
Other Type: POS, CDHP
Model Type: Group
Benefits Offered: Behavioral Health, Dental, Disease
Management, Home Care, Inpatient SNF, Long-Term Care,
Physical Therapy, Podiatry, Prescription, Psychiatric,
Transplant, Vision, Life
Offers Demand Management Patient Information Service: Yes
DMPI Services Offered: Secondary prevention of Coronary
Artery Disease, Pediatric Asthma, Diabetes Mellitius,
Congestive Heart Failure, Hypertension

Type of Coverage
Commercial, Individual, Medicare, Medicare cost
Catastrophic Illness Benefit: Covered

Type of Payment Plans Offered
DFFS, Capitated

Geographic Areas Served
77 counties in the Central, East, North, and West Texas
regions

Subscriber Information
Average Monthly Fee Per Subscriber
(Employee + Employer Contribution):
Employee Only (Self): Varies by plan
Average Annual Deductible Per Subscriber:
Employee Only (Self): $0.00
Employee & 1 Family Member: $0.00
Employee & 2 Family Members: $0.00
Average Subscriber Co-Payment:
Primary Care Physician: $10.00
Prescription Drugs: $5.00/20.00/50.00
Hospital ER: $75.00
Home Health Care: $10.00
Nursing Home: $0

Network Qualifications
Pre-Admission Certification: No

Peer Review Type
Utilization Review: Yes
Second Surgical Opinion: No
Case Management: Yes

Publishes and Distributes Report Card: Yes

Accreditation Certification
NCQA
TJC Accreditation, Medicare Approved, Utilization Review,
State Licensure, Quality Assurance Program

Key Personnel
President/CEO. . . . . Jeff Ingrum
Chief Financial Officer . . . . Stephen Bush
VP, Network Management . . . . Jason Tipton
Vp, Government Programs . . . . Stephanie Rogersl

Average Claim Compensation
Physician's Fees Charged: 57%

Hospital's Fees Charged: 43%

Employer References
Texas A&M, ERS, Wiliamson County

761 Script Care, Ltd.

6380 Folsom Drive
Beaumont, TX 77706
Toll-Free: 800-880-9988
customerservice@scriptcare.com
www.scriptcare.com
Year Founded: 1989
Number of Primary Care Physicians: 60,000

Healthplan and Services Defined
PLAN TYPE: PPO
Other Type: PBM
Plan Specialty: PBM
Benefits Offered: Prescription

Type of Payment Plans Offered
Capitated, FFS

Geographic Areas Served
Nationwide

Subscriber Information
Average Subscriber Co-Payment:
Prescription Drugs: Variable

Peer Review Type
Case Management: Yes

Key Personnel
President. . . . . Jim Brown
VP Sales/Marketing . . . . Tab Bryan

762 Seton Healthcare Family

P.O. Box 14545
Austin, TX 78761
Toll-Free: 866-272-2507
Phone: 512-421-5667
Fax: 512-421-4431
SetonHealthPlan@seton.org
www.seton.net/health-plan/
Subsidiary of: Ascension
Non-Profit Organization: Yes
Year Founded: 1902
Number of Affiliated Hospitals: 100
Total Enrollment: 15,000

Healthplan and Services Defined
PLAN TYPE: HMO
Benefits Offered: Behavioral Health, Disease Management,
Long-Term Care, Physical Therapy, Podiatry, Prescription,
Wellness, Cancer; Cardiac; Orthopedic; Plastic &
Reconstructive Surgery; Pediatric;Dermatology; Trauma &
Emergency

Type of Coverage
Commercial

Geographic Areas Served
Central Texas

Key Personnel
President/CEO . . . . Craig Cordola
CEO, Seton Family of Hos. . . . . Michelle L. Robertson
VP, Human Resources . . . . Joe Canales
Marketing & Communication . . . . Mike Dollen

763 Sterling Insurance

P.O. Box 26580
Austin, TX 78755-0580
Toll-Free: 800-688-0010
Fax: 888-670-0146
www.cigna.com/sterlinginsurance/
Subsidiary of: CIGNA/Sterling Life Insurance
Total Enrollment: 44,000
State Enrollment: 44,000

Healthplan and Services Defined
PLAN TYPE: Medicare
Benefits Offered: Prescription, Life

Type of Coverage
Individual, Medicare, Supplemental Medicare

Geographic Areas Served
39 States

764 TexanPlus Medicare Advantage HMO

P.O. Box 18400
Austin, TX 78760-8400
Toll-Free: 866-249-8668
www.universal-american-medicare.com/texanplus-hmo
Subsidiary of: wellCare
For Profit Organization: Yes
Total Enrollment: 42,000

Healthplan and Services Defined
PLAN TYPE: Multiple
Benefits Offered: Chiropractic, Dental, Disease Management,
Home Care, Inpatient SNF, Physical Therapy, Podiatry,
Prescription, Psychiatric, Vision, Wellness

Type of Coverage
Individual, Medicare

Geographic Areas Served
Statewide

Subscriber Information
Average Monthly Fee Per Subscriber
(Employee + Employer Contribution):
Employee Only (Self): Varies
Medicare: Varies
Average Annual Deductible Per Subscriber:
Employee Only (Self): Varies
Medicare: Varies
Average Subscriber Co-Payment:
Primary Care Physician: Varies
Non-Network Physician: Varies
Prescription Drugs: Varies
Hospital ER: Varies
Home Health Care: Varies
Home Health Care Max. Days/Visits Covered: Varies
Nursing Home: Varies

Nursing Home Max. Days/Visits Covered: Varies

Key Personnel
Chairman/CEO . . . . Richard A. Barasch
Chief Financial Officer . . . . Steven H. Black
SVP, Market Operations. Erin Page
General Counsel/Secretary . . . . Anthony L. Wolk
SVP, Healthcare Services. . . . . Theodore Carpenter

765 Texas HealthSpring

2800 North Loop West
Houston, TX 77092
Phone: 832-553-3300
www.cigna.com/medicare/cigna-healthspring
Subsidiary of: Cigna Corporation
For Profit Organization: Yes
Year Founded: 2000

Healthplan and Services Defined
PLAN TYPE: Medicare

Type of Coverage
Medicare, Medicaid

Geographic Areas Served
Houston, Golden Triangle & Valley, North Texas & Lubbock

Key Personnel
Marketing Manager . . . . Osjetta Gascey
Broker Account Manager. . . . . Ann Gray
Dir., Network Operations . . . . Kim Stuart

766 UniCare Texas

3820 American Drive
Plano, TX 75075
Toll-Free: 800-333-2203
Phone: 972-599-3888
www.unicare.com
Secondary Address: 106 East Sixth Street, Suite 333, Austin, TX 78701
Subsidiary of: Anthem, Inc.
For Profit Organization: Yes
Year Founded: 1995

Healthplan and Services Defined
PLAN TYPE: HMO/PPO
Model Type: Network
Plan Specialty: Dental, EPO, Lab, Radiology
Benefits Offered: Dental, Inpatient SNF, Long-Term Care,
Prescription, Transplant, Wellness, AD&D, Life, LTD,
STD, EAP

Type of Coverage
Individual, Indemnity, Medicare, Supplemental Medicare

Geographic Areas Served
Statewide

Network Qualifications
Pre-Admission Certification: Yes

Peer Review Type
Utilization Review: Yes
Second Surgical Opinion: Yes
Case Management: Yes

Publishes and Distributes Report Card: No

Accreditation Certification
URAC, NCQA
TJC Accreditation, Utilization Review, Pre-Admission
Certification, State Licensure, Quality Assurance Program

Specialty Managed Care Partners
Wellpoint Pharmacy Management, Wellpoint Dental Services,
Wellpoint Behavioral Health
Enters into Contracts with Regional Business Coalitions: No

767 United Concordia of Texas

5546 Merkens Drive
San Antonio, TX 78240
Phone: 210-677-0500
www.unitedconcordia.com
For Profit Organization: Yes
Year Founded: 1971
Total Enrollment: 7,800,000

Healthplan and Services Defined
PLAN TYPE: Dental
Plan Specialty: Dental
Benefits Offered: Dental

Type of Coverage
Commercial, Individual, Military personnel & families

Geographic Areas Served
Nationwide

Accreditation Certification
URAC

Key Personnel
Sales Director. . . . . Christi Harvey
Contact. . . . . Beth Rutherford
717-260-7659
beth.rutherford@ucci.com

768 UnitedHealthcare of Texas

1250 Capital of Texas Highway
Building 1, Suite 400
West Lake Hills, TX 78746
Toll-Free: 888-545-5205
Phone: 512-347-2600
www.uhc.com
Secondary Address: 1311 W President George Bush Highway,
Richardson, TX 75080, 800-458-5653
Subsidiary of: UnitedHealth Group
For Profit Organization: Yes
Year Founded: 1986

Healthplan and Services Defined
PLAN TYPE: HMO/PPO
Model Type: Network
Plan Specialty: Behavioral Health, Dental, Disease
Management, PBM, Vision
Benefits Offered: Behavioral Health, Dental, Disease
Management, Long-Term Care, Prescription, Vision,
Wellness, AD&D, Life, LTD, STD

Type of Coverage
Commercial, Individual, Medicare, Supplemental Medicare, Medicaid, Catastrophic, Family, Military, Veterans, Group,

Geographic Areas Served
Texas and Oklahoma

Network Qualifications
Pre-Admission Certification: Yes

Publishes and Distributes Report Card: Yes

Accreditation Certification
AAPI, NCQA

Key Personnel
CEO, TX/OK . . . . David Milich

Specialty Managed Care Partners
Enters into Contracts with Regional Business Coalitions: Yes

769   USA Managed Care Organization

1250 S Capital of Texas Highway
Bldg 3, Suite 500
Austin, TX 78746
Toll-Free: 800-872-0020
info@usamco.com
www.usamco.com
Secondary Address: 7301 North 16th Street, Suite 201, Phoenix, AZ 85020
For Profit Organization: Yes
Year Founded: 1984
Number of Affiliated Hospitals: 5,000
Number of Primary Care Physicians: 430,000
Total Enrollment: 5,427,579
State Enrollment: 1,118,582

Healthplan and Services Defined
PLAN TYPE: PPO
Model Type: Group
Plan Specialty: Behavioral Health, Chiropractic, Dental, Disease Management, EPO, Lab, PBM, Vision, Radiology, Worker's Compensation, UR
Benefits Offered: Behavioral Health, Chiropractic, Dental, Disease Management, Physical Therapy, Prescription, Vision, Wellness, Worker's Compensation

Type of Coverage
Commercial, Medicare

Type of Payment Plans Offered
POS, DFFS, FFS, Combination FFS & DFFS

Network Qualifications
Pre-Admission Certification: Yes

Peer Review Type
Utilization Review: Yes
Second Surgical Opinion: Yes
Case Management: Yes

Publishes and Distributes Report Card: No

Accreditation Certification
TJC Accreditation, Pre-Admission Certification, State Licensure, Quality Assurance Program

Key Personnel
President and CEO . . . . Michael Bogle

Average Claim Compensation
Physician's Fees Charged: 34%
Hospital's Fees Charged: 32%

770   UTMB HealthCare Systems

301 University Boulevard
Galveston, TX 77555-0915
Toll-Free: 855-256-7876
Phone: 409-766-4064
www.utmbhcs.org
Subsidiary of: The University of Texas Medical Branch
Non-Profit Organization: Yes
Year Founded: 1998
Total Enrollment: 1,000

Healthplan and Services Defined
PLAN TYPE: HMO
Benefits Offered: Disease Management

Type of Coverage
Commercial, Medicare, CHIP

Geographic Areas Served
Statewide

Key Personnel
Chief Executive Officer . . . . Donna Sollenberger
President . . . . David L. Callender

771   Valley Baptist Health Plan

2101 Pease Street
Harlingen, TX 78550
Toll-Free: 855-720-7448
Phone: 956-389-1100
www.valleybaptist.net
Subsidiary of: Valley Baptist Insurance Company
Non-Profit Organization: Yes
Total Enrollment: 22,000
State Enrollment: 12,004

Healthplan and Services Defined
PLAN TYPE: HMO
Plan Specialty: Lab, Surgical and Medical Weight Loss Program
Benefits Offered: Behavioral Health, Chiropractic, Dental, Disease Management, Home Care, Inpatient SNF, Physical Therapy, Podiatry, Prescription, Psychiatric, Transplant, Vision, Wellness, Durable Medical Equipment; Orthopedics; Rehabilitation

Type of Coverage
Commercial

Type of Payment Plans Offered
POS

Geographic Areas Served
Statewide

Subscriber Information
Average Monthly Fee Per Subscriber (Employee + Employer Contribution):

Employee Only (Self): Varies
Employee & 1 Family Member: Varies
Employee & 2 Family Members: Varies
Medicare: Varies
Average Annual Deductible Per Subscriber:
Employee Only (Self): Varies
Employee & 1 Family Member: Varies
Employee & 2 Family Members: Varies
Medicare: Varies
Average Subscriber Co-Payment:
Primary Care Physician: Varies
Non-Network Physician: Varies
Prescription Drugs: Varies
Hospital ER: Varies
Home Health Care: Varies
Home Health Care Max. Days/Visits Covered: Varies
Nursing Home: Varies
Nursing Home Max. Days/Visits Covered: Varies

Key Personnel
Chief Executive Officer . . . . Manny Vela
Chief Financial Officer . . . . Marco Rodriguez
Chief Nursing Officer . . . . Stephen Hill
Chief Operating Officer . . . . Daniel Listi

Specialty Managed Care Partners
Express Scripts

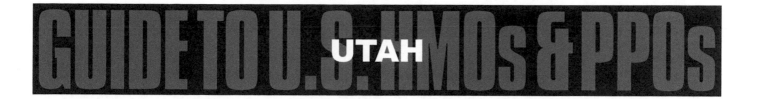
Health Insurance Coverage Status and Type of Coverage by Age

Category	All Persons		Under 18 years		Under 65 years	
	Number	%	Number	%	Number	%
Total population	3,076	-	973	-	2,746	-
Covered by some type of health insurance	2,795 *(12)*	90.8 *(0.4)*	901 *(6)*	92.7 *(0.6)*	2,468 *(12)*	89.9 *(0.4)*
Covered by private health insurance	2,413 *(19)*	78.4 *(0.6)*	746 *(11)*	76.7 *(1.1)*	2,210 *(18)*	80.5 *(0.6)*
Employer-based	1,994 *(22)*	64.8 *(0.7)*	648 *(13)*	66.6 *(1.3)*	1,882 *(21)*	68.5 *(0.8)*
Direct purchase	450 *(16)*	14.6 *(0.5)*	99 *(8)*	10.2 *(0.8)*	351 *(15)*	12.8 *(0.5)*
TRICARE	69 *(6)*	2.3 *(0.2)*	15 *(3)*	1.5 *(0.3)*	43 *(5)*	1.6 *(0.2)*
Covered by public health insurance	657 *(14)*	21.4 *(0.5)*	189 *(10)*	19.4 *(1.0)*	343 *(14)*	12.5 *(0.5)*
Medicaid	333 *(13)*	10.8 *(0.4)*	187 *(10)*	19.2 *(1.0)*	301 *(13)*	11.0 *(0.5)*
Medicare	356 *(4)*	11.6 *(0.1)*	2 *(1)*	0.2 *(0.1)*	42 *(3)*	1.5 *(0.1)*
VA Care	48 *(3)*	1.6 *(0.1)*	1 *(1)*	0.1 *(0.1)*	20 *(2)*	0.7 *(0.1)*
Not covered at any time during the year	282 *(12)*	9.2 *(0.4)*	71 *(6)*	7.3 *(0.6)*	279 *(12)*	10.1 *(0.4)*

Note: Numbers in thousands; Figures cover civilian noninstitutionalized population in 2017; N/A indicates that data was not available; Z represents or rounds to zero; Margin of error appears in parenthesis and is calculated using replicate weights.
Source: U.S. Census Bureau, American Community Survey, Table HIC-4_ACS. Health Insurance Coverage Status and Type of Coverage by State—All People: 2008 to 2017, Table HIC-5_ACS. Health Insurance Coverage Status and Type of Coverage by State—Children Under 18: 2008 to 2017, Table HIC-6_ACS. Health Insurance Coverage Status and Type of Coverage by State—Persons Under 65: 2008 to 2017

Utah

772 Altius Health Plans

10150 S Centennial Parkway
Suite 450
Sandy, UT 84070
Toll-Free: 800-365-1334
coventryhealthcare.com/Altius/index.htm
Subsidiary of: Coventry Health Care
For Profit Organization: Yes
Year Founded: 1998
Number of Affiliated Hospitals: 46
Number of Primary Care Physicians: 3,800
Number of Referral/Specialty Physicians: 1,850
Total Enrollment: 148,000
State Enrollment: 84,000

Healthplan and Services Defined
　PLAN TYPE: Multiple
　Model Type: Group, POS
　Plan Specialty: Behavioral Health, Chiropractic, Disease
　　Management, Lab, PBM, Vision, Radiology, UR
　Benefits Offered: Behavioral Health, Chiropractic, Dental,
　　Disease Management, Home Care, Inpatient SNF, Physical
　　Therapy, Podiatry, Prescription, Psychiatric, Transplant,
　　Vision, Wellness
　Offers Demand Management Patient Information Service:
　　Yes

Type of Coverage
　Commercial, Catastrophic
　Catastrophic Illness Benefit: Unlimited

Type of Payment Plans Offered
　POS, DFFS

Geographic Areas Served
　Utah, Idaho, Wyoming, and Nevada

Subscriber Information
　Average Monthly Fee Per Subscriber
　　(Employee + Employer Contribution):
　　　Employee Only (Self): Varies
　　　Employee & 1 Family Member: Varies
　　　Employee & 2 Family Members: Varies
　　　Medicare: Varies
　Average Annual Deductible Per Subscriber:
　　　Employee Only (Self): Varies
　　　Employee & 1 Family Member: Varies
　　　Employee & 2 Family Members: Varies
　　　Medicare: Varies
　Average Subscriber Co-Payment:
　　　Primary Care Physician: $15.00
　　　Non-Network Physician: 70%
　　　Prescription Drugs: Varies
　　　Hospital ER: Varies
　　　Home Health Care: Varies
　　　Home Health Care Max. Days/Visits Covered: 60 visits
　　　Nursing Home: Varies
　　　Nursing Home Max. Days/Visits Covered: 60 visits

Network Qualifications
　Pre-Admission Certification: Yes

Peer Review Type
　Utilization Review: Yes
　Second Surgical Opinion: Yes
　Case Management: Yes

Publishes and Distributes Report Card: Yes

Accreditation Certification
　URAC
　TJC Accreditation, Medicare Approved, Utilization Review,
　　Pre-Admission Certification, State Licensure, Quality
　　Assurance Program

Key Personnel
　VP, Network Development . . . . Kevin Lawlor

Specialty Managed Care Partners
　Horizon Behavioral Health, ESI

Employer References
　Federal Government, State of Utah, Davis County School
　　District, Wells Fargo, DMBA

773 BridgeSpan Health

2890 E Cottonwood Parkway
Salt Like City, UT 84121
Toll-Free: 855-857-9943
www.bridgespanhealth.com
Subsidiary of: Cambia Health Solutions
Non-Profit Organization: Yes
Year Founded: 2012

Healthplan and Services Defined
　PLAN TYPE: HMO
　Benefits Offered: Behavioral Health, Physical Therapy,
　　Prescription, Wellness, Abulance Care; Hospice; Labs &
　　Imaging; Maternity; Substance Abuse; Rehabilitation;
　　Pediatrics

Geographic Areas Served
　Idaho, Oregon, Utah, and Washington

Key Personnel
　President . . . . Chris Blanton

774 Emi Health

5101 S Commerce Street
Murray, UT 84107
Toll-Free: 800-662-5851
Phone: 801-262-7475
Fax: 801-269-9734
cs@emihealth.com
www.emihealth.com
Subsidiary of: Educators Mutual
Non-Profit Organization: Yes
Year Founded: 1935
Physician Owned Organization: Yes
Federally Qualified: Yes
Number of Affiliated Hospitals: 25
Number of Primary Care Physicians: 3,500
Total Enrollment: 6,000
State Enrollment: 65,000

Healthplan and Services Defined
  PLAN TYPE: HMO/PPO
  Model Type: Network
  Plan Specialty: Behavioral Health, Chiropractic, Disease
    Management, Radiology, UR
  Benefits Offered: Behavioral Health, Chiropractic,
    Complementary Medicine, Dental, Disease Management,
    Home Care, Inpatient SNF, Physical Therapy, Podiatry,
    Prescription, Psychiatric, Transplant, Vision, Wellness,
    AD&D, Life, LTD, STD
  Offers Demand Management Patient Information Service:
    Yes
  DMPI Services Offered: Wellness Web

Type of Coverage
  Commercial, Individual

Type of Payment Plans Offered
  POS

Geographic Areas Served
  counties: Box Elder; Cache; Davis; Salt Lake; Weber

Subscriber Information
  Average Monthly Fee Per Subscriber
    (Employee + Employer Contribution):
      Employee Only (Self): Varies by plan
  Average Annual Deductible Per Subscriber:
    Employee Only (Self): $0
    Employee & 1 Family Member: $0
    Employee & 2 Family Members: $0
    Medicare: $0
  Average Subscriber Co-Payment:
    Primary Care Physician: $5.00
    Prescription Drugs: 30%
    Hospital ER: $25.00
    Home Health Care: $0
    Nursing Home: $0

Network Qualifications
  Pre-Admission Certification: Yes

Peer Review Type
  Utilization Review: Yes
  Second Surgical Opinion: No
  Case Management: Yes

Publishes and Distributes Report Card: Yes

Accreditation Certification
  TJC Accreditation, Utilization Review, Pre-Admission
    Certification, State Licensure, Quality Assurance Program

Key Personnel
  President/CEO . . . . Steven C. Morrison
  EVP/CFO/Treasurer. . . . . Mike Greenhalgh
  EVP/COO/Secretary . . . . Ryan Lowther
  SVP/CCO/Legal Officer . . . . Brandon L. Smart, Esq.
  Chief Actuary . . . . David Wood
  EVP, IT . . . . Joe Campbell
  SVP, Comm./Provider Rel. . . . . Christie Hawkes
  Sales & Marketing. . . . . Cindy Dunnavant

Specialty Managed Care Partners
  Enters into Contracts with Regional Business Coalitions: No

---

775   # Humana Health Insurance of Utah
9815 South Monroe Street
Suite 300
Sandy, UT 84070
Toll-Free: 800-884-8328
Phone: 801-256-6200
Fax: 801-256-0782
www.humana.com
Subsidiary of: Humana
For Profit Organization: Yes

Healthplan and Services Defined
  PLAN TYPE: HMO/PPO
  Model Type: Network
  Plan Specialty: Dental, Vision
  Benefits Offered: Dental, Vision, Life, LTD, STD

Type of Coverage
  Commercial, Individual

Geographic Areas Served
  Statewide

Accreditation Certification
  URAC, NCQA, CORE

Key Personnel
  Market Manager . . . . Nathan Brown

---

776   # Intermountain Healthcare
36 S State Street
Salt Lake City, UT 84111
Phone: 801-442-2000
www.intermountainhealthcare.org
Non-Profit Organization: Yes
Year Founded: 1975
Number of Affiliated Hospitals: 22
Number of Primary Care Physicians: 1,600
Total Enrollment: 750,000

Healthplan and Services Defined
  PLAN TYPE: HMO
  Benefits Offered: Chiropractic, Complementary Medicine,
    Dental, Home Care, Inpatient SNF, Long-Term Care,
    Podiatry, Prescription, Psychiatric, Transplant, Vision,
    Wellness, Worker's Compensation

Type of Coverage
  Commercial, Individual, Medicare, Medicaid

Geographic Areas Served
  Utah and SE Idaho

Accreditation Certification
  NCQA

Key Personnel
  President/CEO. . . . . A. Marc Harrison, MD
  Chief Operating Officer. . . . . Robert W. Allen
  Chief Physician Executive . . . . Mark Briesacher
  Chief Development Officer . . . . David L. Flood
  Chief Financial Officer . . . . Bert Zimmerli

777 Molina Healthcare of Utah
7050 Union Park Center
Suite 200
Midvale, UT 84047
Toll-Free: 866-449-6817
Phone: 801-858-0400
www.molinahealthcare.com
Subsidiary of: Molina Healthcare, Inc.
For Profit Organization: Yes
Year Founded: 1980
Physician Owned Organization: Yes

Healthplan and Services Defined
  PLAN TYPE: Medicare
  Model Type: Network
  Plan Specialty: Integrated Medicare/Medicaid (Duals)
  Benefits Offered: Chiropractic, Dental, Home Care, Inpatient
    SNF, Long-Term Care, Podiatry, Vision

Type of Coverage
  Commercial, Medicare, Supplemental Medicare, Medicaid

Accreditation Certification
  URAC, NCQA

Key Personnel
  President, ID/UT . . . . Brandon Hendrickson
  Dir., Customer Services . . . . Diane McWilliams

778 Opticare of Utah
1901 W Parkway Boulevard
Salt Lake City, UT 84119
Toll-Free: 800-363-0950
Phone: 801-869-2020
service@opticareofutah.com
www.opticareofutah.com
For Profit Organization: Yes
Year Founded: 1985
Number of Referral/Specialty Physicians: 40
Total Enrollment: 150,000
State Enrollment: 150,000

Healthplan and Services Defined
  PLAN TYPE: Vision
  Other Type: Optical
  Model Type: Network
  Plan Specialty: Vision
  Benefits Offered: Vision

Type of Payment Plans Offered
  POS, Capitated, FFS

Geographic Areas Served
  Statewide

Subscriber Information
  Average Subscriber Co-Payment:
    Primary Care Physician: Varies

Network Qualifications
  Pre-Admission Certification: Yes

Peer Review Type
  Utilization Review: Yes
  Second Surgical Opinion: Yes
  Case Management: Yes

Key Personnel
  CEO/ABO . . . . Aaron Schubach
    800-363-0950
    aaron@standardoptical.net
  President . . . . Stephen Schubach
    stephen@standardoptical.net
  Account Manager . . . . Jessica Boss
    801-910-3978
    jboss@opticareofutah.com
  National Sales Director . . . . Camille Williams
    801-360-5448
    cwilliams@opticareofutah.com
  Office Manager . . . . CarlieDane Livingston
    801-869-2021
    carlie@opticareofutah.com

Specialty Managed Care Partners
  Enters into Contracts with Regional Business Coalitions: Yes

Employer References
  State of Utah Employees

779 Premier Access Insurance/Access Dental
P.O. Box 659010
Sacramento, CA 95865-9010
Toll-Free: 888-634-6074
Phone: 916-920-2500
Fax: 916-563-9000
info@premierlife.com
www.premierppo.com
Subsidiary of: Guardian Life Insurance Co.
For Profit Organization: Yes
Year Founded: 1989
Number of Primary Care Physicians: 1,000

Healthplan and Services Defined
  PLAN TYPE: PPO
  Other Type: Dental
  Plan Specialty: Dental
  Benefits Offered: Dental

Key Personnel
  President & CEO . . . . Deanna M. Mulligan

780 Public Employees Health Program
560 East 200 South
Salt Lake City, UT 84102-2099
Toll-Free: 800-765-7347
Phone: 801-366-7555
www.pehp.org
Subsidiary of: Utah Retirement Systems
Non-Profit Organization: Yes
Year Founded: 1977
Number of Affiliated Hospitals: 49
Number of Primary Care Physicians: 12,000
Number of Referral/Specialty Physicians: 2,900
Total Enrollment: 177,854
State Enrollment: 177,854

Healthplan and Services Defined
  PLAN TYPE: PPO
  Model Type: Network

Plan Specialty: Dental, Disease Management, Lab, PBM, Radiology, UR
Benefits Offered: Dental, Disease Management, Home Care, Prescription, Transplant, Wellness, AD&D, Life, LTD

Type of Coverage
Supplemental Medicare, Children's Health Insurance Program
Catastrophic Illness Benefit: None

Type of Payment Plans Offered
FFS

Subscriber Information
Average Monthly Fee Per Subscriber
(Employee + Employer Contribution):
Employee Only (Self): Varies by plan
Employee & 1 Family Member: $583.00
Average Annual Deductible Per Subscriber:
Employee Only (Self): $0
Employee & 1 Family Member: $0
Employee & 2 Family Members: $0
Medicare: $0
Average Subscriber Co-Payment:
Primary Care Physician: $15.00
Non-Network Physician: 15.00 + 30%
Prescription Drugs: 20%
Hospital ER: $80.00
Home Health Care Max. Days/Visits Covered: Unlimited

Network Qualifications
Pre-Admission Certification: No

Peer Review Type
Utilization Review: Yes
Second Surgical Opinion: Yes
Case Management: Yes

Publishes and Distributes Report Card: Yes

Accreditation Certification
TJC Accreditation, Medicare Approved, State Licensure

Key Personnel
Managing Director . . . . R. Chet Loftis
Provider Relations . . . . Cortney Larson
Marketing Director . . . . Joel Sheppard

Average Claim Compensation
Physician's Fees Charged: 70%
Hospital's Fees Charged: 80%

Specialty Managed Care Partners
Managed Mental Healthcare, Chiropratic Health Plan, IHC Auesst
Enters into Contracts with Regional Business Coalitions: Yes

Employer References
State of Utah, Jordon School District, Salt Lake County, Salt Lake City, Utah School Boards Association

781   Regence BlueCross BlueShield of Utah
P.O. Box 1071
Portland, OR 97207
Toll-Free: 888-367-2117
www.regence.com
Subsidiary of: Regence

Non-Profit Organization: Yes
Total Enrollment: 2,400,000
State Enrollment: 330,000

Healthplan and Services Defined
PLAN TYPE: Multiple
Model Type: Network
Benefits Offered: Dental, Prescription, Vision, Wellness, Life, Preventive Care

Type of Coverage
Commercial, Individual, Supplemental Medicare

Key Personnel
President/Revenue Officer . . . . Angela Dowling
Chief Medical Officer . . . . Richard Popiel

782   SelectHealth
5381 S Green Street
Murray, UT 84123
Toll-Free: 800-538-5038
selecthealth.org
Non-Profit Organization: Yes

Healthplan and Services Defined
PLAN TYPE: HMO

Type of Coverage
Commercial, Individual

Geographic Areas Served
Utah and Idaho

Accreditation Certification
NCQA

783   Total Dental Administrators
6985 Union Park Center
Suite 675
Cottonwood Heights, UT 84047
Toll-Free: 800-880-3536
Phone: 801-268-9840
Fax: 801-268-9873
www.tdadental.com
Secondary Address: 2111 E. Highland Avenue, Suite 250, Phoenix, AZ 85016-4735, 602-266-1995
Subsidiary of: Companion Life Insurance Co.

Healthplan and Services Defined
PLAN TYPE: Dental

Key Personnel
President & CEO . . . . Jeremy Spencer

784   UnitedHealthcare of Utah

Salt Lake City, UT 84120
Toll-Free: 888-545-5205
www.uhc.com
Subsidiary of: UnitedHealth Group
For Profit Organization: Yes

Healthplan and Services Defined
PLAN TYPE: HMO/PPO

Model Type: Network
Plan Specialty: Behavioral Health, Dental, Disease
 Management, PBM, Vision
Benefits Offered: Behavioral Health, Dental, Disease
 Management, Long-Term Care, Prescription, Vision,
 Wellness, Life, LTD, STD

Type of Coverage
 Individual, Medicare, Supplemental Medicare, Medicaid,
 Catastrophic, Family, Military, Veterans, Group,

Geographic Areas Served
 Statewide

Key Personnel
 Chief Operating Officer . . . . Chris Hard

785 University Health Plans
6053 Fashion Square Drive
Suite 110
Murray, UT 84107
Toll-Free: 888-271-5870
Phone: 801-587-6480
Fax: 801-281-6121
uuhp@hsc.utah.edu
uhealthplan.utah.edu
Mailing Address: P.O. Box 45180, Salt Lake City, UT
 84145-0180
Non-Profit Organization: Yes
Number of Affiliated Hospitals: 28
Number of Primary Care Physicians: 1,750
Total Enrollment: 86,000
State Enrollment: 50,000

Healthplan and Services Defined
 PLAN TYPE: HMO/PPO
 Benefits Offered: Disease Management, Wellness

Type of Coverage
 Commercial, Medicare, Medicaid

Geographic Areas Served
 Statewide

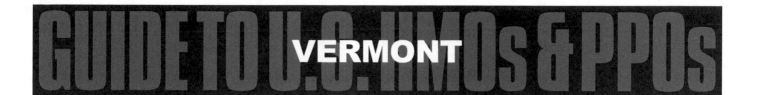

Health Insurance Coverage Status and Type of Coverage by Age

Category	All Persons		Under 18 years		Under 65 years	
	Number	%	Number	%	Number	%
Total population	618	-	127	-	504	-
Covered by some type of health insurance	589 (3)	95.4 (0.4)	125 (1)	98.4 (0.6)	476 (3)	94.5 (0.5)
Covered by private health insurance	411 (8)	66.5 (1.3)	69 (3)	54.1 (2.4)	338 (7)	67.1 (1.5)
Employer-based	327 (8)	53.0 (1.3)	62 (3)	49.1 (2.3)	291 (7)	57.7 (1.5)
Direct purchase	92 (5)	14.9 (0.9)	7 (1)	5.3 (1.1)	51 (4)	10.2 (0.9)
TRICARE	15 (2)	2.5 (0.4)	2 (1)	1.5 (0.7)	9 (2)	1.8 (0.4)
Covered by public health insurance	273 (7)	44.2 (1.1)	64 (3)	50.7 (2.3)	162 (7)	32.2 (1.4)
Medicaid	166 (7)	26.8 (1.1)	64 (3)	50.5 (2.3)	150 (7)	29.8 (1.3)
Medicare	130 (2)	21.1 (0.4)	1 (1)	1.2 (0.8)	20 (2)	4.0 (0.4)
VA Care	17 (2)	2.7 (0.3)	Z (Z)	0.1 (0.2)	6 (1)	1.2 (0.2)
Not covered at any time during the year	28 (3)	4.6 (0.4)	2 (1)	1.6 (0.6)	28 (3)	5.5 (0.5)

Note: Numbers in thousands; Figures cover civilian noninstitutionalized population in 2017; N/A indicates that data was not available; Z represents or rounds to zero; Margin of error appears in parenthesis and is calculated using replicate weights.
Source: U.S. Census Bureau, American Community Survey, Table HIC-4_ACS. Health Insurance Coverage Status and Type of Coverage by State—All People: 2008 to 2017, Table HIC-5_ACS. Health Insurance Coverage Status and Type of Coverage by State—Children Under 18: 2008 to 2017, Table HIC-6_ACS. Health Insurance Coverage Status and Type of Coverage by State—Persons Under 65: 2008 to 2017

Vermont

786 Blue Cross & Blue Shield of Vermont
445 Industrial Lane
Berlin, VT 05602
Phone: 802-223-6131
www.bcbsvt.com
Mailing Address: P.O. Box 186, Montpelier, VT 05601-0186
Subsidiary of: Blue Cross Blue Shield Association
Non-Profit Organization: Yes
Year Founded: 1944
Total Enrollment: 180,000
State Enrollment: 54,023

Healthplan and Services Defined
PLAN TYPE: PPO
Model Type: Network
Plan Specialty: Behavioral Health, Chiropractic, Disease
Management, PBM, Vision, UR
Benefits Offered: Behavioral Health, Chiropractic, Physical
Therapy, Prescription, Psychiatric, Vision, AD&D, Life,
LTD, STD, Alternative Healthcare discounts, Vermont
Medigap Blue

Type of Coverage
Commercial, Individual, Indemnity, Medicare, Supplemental
Medicare, Catastrophic
Catastrophic Illness Benefit: Maximum $1M

Type of Payment Plans Offered
Capitated

Geographic Areas Served
Statewide

Subscriber Information
Average Monthly Fee Per Subscriber
(Employee + Employer Contribution):
Employee Only (Self): Varies by plan
Average Annual Deductible Per Subscriber:
Employee Only (Self): $400.00
Employee & 1 Family Member: $400.00
Employee & 2 Family Members: $200.00
Average Subscriber Co-Payment:
Primary Care Physician: $10.00
Prescription Drugs: $10.00/20.00/35.00
Hospital ER: $50.00
Home Health Care: $40.00

Network Qualifications
Pre-Admission Certification: Yes

Peer Review Type
Utilization Review: Yes
Second Surgical Opinion: No
Case Management: Yes

Publishes and Distributes Report Card: No

Accreditation Certification
Utilization Review, State Licensure, Quality Assurance
Program

Key Personnel
President and CEO . . . . Don George
VP, Con Svcs & Planning . . . . Catherine Hamilton, PhD

Chief Marketing Executive . . . . Ellen Yakubik
VP, Finance/CFO . . . . Ruth K Greene

Average Claim Compensation
Physician's Fees Charged: 85%
Hospital's Fees Charged: 92%

Specialty Managed Care Partners
Magellan, Restat
Enters into Contracts with Regional Business Coalitions: Yes

787 Coventry Health Care of Vermont
6720-B Rockledge Drive
Suite 800
Bethesda, MD 20817
Phone: 301-581-0600
www.coventryhealthcare.com
Subsidiary of: Aetna Inc.
For Profit Organization: Yes

Healthplan and Services Defined
PLAN TYPE: HMO/PPO
Model Type: Network
Plan Specialty: Behavioral Health, Dental, Worker's
Compensation
Benefits Offered: Behavioral Health, Dental, Prescription,
Wellness, Worker's Compensation

Type of Coverage
Commercial, Medicare, Medicaid

Geographic Areas Served
Statewide

Key Personnel
Applications Development . . . . Chris Leavitt

788 Northeast Delta Dental Vermont
12 Bacon Street
Suite B
Burlington, VT 05401-6140
Phone: 802-658-7839
Fax: 802-865-4430
nedelta@nedelta.com
www.nedelta.com
Non-Profit Organization: Yes
Year Founded: 1961

Healthplan and Services Defined
PLAN TYPE: Dental
Other Type: Dental PPO
Plan Specialty: ASO, Dental
Benefits Offered: Dental

Type of Coverage
Commercial, Individual

Geographic Areas Served
Maine, New Hampshire, and Vermont

Key Personnel
President/CEO . . . . Thomas Raffio
Chair . . . . David A. Baasch, DDS
Vice Chair . . . . David Solomon, DDS
Treasurer . . . . Katherine A. O'Connell, CPA

Secretary . . . . Richard W. Park
Legal Counsel . . . . William Mason, Esq.
Senior Vice President . . . . William H. Lambrukos

---

789   UnitedHealthcare of Vermont

Warwick, VT 02886
Toll-Free: 888-545-5205
www.uhc.com
Subsidiary of: UnitedHealth Group
For Profit Organization: Yes
Year Founded: 1986

Healthplan and Services Defined
   PLAN TYPE: HMO/PPO
   Model Type: Network
   Plan Specialty: Behavioral Health, Dental, Disease
      Management, MSO, PBM, Vision
   Benefits Offered: Behavioral Health, Chiropractic,
      Complementary Medicine, Dental, Disease Management,
      Home Care, Inpatient SNF, Long-Term Care, Physical
      Therapy, Podiatry, Prescription, Psychiatric, Transplant,
      Vision, Wellness, AD&D, Life, LTD, STD

Type of Coverage
   Commercial, Individual, Medicare, Supplemental Medicare,
      Medicaid, Catastrophic, Family, Military, Veterans, Group,

Type of Payment Plans Offered
   DFFS, FFS, Combination FFS & DFFS

Geographic Areas Served
   Statewide. Vermont is covered by the Rhode Island branch

Subscriber Information
   Average Monthly Fee Per Subscriber
      (Employee + Employer Contribution):
         Employee Only (Self): Varies
   Average Subscriber Co-Payment:
         Primary Care Physician: $10
         Prescription Drugs: $10/15/30
         Hospital ER: $50

Network Qualifications
   Pre-Admission Certification: Yes

Peer Review Type
   Case Management: Yes

Publishes and Distributes Report Card: Yes

Accreditation Certification
   URAC, NCQA
   State Licensure, Quality Assurance Program

Average Claim Compensation
   Physician's Fees Charged: 70%
   Hospital's Fees Charged: 55%

Specialty Managed Care Partners
   United Behavioral Health
   Enters into Contracts with Regional Business Coalitions: No

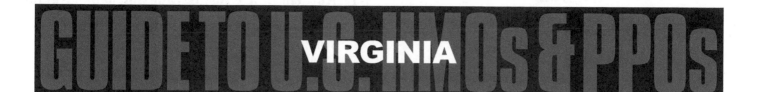

Health Insurance Coverage Status and Type of Coverage by Age

Category	All Persons		Under 18 years		Under 65 years	
	Number	%	Number	%	Number	%
Total population	8,257	-	1,983	-	7,013	-
Covered by some type of health insurance	7,528 (22)	91.2 (0.3)	1,882 (8)	94.9 (0.4)	6,295 (21)	89.8 (0.3)
Covered by private health insurance	6,293 (34)	76.2 (0.4)	1,403 (15)	70.7 (0.8)	5,431 (31)	77.5 (0.4)
Employer-based	4,920 (35)	59.6 (0.4)	1,131 (15)	57.0 (0.8)	4,443 (33)	63.4 (0.5)
Direct purchase	1,229 (23)	14.9 (0.3)	166 (9)	8.4 (0.4)	805 (22)	11.5 (0.3)
TRICARE	657 (16)	8.0 (0.2)	168 (9)	8.5 (0.5)	496 (16)	7.1 (0.2)
Covered by public health insurance	2,295 (24)	27.8 (0.3)	542 (15)	27.4 (0.7)	1,113 (23)	15.9 (0.3)
Medicaid	975 (22)	11.8 (0.3)	523 (15)	26.4 (0.7)	863 (21)	12.3 (0.3)
Medicare	1,375 (10)	16.6 (0.1)	17 (3)	0.9 (0.2)	194 (8)	2.8 (0.1)
VA Care	237 (7)	2.9 (0.1)	8 (2)	0.4 (0.1)	140 (6)	2.0 (0.1)
Not covered at any time during the year	729 (21)	8.8 (0.3)	101 (7)	5.1 (0.4)	718 (21)	10.2 (0.3)

Note: Numbers in thousands; Figures cover civilian noninstitutionalized population in 2017; N/A indicates that data was not available; Z represents or rounds to zero; Margin of error appears in parenthesis and is calculated using replicate weights.
Source: U.S. Census Bureau, American Community Survey, Table HIC-4_ACS. Health Insurance Coverage Status and Type of Coverage by State—All People: 2008 to 2017, Table HIC-5_ACS. Health Insurance Coverage Status and Type of Coverage by State—Children Under 18: 2008 to 2017, Table HIC-6_ACS. Health Insurance Coverage Status and Type of Coverage by State—Persons Under 65: 2008 to 2017

Virginia

790 Aetna Health of Virginia

9881 Mayland Drive
Richmond, CT 23233
Toll-Free: 855-463-0933
www.aetnabetterhealth.com/virginia
Mailing Address: P.O. Box 63518, Phoenix, AZ 85082-3518
Subsidiary of: Aetna Inc.
For Profit Organization: Yes
Year Founded: 1984

Healthplan and Services Defined
PLAN TYPE: HMO/PPO
Other Type: POS
Model Type: Network
Plan Specialty: Behavioral Health, Dental, EPO, Lab, PBM, Vision, Radiology
Benefits Offered: Behavioral Health, Dental, Disease Management, Long-Term Care, Physical Therapy, Podiatry, Prescription, Psychiatric, Vision, Wellness, Life, LTD, STD

Type of Coverage
Commercial, Medicaid, Catastrophic, Student health

Type of Payment Plans Offered
POS, DFFS

Geographic Areas Served
Alexandria City, Arlington, Fairfax, Fairfax City, Falls Church City, Loudoun, Stafford, Spotsylvania, Fredericksburg City, Prince William County, Manassas City, Manassas Park City, Winchester City, Frederick County, Clarke County, Shenandoah County, Warren County and Page County

Subscriber Information
Average Annual Deductible Per Subscriber:
Employee Only (Self): Varies
Employee & 1 Family Member: Varies
Employee & 2 Family Members: Varies
Medicare: Varies

Network Qualifications
Pre-Admission Certification: Yes

Peer Review Type
Utilization Review: No
Second Surgical Opinion: Yes
Case Management: Yes

Publishes and Distributes Report Card: Yes

Accreditation Certification
NCQA
TJC Accreditation, Utilization Review, Pre-Admission Certification, State Licensure, Quality Assurance Program

Key Personnel
CEO . . . . Todd White
CEO, Virginia Medicaid . . . . Roger Gunter
Dir., Medicaid Business . . . . Jann Anderson

Specialty Managed Care Partners
Enters into Contracts with Regional Business Coalitions: Yes

791 Anthem Blue Cross & Blue Shield of Virginia

2015 Staples Mill Road
Richmond, VA 23230
Toll-Free: 866-755-2680
Phone: 804-354-7000
www.anthem.com
For Profit Organization: Yes
Year Founded: 1980
Total Enrollment: 2,800,000
State Enrollment: 2,800,000

Healthplan and Services Defined
PLAN TYPE: HMO
Model Type: Network
Plan Specialty: ASO, Behavioral Health, Chiropractic, Dental, Disease Management, Lab, PBM, Vision, Radiology, Worker's Compensation, UR
Benefits Offered: Behavioral Health, Chiropractic, Dental, Disease Management, Home Care, Inpatient SNF, Physical Therapy, Podiatry, Prescription, Psychiatric, Transplant, Vision, Wellness, Worker's Compensation, Life

Type of Coverage
Commercial, Individual, Medicare, Catastrophic
Catastrophic Illness Benefit: Unlimited

Type of Payment Plans Offered
Capitated

Geographic Areas Served
All of Virginia except for the City of Fairfax, the Town of Vienna and the area east of State Route 123

Subscriber Information
Average Subscriber Co-Payment:
Primary Care Physician: $5.00/10.00
Prescription Drugs: $5.00/10.00
Hospital ER: $25.00
Home Health Care Max. Days/Visits Covered: 100 days

Peer Review Type
Case Management: Yes

Publishes and Distributes Report Card: Yes

Accreditation Certification
URAC, NCQA
TJC Accreditation, Medicare Approved, Utilization Review, Pre-Admission Certification, State Licensure, Quality Assurance Program

Key Personnel
President . . . . Jeff Ricketts
Corperate Communications . . . . Scott Golden
804-354-5252
scott.golden@anthem.com

Specialty Managed Care Partners
Enters into Contracts with Regional Business Coalitions: Yes

Employer References
Commonwealth of Virginia, GE

792 CareFirst Blue Cross & Blue Shield of Virginia

10780 Parkridge Boulevard
Suite 300
Reston, VA 20191
Toll-Free: 800-544-8703
www.carefirst.com
Non-Profit Organization: Yes
Year Founded: 1985
Number of Affiliated Hospitals: 165
Number of Primary Care Physicians: 4,500
Number of Referral/Specialty Physicians: 15,068
Total Enrollment: 3,400,000

Healthplan and Services Defined
PLAN TYPE: HMO/PPO
Model Type: IPA
Plan Specialty: ASO, Behavioral Health, Dental, Vision
Benefits Offered: Behavioral Health, Chiropractic, Dental, Disease Management, Home Care, Physical Therapy, Podiatry, Prescription, Psychiatric, Transplant, Vision, Wellness

Type of Coverage
Commercial, Individual

Type of Payment Plans Offered
POS

Geographic Areas Served
Arlington County and portions of Fairfax and Prince William counties east of State Route 123

Accreditation Certification
NCQA

793 Delta Dental of Virginia

4818 Starkey Road
Roanoke, VA 24018
Toll-Free: 800-237-6060
Phone: 540-989-8000
www.deltadentalva.com
Secondary Address: 4860 Cox Road, Suite 130, Glen Allen, VA 23060
Non-Profit Organization: Yes
Year Founded: 1964
Total Enrollment: 68,000,000
State Enrollment: 2,000,000

Healthplan and Services Defined
PLAN TYPE: Dental
Other Type: Dental PPO/POS
Plan Specialty: Dental
Benefits Offered: Dental

Type of Coverage
Commercial, Individual

Type of Payment Plans Offered
FFS

Geographic Areas Served
Statewide

Accreditation Certification
TJC

Key Personnel
President & CEO . . . . Frank Lucia
Chairman . . . . Lyn Brooks

794 Dominion Dental Services

251 18th Street South
Suite 900
Arlington, VA 22202
Toll-Free: 888-518-5338
www.dominionnational.com
Mailing Address: P.O. Box 1126, Claims/Utilization, Elk Grove Village, IL 60009
For Profit Organization: Yes
Year Founded: 1996
Physician Owned Organization: Yes
Total Enrollment: 24,000,000
State Enrollment: 490,000

Healthplan and Services Defined
PLAN TYPE: Dental
Plan Specialty: Dental
Benefits Offered: Dental

Type of Coverage
Commercial, Individual

Type of Payment Plans Offered
DFFS, Capitated, Combination FFS & DFFS

Geographic Areas Served
Maryland; Delaware; Pennsylvania; District of Columbia; Virginia and New Jersey

Network Qualifications
Pre-Admission Certification: Yes

Peer Review Type
Utilization Review: Yes
Case Management: Yes

Publishes and Distributes Report Card: No

Accreditation Certification
NCQA

Key Personnel
President and COO . . . . Mike Davis
VP of Business Management. . . . . Jay Rausch
VP of Operations. . . . . Ann Quinlan
VP of Accounting . . . . Dee Dee Brooks
Dental Director . . . . Wayne Silverman, DDS
Director of Marketing . . . . Jeff Schwab
Member Services . . . . Pete Harris

Specialty Managed Care Partners
Enters into Contracts with Regional Business Coalitions: Yes

795 EPIC Pharmacy Network

8703 Studley Road
Suite B
Mechanicsville, VA 23116-2016
Toll-Free: 800-876-3742
Phone: 804-559-4597
Fax: 804-559-2038
www.epicrx.com
Subsidiary of: EPIC Pharmacies, Inc.
For Profit Organization: Yes
Year Founded: 1992
Number of Primary Care Physicians: 1,400

Healthplan and Services Defined
PLAN TYPE: Multiple
Plan Specialty: PBM
Benefits Offered: Prescription

Geographic Areas Served
Mid-Atlantic states

Key Personnel
Chief Executive Officer . . . . Jay Romero
VP of Contracts . . . . Thomas E. Scono
Executive Vice President. . . . . Mark P Barwig

796 Evolent Health

800 N Gelebe Road
Suite 500
Arlington, VA 22203
Phone: 571-389-6000
Fax: 571-389-6001
info@evolenthealth.com
www.evolenthealth.com
For Profit Organization: Yes
Year Founded: 2011

Healthplan and Services Defined
PLAN TYPE: Multiple
Benefits Offered: Prescription

Type of Coverage
Commercial, Medicare, Medicaid

Geographic Areas Served
Virgina, California, and Illinois

Key Personnel
Co-Founder/CEO . . . . Frank Williams
Co-Founder/President . . . . Seth Blackley
Co-Founder/COO . . . . Tom Peterson
CIO. . . . . Anita Cattrell, PhD
CFO. . . . . Nicky McGrane
CMO. . . . . Andrew Snyder, MD
VP/CCO . . . . Jordan Flynn
Chief Customer Officer . . . . Robin Glass
Medical Info Officer. . . . . Jesse James, MD
Chief Technology Officer . . . . Chad Pomeroy
Chief Accounting Officer. . . . . Lydia Stone
EVP, Strategy. . . . . John Tam, MD
General Counsel . . . . Jonathan Weinberg

797 Humana Health Insurance of Virginia

4191 Innslake Drive
Suite 100
Glen Allen, VA 23060
Toll-Free: 800-350-7213
Phone: 804-253-0060
Fax: 804-217-6514
www.humana.com
Secondary Address: 3800 Electric Road, Suite 406, Roanoke, VA 24018, 540-772-5762
Subsidiary of: Humana
For Profit Organization: Yes

Healthplan and Services Defined
PLAN TYPE: HMO/PPO
Model Type: Network
Plan Specialty: Dental, Vision
Benefits Offered: Dental, Vision, Life, LTD, STD

Type of Coverage
Commercial, Individual

Geographic Areas Served
Statewide

Accreditation Certification
URAC, NCQA, CORE

Key Personnel
Market Manager . . . . Jose L. Cabrera, Jr.

798 MedCost Virginia

812 Moorefield Park Drive
Suite 204
Richmond, VA 23236
Phone: 804-320-3837
Fax: 804-320-5984
jhoover@vhn.com
www.vhn.com
For Profit Organization: Yes
Year Founded: 1988
Physician Owned Organization: No
Federally Qualified: No
Number of Primary Care Physicians: 75,000
Total Enrollment: 88,366
State Enrollment: 88,366

Healthplan and Services Defined
PLAN TYPE: PPO
Model Type: Network
Plan Specialty: Worker's Compensation, Medical PPO
Offers Demand Management Patient Information Service: No

Type of Coverage
Commercial

Geographic Areas Served
Virginia, North and South Carolina

Network Qualifications
Pre-Admission Certification: Yes

Publishes and Distributes Report Card: No

Accreditation Certification
Medicare; State License

TJC Accreditation, Medicare Approved, Utilization Review, State Licensure

Average Claim Compensation
Physician's Fees Charged: 79%
Hospital's Fees Charged: 67%

Specialty Managed Care Partners
Enters into Contracts with Regional Business Coalitions: Yes

---

799 Optima Health Plan

4417 Corporation Lane
Virginia Beach, VA 23462-3162
Toll-Free: 877-552-7401
Phone: 757-552-7401
members@optimahealth.com
www.optimahealth.com
Secondary Address: 1604 Santa Rosa Road, Suite 100, Richmond, VA 23229
Subsidiary of: Sentara Health Plans
Non-Profit Organization: Yes
Year Founded: 1984
Federally Qualified: Yes
Number of Affiliated Hospitals: 12
Number of Primary Care Physicians: 15,000
Number of Referral/Specialty Physicians: 3,870
Total Enrollment: 430,000
State Enrollment: 430,000

Healthplan and Services Defined
PLAN TYPE: HMO/PPO
Other Type: POS
Model Type: Network
Plan Specialty: ASO, Behavioral Health, Chiropractic, Dental, PBM, Vision
Benefits Offered: Behavioral Health, Chiropractic, Complementary Medicine, Dental, Disease Management, Home Care, Inpatient SNF, Long-Term Care, Physical Therapy, Podiatry, Prescription, Psychiatric, Transplant, Vision, Wellness
Offers Demand Management Patient Information Service: Yes
DMPI Services Offered: After hours nurse triage

Type of Coverage
Commercial, Individual, Medicare, Medicaid
Catastrophic Illness Benefit: Covered

Type of Payment Plans Offered
FFS

Geographic Areas Served
Selected counties in Virginia

Subscriber Information
Average Monthly Fee Per Subscriber
(Employee + Employer Contribution):
Employee Only (Self): Varies by plan
Medicare: Varies
Average Annual Deductible Per Subscriber:
Employee Only (Self): $0
Employee & 1 Family Member: $0
Employee & 2 Family Members: $0
Medicare: Varies

Average Subscriber Co-Payment:
Primary Care Physician: $15.00
Non-Network Physician: 70 %
Prescription Drugs: 50/20%
Hospital ER: 80%
Home Health Care: 80%

Network Qualifications
Pre-Admission Certification: Yes

Peer Review Type
Utilization Review: Yes
Second Surgical Opinion: No
Case Management: Yes

Accreditation Certification
URAC, NCQA

Key Personnel
President . . . . Dennis A. Matheis
SVP/CFO . . . . Andy Hilbert
SVP, Sales & Marketing . . . . John E. DeGruttola
SVP/CMO . . . . Thomas Lundquist, MD, FAAP

Specialty Managed Care Partners
Cole Vision, American Specialty Health, Doral Dental, Sentara Mental Health
Enters into Contracts with Regional Business Coalitions: Yes

Employer References
City of Virginia Beach, City of Norfolk, Bank of America, Nexcom, CHKD

---

800 Piedmont Community Health Plan

2316 Atherholt Road
Lynchburg, VA 24501
Toll-Free: 800-400-7247
Phone: 434-947-4463
www.pchp.net
Subsidiary of: Centra Health System
For Profit Organization: Yes
Year Founded: 1995
Physician Owned Organization: Yes
Total Enrollment: 30,000
State Enrollment: 30,000

Healthplan and Services Defined
PLAN TYPE: Multiple
Other Type: POS
Benefits Offered: Disease Management, Prescription, Wellness

Type of Payment Plans Offered
POS

Geographic Areas Served
Cities of Lynchburg and Bedford and the counties of Albemarle, Amherst, Appomattox, Bedford, Buchkingham, Campbell, Cumberland, Lunenburg, Nottoway and Price Edward

Key Personnel
Marketing Executive . . . . Lori Carter
434-947-4463

Specialty Managed Care Partners
Caremark Rx

801   United Concordia of Virginia
4860 Cox Road
Suite 200
Glen Allen, VA 23060
Phone: 804-217-8336
www.unitedconcordia.com
For Profit Organization: Yes
Year Founded: 1971
Total Enrollment: 7,800,000

Healthplan and Services Defined
  PLAN TYPE: Dental
  Plan Specialty: Dental
  Benefits Offered: Dental

Type of Coverage
  Commercial, Individual, Military personnel & families

Geographic Areas Served
  Nationwide

Accreditation Certification
  URAC

Key Personnel
  Contact. . . . . Beth Rutherford
    717-260-7659
    beth.rutherford@ucci.com

802   UnitedHealthcare of Virginia
9020 Stony Point Parkway
Richmond, VA 23235
Toll-Free: 888-545-5205
Phone: 804-267-5200
www.uhc.com
Subsidiary of: UnitedHealth Group
For Profit Organization: Yes

Healthplan and Services Defined
  PLAN TYPE: HMO/PPO
  Model Type: Network
  Plan Specialty: Behavioral Health, Dental, Disease
    Management, PBM, Vision
  Benefits Offered: Behavioral Health, Dental, Disease
    Management, Long-Term Care, Prescription, Vision,
    Wellness, Life, LTD, STD

Type of Coverage
  Individual, Medicare, Supplemental Medicare, Medicaid,
    Catastrophic, Family, Military, Veterans, Group,

Geographic Areas Served
  Statewide, and West Virgnia

Accreditation Certification
  TJC

Key Personnel
  VP, Sales & Marketing . . . . Chuck Rose, III

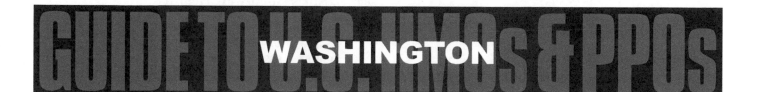
Health Insurance Coverage Status and Type of Coverage by Age

Category	All Persons		Under 18 years		Under 65 years	
	Number	%	Number	%	Number	%
Total population	7,300	-	1,740	-	6,202	-
Covered by some type of health insurance	6,854 *(15)*	93.9 *(0.2)*	1,694 *(7)*	97.4 *(0.3)*	5,763 *(15)*	92.9 *(0.2)*
Covered by private health insurance	5,169 *(34)*	70.8 *(0.5)*	1,093 *(17)*	62.8 *(1.0)*	4,466 *(32)*	72.0 *(0.5)*
Employer-based	4,168 *(34)*	57.1 *(0.5)*	937 *(17)*	53.9 *(0.9)*	3,826 *(32)*	61.7 *(0.5)*
Direct purchase	984 *(18)*	13.5 *(0.3)*	122 *(8)*	7.0 *(0.5)*	600 *(16)*	9.7 *(0.3)*
TRICARE	317 *(13)*	4.3 *(0.2)*	75 *(6)*	4.3 *(0.3)*	222 *(11)*	3.6 *(0.2)*
Covered by public health insurance	2,615 *(28)*	35.8 *(0.4)*	680 *(17)*	39.1 *(1.0)*	1,560 *(27)*	25.2 *(0.4)*
Medicaid	1,534 *(28)*	21.0 *(0.4)*	675 *(17)*	38.8 *(1.0)*	1,403 *(27)*	22.6 *(0.4)*
Medicare	1,211 *(9)*	16.6 *(0.1)*	9 *(2)*	0.5 *(0.1)*	158 *(7)*	2.6 *(0.1)*
VA Care	193 *(8)*	2.6 *(0.1)*	2 *(1)*	0.1 *(0.1)*	98 *(7)*	1.6 *(0.1)*
Not covered at any time during the year	446 *(15)*	6.1 *(0.2)*	46 *(5)*	2.6 *(0.3)*	439 *(15)*	7.1 *(0.2)*

Note: Numbers in thousands; Figures cover civilian noninstitutionalized population in 2017; N/A indicates that data was not available; Z represents or rounds to zero; Margin of error appears in parenthesis and is calculated using replicate weights.
Source: U.S. Census Bureau, American Community Survey, Table HIC-4_ACS. Health Insurance Coverage Status and Type of Coverage by State—All People: 2008 to 2017, Table HIC-5_ACS. Health Insurance Coverage Status and Type of Coverage by State—Children Under 18: 2008 to 2017, Table HIC-6_ACS. Health Insurance Coverage Status and Type of Coverage by State—Persons Under 65: 2008 to 2017

Washington

803 Aetna Health of Washington
151 Farmington Avenue
Hartford, CT 06156
Toll-Free: 800-872-3862
Phone: 860-273-0123
www.aetna.com
Subsidiary of: Aetna Inc.
For Profit Organization: Yes

Healthplan and Services Defined
PLAN TYPE: PPO
Other Type: POS
Model Type: Network
Plan Specialty: Behavioral Health, EPO, Lab, PBM,
   Radiology
Benefits Offered: Chiropractic, Dental, Disease Management,
   Home Care, Long-Term Care, Physical Therapy, Podiatry,
   Prescription, Vision

Type of Coverage
Commercial, Student Health

Type of Payment Plans Offered
Capitated

Geographic Areas Served
Statewide

Publishes and Distributes Report Card: Yes

Accreditation Certification
AAAHC

Key Personnel
Regional Head of Sales . . . . Clarence Williams

804 Amerigroup Washington
705 5th Avenue S
Suite 300
Seattle, WA 98104
Toll-Free: 800-600-4441
Phone: 206-623-1756
www.myamerigroup.com/wa
Subsidiary of: Anthem, Inc.
For Profit Organization: Yes

Healthplan and Services Defined
PLAN TYPE: Other
Model Type: Network
Plan Specialty: Disease Management, Managed health care
   for people in public programs.
Benefits Offered: Disease Management, Prescription

Type of Coverage
Medicaid

Geographic Areas Served
Statewide

Key Personnel
Plan President. . . . . Daryl Edmonds
Dir., Medicaid Operations . . . . Donnell Barnette

805 Asuris Northwest Health
528 E Spokane Falls Boulevard
Suite 301
Spokane, WA 99202
Toll-Free: 888-367-2109
www.asuris.com
Subsidiary of: Cambia Health Solutions
Non-Profit Organization: Yes
Year Founded: 1998
Total Enrollment: 71,000

Healthplan and Services Defined
PLAN TYPE: Multiple
Model Type: Network, TPA
Plan Specialty: ASO, Behavioral Health, Chiropractic,
   Disease Management, Lab, Vision, Radiology
Benefits Offered: Chiropractic, Dental, Disease Management,
   Home Care, Inpatient SNF, Physical Therapy, Podiatry,
   Prescription, Psychiatric, Vision, Wellness, AD&D, Life,
   LTD, STD

Type of Coverage
Individual, Medicare, Supplemental Medicare, Medicaid

Geographic Areas Served
Eastern Washington

Peer Review Type
Utilization Review: Yes
Second Surgical Opinion: Yes

Accreditation Certification
URAC
TJC Accreditation, Medicare Approved, State Licensure

Key Personnel
President . . . . Brady Cass

Average Claim Compensation
Physician's Fees Charged: 80%
Hospital's Fees Charged: 80%

806 Community Health Plan of Washington
1111 3rd Avenue
Suite 400
Seattle, WA 98101
Toll-Free: 800-440-1561
Phone: 206-652-7213
customercare@chpw.org
www.chpw.org
Non-Profit Organization: Yes
Year Founded: 1992
Number of Affiliated Hospitals: 100
Number of Primary Care Physicians: 2,500
Number of Referral/Specialty Physicians: 14,000
Total Enrollment: 300,000
State Enrollment: 300,000

Healthplan and Services Defined
PLAN TYPE: Multiple
Benefits Offered: Disease Management, Prescription,
   Wellness

Type of Coverage
Commercial, Individual, Medicare, Medicaid

Geographic Areas Served
38 counties in Washington State

Subscriber Information
Average Monthly Fee Per Subscriber
(Employee + Employer Contribution):
Employee Only (Self): Varies
Employee & 1 Family Member: Varies
Employee & 2 Family Members: Varies
Medicare: Varies
Average Annual Deductible Per Subscriber:
Employee Only (Self): Varies
Employee & 1 Family Member: Varies
Employee & 2 Family Members: Varies
Medicare: Varies
Average Subscriber Co-Payment:
Primary Care Physician: Varies
Non-Network Physician: Varies
Prescription Drugs: Varies
Hospital ER: Varies
Home Health Care: Varies
Home Health Care Max. Days/Visits Covered: Varies
Nursing Home: Varies
Nursing Home Max. Days/Visits Covered: Varies

Key Personnel
Chief Executive Officer . . . . Leanne Berge, Esq.
Chief Operating Officer . . . . Alan Lederman
Chief Financial Officer . . . . Stacy Kessel
Chief Medical Officer. . . . . Keith Brown, MD
Chief of Health Services . . . . Patty Jones
External Relations . . . . Abie Castillo
Media Contact . . . . Jackie Micucci
206-652-7213
jackie.micucci@chpw.org

Specialty Managed Care Partners
Express Scripts

---

807   Coventry Health Care of Washington
319 7th Avenue SE
Olympia, WA 98501
Phone: 360-787-2662
www.coventryhealthcare.com
Secondary Address: 5905 Pacific Highway East, Fife, WA
98424, 253-455-7193
Subsidiary of: Aetna Inc.
For Profit Organization: Yes

Healthplan and Services Defined
PLAN TYPE: HMO/PPO
Model Type: Network
Plan Specialty: Behavioral Health, Dental, Worker's
Compensation
Benefits Offered: Behavioral Health, Dental, Prescription,
Wellness, Worker's Compensation

Type of Coverage
Commercial, Medicare, Medicaid

Geographic Areas Served
Statewide

---

808   Delta Dental of Washington
P.O. Box 75688
Seattle, WA 98175
Toll-Free: 800-554-1907
www.deltadentalwa.com
Non-Profit Organization: Yes
Year Founded: 1954

Healthplan and Services Defined
PLAN TYPE: Dental
Other Type: Dental PPO
Model Type: Network
Plan Specialty: ASO, Dental
Benefits Offered: Dental

Type of Coverage
Commercial, Individual
Catastrophic Illness Benefit: None

Geographic Areas Served
Statewide

Key Personnel
President & CEO . . . . Jim Dwyer
COO & CFO . . . . Brad Berg
Human Resources . . . . Karen Aliabadi
VP, Underwriting. . . . . Eric Lo
Marketing & Sales Officer. . . . . Kristin Merlo

---

809   Dental Health Services of Washington
100 West Harrison Street
Suite S-440, South Tower
Seattle, WA 98119
Toll-Free: 800-637-6453
Phone: 206-633-2300
Fax: 206-624-8755
www.dentalhealthservices.com
For Profit Organization: Yes
Year Founded: 1974
Physician Owned Organization: Yes
Federally Qualified: Yes
Number of Primary Care Physicians: 1,000
Number of Referral/Specialty Physicians: 400
Total Enrollment: 90,000

Healthplan and Services Defined
PLAN TYPE: Dental
Model Type: Network
Plan Specialty: Dental
Benefits Offered: Dental

Type of Coverage
Commercial, Individual
Catastrophic Illness Benefit: None

Geographic Areas Served
california, Washington, and Oregon

Subscriber Information
Average Monthly Fee Per Subscriber
(Employee + Employer Contribution):
Employee Only (Self): Varies
Employee & 1 Family Member: Varies
Employee & 2 Family Members: Varies

Network Qualifications
Pre-Admission Certification: Yes

Key Personnel
Founder . . . . Godfrey Pernell

810   First Choice Health

600 Univeristy Street
Suite 1400
Seattle, WA 98101-3129
Toll-Free: 800-467-5281
Fax: 206-667-8062
contact@fchn.com
www.fchn.com
Secondary Address: 120 W Cataldo Avenue, Suite 200,
Spokane, WA 99201, 509-227-5700
For Profit Organization: Yes
Year Founded: 1996
Number of Affiliated Hospitals: 94
Number of Primary Care Physicians: 980
Number of Referral/Specialty Physicians: 1,793

Healthplan and Services Defined
PLAN TYPE: PPO
Benefits Offered: Wellness

Type of Coverage
Commercial, Individual, Private & Public Plans, Geo-specifi

Geographic Areas Served
Washington, Oregon, Alaska, Idaho, Montana, Wyoming, and
select areas of North Dakota and South Dakota

Key Personnel
Marketing/Sales Officer . . . . Curtis Taylor

811   Humana Health Insurance of Washington

1498 SE Tech Center Place
Suite 300
Vancouver, WA 98683
Toll-Free: 800-781-4203
Phone: 360-253-7523
Fax: 360-253-7524
www.humana.com
Subsidiary of: Humana
For Profit Organization: Yes

Healthplan and Services Defined
PLAN TYPE: HMO/PPO
Model Type: Network
Plan Specialty: Dental, Vision
Benefits Offered: Dental, Disease Management, Prescription,
Vision, Wellness, Life, LTD, STD

Type of Coverage
Commercial, Medicare

Geographic Areas Served
Statewide

Accreditation Certification
URAC, NCQA, CORE

Key Personnel
Market President. . . . . Catherine Field

812   LifeWise

7001 220th Street SW
Building 1
Mountlake Terrace, WA 98043
Toll-Free: 800-592-6804
www.lifewisewa.com
Mailing Address: P.O. Box 91059, Seattle, WA 98111-9159
For Profit Organization: Yes
Year Founded: 1986
Number of Primary Care Physicians: 9,000
Total Enrollment: 1,900,000

Healthplan and Services Defined
PLAN TYPE: PPO
Benefits Offered: Acupuncture, Naturopathy

Geographic Areas Served
Washington and Alaska

Accreditation Certification
NCQA

Key Personnel
President & CEO . . . . Jim Havens

813   Molina Healthcare of Washington

21540 30th Drive SE
Suite 400
Bothell, WA 98021
Toll-Free: 800-869-7175
www.molinahealthcare.com
Mailing Address: P.O. Box 4004, Bothell, WA 98041-4004
Subsidiary of: Molina Healthcare, Inc.
For Profit Organization: Yes

Healthplan and Services Defined
PLAN TYPE: Medicare
Model Type: Network
Plan Specialty: Dental, PBM, Vision, Integrated
Medicare/Medicaid (Duals)
Benefits Offered: Dental, Prescription, Vision, Wellness, Life

Type of Coverage
Individual, Medicare, Supplemental Medicare, Medicaid

Geographic Areas Served
Statewide

Key Personnel
Chief Medical Officer . . . . Frances Gough
VP, Network Management . . . . Laurel Lee
Strategic Initiatives. . . . . Mark Bigelow

814   Soundpath Health

33820 Weyerhaeuser Way S
Suite 200
Federal Way, WA 98001
Toll-Free: 866-789-7747
Fax: 844-612-4062
www.soundpathhealth.com
Mailing Address: P.O. Box 27510, Federal Way, WA 98093
Subsidiary of: Catholic Health Initiatives
Year Founded: 2007
Number of Affiliated Hospitals: 76

Total Enrollment: 17,000
State Enrollment: 17,000

Healthplan and Services Defined
PLAN TYPE: Medicare

Type of Coverage
Medicare

Accreditation Certification
TJC, URAC

Key Personnel
President/CEO .... Steve Schramm

815 United Concordia of Washington
4401 Deer Path Road
Harrisburg, PA 17110
Phone: 717-260-6800
www.unitedconcordia.com
For Profit Organization: Yes
Year Founded: 1971
Total Enrollment: 7,800,000

Healthplan and Services Defined
PLAN TYPE: Dental
Plan Specialty: Dental
Benefits Offered: Dental

Type of Coverage
Commercial, Individual, Military personnel & families

Geographic Areas Served
Nationwide

Accreditation Certification
URAC

Key Personnel
Contact............................ Beth Rutherford
717-260-7659
beth.rutherford@ucci.com

816 UnitedHealthcare of Washington
1212 N Washington Street
Suite 307
Spokane, WA 99201
Toll-Free: 888-545-5205
Phone: 509-324-7172
www.uhc.com
Secondary Address: 7525 SE 24th Street, Mercer Island, WA
98040, 206-519-6472
Subsidiary of: UnitedHealth Group
For Profit Organization: Yes

Healthplan and Services Defined
PLAN TYPE: HMO/PPO
Model Type: Network
Plan Specialty: Behavioral Health, Dental, Disease
Management, PBM, Vision
Benefits Offered: Behavioral Health, Dental, Disease
Management, Long-Term Care, Prescription, Vision,
Wellness, Life, LTD, STD

Type of Coverage
Individual, Medicare, Supplemental Medicare, Medicaid,
Catastrophic, Family, Military, Veterans, Group,

Geographic Areas Served
Washington and Montana

Accreditation Certification
URAC

Key Personnel
VP, Sales & Marketing .... David Hansen

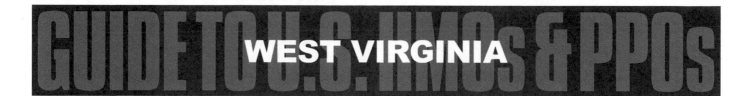
Health Insurance Coverage Status and Type of Coverage by Age

Category	All Persons		Under 18 years		Under 65 years	
	Number	%	Number	%	Number	%
Total population	1,787	-	399	-	1,445	-
Covered by some type of health insurance	1,678 *(7)*	93.9 *(0.4)*	389 *(4)*	97.4 *(0.5)*	1,337 *(7)*	92.5 *(0.5)*
Covered by private health insurance	1,108 *(16)*	62.0 *(0.9)*	214 *(6)*	53.5 *(1.6)*	891 *(15)*	61.6 *(1.0)*
Employer-based	937 *(16)*	52.4 *(0.9)*	196 *(6)*	49.1 *(1.6)*	802 *(15)*	55.5 *(1.0)*
Direct purchase	185 *(7)*	10.4 *(0.4)*	16 *(3)*	3.9 *(0.6)*	93 *(6)*	6.4 *(0.4)*
TRICARE	37 *(4)*	2.1 *(0.2)*	6 *(2)*	1.6 *(0.5)*	20 *(3)*	1.4 *(0.2)*
Covered by public health insurance	852 *(14)*	47.6 *(0.8)*	196 *(8)*	49.1 *(1.8)*	516 *(14)*	35.7 *(1.0)*
Medicaid	498 *(14)*	27.9 *(0.8)*	196 *(8)*	49.0 *(1.8)*	457 *(14)*	31.6 *(0.9)*
Medicare	411 *(5)*	23.0 *(0.3)*	1 *(Z)*	0.2 *(0.1)*	76 *(4)*	5.3 *(0.3)*
VA Care	60 *(4)*	3.3 *(0.2)*	Z *(Z)*	0.1 *(0.1)*	24 *(3)*	1.6 *(0.2)*
Not covered at any time during the year	109 *(7)*	6.1 *(0.4)*	11 *(2)*	2.6 *(0.5)*	108 *(7)*	7.5 *(0.5)*

Note: Numbers in thousands; Figures cover civilian noninstitutionalized population in 2017; N/A indicates that data was not available; Z represents or rounds to zero; Margin of error appears in parenthesis and is calculated using replicate weights.
Source: U.S. Census Bureau, American Community Survey, Table HIC-4_ACS. Health Insurance Coverage Status and Type of Coverage by State—All People: 2008 to 2017, Table HIC-5_ACS. Health Insurance Coverage Status and Type of Coverage by State—Children Under 18: 2008 to 2017, Table HIC-6_ACS. Health Insurance Coverage Status and Type of Coverage by State—Persons Under 65: 2008 to 2017

West Virginia

817 Aetna Health of West Virginia
500 Virginia Street East
Suite 400
Charleston, WV 25301
Toll-Free: 888-348-2922
Fax: 844-255-7027
www.aetnabetterhealth.com/westvirginia
Mailing Address: P.O. Box 67450, Phoenix, AZ 85082-7450
Subsidiary of: Aetna Inc.
For Profit Organization: Yes

Healthplan and Services Defined
PLAN TYPE: PPO
Other Type: POS
Model Type: Network
Plan Specialty: Behavioral Health, EPO, Lab, PBM, Radiology
Benefits Offered: Behavioral Health, Dental, Disease Management, Long-Term Care, Physical Therapy, Podiatry, Prescription, Psychiatric, Vision, Wellness, Life, LTD, STD

Type of Coverage
Commercial, Student health

Geographic Areas Served
Statewide

Key Personnel
CEO . . . . Todd White
Senior Compliance Lead. . . . . Fuzzy Page

818 CareSource West Virginia
230 N Main Street
Dayton, OH 45402
Phone: 937-224-3300
www.caresource.com
Non-Profit Organization: Yes
Total Enrollment: 1,000,000

Healthplan and Services Defined
PLAN TYPE: Medicare

Type of Coverage
Medicare, Medicaid

Geographic Areas Served
West Virginia counties: Barbour, Boone, Calhoun, Clay, Doddridge, Fayette, Gilmer, Harrison, Jackson, Logan, Marion, Monongalia, Pleasants, Preston, Raleigh, Ritchie, Roane, Taylor, Tyler, Wetzel, Wirt and Wood

819 Delta Dental of West Virginia
One Delta Drive
Mechanicsburg, PA 17055-6999
Toll-Free: 800-932-0783
www.deltadentalins.com
Mailing Address: P.O. Box 1803, Alpharetta, GA 30023
Non-Profit Organization: Yes

Healthplan and Services Defined
PLAN TYPE: Dental
Other Type: Dental PPO
Plan Specialty: Dental
Benefits Offered: Dental

Type of Coverage
Commercial, Individual

Geographic Areas Served
Statewide

Key Personnel
President/CEO. . . . . Tony Barth
Chief Financial Officer . . . . Mike Castro
Chief Legal Officer. . . . . Mike Hankinson
Chief Operating Officer . . . . Nilesh Patel
EVP, Sales & Marketing . . . . Belinda Martinez

820 Highmark BCBS West Virginia
300 Wharton Circle
Suite 150
Triadelphia, WV 26059
Toll-Free: 800-876-7639
Phone: 412-544-0100
www.highmarkbcbswv.com
Secondary Address: Fifth Avenue Place, 120 Fifth Avenue, Pittsburgh, PA 15222-3099, 412-544-7000
Subsidiary of: Highmark, Inc.
For Profit Organization: Yes
Year Founded: 1932
Number of Affiliated Hospitals: 65
Number of Primary Care Physicians: 1,400
Number of Referral/Specialty Physicians: 3,200
Total Enrollment: 5,300,000
State Enrollment: 500,000

Healthplan and Services Defined
PLAN TYPE: PPO
Model Type: Network, PPO, POS, TPA
Plan Specialty: ASO, Behavioral Health, Chiropractic, EPO, Lab, Radiology, UR, Case Management
Benefits Offered: Behavioral Health, Chiropractic, Home Care, Inpatient SNF, Long-Term Care, Physical Therapy, Podiatry, Prescription, Psychiatric, Transplant

Type of Coverage
Commercial, Individual, Supplemental Medicare

Type of Payment Plans Offered
POS, DFFS

Geographic Areas Served
West Virginia and Washington County, Ohio

Network Qualifications
Pre-Admission Certification: Yes

Peer Review Type
Utilization Review: Yes
Second Surgical Opinion: Yes
Case Management: Yes

Publishes and Distributes Report Card: No

Accreditation Certification
URAC

Key Personnel
President . . . . Deborah L. Rice-Johnson
Chief Medical Officer . . . . Charles Deshazer
Chief Executive Officer . . . . David L. Holmberg

Specialty Managed Care Partners
WV University, Charleston Area Medical Center (CAMC)
Enters into Contracts with Regional Business Coalitions: No

821 Humana Health Insurance of West Virginia

Toll-Free: 800-951-0130
Phone: 304-925-0972
Fax: 304-925-0976
www.humana.com
Subsidiary of: Humana
For Profit Organization: Yes

Healthplan and Services Defined
PLAN TYPE: HMO/PPO
Model Type: Network
Plan Specialty: Dental, Vision
Benefits Offered: Dental, Vision, Life, LTD, STD

Type of Coverage
Commercial

Geographic Areas Served
Statewide

Accreditation Certification
URAC, NCQA

Key Personnel
Director of Sales, KY/WV . . . . Gary Wilson

822 Molina Medicaid Solutions

1600 Pennsylvania Avenue
Charleston, WV 25302
Phone: 304-348-3200
molinahealthcare.com
Subsidiary of: Molina Healthcare, Inc.
For Profit Organization: Yes
Year Founded: 1980

Healthplan and Services Defined
PLAN TYPE: Medicare
Plan Specialty: Dental, PBM, Vision, Intergrated
Medicaid/Medicare (Duals)
Benefits Offered: Dental, Prescription, Vision, Wellness, Life

Geographic Areas Served
Statewide

Key Personnel
Plan President. . . . . Robert Hager
Regional CEO . . . . Karen Hoylman
Business Development. . . . . Michael Culleton

823 Mountain Health Trust/Physician Assured Access System

231 Capitol Street
Suite 310
Charleston, WV 25301
Toll-Free: 800-449-8466
Fax: 304-345-1581
www.mountainhealthtrust.com
Year Founded: 1996

Healthplan and Services Defined
PLAN TYPE: HMO
Benefits Offered: Dental, Disease Management, Home Care,
Inpatient SNF, Prescription, Vision, Wellness, Hearing;
Durable Medical Equipment; Midwife Services

Type of Coverage
Medicaid

Geographic Areas Served
Statewide

824 UniCare West Virginia

200 Association Drive
Suite 200
Charleston, WV 25311
Toll-Free: 888-611-9958
www.unicare.com
Subsidiary of: Anthem, Inc.
For Profit Organization: Yes
Year Founded: 1985
Number of Affiliated Hospitals: 102
Number of Primary Care Physicians: 3,500
Number of Referral/Specialty Physicians: 8,000
Total Enrollment: 80,000

Healthplan and Services Defined
PLAN TYPE: Multiple
Model Type: Network
Plan Specialty: Dental, Vision
Benefits Offered: Chiropractic, Dental, Physical Therapy,
Prescription, Vision, Life

Type of Coverage
Medicare, Supplemental Medicare, Medicaid

Geographic Areas Served
Statewide

Subscriber Information
Average Monthly Fee Per Subscriber
(Employee + Employer Contribution):
Employee Only (Self): Varies
Employee & 1 Family Member: Varies
Employee & 2 Family Members: Varies
Medicare: Varies
Average Annual Deductible Per Subscriber:
Employee Only (Self): Varies
Employee & 1 Family Member: Varies
Employee & 2 Family Members: Varies
Medicare: Varies
Average Subscriber Co-Payment:
Primary Care Physician: Varies
Non-Network Physician: Varies

Prescription Drugs: Varies
Hospital ER: Varies
Home Health Care: Varies
Home Health Care Max. Days/Visits Covered: Varies
Nursing Home: Varies
Nursing Home Max. Days/Visits Covered: Varies

Network Qualifications
Pre-Admission Certification: Yes

Peer Review Type
Utilization Review: Yes
Second Surgical Opinion: Yes
Case Management: Yes

Publishes and Distributes Report Card: No

Accreditation Certification
URAC
TJC Accreditation, Medicare Approved, Utilization Review,
Pre-Admission Certification, State Licensure, Quality
Assurance Program

Key Personnel
President . . . . John Mitch Collins
Chief Operating Officer . . . . Tadd Haynes
Dir., Medicaid Plan Mkt . . . . Billie Moore

---

825   UnitedHealthcare of West Virginia
9020 Stony Point Parkway
Richmond, VA 23235
Toll-Free: 888-545-5202
Phone: 804-267-5200
www.uhc.com
Subsidiary of: UnitedHealth Group
Year Founded: 1977

Healthplan and Services Defined
PLAN TYPE: HMO/PPO
Model Type: Network
Plan Specialty: Behavioral Health, Dental, Disease
Management, Lab, PBM, Vision, Radiology
Benefits Offered: Behavioral Health, Chiropractic, Dental,
Disease Management, Long-Term Care, Physical Therapy,
Prescription, Vision, Wellness, AD&D, Life, LTD, STD

Type of Coverage
Commercial, Individual, Indemnity, Medicare, Supplemental
Medicare, Medicaid, Catastrophic, Family, Military,
Veterans, Group,

Geographic Areas Served
Statewide. West Virginia is covered by the Virginia branch

Network Qualifications
Pre-Admission Certification: Yes

Peer Review Type
Utilization Review: Yes
Second Surgical Opinion: Yes
Case Management: Yes

Publishes and Distributes Report Card: Yes

Accreditation Certification
TJC, NCQA

Key Personnel
VP, Sales & Marketing . . . . Chuck Rose

Specialty Managed Care Partners
Enters into Contracts with Regional Business Coalitions: Yes

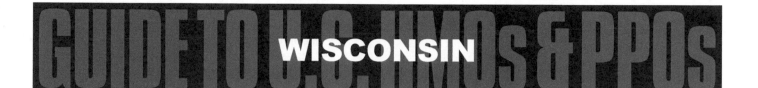
Health Insurance Coverage Status and Type of Coverage by Age

Category	All Persons		Under 18 years		Under 65 years	
	Number	%	Number	%	Number	%
Total population	5,724	-	1,362	-	4,796	-
Covered by some type of health insurance	5,415 *(11)*	94.6 *(0.2)*	1,309 *(6)*	96.1 *(0.3)*	4,490 *(11)*	93.6 *(0.2)*
Covered by private health insurance	4,306 *(23)*	75.2 *(0.4)*	952 *(12)*	69.9 *(0.9)*	3,714 *(22)*	77.4 *(0.5)*
Employer-based	3,569 *(25)*	62.4 *(0.4)*	882 *(12)*	64.8 *(0.8)*	3,321 *(25)*	69.2 *(0.5)*
Direct purchase	833 *(15)*	14.5 *(0.3)*	75 *(5)*	5.5 *(0.4)*	449 *(13)*	9.4 *(0.3)*
TRICARE	81 *(5)*	1.4 *(0.1)*	12 *(2)*	0.9 *(0.1)*	48 *(4)*	1.0 *(0.1)*
Covered by public health insurance	1,873 *(21)*	32.7 *(0.4)*	429 *(13)*	31.5 *(0.9)*	969 *(21)*	20.2 *(0.4)*
Medicaid	978 *(21)*	17.1 *(0.4)*	424 *(13)*	31.1 *(0.9)*	864 *(21)*	18.0 *(0.4)*
Medicare	1,038 *(7)*	18.1 *(0.1)*	9 *(2)*	0.7 *(0.1)*	135 *(6)*	2.8 *(0.1)*
VA Care	136 *(5)*	2.4 *(0.1)*	1 *(Z)*	0.1 *(Z)*	54 *(3)*	1.1 *(0.1)*
Not covered at any time during the year	309 *(11)*	5.4 *(0.2)*	53 *(4)*	3.9 *(0.3)*	306 *(11)*	6.4 *(0.2)*

Note: Numbers in thousands; Figures cover civilian noninstitutionalized population in 2017; N/A indicates that data was not available; Z represents or rounds to zero; Margin of error appears in parenthesis and is calculated using replicate weights.
Source: U.S. Census Bureau, American Community Survey, Table HIC-4_ACS. Health Insurance Coverage Status and Type of Coverage by State—All People: 2008 to 2017, Table HIC-5_ACS. Health Insurance Coverage Status and Type of Coverage by State—Children Under 18: 2008 to 2017, Table HIC-6_ACS. Health Insurance Coverage Status and Type of Coverage by State—Persons Under 65: 2008 to 2017

Wisconsin

826 Aetna Health of Wisconsin
151 Farmington Avenue
Hartford, CT 06156
Toll-Free: 800-872-3862
Phone: 860-273-0123
www.aetna.com
Subsidiary of: Aetna Inc.
For Profit Organization: Yes

Healthplan and Services Defined
PLAN TYPE: PPO
Other Type: POS
Plan Specialty: Behavioral Health, EPO, Lab, PBM,
Radiology
Benefits Offered: Behavioral Health, Dental, Disease
Management, Long-Term Care, Physical Therapy,
Podiatry, Prescription, Psychiatric, Wellness, Life, LTD,
STD

Type of Coverage
Commercial, Student health

Type of Payment Plans Offered
POS, FFS

Geographic Areas Served
Statewide

Key Personnel
Sales Director . . . . Syd Warner

827 American Family Insurance
6000 Madison Parkway
Madison, WI 53783
Toll-Free: 800-692-6326
www.amfam.com

Healthplan and Services Defined
PLAN TYPE: Multiple
Benefits Offered: Life

Type of Coverage
Commercial, Individual, Supplemental Medicare, Short-term

Geographic Areas Served
Arizona, Colorado, Georgia, Idaho, Illinois, Indiana, Iowa,
Kansas, Minnesota, Missouri, Nebraska, Nevada, North
Dakota, Ohio, Oregon, South Dakota, Utah, Washington,
Wisconsin

Key Personnel
Chairman, President & CEO . . . . Jack Salzwedel

828 Anthem Blue Cross & Blue Shield of Wisconsin
6775 W Washington Street
Milwaukee, WI 53214
Phone: 414-459-5057
www.anthem.com
Secondary Address: 480 Pilgrim Way, Green Bay, WI 54304
Subsidiary of: Anthem, Inc.
For Profit Organization: Yes

Healthplan and Services Defined
PLAN TYPE: HMO/PPO
Model Type: Network
Plan Specialty: ASO, Behavioral Health, Chiropractic, Dental,
Disease Management, Lab, PBM, Vision, Radiology,
Worker's Compensation, UR
Benefits Offered: Behavioral Health, Chiropractic, Dental,
Disease Management, Home Care, Inpatient SNF, Physical
Therapy, Podiatry, Prescription, Psychiatric, Transplant,
Vision, Wellness, Worker's Compensation, Life

Type of Coverage
Commercial, Individual, Medicare, Supplemental Medicare,
Medicaid, Catastrophic

Geographic Areas Served
Statewide

Accreditation Certification
URAC, NCQA

Key Personnel
President . . . . Paul Nobile

829 Ascension At Home
Affinity Home Care Plus
2074 American Drive, Suite A
Neenah, WI 54956
Phone: 920-735-8100
Fax: 920-735-8101
ascensionathome.com
Subsidiary of: Ascension
Non-Profit Organization: Yes

Healthplan and Services Defined
PLAN TYPE: Other
Plan Specialty: Disease Management
Benefits Offered: Dental, Disease Management, Home Care,
Wellness, Ambulance & Transportation; Nursing Service;
Short-and-long-term care management planning; Hospice

Geographic Areas Served
Texas, Alabama, Indiana, Kansas, Michigan, Mississippi,
Oklahoma, wisconsin

Key Personnel
President . . . . Kirk Allen
Dir., Home Health Service . . . . Darcy Burthay

830 Assurant Employee Benefits Wisconsin
125 N Executive Drive
Brookfield, WI 53005
Phone: 262-798-0280
www.assurantemployeebenefits.com
Subsidiary of: Sun Life Financial, US
For Profit Organization: Yes

Healthplan and Services Defined
PLAN TYPE: Multiple
Plan Specialty: Dental, Vision
Benefits Offered: Dental, Disease Management, Vision,
Wellness, AD&D, Life, LTD, STD

Type of Coverage
Commercial, Individual

Geographic Areas Served
Statewide

Subscriber Information
Average Monthly Fee Per Subscriber
(Employee + Employer Contribution):
Employee Only (Self): Varies by plan

Accreditation Certification
URAC, NCQA

Key Personnel
President.............................. Dan Fishbein
Senior Vice President .... Kevin Krzeminski
Human Resources..................... Kathy deCastro
Marketing............................. Ed Milano
Chairman .... William Anderson

---

831 Care Plus Dental Plans

205 E Wisconsin Avenue
Milwaukee, WI 53202
Toll-Free: 800-318-7007
Phone: 414-778-3600
www.careplusdentalplans.com
Subsidiary of: Dental Associates Ltd
Non-Profit Organization: Yes
Year Founded: 1983
Physician Owned Organization: Yes
Total Enrollment: 200,000

Healthplan and Services Defined
PLAN TYPE: Dental
Model Type: Staff
Plan Specialty: Dental
Benefits Offered: Dental, Prescription

Type of Coverage
Commercial, Individual

Type of Payment Plans Offered
Capitated

Geographic Areas Served
Appleton, Fond Du Lac, Green Bay, Greenville, Kenosha, Milwaukee & Waukesha

Peer Review Type
Utilization Review: Yes

Accreditation Certification
AAAHC

Key Personnel
Sales Account Executive .... Eileen Murphy
Business Development.................. James Schmitz
Sr. Client Service Mgn .... Branda Boyd

---

832 ChiroCare of Wisconsin

3300 Fernbrook Lane
Suite 150
Plymouth, WI 55447
Toll-Free: 800-397-1541
Phone: 414-476-4733
www.chirocare.com
Subsidiary of: Fulcrum Health, Inc.

Non-Profit Organization: Yes
Year Founded: 1986
Total Enrollment: 150,000

Healthplan and Services Defined
PLAN TYPE: PPO
Model Type: IPA, Network
Plan Specialty: Chiropractic, Complimentary Medicine Networks
Benefits Offered: Chiropractic

Type of Coverage
Commercial, Indemnity, Medicare, Supplemental Medicare, Medicaid

Type of Payment Plans Offered
POS, DFFS, Capitated, FFS, Combination FFS & DFFS

Geographic Areas Served
Statewide

Network Qualifications
Pre-Admission Certification: Yes

Peer Review Type
Utilization Review: Yes
Second Surgical Opinion: Yes
Case Management: Yes

Accreditation Certification
URAC, NCQA
Quality Assurance Program

Key Personnel
CEO .... Patricia Dennis

---

833 Coventry Health Care of Wisconsin

1238 Market Place
Waukesha, WI 53189
Phone: 262-650-9221
www.coventryhealthcare.com
Secondary Address: 242 N Broadway, Milwaukee, MI 53202, 414-395-8643
Subsidiary of: Aetna Inc.
For Profit Organization: Yes

Healthplan and Services Defined
PLAN TYPE: HMO/PPO
Model Type: Network
Plan Specialty: Behavioral Health, Dental, Worker's Compensation
Benefits Offered: Behavioral Health, Dental, Prescription, Wellness, Worker's Compensation

Type of Coverage
Commercial, Medicare, Medicaid

Geographic Areas Served
Statewide

---

834 Dean Health Plan

1277 Deming Way
Madison, WI 53717
Toll-Free: 866-794-3326
www.deancare.com
Mailing Address: P.O. Box 56099, Madison, WI 53705

For Profit Organization: Yes
Year Founded: 1983
Physician Owned Organization: Yes
Federally Qualified: Yes
Number of Affiliated Hospitals: 26
Number of Primary Care Physicians: 1,500
Total Enrollment: 247,881

Healthplan and Services Defined
  PLAN TYPE: Multiple
  Model Type: Network
  Benefits Offered: Behavioral Health, Chiropractic, Dental,
    Disease Management, Home Care, Inpatient SNF, Physical
    Therapy, Podiatry, Prescription, Psychiatric, Transplant,
    Vision, Wellness
  Offers Demand Management Patient Information Service:
    Yes
  DMPI Services Offered: On Call Nurse Line

Type of Coverage
  Commercial, Individual, Indemnity, Medicare, Supplemental
    Medicare, Medicaid

Type of Payment Plans Offered
  Capitated

Geographic Areas Served
  20 counties in Southern Wisconsin

Subscriber Information
  Average Monthly Fee Per Subscriber
    (Employee + Employer Contribution):
      Employee Only (Self): Varies
      Employee & 1 Family Member: Varies
      Employee & 2 Family Members: Varies
      Medicare: Varies
  Average Annual Deductible Per Subscriber:
      Employee Only (Self): Varies
      Employee & 1 Family Member: Varies
      Employee & 2 Family Members: Varies
      Medicare: Varies
  Average Subscriber Co-Payment:
      Primary Care Physician: Varies
      Non-Network Physician: Varies
      Prescription Drugs: Varies
      Hospital ER: Varies
      Home Health Care: Varies
      Home Health Care Max. Days/Visits Covered: Varies
      Nursing Home: Varies
      Nursing Home Max. Days/Visits Covered: Varies

Network Qualifications
  Pre-Admission Certification: Yes

Peer Review Type
  Utilization Review: Yes

Publishes and Distributes Report Card: Yes

Accreditation Certification
  NCQA

Key Personnel
  President . . . . David Fields
  Executive Director . . . . David Docherty
  Director of Compliance . . . . Stephanie Cook
  VP of Operations. . . . . Marcus Julian

Chief Medical Offier . . . . Dr. Julia Wright
Chief Financial Officer. . . . . Randy Ruplinger

Specialty Managed Care Partners
  Enters into Contracts with Regional Business Coalitions: No

Employer References
  State of Wisconsin Employees

---

835 Delta Dental of Wisconsin
P.O. Box 828
Stevens Point, WI 54481-0828
Toll-Free: 800-236-3712
www.deltadentalwi.com
Non-Profit Organization: Yes
Year Founded: 1962

Healthplan and Services Defined
  PLAN TYPE: Dental
  Other Type: Dental PPO
  Model Type: Network
  Plan Specialty: Dental, Vision
  Benefits Offered: Dental, Vision

Type of Coverage
  Commercial, Individual

Type of Payment Plans Offered
  POS, FFS

Geographic Areas Served
  Statewide

Peer Review Type
  Case Management: Yes

Publishes and Distributes Report Card: No

Accreditation Certification
  TJC

Key Personnel
  Executive VP. . . . . Dennis Peterson
  Director of Sales . . . . Kim Christophersen
  Chief Actuary. . . . . Scott Meyer
  Director, IT . . . . Michael Upright

Specialty Managed Care Partners
  Enters into Contracts with Regional Business Coalitions: No

---

836 Dental Protection Plan
7130 W Greenfield Avenue
West Allis, WI 53214-4708
Phone: 414-259-9522
www.bayviewdentalcare.com
Subsidiary of: Bayview Dental Care
Year Founded: 1987

Healthplan and Services Defined
  PLAN TYPE: Dental
  Other Type: Dental HMO
  Plan Specialty: Dental
  Benefits Offered: Dental

Geographic Areas Served
  Nationwide

Subscriber Information
Average Monthly Fee Per Subscriber
(Employee + Employer Contribution):
Employee Only (Self): $35/year

Peer Review Type
Case Management: Yes

Publishes and Distributes Report Card: Yes

---

837 Group Health Cooperative of Eau Claire

2503 N Hillcrest Parkway
Altoona, WI 54702
Toll-Free: 888-203-7770
Phone: 715-552-4300
Fax: 715-836-7683
www.group-health.com
Non-Profit Organization: Yes
Year Founded: 1976
Number of Primary Care Physicians: 7,700
Total Enrollment: 75,000

Healthplan and Services Defined
PLAN TYPE: HMO
Model Type: Network
Benefits Offered: Dental, Disease Management, Prescription,
Wellness, Comprehensive Health
Offers Demand Management Patient Information Service:
Yes
DMPI Services Offered: FirstCare Nurseline

Type of Coverage
Commercial, Medicaid, SSI
Catastrophic Illness Benefit: Varies per case

Geographic Areas Served
Barron, Buffalo, Chippewa, Clark, Dunn, Eau Claire,
Jackson, Pepin, Rusk, Sawyer, Taylor, Trempealeau,
Washburn, Ashland, Bayfield, Douglas, Burnett, Polk, St.
Croix, Pierce, LaCrosse, Monroe, Juneau, Veronn, Crawford,
Richland, Sauk, Columbia, Grant, Iowa, Lafayette, Green
counties

Peer Review Type
Utilization Review: Yes
Second Surgical Opinion: Yes
Case Management: Yes

Publishes and Distributes Report Card: Yes

Accreditation Certification
AAAHC
TJC Accreditation, Medicare Approved, Utilization Review,
State Licensure, Quality Assurance Program

Key Personnel
General Manager & CEO . . . . Peter Farrow
Chief Medical Officer . . . . Michele Bauer, MD
Chief Financial Officer . . . . Bob Tanner

Specialty Managed Care Partners
CMS, OMNE
Enters into Contracts with Regional Business Coalitions: Yes

---

838 Group Health Cooperative of South Central Wisconsin

1265 John Q Hammons Drive
Madison, WI 53717-1962
Toll-Free: 800-605-4327
Phone: 608-828-4853
member_services@ghcscw.com
www.ghcscw.com
Non-Profit Organization: Yes
Year Founded: 1976
Owned by an Integrated Delivery Network (IDN): Yes
Federally Qualified: Yes
Total Enrollment: 80,000

Healthplan and Services Defined
PLAN TYPE: HMO
Model Type: Staff
Plan Specialty: Dental, Lab, Vision, Radiology
Benefits Offered: Chiropractic, Disease Management,
Physical Therapy, Prescription, Vision, Wellness,
Acupuncture
Offers Demand Management Patient Information Service: Yes

Type of Coverage
Commercial, Medicare, Medicaid

Type of Payment Plans Offered
DFFS, Capitated

Geographic Areas Served
Dane County

Publishes and Distributes Report Card: Yes

Accreditation Certification
AAAHC, NCQA
Medicare Approved, Utilization Review, Pre-Admission
Certification, State Licensure, Quality Assurance Program

Key Personnel
Chair . . . . Ann Hoyt
Vice Chair . . . . Henry Sanders
Treasurer . . . . Bill Oemichen
Secretary . . . . Donna Twining
President/CEO . . . . Mark Huth, MD
CMO . . . . Chris Kastman, MD
CFO . . . . Bruce Quade
CIO . . . . Annette Fox

Specialty Managed Care Partners
UW Hospitals
Enters into Contracts with Regional Business Coalitions: Yes

---

839 Gundersen Lutheran Health Plan

2651 Midwest Drive
Onalaska, WI 54650
Toll-Free: 800-362-3310
customerservice@quartzbenefits.com
www.gundersenhealthplan.org
Secondary Address: 840 Carolina Street, Sauk City, WI 53583
Subsidiary of: Quartz Health Solutions, Inc
Non-Profit Organization: Yes
Year Founded: 1995
Physician Owned Organization: Yes

Federally Qualified: Yes
Number of Affiliated Hospitals: 14
Number of Primary Care Physicians: 850
Number of Referral/Specialty Physicians: 200
Total Enrollment: 90,000
State Enrollment: 90,000

Healthplan and Services Defined
  PLAN TYPE: HMO
  Other Type: POS
  Model Type: Network
  Plan Specialty: ASO, Behavioral Health, Chiropractic,
    Disease Management, Lab, PBM, Radiology, UR
  Benefits Offered: Behavioral Health, Chiropractic, Disease
    Management, Home Care, Inpatient SNF, Physical
    Therapy, Podiatry, Prescription, Psychiatric, Transplant,
    Vision, Wellness, AD&D
  Offers Demand Management Patient Information Service:
    Yes
  DMPI Services Offered: Nurse Advisor Line

Type of Coverage
  Commercial, Individual, Medicare

Geographic Areas Served
  Western Wisconsin

Subscriber Information
  Average Monthly Fee Per Subscriber
    (Employee + Employer Contribution):
      Employee Only (Self): Varies
  Average Annual Deductible Per Subscriber:
    Employee & 2 Family Members: Varies

Accreditation Certification
  TJC, URAC, NCQA
  Pre-Admission Certification

---

840   Health Tradition

1808 East Main Street
Onalaska, WI 54650
Toll-Free: 888-459-3020
Phone: 608-781-9692
www.healthtradition.com
For Profit Organization: Yes
Year Founded: 1986
Number of Affiliated Hospitals: 17
Number of Primary Care Physicians: 800
Number of Referral/Specialty Physicians: 100
Total Enrollment: 34,000
State Enrollment: 40,000

Healthplan and Services Defined
  PLAN TYPE: HMO
  Model Type: Group
  Benefits Offered: Disease Management, Prescription,
    Wellness
  Offers Demand Management Patient Information Service:
    Yes
  DMPI Services Offered: 24 hour nurse line

Type of Coverage
  Medicare, Medicaid
  Catastrophic Illness Benefit: Maximum $2M

Type of Payment Plans Offered
  POS, Combination FFS & DFFS

Geographic Areas Served
  Iowa: Allamakee; Minnesota: Houston; Buffalo, Crawford,
  Fillmore, Jackson, La Crosse, Monroe, Trempealeau, Vernon,
  Winneshiek, Winona counties

Subscriber Information
  Average Monthly Fee Per Subscriber
    (Employee + Employer Contribution):
      Employee Only (Self): Varies by plan
  Average Annual Deductible Per Subscriber:
    Employee Only (Self): $50.00
    Employee & 1 Family Member: $100.00
    Employee & 2 Family Members: $150.00
  Average Subscriber Co-Payment:
    Primary Care Physician: $0
    Prescription Drugs: $11.00
    Hospital ER: $25.00-50.00
    Home Health Care: $0
    Home Health Care Max. Days/Visits Covered: 345 days
    Nursing Home: $0
    Nursing Home Max. Days/Visits Covered: 60 days

Network Qualifications
  Pre-Admission Certification: Yes

Peer Review Type
  Utilization Review: Yes
  Second Surgical Opinion: Yes
  Case Management: Yes

Publishes and Distributes Report Card: No

Accreditation Certification
  TJC Accreditation, Medicare Approved, Utilization Review,
    Pre-Admission Certification, State Licensure, Quality
    Assurance Program

Key Personnel
  Director/Sales & Market . . . . Michael Eckstein

Average Claim Compensation
  Physician's Fees Charged: 85%
  Hospital's Fees Charged: 85%

Specialty Managed Care Partners
  Franciscon Scam Health Care
  Enters into Contracts with Regional Business Coalitions: No

---

841   Humana Health Insurance of Wisconsin

N19W24133 Riverwood Drive
Suite 300
Waukesha, WI 53188
Toll-Free: 800-289-0260
Phone: 262-408-4300
Fax: 920-632-9508
www.humana.com
For Profit Organization: Yes
Year Founded: 1985
Physician Owned Organization: Yes

Healthplan and Services Defined
  PLAN TYPE: HMO/PPO
  Model Type: IPA, Network

Plan Specialty: UR
Benefits Offered: Behavioral Health, Chiropractic, Dental, Disease Management, Home Care, Inpatient SNF, Physical Therapy, Podiatry, Prescription, Psychiatric, Transplant, Vision, Wellness, Worker's Compensation, AD&D, Life, LTD
Offers Demand Management Patient Information Service: Yes

Type of Coverage
Commercial, Individual

Type of Payment Plans Offered
POS, DFFS, Capitated, FFS, Combination FFS & DFFS

Geographic Areas Served
Dodge, Jefferson, Kenosha, Milwaukee, Ozaukee, Racine, Sheboygan, Walworth, Washington, Fond du Luc, Green, Montowoe, Rock & Waukesha counties

Peer Review Type
Utilization Review: Yes
Second Surgical Opinion: Yes
Case Management: Yes

Accreditation Certification
AAAHC, URAC, NCQA, CORE

Key Personnel
VP, Provider Development . . . . Mark Wernicke

Specialty Managed Care Partners
Aurora Behavioral, Chirotech, Accordant, Health Service

842 Managed Health Services
10700 W Research Drive
Wauwatosa, WI 53226
Toll-Free: 888-713-6180
www.mhswi.com
For Profit Organization: Yes
Year Founded: 1984
Number of Affiliated Hospitals: 57
Number of Primary Care Physicians: 5,500
Number of Referral/Specialty Physicians: 1,255
Total Enrollment: 130,000
State Enrollment: 164,700

Healthplan and Services Defined
PLAN TYPE: HMO
Model Type: IPA, Network
Benefits Offered: Disease Management, Prescription, Wellness
Offers Demand Management Patient Information Service: Yes

Type of Coverage
Medicare, Medicaid
Catastrophic Illness Benefit: Varies per case

Type of Payment Plans Offered
POS, FFS

Geographic Areas Served
22 counties in Wisconsin, Northern Indiana, and Illinois, Racine, Kenosha; Indiana: Indianapolis; Illinois: Chicago

Subscriber Information
Average Monthly Fee Per Subscriber
(Employee + Employer Contribution):
Employee Only (Self): Varies
Employee & 1 Family Member: Varies
Employee & 2 Family Members: Varies
Medicare: Varies
Average Annual Deductible Per Subscriber:
Employee Only (Self): Varies
Employee & 1 Family Member: Varies
Employee & 2 Family Members: Varies
Medicare: Varies
Average Subscriber Co-Payment:
Primary Care Physician: $10.00/15.00
Non-Network Physician: 100%
Prescription Drugs: $5.00/10.00
Hospital ER: $25.00
Home Health Care: $0

Network Qualifications
Pre-Admission Certification: Yes

Peer Review Type
Utilization Review: Yes

Publishes and Distributes Report Card: Yes

Accreditation Certification
NCQA
TJC Accreditation, Medicare Approved, Utilization Review, Pre-Admission Certification, State Licensure, Quality Assurance Program

Key Personnel
Chairman . . . . John Finerty, Jr.
President & CEO . . . . Sherry Husa

Specialty Managed Care Partners
Enters into Contracts with Regional Business Coalitions: Yes

843 MercyHealth System
1000 Mineral Point Avenue
Janesville, WI 53547
Toll-Free: 888-396-3729
Phone: 815-971-5000
mercyhealthsystem.org
Non-Profit Organization: Yes
Year Founded: 1889
Number of Affiliated Hospitals: 5
Number of Primary Care Physicians: 650

Healthplan and Services Defined
PLAN TYPE: HMO
Benefits Offered: Disease Management, Orthopedic surgery; neurosurgery; cancer care; plastic/reconstructive sergery; trauma centers

Geographic Areas Served
Southern Wisconsin and Northern Illinois counties

Key Personnel
President & CEO . . . . Javon R. Bea

844 Molina Healthcare of Wisconsin

11200 W Parkland Avenue
Milwaukee, WI 53224
Toll-Free: 888-999-2404
www.molinahealthcare.com
Subsidiary of: Molina Healthcare, Inc.
For Profit Organization: Yes

Healthplan and Services Defined
PLAN TYPE: Medicare
Model Type: Network
Plan Specialty: Dental, PBM, Vision, Integrated
    Medicare/Medicaid (Duals)
Benefits Offered: Dental, Prescription, Vision, Wellness, Life

Type of Coverage
Individual, Medicare, Supplemental Medicare, Medicaid

Geographic Areas Served
Statewide

Key Personnel
Healthcare Services Mgr. . . . . Linda Murphy
Chief Medical Officer . . . . Raymond Zastrow
VP, Provider Network . . . . Melissa Henderson
Dir., Provider Contracts . . . . Christina Weickardt

845 Network Health Plan of Wisconsin

1570 Midway Place
Menasha, WI 54952
Toll-Free: 800-826-0940
Phone: 920-720-1300
www.networkhealth.com
Subsidiary of: Affinity Health System
For Profit Organization: Yes
Year Founded: 1982
Total Enrollment: 118,000
State Enrollment: 67,812

Healthplan and Services Defined
PLAN TYPE: HMO
Model Type: Group, Network
Plan Specialty: Behavioral Health, Chiropractic, Disease
    Management, Lab
Benefits Offered: Chiropractic, Disease Management,
    Prescription, Wellness, Maternity care

Type of Coverage
Commercial, Medicare, Medicaid

Type of Payment Plans Offered
POS, Combination FFS & DFFS

Geographic Areas Served
Brown, Calumet, Dodge, Door, Fond du Lac, Green Lake,
Kewaunee, Manitowoc, Marquette, Outagamie, Portage,
Shawano, Sheboygan, Waupaca, Waushara, Winnebago
counties

Subscriber Information
Average Monthly Fee Per Subscriber
    (Employee + Employer Contribution):
        Employee Only (Self): Varies
        Employee & 1 Family Member: Varies
        Employee & 2 Family Members: Varies

Medicare: Varies
Average Annual Deductible Per Subscriber:
    Employee Only (Self): Varies
    Employee & 1 Family Member: Varies
    Employee & 2 Family Members: Varies
    Medicare: Varies
Average Subscriber Co-Payment:
    Primary Care Physician: $10.00
    Prescription Drugs: $5.00-7.00
    Home Health Care: $0

Network Qualifications
Pre-Admission Certification: Yes

Peer Review Type
Utilization Review: Yes
Second Surgical Opinion: No
Case Management: Yes

Publishes and Distributes Report Card: Yes

Accreditation Certification
NCQA
TJC Accreditation, Medicare Approved, Utilization Review,
    Pre-Admission Certification, State Licensure, Quality
    Assurance Program

Key Personnel
President/CEO . . . . Coreen Dicus-Johnson
CFO. . . . . Brian Ollech
CAO. . . . . Penny Ransom
General Counsel. . . . . Kathryn Finerty
CMO . . . . Gregory Buran, MD
Chief Actuary . . . . Kevin Borchert

Specialty Managed Care Partners
Enters into Contracts with Regional Business Coalitions: Yes

846 Physicians Plus Insurance Corporation

2650 Novation Parkway
Madison, WI 53713
Toll-Free: 800-545-5015
Phone: 608-282-8900
ppicinfo@QuartzBenefits.com
www.pplusic.com
Mailing Address: P.O. Box 2078, Madison, WI 53701
Subsidiary of: Quartz Health Solutions Inc
For Profit Organization: Yes
Year Founded: 1986
Physician Owned Organization: Yes
Number of Primary Care Physicians: 4,900
Total Enrollment: 112,000
State Enrollment: 112,000

Healthplan and Services Defined
PLAN TYPE: HMO/PPO
Other Type: POS
Model Type: Network
Plan Specialty: Behavioral Health, Chiropractic, Dental,
    Disease Management, Lab, X-Ray
Benefits Offered: Behavioral Health, Chiropractic, Dental,
    Disease Management, Home Care, Inpatient SNF, Physical
    Therapy, Podiatry, Prescription, Transplant, Vision,
    Wellness, Durable Medical Equipment

Type of Coverage
Individual, Supplemental Medicare, Commercial Small
Group, Large Group
Catastrophic Illness Benefit: Covered

Type of Payment Plans Offered
Capitated, FFS, Combination FFS & DFFS

Geographic Areas Served
South Central Wisconsin

Subscriber Information
Average Monthly Fee Per Subscriber
(Employee + Employer Contribution):
Employee Only (Self): Varies by plan
Average Annual Deductible Per Subscriber:
Employee Only (Self): Varies by plan
Employee & 1 Family Member: $0
Employee & 2 Family Members: $0
Medicare: $0
Average Subscriber Co-Payment:
Primary Care Physician: Varies by plan
Hospital ER: $100.00
Home Health Care Max. Days/Visits Covered: 100 visits
Nursing Home Max. Days/Visits Covered: 100 days

Network Qualifications
Pre-Admission Certification: Yes

Peer Review Type
Utilization Review: Yes
Second Surgical Opinion: Yes
Case Management: Yes

Publishes and Distributes Report Card: Yes

Accreditation Certification
NCQA
State Licensure, Quality Assurance Program

Key Personnel
Medical Director . . . . Jason Yelk
Assistant VP, Marketing . . . . Jennifer Woomer Dinehart
608-821-1082

Average Claim Compensation
Physician's Fees Charged: 70%
Hospital's Fees Charged: 75%

Specialty Managed Care Partners
Enters into Contracts with Regional Business Coalitions: No

---

847 Prevea Health Network
P.O. Box 19070
Green Bay, WI 54307
Toll-Free: 888-277-3832
Phone: 920-496-4700
www.prevea.com
For Profit Organization: Yes
Year Founded: 1996
Number of Affiliated Hospitals: 14
Number of Primary Care Physicians: 1,602
Total Enrollment: 119,712
State Enrollment: 15,706

Healthplan and Services Defined
PLAN TYPE: PPO

Model Type: Group
Plan Specialty: UR
Benefits Offered: Behavioral Health, Chiropractic, Disease
Management, Home Care, Prescription, Transplant,
Wellness, Allergy; Asthma; Cancer Rehab; Cardiac;
Dermatology; Lab & Pathology; Pediatric; Reconstructive
Plastic Surgery

Type of Coverage
Commercial, Supplemental Medicare

Geographic Areas Served
Northeast Wisconsin and Western Wisconsin's Chippewa
Valley region

Subscriber Information
Average Annual Deductible Per Subscriber:
Employee Only (Self): $0
Employee & 1 Family Member: $0
Employee & 2 Family Members: $0
Medicare: $0
Average Subscriber Co-Payment:
Primary Care Physician: $0

Accreditation Certification
TJC
Pre-Admission Certification

Key Personnel
President/CEO . . . . Ashok Rai, MD
VP/CMO . . . . Gregory Grose, MD
SVP/CFO . . . . Lorrie Jacobetti
SVP/COO . . . . Brian Charlier
SVP/HR/Risk Management . . . . Samantha Tonn
SVP/General Counsel . . . . Larry Gille
VP, Chief Quality Officer . . . . Paul Pritchard, MD
VP, Strategy/Development . . . . Kaitlin Brice
CIO . . . . Shane Miller

Specialty Managed Care Partners
Express Scripts

---

848 Security Health Plan of Wisconsin
1515 Saint Joseph Avenue
P.O. Box 8000
Marshfield, WI 54449-8000
Toll-Free: 800-472-2363
Phone: 715-221-9555
Fax: 715-221-9500
www.securityhealth.org
Non-Profit Organization: Yes
Year Founded: 1986
Physician Owned Organization: Yes
Total Enrollment: 187,000
State Enrollment: 187,000

Healthplan and Services Defined
PLAN TYPE: Multiple
Model Type: Network
Plan Specialty: Behavioral Health, Chiropractic, Disease
Management, EPO, Lab, PBM, Vision, Radiology, Worker's
Compensation, UR
Benefits Offered: Behavioral Health, Chiropractic,
Complementary Medicine, Dental, Disease Management,

Home Care, Inpatient SNF, Long-Term Care, Podiatry, Prescription, Psychiatric, Transplant, Vision, Wellness, Worker's Compensation, AD&D, Durable Medical Equipment

Offers Demand Management Patient Information Service: Yes

DMPI Services Offered: Nurse Line, Health Information Line

Type of Coverage
Commercial, Individual, Indemnity, Medicare, Supplemental Medicare, Medicaid, TPA
Catastrophic Illness Benefit: Covered

Type of Payment Plans Offered
Capitated, FFS

Geographic Areas Served
Northern, Western and Central Wisconsin

Subscriber Information
Average Monthly Fee Per Subscriber
(Employee + Employer Contribution):
Employee Only (Self): Varies by plan
Average Annual Deductible Per Subscriber:
Employee Only (Self): $200.00
Employee & 2 Family Members: $100.00
Medicare: $0
Average Subscriber Co-Payment:
Primary Care Physician: $20.00
Non-Network Physician: $20.00
Prescription Drugs: $3.00
Hospital ER: $50.00
Home Health Care: $0
Home Health Care Max. Days/Visits Covered: 40 days
Nursing Home: $0
Nursing Home Max. Days/Visits Covered: 30 days

Network Qualifications
Pre-Admission Certification: No

Peer Review Type
Utilization Review: Yes

Publishes and Distributes Report Card: Yes

Accreditation Certification
NCQA
Medicare Approved, Pre-Admission Certification

Key Personnel
Medical Director . . . . Robert Steiner, MD
Chief Medical Officer . . . . Eric Quivers
Dir., Population Health . . . . Melissa DeGoede
Asst. Director of Claims . . . . Stephanie Bauer
Applications Development . . . . Roshan Lenora
Communications Manager . . . . Rebecca Normington
715-221-9726
normington.rebecca@securityhealth.org

Specialty Managed Care Partners
Enters into Contracts with Regional Business Coalitions: Yes

849 Trilogy Health Insurance
18000 West Sarah Lane
Suite 310
Brookfield, WI 53045
Toll-Free: 866-429-3241
Phone: 262-432-9140
www.trilogycares.com
For Profit Organization: Yes
Number of Affiliated Hospitals: 86
Number of Primary Care Physicians: 3,700
Total Enrollment: 5,000

Healthplan and Services Defined
PLAN TYPE: PPO
Other Type: HSA
Benefits Offered: Disease Management, Prescription, Wellness
Offers Demand Management Patient Information Service: Yes
DMPI Services Offered: 24-Hour Nurse Line

Type of Coverage
Commercial

Accreditation Certification
URAC

850 UnitedHealthcare of Wisconsin
3100 Ams Boulevard
Green Bay, WI 54313
Toll-Free: 800-291-2634
www.uhc.com
Secondary Address: 10701 Research Drive, Wauwatosa, WI 53226, 414-443-4000
Subsidiary of: UnitedHealth Group
For Profit Organization: Yes

Healthplan and Services Defined
PLAN TYPE: HMO/PPO
Model Type: Network
Plan Specialty: Behavioral Health, Dental, Disease Management, PBM, Vision
Benefits Offered: Behavioral Health, Dental, Disease Management, Long-Term Care, Prescription, Vision, Wellness, Life, LTD, STD

Type of Coverage
Commercial, Individual, Medicare, Supplemental Medicare, Medicaid, Catastrophic, Family, Military, Veterans, Group,

Geographic Areas Served
Statewide

Key Personnel
President/CEO, WI/MI . . . . Dustin Hinton

851 Unity Health Insurance
840 Carolina Street
Sauk City, WI 53583
Toll-Free: 800-362-3310
Phone: 608-644-3430
unityhealth.com
Subsidiary of: Quartz Health Solutions, Inc
For Profit Organization: Yes

Year Founded: 1994
Number of Affiliated Hospitals: 44
Number of Primary Care Physicians: 908
Number of Referral/Specialty Physicians: 3,227
Total Enrollment: 90,000
State Enrollment: 75,000

Healthplan and Services Defined
  PLAN TYPE: Multiple
  Model Type: Network
  Benefits Offered: Behavioral Health, Chiropractic, Dental,
    Disease Management, Home Care, Inpatient SNF, Physical
    Therapy, Podiatry, Prescription, Psychiatric, Transplant,
    Vision, Wellness

Type of Coverage
  Commercial, Individual, Medicare, Medicaid

Type of Payment Plans Offered
  POS, DFFS, FFS, Combination FFS & DFFS

Geographic Areas Served
  20 counties in Southwestern and South Central Wisconsin

Network Qualifications
  Pre-Admission Certification: Yes

Peer Review Type
  Utilization Review: Yes
  Second Surgical Opinion: Yes
  Case Management: Yes

Publishes and Distributes Report Card: Yes

Accreditation Certification
  NCQA
  Medicare Approved, Utilization Review, Pre-Admission
    Certification, State Licensure, Quality Assurance Program

Key Personnel
  President/CEO .... Terry Bolz
  Chief Operating Office .... Gail Midlikowski
  Chief Medical Officer .... Gary Lenth
  VP/CFO/Treasurer .... Jim Hiveley

Specialty Managed Care Partners
  Behavioral Health Consultation System, UW Hospital and
    Clinics, APS Healthcare
  Enters into Contracts with Regional Business Coalitions: No

Employer References
  University of Wisconsin Medical Foundation, Middleton
    Cross Plains School District, Rockwell Automation,
    Brakebush Brothers, Epic Systemss Corporation

---

852 Wisconsin Physician's Service
1717 West Broadway
P.O. Box 8190
Madison, WI 53708-8190
Toll-Free: 888-915-4001
Fax: 608-223-3639
www.wpshealth.com
Non-Profit Organization: Yes
Year Founded: 1946
Owned by an Integrated Delivery Network (IDN): Yes
Number of Affiliated Hospitals: 129

Number of Primary Care Physicians: 14,500
Total Enrollment: 175,000
State Enrollment: 223,000

Healthplan and Services Defined
  PLAN TYPE: Multiple
  Model Type: Network
  Plan Specialty: ASO, Behavioral Health, Chiropractic, Dental,
    Disease Management, EPO, Lab, PBM, Vision, Radiology,
    Worker's Compensation, UR, Rational Med
  Benefits Offered: Behavioral Health, Chiropractic, Dental,
    Disease Management, Home Care, Inpatient SNF, Physical
    Therapy, Podiatry, Prescription, Psychiatric, Transplant,
    Vision, Wellness, AD&D, Life, LTD, STD
  Offers Demand Management Patient Information Service: Yes

Type of Coverage
  Commercial, Individual, Indemnity, Medicare, Supplemental
    Medicare, Catastrophic
  Catastrophic Illness Benefit: Varies per case

Type of Payment Plans Offered
  POS, DFFS

Subscriber Information
  Average Annual Deductible Per Subscriber:
    Employee Only (Self): $0
    Employee & 1 Family Member: $0
    Employee & 2 Family Members: $0
    Medicare: $0

Peer Review Type
  Case Management: Yes

Publishes and Distributes Report Card: Yes

Accreditation Certification
  AAAHC, URAC
  Medicare Approved, Utilization Review, State Licensure,
    Quality Assurance Program

Key Personnel
  President and CEO .... Mike Hamerlik
  Chief Financial Officer .... Vicki Bernards
  Administrative Officer .... Craig Campbell
  VP, Government Relations .... Rob Palmer

Specialty Managed Care Partners
  Delta Dental
  Enters into Contracts with Regional Business Coalitions: Yes

Employer References
  US Department of Defense

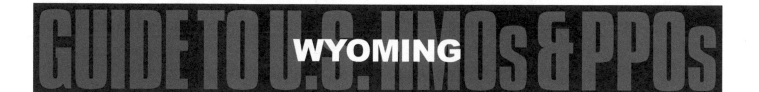
Health Insurance Coverage Status and Type of Coverage by Age

Category	All Persons		Under 18 years		Under 65 years	
	Number	%	Number	%	Number	%
Total population	569	-	146	-	481	-
Covered by some type of health insurance	499 (7)	87.7 (1.2)	132 (3)	90.5 (2.0)	411 (7)	85.5 (1.4)
Covered by private health insurance	412 (9)	72.5 (1.7)	102 (5)	70.1 (3.0)	354 (9)	73.6 (1.9)
Employer-based	325 (9)	57.2 (1.6)	88 (5)	60.5 (3.1)	301 (9)	62.5 (1.8)
Direct purchase	89 (5)	15.6 (0.9)	12 (2)	8.4 (1.5)	53 (5)	11.0 (0.9)
TRICARE	20 (3)	3.6 (0.6)	5 (2)	3.3 (1.1)	14 (3)	2.9 (0.6)
Covered by public health insurance	161 (6)	28.3 (1.1)	35 (4)	23.7 (2.6)	75 (6)	15.5 (1.2)
Medicaid	69 (6)	12.2 (1.0)	34 (4)	23.5 (2.6)	62 (6)	12.8 (1.2)
Medicare	98 (2)	17.3 (0.4)	Z (Z)	0.3 (0.3)	12 (2)	2.6 (0.4)
VA Care	19 (2)	3.4 (0.3)	Z (Z)	0.1 (0.1)	8 (2)	1.8 (0.3)
Not covered at any time during the year	70 (7)	12.3 (1.2)	14 (3)	9.5 (2.0)	70 (7)	14.5 (1.4)

Note: Numbers in thousands; Figures cover civilian noninstitutionalized population in 2017; N/A indicates that data was not available; Z represents or rounds to zero; Margin of error appears in parenthesis and is calculated using replicate weights.
Source: U.S. Census Bureau, American Community Survey, Table HIC-4_ACS. Health Insurance Coverage Status and Type of Coverage by State—All People: 2008 to 2017, Table HIC-5_ACS. Health Insurance Coverage Status and Type of Coverage by State—Children Under 18: 2008 to 2017, Table HIC-6_ACS. Health Insurance Coverage Status and Type of Coverage by State—Persons Under 65: 2008 to 2017

Wyoming

853 Aetna Health of Wyoming

151 Farmington Avenue
Hartford, CT 06156
Toll-Free: 800-872-3862
Phone: 860-273-0123
www.aetna.com
Subsidiary of: Aetna Inc.
For Profit Organization: Yes

Healthplan and Services Defined
PLAN TYPE: PPO
Other Type: POS
Model Type: Network
Plan Specialty: Behavioral Health, EPO, Lab, PBM, Radiology
Benefits Offered: Behavioral Health, Dental, Disease Management, Long-Term Care, Physical Therapy, Podiatry, Prescription, Psychiatric, Wellness, Life, LTD, STD

Type of Coverage
Commercial, Student health

Type of Payment Plans Offered
POS, FFS

Geographic Areas Served
Statewide

Key Personnel
Director, Underwriting . . . . Brad Gunnell

854 Blue Cross & Blue Shield of Wyoming

4000 House Avenue
Cheyenne, WY 82001
Toll-Free: 800-442-2376
www.bcbswy.com
Non-Profit Organization: Yes
Year Founded: 1976
Total Enrollment: 100,000
State Enrollment: 100,000

Healthplan and Services Defined
PLAN TYPE: HMO
Benefits Offered: Disease Management, Physical Therapy, Wellness

Type of Coverage
Commercial, Individual, Medicare, Medicaid

Type of Payment Plans Offered
FFS

Geographic Areas Served
Statewide

Key Personnel
President/CEO . . . . Rick Schum
CFO. . . . . Diane Gore
VP, Marketing/Sales . . . . Lee Shannon

Specialty Managed Care Partners
Prime Therapeutics

Employer References
Tricare

855 Delta Dental of Wyoming

6234 Yellowstone Road
P.O. Box 29
Cheyenne, WY 82009
Toll-Free: 800-735-3379
Phone: 307-632-3313
Fax: 307-632-7309
customerservice@deltadentalwy.org
www.deltadentalwy.org
Non-Profit Organization: Yes

Healthplan and Services Defined
PLAN TYPE: Dental
Other Type: Dental PPO
Model Type: Network
Plan Specialty: ASO, Dental
Benefits Offered: Dental

Type of Coverage
Commercial, Individual
Catastrophic Illness Benefit: None

Geographic Areas Served
Statewide

Accreditation Certification
URAC, NCQA

Key Personnel
President & CEO . . . . Kerry P. Hall
VP, Admin./Gov. Relations . . . . Patricia J. Guzman
Director of Accounting . . . . Jennifer R. Hanrahan

856 Humana Health Insurance of Wyoming

12300 Whitewater Drive
Suite 150
Minnetonka, MN 55343
Toll-Free: 877-367-6990
Phone: 952-253-3540
Fax: 952-938-2787
www.humana.com
Subsidiary of: Humana
For Profit Organization: Yes

Healthplan and Services Defined
PLAN TYPE: HMO/PPO
Model Type: Network
Plan Specialty: Dental, Vision
Benefits Offered: Dental, Vision, Life, LTD, STD

Type of Coverage
Commercial

Geographic Areas Served
Statewide. Wyoming is covered by the Minnesota branch

Accreditation Certification
URAC, NCQA, CORE

Key Personnel
Executive Director . . . . Steve Dwyer

857 UnitedHealthcare of Wyoming

6465 S Greenwood Plaza Boulevard
Suite 300
Centennial, CO 80111
Toll-Free: 866-574-6088
www.uhc.com
Subsidiary of: UnitedHealth Group

Healthplan and Services Defined
PLAN TYPE: HMO/PPO
Model Type: Network
Plan Specialty: Behavioral Health, Dental, Disease
Management, MSO, PBM, Vision
Benefits Offered: Behavioral Health, Chiropractic,
Complementary
Medicine, Dental, Disease Management, Home Care,
Inpatient SNF, Long-Term Care, Physical Therapy,
Podiatry, Prescription, Psychiatric, Transplant,
Vision, Wellness, AD&D, Life, Benefits vary
according to plan

Type of Coverage
Commercial, Individual, Medicare, Medicaid, Family,
Military, Veterans, Group,

Type of Payment Plans Offered
DFFS, FFS, Combination FFS & DFFS

Geographic Areas Served
Statewide. Wyoming is covered by the Colorado branch

Subscriber Information
Average Monthly Fee Per Subscriber
(Employee + Employer Contribution):
Employee Only (Self): Varies

Network Qualifications
Pre-Admission Certification: Yes

Peer Review Type
Case Management: Yes

Publishes and Distributes Report Card: Yes

Accreditation Certification
URAC, NCQA
State Licensure, Quality Assurance Program

Key Personnel
President/CEO, CO/WY . . . . Marc Neely

Average Claim Compensation
Physician's Fees Charged: 70%
Hospital's Fees Charged: 55%

Specialty Managed Care Partners
United Behavioral Health
Enters into Contracts with Regional Business Coalitions: No

Appendix A: Glossary of Terms

A

Access

A person's ability to obtain healthcare services.

Acute Care

Medical treatment rendered to people whose illnesses or medical problems are short-term or don't require long-term continuing care. Acute care facilities are hospitals that mainly treat people with short-term health problems.

Aggregate Indemnity

The maximum amount of payment provided by an insurer for each covered service for a group of insured people.

Aid to Families with Dependent Children (AFDC)

A state-based federal assistance program that provided cash payments to needy children (and their caretakers), who met certain income requirements. AFDC has now been replaced by a new block grant program, but the requirements, or criteria, can still be used for determining eligibility for Medicaid.

Alliance

Large businesses, small businesses, and individuals who form a group for insurance coverage.

All-payer System

A proposed healthcare system in which, no matter who is paying, prices for health services and payment methods are the same. Federal or state government, a private insurance company, a self-insured employer plan, an individual, or any other payer would pay the same rates. Also called Multiple Payer system.

Ambulatory Care

All health services that are provided on an out-patient basis, that don't require overnight care. Also called out-patient care.

Ancillary Services

Supplemental services, including laboratory, radiology and physical therapy, that are provided along with medical or hospital care.

B

Beneficiary

A person who is eligible for or receiving benefits under an insurance policy or plan.

Benefits

The services that members are entitled to receive based on their health plan.

Blue Cross/Blue Shield

Non-profit, tax-exempt insurance service plans that cover hospital care, physician care and related services. Blue Cross and Blue Shield are separate organizations that have different benefits, premiums and policies. These organizations are in all states, and The Blue Cross and Blue Shield Association of America is their national organization.

Board Certified

Status granted to a medical specialist who completes required training and passes and examination in his/her specialized area. Individuals who have met all requirements, but have not completed the exam are referred to as "board eligible."

Board Eligible

Reference to medical specialists who have completed all required training but have not completed the exam in his/her specialized area.

C

Cafeteria Plan

This benefit plan gives employees a set amount of funds that they can choose to spend on a different benefit options, such as health insurance or retirement savings

Capitation

A fixed prepayment, per patient covered, to a healthcare provider to deliver medical services to a particular group of patients. The payment is the same no matter how many services or what type of services each patient actually gets. Under capitation, the provider is financially responsible.

Care Guidelines

A set of medical treatments for a particular condition or group of patients that has been reviewed and endorsed by a national organization, such as the Agency for Healthcare Policy Research.

Carrier

A private organization, usually an insurance company, that finances healthcare.

Carve-out

Medical services that are separated out and contracted for independently from any other benefits.

Case management

Intended to improve health outcomes or control costs, services and education are tailored to a patient's needs, which are designed to improve health outcomes and/or control costs

Catastrophic Health Insurance

Health insurance that provides coverage for treating severe or lengthy illnesses or disability.

CHAMPUS

(Civilian Health and Medical Program of the Uniformed Services) A health plan that serves the dependents of active duty military personnel and retired military personnel and their dependents.

Chronic Care

Treatment given to people whose health problems are long-term and continuing. Nu nursing homes, mental hospitals and rehabilitation facilities are chronic care facilities.

Chronic Disease
A medical problem that will not improve, that lasts a lifetime, or recurs.

Claims
Bills for services. Doctors, hospitals, labs and other providers send billed claims to health insurance plans, and what the plans pay are called paid claims.

COBRA
(Consolidated Omnibus Budget Reconciliation Act of 1985) Designed to provide health coverage to workers between jobs, this legal act lets workers who leave a company buy health insurance from that company at the employer's group rate rather than an individual rate.

Co-insurance
A cost-sharing requirement under some health insurance policies in which the insured person pays some of the costs of covered services.

Cooperatives/Co-ops
HMOs that are managed by the members of the health plan or insurance purchasing arrangements in which businesses or other groups join together to gain the buying power of large employers or groups.

Co-pay
Flat fees or payments (often $5-10) that a patient pays for each doctor visit or prescription.

Cost Containment
The method of preventing healthcare costs from increasing beyond a set level by controlling or reducing inefficiency and waste in the healthcare system.

Cost Sharing
An insurance policy requires the insured person to pay a portion of the costs of covered services. Deductibles, co-insurance and co-payments are cost sharing.

Cost Shifting
When one group of patients does not pay for services, such as uninsured or Medicare patients, healthcare providers pass on the costs for these health services to other groups of patients.

Coverage
A person's healthcare costs are paid by their insurance or by the government..

Covered services
Treatments or other services for which a health plan pays at least part of the charge.

D

Deductible
The amount of money, or value of certain services (such as one physician visit), a patient or family must pay before costs (or percentages of costs) are covered by the health plan or insurance company, usually per year.

Diagnostic related groups (DRGs)
A system for classifying hospital stays according to the diagnosis of the medical problem being treated, for the purposes of payment.

Direct access
The ability to see a doctor or receive a medical service without a referral from your primary care physician.

Disease management
Programs for people who have chronic illnesses, such as asthma or diabetes, that try to encourage them to have a healthy lifestyle, to take medications as prescribed, and that coordinate care.

Disposable Personal Income
The amount of a person's income that is left over after money has been spent on basic necessities such as rent, food, and clothing.

E

Early and Periodic Screening, Diagnosis, and Treatment Program (EPSDT)
As part of the Medicaid program, the law requires that all states have a program for eligible children under age 21 to receive a medical assessment, medical treatments and other measures to correct any problems and treat chronic conditions.

Elective
A healthcare procedure that is not an emergency and that the patient and doctor plan in advance.

Emergency
A medical condition that starts suddenly and requires immediate care.

Employee Retirement Income Security Act (ERISA)
A Federal act, passed in 1974, that established new standards for employer-funded health benefit and pension programs. Companies that have self-funded health benefit plans operating under ERISA are not subject to state insurance regulations and healthcare legislation.

Employer Contribution
The contribution is the money a company pays for its employees' healthcare. Exclusions
Health conditions that are explicitly not covered in an insurance package and that your insurance will not pay for.

Exclusive Provider Organizations (EPO)/Exclusive Provider Arrangement (EPA)
An indemnity or service plan that provides benefits only if those hospitals or doctors with which it contracts provide the medical services, with some exceptions for emergency and out-of-area services.

F

Federal Employee Health Benefit Program (FEP)
Health insurance program for Federal workers and their dependents, established in 1959 under the Federal Employees Health Benefits Act. Federal employees may choose to participate in one of two or more plans.

Fee-for-Service

Physicians or other providers bill separately for each patient encounter or service they provide. This method of billing means the insurance company pays all or some set percentage of the fees that hospitals and doctors set and charge. Expenditures increase if the increaseThis is still the main system of paying for healthcare services in the United States.

First Dollar Coverage

A system in which the insurer pays for all employee out-of-pocket healthcare costs. Under first dollar coverage, the beneficiary has no deductible and no co-payments.

Flex plan

An account that lets workers set aside pretax dollars to pay for medical benefits, childcare, and other services.

Formulary

A list of medications that a managed care company encourages or requires physicians to prescribe as necessary in order to reduce costs.

G

Gag clause

A contractual agreement between a managed care organization and a provider that restricts what the provider can say about the managed care company

Gatekeeper

The person in a managed care organization, often a primary care provider, who controls a patient's access to healthcare services and whose approval is required for referrals to other services or other specialists.

General Practice

Physicians without specialty training who provide a wide range of primary healthcare services to patients.

Global Budgeting

A way of containing hospital costs in which participating hospitals share a budget, agreeing together to set the maximum amount of money that will be paid for healthcare.

Group Insurance

Health insurance offered through business, union trusts or other groups and associations. The most common system of health insurance in the United States, in which the cost of insurance is based on the age, sex, health status and occupation of the people in the group.

Group model HMO

An HMO that contracts with an independent group practice to provide medical services

Guaranteed Issue

The requirement that an insurance plan accept everyone who applies for coverage and guarantee the renewal of that coverage as long as the covered person pays the policy premium.

H

Healthcare Benefits

The specific services and procedures covered by a health plan or insurer.

Healthcare Financing Administration (HCFA)

The federal government agency within the Department of Health and Human Services that directs the Medicare and Medicaid programs. HCFA also does research to support these programs and oversees more than a quarter of all healthcare costs in the United States.

Health Insurance

Financial protection against the healthcare costs caused by treating disease or accidental injury.

Health Insurance Portability and Accountability Act (HIPAA)

Also known as Kennedy-Kassebaum law, this guarantees that people who lose their group health insurance will have access to individual insurance, regardless of pre-existing medical problems. The law also allows employees to secure health insurance from their new employer when they switch jobs even if they have a pre-existing medical condition.

Health Insurance Purchasing Cooperatives (HIPCs)

Public or private organizations that get health insurance coverage for certain populations of people, combining everyone in a specific geographic region and basing insurance rates on the people in that area.

Health Maintenance Organization (HMO)

A health plan provides comprehensive medical services to its members for a fixed, prepaid premium. Members must use participating providers and are enrolled for a fixed period of time. HMOs can do business either on a for-profit or not-for-profit basis.

Health Plan Employer Data and Information Set (HEDIS)

Performance measures designed by the National Committee for Quality Assurance to give participating managed health plans and employers to information about the value of their healthcare and trends in their health plan performance compared with other health plans.

Home healthcare

Skilled nurses and trained aides who provide nursing services and related care to someone at home.

Hospice Care

Care given to terminally ill patients. Hospital Alliances Groups of hospitals that join together to cut their costs by purchasing services and equipment in volume.

I

Indemnity Insurance

A system of health insurance in which the insurer pays for the costs of covered services after care has been given, and which usually defines the maximum amounts which will be paid for covered services. This is the most common type of insurance in the United States.

Independent Practice Association (IPA)
A group of private physicians who join together in an association to contract with a managed care organization.

Indigent Care
Care provided, at no cost, to people who do not have health insurance or are not covered by Medicare, Medicaid, or other public programs.

In-patient
A person who has been admitted to a hospital or other health facility, for a period of at least 24 hours.

Integrated Delivery System (IDS)
An organization that usually includes a hospital, a large medical group, and an insurer such as an HMO or PPO.

Integrated Provider (IP)
A group of providers that offer comprehensive and coordinated care, and usually provides a range of medical care facilities and service plans including hospitals, group practices, a health plan and other related healthcare services.

J

Joint Commission on the Accreditation of Healthcare Organizations (JCAHO)
A national private, non-profit organization that accredits healthcare organizations and agencies and sets guidelines for operation for these facilities.

L

Limitations
A "cap" or limit on the amount of services that may be provided. It may be the maximum cost or number of days that a service or treatment is covered.

Limited Service Hospital
A hospital, often located in a rural area, that provides a limited set of medical and surgical services.

Long-term Care
Healthcare, personal care and social services provided to people who have a chronic illness or disability and do not have full functional capacity. This care can take place in an institution or at home, on a long-term basis.

M

Malpractice Insurance
Coverage for medical professionals which pays the costs of legal fees and/or any damages assessed by the court in a lawsuit brought against a professional who has been charged with negligence.

Managed care
This term describes many types of health insurance, including HMOs and PPOs. They control the use of health services by their members so that they can contain healthcare costs and/or improve the quality of care.

Mandate
Law requiring that a health plan or insurance carrier must offer a particular procedure or type of coverage.

Means Test
An assessment of a person's or family's income or assets so that it can be determined if they are eligible to receive public support, such as Medicaid.

Medicaid
An insurance program for people with low incomes who are unable to afford healthcare. Although funded by the federal government, Medicaid is administered by each state. Following very broad federal guidelines, states determine specific benefits and amounts of payment for providers.

Medical IRAs
Personal accounts which, like individual retirement plans, allow a person to accumulate funds for future use. The money in these accounts must be used to pay for medical services. The employee decides how much money he or she will spend on healthcare.

Medically Indigent
A person who does not have insurance and is not covered by Medicaid, Medicare or other public programs.

Medicare
A federal program of medical care benefits created in 1965 designed for those over age 65 or permanently disabled. Medicare consists of two separate programs: A and B. Medicare Part A, which is automatic at age 65, covers hospital costs and is financed largely by employer payroll taxes. Medicare Part B covers outpatient care and is financed through taxes and individual payments toward a premium.

Medicare Supplements or Medigap
A privately-purchased health insurance policy available to Medicare beneficiaries to cover costs of care that Medicare does not pay. Some policies cover additional costs, such as preventive care, prescription drugs, or at-home care.

Member
The person enrolled in a health plan.

N

National Committee on Quality Assurance (NCQA)
An independent national organization that reviews and accredits managed care plans and measures the quality of care offered by managed care plans.

Network

A group of affiliated contracted healthcare providers (physicians, hospitals, testing centers, rehabilitation centers etc.), such as an HMO, PPO, or Point of Service plan.

Non-contributory Plan

A group insurance plan that requires no payment from employees for their healthcare coverage.

Non-participating Provider

A healthcare provider who is not part of a health plan. Usually patients must pay their own healthcare costs to see a non-participating provider.

Nurse practitioner

A nurse specialist who provides primary and/or specialty care to patients. In some states nurse practitioners do not have to be supervised by a doctor.

O

Open Enrollment Period

A specified period of time during which people are allowed to change health plans.

Open Panel

A right included in an HMO, which allows the covered person to get non-emergency covered services from a specialist without getting a referral from the primary care physician or gatekeeper.

Out of Pocket costs or expenditures

The amount of money that a person must pay for his or her healthcare, including: deductibles, co-pays, payments for services that are not covered, and/or health insurance premiums that are not paid by his or her employer.

Outcomes

Measures of the effectiveness of particular kinds of medical treatment. This refers to what is quantified to determine if a specific treatment or type of service works.

Out of Pocket Maximum

The maximum amount that a person must pay under a plan or insurance contract.

Outpatient Care

Healthcare services that do not require a patient to receive overnight care in a hospital.

P

Participating Physician or Provider

Healthcare providers who have contracted with a managed care plan to provide eligible healthcare services to members of that plan.

Payer

The organization responsible for the costs of healthcare services. A payer may be private insurance, the government, or an employer's self-funded plan.

Peer Review Organization (PRO or PSRO)

An agency that monitors the quality and appropriateness of medical care delivered to Medicare and Medicaid patients. Healthcare professionals in these agencies review other professionals with similar training and experience. [See Quality Improvement Organizations]

Percent of Poverty

A term that describes the income level a person or family must have to be eligible for Medicaid.

Physician Assistant

A health professional who provides primary and/or specialty care to patients under the supervision of a physician.

Physician Hospital Organizations (PHOs)

An organization that contracts with payers on behalf of one or more hospitals and affiliated physicians. Physicians still own their practices.

Play or Pay

This system would provide coverage for all people by requiring employers either to provide health insurance for their employees and dependents (play) or pay a contribution to a publicly-provided system that covers uninsured or unemployed people without private insurance (pay).

Point of Service (POS)

A type of insurance where each time healthcare services are needed, the patient can choose from different types of provider systems (indemnity plan, PPO or HMO). Usually, members are required to pay more to see PPO or non-participating providers than to see HMO providers.

Portability

A person's ability to keep his or her health coverage during times of change in health status or personal situation (such as change in employment or unemployment, marriage or divorce) or while moving between health plans.

Postnatal Care

Healthcare services received by a woman immediately following the delivery of her child

Pre-authorization

The process where, before a patient can be admitted to the hospital or receive other types of specialty services, the managed care company must approve of the proposed service in order to cover it.

Pre-existing Condition

A medical condition or diagnosis that began before coverage began under a current plan or insurance contract. The insurance company may provide coverage but will specifically exclude treatment for such a condition from that person's coverage for a certain period of time, often six months to a year.

Preferred Provider Organization (PPO)

A type of insurance in which the managed care company pays a higher percentage of the costs when a preferred (in-plan) provider is used. The participating providers have agreed to provide their services at negotiated discount fees.

Premium
The amount paid periodically to buy health insurance coverage. Employers and employees usually share the cost of premiums.

Premium Cap
The maximum amount of money an insurance company can charge for coverage.

Premium Tax
A state tax on insurance premiums.

Prepaid Group Practice
A type of HMO where participating providers receive a fixed payment in advance for providing particular healthcare services.

Preventive Care
Healthcare services that prevent disease or its consequences. It includes primary prevention to keep people from getting sick (such as immunizations), secondary prevention to detect early disease (such as Pap smears) and tertiary prevention to keep ill people or those at high risk of disease from getting sicker (such as helping someone with lung disease to quit smoking).

Primary Care
Basic or general routine office medical care, usually from an internist, obstetrician-gynecologist, family practitioner, or pediatrician.

Primary care provider (PCP)
The health professional who provides basic healthcare services. The PCP may control patients' access to the rest of the healthcare system through referrals.

Private Insurance
Health insurance that is provided by insurance companies such as commercial insurers and Blue Cross plans, self-funded plans sponsored by employers, HMOs or other managed care arrangements.

Provider
An individual or institution who provides medical care, including a physician, hospital, skilled nursing facility, or intensive care facility.

Provider-Sponsored Organization (PSO)
Healthcare providers (physicians and/or hospitals) who form an affiliation to act as insurer for an enrolled population.

Q

Quality Assessment
Measurement of the quality of care.

Quality Assurance and Quality Improvement
A systematic process to improve quality of healthcare by monitoring quality, finding out what is not working, and fixing the problems of healthcare delivery.

Quality Improvement Organization (QIO)
An organization contracting with HCFA to review the medical necessity and quality of care provided to Medicare beneficiaries.

Quality of care
How well health services result in desired health outcomes.

R

Rate Setting
These programs were developed by several states in the 1970's to establish in advance the amount that hospitals would be paid no matter how high or low their costs actually were in any particular year. (Also known as hospital rate setting or prospective reimbursement programs)

Referral system
The process through which a primary care provider authorizes a patient to see a specialist to receive additional care.

Reimbursement
The amount paid to providers for services they provide to patients.

Risk
The responsibility for profiting or losing money based on the cost of healthcare services provided. Traditionally, health insurance companies have carried the risk. Under capitation, healthcare providers bear risk.

S

Self-insured
A type of insurance arrangement where employers, usually large employers, pay for medical claims out of their own funds rather than contracting with an insurance company for coverage. This puts the employer at risk for its employees' medical expenses rather than an insurance company.

Single Payer System
A healthcare reform proposal in which healthcare costs are paid by taxes rather than by the employer and employee. All people would have coverage paid by the government.

Socialized Medicine
A healthcare system in which providers are paid by the government, and healthcare facilities are run by the government.

Staff Model HMO
A type of managed care where physicians are employees of the health plan, usually in the health plan's own health center or facility.

Standard Benefit Package
A defined set of benefits provided to all people covered under a health plan.

T

Third Party Administrator (TPA)
An organization that processes health plan claims but does not carry any insurance risk.

Third Party Payer
An organization other than the patient or healthcare provider involved in the financing of personal health services.

U

Uncompensated Care
Healthcare provided to people who cannot pay for it and who are not covered by any insurance. This includes both charity care which is not billed and the cost of services that were billed but never paid.

Underinsured
People who have some type of health insurance but not enough insurance to cover their the cost of necessary healthcare. This includes people who have very high deductibles of $1000 to $5000 per year, or insurance policies that have specific exclusions for costly services.

Underwriting
This process is the basis of insurance. It analyzes the health status and history, claims experience (cost), age and general health risks of the individual or group who is applying for insurance coverage.

Uninsured
People who do not have health insurance of any type. Over 80 percent of the uninsured are working adults and their family members.

Universal Coverage
This refers to the proposal that all people could get health insurance, regardless of the way that the system is financed.

Utilization Review
A program designed to help reduce unnecessary medical expenses by studying the appropriateness of when certain services are used and by how many patients they are used.

Utilization
How many times people use particular healthcare services during particular periods of time.

V

Vertical Integration
A healthcare system that includes the entire range of healthcare services from out-patient to hospital and long-term care.

W

Waiting Period
The amount of time a person must wait from the date he or she is accepted into a health plan (or from when he or she applies) until the insurance becomes effective and he or she can receive benefits.

Withhold
A percentage of providers' fees that managed care companies hold back from providers which is only given to them if the amount of care they provide (or that the entire plan provides) is under a budgeted amount for each quarter or the whole year.

Worker's Compensation Coverage
States require employers to provide coverage to compensate employees for work-related injuries or disabilities.

Source: Public Broadcasting Service, http://www.pbs.org/ healthcarecrisis/glossary.htm. Reprinted with permission of www.issuestv.com and www.pbs.com.

Appendix B: Industry Websites

Alliance of Community Health Plans (ACHP)

http://www.achp.org

Offers information on health care so that it is safe, effective, patient-centered, timely, efficient and equitable. Members use this web site to collaborate, share strategies and work toward solutions to some of health care's biggest challenges.

America's Health Insurance Plans (AHIP)

http://www.ahip.org

AHIP is a national trade association representing nearly 1,300 member companies providing health insurance coverage to more than 200 million Americans.

American Academy of Medical Administrators (AAMA)

http://www.aameda.org

Supports individuals involved in medical administration at the executive - or middle-management levels. Promotes educational courses for the training of persons in medical administration. Conducts research. Offers placement service.

American Accreditation Healthcare Commission/URAC

http://www.urac.org

URAC (Utilization Review Accreditation Commission) is a 501(c)(3) non-profit charitable organization founded in 1990 to establish standards for the managed care industry. URAC's broad-based membership includes representation from all the constituencies affected by managed care - employers, consumers, regulators, health care providers, and the workers' compensation and managed care industries.

American Association of Healthcare Administrative Management (AAHAM)

http://www.aaham.org

A professional organization in healthcare administrative management that offers information, education and advocacy in the areas of reimbursement, admitting and registration, data management, medical records, patient relations and more. Founded in 1968, AAHAM represents a broad-based constituency of healthcare professionals through a comprehensive program of legislative and regulatory monitoring and its participation in industry groups such as ANSI, DISA and NUBC.

American Association of Integrated Healthcare Delivery Systems (AAIHDS)

http://www.aaihds.org

AAIHDS was founded in 1993 as a non-profit organization dedicated to the educational advancement of provider-based managed care professionals involved in integrated healthcare delivery.

American Association of Preferred Provider Organizations (AAPPO)

http://www.aappo.org

A national association of preferred provider organizations (PPOs) and affiliate organizations, established in 1983 to advance awareness of the benefits - greater access, choice and flexibility - that PPOs bring to American health care.

American College of Health Care Administrators (ACHCA)

http://achca.org

Founded in 1962, ACHCA provides superior educational programming, professional certification, and career development opportunities for its members. It identifies, recognizes, and supports long term care leaders, advocating for their mission and promoting excellence in their profession.

American College of Healthcare Executives (ACHE)

http://www.ache.org

International professional society of more than 30,000 healthcare executives, including credentialing and educational programs and sponsors the Congress on Healthcare Management. ACHE's publishing division, Health Administration Press, is one of the largest publishers of books.

American College of Physician Executives (ACPE)

http://www.acpe.org

Supports physicians whose primary professional responsibility is the management of healthcare organizations. Provides for continuing education and certification of the physician executive. Offers specialized career planning, counseling, recruitment and placement services, and research and information data on physician managers.

American Health Care Association (AHCA)

http://www.ahcancal.org

A non-profit federation of affiliated state health organizations, representing more than 10,000 non-profit and for-profit assisted living, nursing facility, developmentally-disabled, and subacute care providers that care for more than 1.5 million elderly and disabled individuals nationally.

American Health Planning Association (AHPA)

http://www.ahpanet.org

A non-profit public interest organization that brings together individuals and organizations interested in the availability, affordability and equitable distribution of health services. AHPA supports community participation in health policy formulation and in the organization and operation of local health services.

American Health Quality Association (AHQA)

http://www.ahqa.org

The American Health Quality Association represents Quality Improvement Organizations (QIOs) and professionals working to improve the quality of health care in communities across America. QIOs share information about best practices with physicians, hospitals, nursing homes, home health agencies, and others. Working together with health care providers, QIOs identify opportunities and provide assistance for improvement.

American Medical Association (AMA)

http://www.ama-assn.org

Founded more than 150 years ago, the AMA's work includes the development and promotion of standards in medical practice, research, and education. This site offers medical information for physicians, medical students, other health professionals, and patients.

American Medical Directors Association (AMDA)
http://www.amda.com
A professional association of medical directors, attending
physicians, and others practicing in the long term care continuum,
that provides education, advocacy, information, and professional
development to promote the delivery of quality long term care
medicine.

American Medical Group Association (AMGA)
http://www.amga.org
Association that supports various medical groups and organized
systems of care at the national level.

Association of Family Medicine Residency Directors (AFMRD)
http://www.afmrd.org
Provides representation for residency directors at a national level
and provides a political voice for them to appropriate arenas.
Promotes cooperation and communication between residency
programs and different branches of the family medicine specialty.
Dedicated to improving of education of family physicians. Provides
a network for mutual assistance among FP, residency directors.

Association of Family Practice Administrators (AFPA)
http://www.uams.edu/afpa/afpa1.htm
Promotes professionalism in family practice administration. Serves
as a network for sharing of information and fellowship among
members. Provides technical assistance to members and functions as
a liaison to related professional organizations.

Association of Healthcare Internal Auditors (AHIA)
http://www.ahia.org
Promotes cost containment and increased productivity in health care
institutions through internal auditing. Serves as a forum for the
exchange of experience, ideas, and information among members;
provides continuing professional education courses and informs
members of developments in health care internal auditing. Offers
employment clearinghouse services.

Case Management Society of America (CMSA)
http://www.cmsa.org
Information for the case management profession.

Centers for Medicare and Medicaid Services (CMS)
http://cms.hhs.gov
Formerly known as the Health Care Financing Administration
(HCFA), this is the federal agency that administers Medicare,
Medicaid and the State Children's Health Insurance Program
(SCHIP). CMS provides health insurance for over 74 million
Americans through these programs.

**College of Healthcare Information Management Executives
(CHIME)**
http://www.cio-chime.org
Serves the professional development needs of healthcare CIOs, and
advocating the more effective use of information management
within healthcare.

**Electronic Healthcare Network Accreditation Commission
(EHNAC)**
http://www.ehnac.org

A federally-recognized standards development organization and
non-profit accrediting body designed to improve transactional
quality, operational efficiency and data security in healthcare.

Healthcare Financial Management Association (HFMA)
http://www.hfma.org
HFMA is a membership organization for healthcare financial
management executives and leaders. The association brings
perspective and clarity to the industry's complex issues for the
purpose of preparing members to succeed. Programs, publications
and partnerships enhance the capabilities that strengthen not only
individuals careers, but also the organizations from which members
come.

**Healthcare Information and Management Systems Society
(HIMSS)**
http://www.himss.org
The healthcare industry's membership organization exclusively
focused on providing global leadership for the optimal use of
healthcare information technology (IT) and management systems.
HIMSS represents more than 20,000 individual members and over
300 corporate members leads healthcare public policy and industry
practices through its advocacy, educational and professional
development initiatives designed to promote information and
management systems' contributions to ensuring quality patient care.

Healthfinder.gov
http://www.healthfinder.gov
A comprehensive guide to resources for health information from the
federal government and related agencies.

The Joint Commission (JC)
http://www.jointcommission.org
An independent, not-for-profit organization, JC accredits and
certifies more than 15,000 health care organizations and programs in
the United States which is recognized nationwide as a symbol of
quality that reflects an organization's commitment to meeting certain
performance standards.

Managed Care Information Center (MCIC)
http://www.managedcaremarketplace.com
An online yellow pages for companies providing services to
Managed Care Organizations (MCO), hospitals and physician
groups. There are more than three dozen targeted categories,
offering information on vendors from claims processing to
transportation services to health care compliance.

National Association for Healthcare Quality (NAHQ)
http://www.nahq.org
Provides vital research, education, networking, certification and
professional practice resources, designed to empower healthcare
quality professionals from every specialty. This leading resource for
healthcare quality professionals is an essential connection for
leadership, excellence and innovation in healthcare quality.

National Association for Health Care Recruitment (NAHCR)
http://www.nahcr.com

Supports individuals employed directly by hospitals and other health care organizations which are involved in the practice of professional health care recruitment. Promotes sound principles of professional healthcare recruitment. Provides financial assistance to aid members in planning and implementing regional educational programs. Offers technical assistance and consultation services. Compiles statistics.

National Association Medical Staff Services (NAMSS)
http://www.namss.org
Supports individuals involved in the management and administration of health care provider services. Seeks to enhance the knowledge and experience of medical staff services professionals and promote the certification of those involved in the profession.

National Association of Dental Plans (NADP)
http://www.nadp.org
Promotes and advances the dental benefits industry to improve consumer access to affordable, quality dental care.

National Association of Insurance Commissoners (NAIC)
http://www.naic.org
The mission of the NAIC is to assist state insurance regulators, individually and collectively, in serving the public interest and achieving the following fundamental insurance regulatory goals in a responsive, efficient and cost effective manner, consistent with the wishes of its members: protect the public interest; promote competitive markets; facilitate the fair and equitable treatment of insurance consumers; promote the reliability, solvency and financial solidity of insurance institutions; and support and improve state regulation of insurance.
The NAIC also provides links to State Insurance Department web sites *(http://www.naic.org/state_web_map.htm)*.

The National Association of Managed Care Regulators (NAMCR)
http://www.namcr.org
Includes both regulator members and associate industry members. Established in 1975, NAMCR provides expertise and a forum for discussion to state regulators and managed care companies about current issues facing managed care. NAMCR has also provided expertise to the National Association of Insurance Commissioners (NAIC) in preparation of NAIC Model Acts used by many states.

National Association of State Medicaid Directors (NASMD)
http://www.nasmd.org
Promotes effective Medicaid policy and program administration; works with the federal government on issues through technical advisory groups. Conducts forums on policy and technical issues.

National Committee for Quality Assurance (NCQA)
http://www.ncqa.org

The National Committee for Quality Assurance (NCQA) is a private, not-for-profit organization dedicated to assessing and reporting on the quality of managed care plans. Their efforts are organized around two activities, accreditation and performance measurement, which are complementary strategies for producing information to guide choice.

National Institute for Health Care Management Research and Educational Foundation (NIHCM Foundation)
http://www.nihcm.org
A nonprofit, nonpartisan group that conducts research on health care issues. The Foundation disseminates research findings and analysis and holds forums and briefings for policy makers, the health care industry, consumers, the government, and the media to increase understanding of issues affecting the health care system.

National Quality Forum (NQF)
http://www.qualityforum.org
A not-for-profit membership organization created to develop and implement a national strategy for health care quality measurement and reporting, Prompted by the impact of health care quality on patient outcomes, workforce productivity, and health care costs. NQF has broad participation from all parts of the health care system, including national, state, regional, and local groups representing consumers, public and private purchasers, employers, health care professionals, provider organizations.,health plans, accrediting bodies, labor unions, supporting industries, and organizations.

National Society of Certified Healthcare Business Consultants (NSCHBC)
http://www.ichbc.org
The NSCHBC is a national organization dedicated to serving the needs of consultants who provide ethical, confidential and professional advice to the healthcare industry. Membership by successful completion of certification examination only.

Professional Association of Health Care Office Management (PAHCOM)
http://www.pahcom.com
Supports office managers of small group and solo medical practices. Operates certification program for healthcare office managers.

U.S. Food and Drug Administration (USFDA)
http://www.fda.gov
A department of the U.S. Department of Health and Human Services, the Food and Drug Administration provides information regarding health, medicine and nutrition. Their MedWatch Safety Information and Adverse Event Reporting Program serves both healthcare professionals and the public. MedWatch provides clinical information about safety issues involving medical products, including prescription and over-the-counter drugs, biologics, dietary supplements, and medical devices *(http://www.fda.gov/medwatch)*.

Plan Index

United Concordia of Washington Harrisburg, PA, 815

Western Dental Services Orange, CA, 142

Willamette Dental Group Hillsboro, OR, 655

HMO

Aetna Better Health of Kentucky Louisville, KY, 335

Aetna Health of Arizona Hartford, CT, 17

Aetna Health of California San Diego, CA, 54

Aetna Health of Colorado Hartford, CT, 144

Aetna Health of Connecticut Hartford, CT, 165

Aetna Health of District of Columbia Hartford, CT, 186

Aetna Health of Florida Sunrise, CT, 192

Aetna Health of Georgia Hartford, CT, 227

Aetna Health of Illinois Chicago, IL, 260

Aetna Health of Indiana Hartford, CT, 284

Aetna Health of Kansas Hartford, CT, 319

Aetna Health of Kansas Kansas City, KS, 320

Aetna Health of Kentucky Louisville, KY, 336

Aetna Health of Maine Hartford, CT, 357

Aetna Health of Maryland Linthicum, MD, 366

Aetna Health of Massachusetts Hartford, CT, 383

Aetna Health of Michigan Detroit, MI, 401

Aetna Health of Nevada Hartford, CT, 494

Aetna Health of New Jersey Princeton, NJ, 515

Aetna Health of New York Hartford, CT, 542

Aetna Health of North Carolina Hartford, CT, 583

Aetna Health of Ohio New Albany, OH, 602

Aetna Health of Oklahoma Hartford, CT, 626

Aetna Health of Pennsylvania Philadelphia, PA, 656

Aetna Health of Tennessee Hartford, CT, 718

Aetna Health of Texas Dallas, TX, 729

Aetna Health of Virginia Richmond, CT, 790

Aetna of Illinois , IL, 261

Aetna Student Health Hartford, CT, 168

Affinity Health Plan Bronx, NY, 543

Alameda Alliance for Health Alameda, CA, 55

Allegiance Life & Health Insurance Company Missoula, MT, 451

Alliant Health Plans Dalton, GA, 228

Allied Pacific IPA Alhambra, CA, 58

AlohaCare Honolulu, HI, 243

American Specialty Health San Diego, CA, 59

American Specialty Health Carmel, IN, 286

Amerigroup Georgia Atlanta, GA, 229

Amerigroup Iowa Clive, IA, 307

Amerigroup Maryland Hanover, MD, 368

Amerigroup Tennessee Nashville, TN, 719

Amerigroup Texas Grand Prairie, TX, 733

AmeriHealth New Jersey Cranbury, NJ, 516

AmeriHealth Pennsylvania Philadelphia, PA, 658

Anthem Blue Cross & Blue Shield of Colorado Denver, CO, 146

Anthem Blue Cross & Blue Shield of Connecticut Wallingford, CT, 169

Anthem Blue Cross & Blue Shield of Georgia Atlanta, GA, 230

Anthem Blue Cross & Blue Shield of Indiana Lafayette, IN, 287

Anthem Blue Cross & Blue Shield of Kentucky Lexington, KY, 337

Anthem Blue Cross & Blue Shield of Maine South Portland, ME, 358

Anthem Blue Cross & Blue Shield of Missouri St Louis, MO, 458

Anthem Blue Cross & Blue Shield of Nevada Las Vegas, NV, 495

Anthem Blue Cross & Blue Shield of New Hampshire Manchester, NH, 508

Anthem Blue Cross & Blue Shield of New Hampshire Manchester, NH, 508

Anthem Blue Cross & Blue Shield of Virginia Richmond, VA, 791

Anthem Blue Cross & Blue Shield of Wisconsin Milwaukee, WI, 828

Anthem Blue Cross of California Newbury Park, CA, 60

Anthem, Inc. Indianapolis, IN, 288

Atlanticare Health Plans Egg Harbor Township, NJ, 517

Aultcare Corporation Canton, OH, 604

Avera Health Plans Sioux Falls, SD, 711

AvMed Gainesville Gainesville, FL, 196

AvMed Orlando Orlando, FL, 197

Baptist Health Plan Lexington, KY, 338

Blue Care Network of Michigan Southfield, MI, 403, 404

Blue Cross & Blue Shield of Arizona Phoenix, AZ, 21

Blue Cross & Blue Shield of Illinois Chicago, IL, 262

Blue Cross & Blue Shield of Massachusetts Boston, MA, 386

Blue Cross & Blue Shield of Minnesota Minneapolis, MN, 437

Blue Cross & Blue Shield of Montana Helena, MT, 476

Blue Cross & Blue Shield of New Mexico Albuquerque, NM, 531

Blue Cross & Blue Shield of Oklahoma Tulsa, OK, 628

Blue Cross & Blue Shield of Rhode Island Providence, RI, 694

Blue Cross & Blue Shield of South Carolina Columbia, SC, 702

Blue Cross & Blue Shield of Texas Richardson, TX, 736

Blue Cross & Blue Shield of Wyoming Cheyenne, WY, 854

Blue Cross and Blue Shield of Alabama Birmingham, AL, 4

Blue Cross and Blue Shield of Kansas Topeka, KS, 322

Blue Cross and Blue Shield of Louisiana Baton Rouge, LA, 347

Blue Cross Blue Shield Nevada Las Vegas, NV, 497

Blue Cross Blue Shield of Georgia Atlanta, GA, 231

Blue Cross Blue Shield of North Carolina Durham, NC, 584

Blue Cross of Idaho Health Service, Inc. Meridian, ID, 252

Blue Shield of California San Francisco, CA, 62

BlueCross BlueShield of Western New York Buffalo, NY, 545

BlueShield of Northeastern New York Latham, NY, 546

Brand New Day HMO Westminster, CA, 63

BridgeSpan Health Salt Like City, UT, 773

Bright Health Alabama Minneapolis, MN, 5

Bright Health Colorado Minneapolis, MN, 150

CalOptima Orange, CA, 67

Capital BlueCross Harrisburg, PA, 660

Capital Health Plan Tallahassee, FL, 198

Care1st Health Plan Arizona Phoenix, AZ, 22

Care1st Health Plan Blue Shield of California Promise Monterey Park, CA, 69

CareCentrix Hartford, CT, 170

CareCentrix: Arizona Phoenix, AZ, 23

CareCentrix: Florida Tampa, FL, 199

CareCentrix: Kansas Overland Park, KS, 323

CareCentrix: New York Melville, NY, 547

CareFirst Blue Cross & Blue Shield of Virginia Reston, VA, 792

CareFirst BlueCross BlueShield Baltimore, MD, 370

CDPHP: Capital District Physicians' Health Plan Albany, NY, 549

CenCal Health Santa Barbara, CA, 72

Centene Corporation St. Louis, MO, 460

Central California Alliance for Health Scotts Valley, CA, 73

Total Health Care Detroit, MI, 426

UniCare Illinois Chicago, IL, 282
UniCare Kansas Topeka, KS, 333
UniCare Massachusetts Andover, MA, 399
UniCare Michigan Dearborn, MI, 429
UniCare Texas Plano, TX, 766
UnitedHealthcare Community Plan Delaware Hot Springs, AR, 185
UnitedHealthcare Great Lakes Health Plan Southfield, MI, 431
UnitedHealthcare of Alabama Birmingham, AL, 10
UnitedHealthcare of Alaska Cypress, CA, 16
UnitedHealthcare of Arizona Phoenix, AZ, 42
UnitedHealthcare of Arkansas Little Rock, AR, 52
UnitedHealthcare of Colorado Centennial, CO, 164
UnitedHealthcare of Connecticut Hartford, CT, 179
UnitedHealthcare of Florida Maitland, FL, 224
UnitedHealthcare of Georgia Norcross, GA, 242
UnitedHealthcare of Hawaii Minneapolis, MN, 250
UnitedHealthcare of Idaho Meridian, ID, 259
UnitedHealthcare of Illinois Chicago, IL, 283
UnitedHealthcare of Indiana Indianapolis, IN, 306
UnitedHealthcare of Iowa West Des Moines, IA, 316
UnitedHealthcare of Kansas Overland Park, KS, 334
UnitedHealthcare of Kentucky Louisville, KY, 345
UnitedHealthcare of Louisiana Metairie, LA, 354
UnitedHealthcare of Maine Warwick, RI, 365
UnitedHealthcare of Maryland Columbia, MD, 382
UnitedHealthcare of Massachusetts Warwick, RI, 400
UnitedHealthcare of Michigan Kalamazoo, MI, 432
UnitedHealthcare of Minnesota Minnetonka, MN, 450
UnitedHealthcare of Mississippi Hattiesburg, MS, 456
UnitedHealthcare of Missouri Maryland Heights, MO, 475
UnitedHealthcare of Montana Spokane, WA, 482
UnitedHealthcare of Nebraska Omaha, NE, 493
UnitedHealthcare of Nevada Las Vegas, NV, 506
UnitedHealthcare of New Hampshire Warwick, RI, 513
UnitedHealthcare of New Jersey Iselin, NJ, 529
UnitedHealthcare of New Mexico Albuquerque, NM, 541
UnitedHealthcare of New York New York, NY, 580
UnitedHealthcare of North Carolina Raleigh, NC, 594
UnitedHealthcare of North Dakota Minnetonka, MN, 601
UnitedHealthcare of Northern California Concord, CA, 136
UnitedHealthcare of Ohio Columbus, OH, 625
UnitedHealthcare of Oklahoma Plano, TX, 635
UnitedHealthcare of Oregon Lake Oswego, OR, 654
UnitedHealthcare of Pennsylvania Pittsburgh, PA, 679
UnitedHealthcare of Puerto Rico Minnetonka, MN, 692
UnitedHealthcare of Rhode Island Warwick, RI, 700
UnitedHealthcare of South Carolina Columbia, SC, 710
UnitedHealthcare of South Dakota Minnetonka, MN, 716
UnitedHealthcare of South Florida Miramar, FL, 225
UnitedHealthcare of Southern California Anaheim, CA, 137
UnitedHealthcare of Tennessee Brentwood, TN, 728
UnitedHealthcare of Texas West Lake Hills, TX, 768
UnitedHealthcare of the District of Columbia Washington, DC, 191
UnitedHealthcare of Utah Salt Lake City, UT, 784

UnitedHealthcare of Vermont Warwick, VT, 789
UnitedHealthcare of Virginia Richmond, VA, 802
UnitedHealthcare of Washington Spokane, WA, 816
UnitedHealthcare of West Virginia Richmond, VA, 825
UnitedHealthcare of Wisconsin Green Bay, WI, 850
UnitedHealthcare of Wyoming Centennial, CO, 857
Univera Healthcare Buffalo, NY, 581
University Care Advantage Tuscon, AZ, 43
University Family Care Health Plan Tucson, AZ, 44
University Health Plans Murray, UT, 785
Upper Peninsula Health Plan Marquette, MI, 433
UTMB HealthCare Systems Galveston, TX, 770

Valley Baptist Health Plan Harlingen, TX, 771
Vantage Health Plan Monroe, LA, 355
Ventura County Health Care Plan Oxnard, CA, 139
VIVA Health Birmingham, AL, 11

Wellmark Blue Cross Blue Shield Des Moines, IA, 317
Western Health Advantage Sacramento, CA, 143

Medicare

Alignment Health Plan Orange, CA, 57
AllCare Health Grants Pass, OR, 637
AlohaCare Advantage Plus Honolulu, HI, 244
Atrio Health Plans Roseburg, OR, 638
AvMed Miami, FL, 194
AvMed Ft. Lauderdale Ft. Lauderdale, FL, 195

BlueCross BlueShield Association Chicago, IL, 263

Care N' Care Fort Worth, TX, 737
Care1st Medicare Advantage Plan Monterey Park, CA, 70
Care1st Medicare Advantage Plan Texas Monterey Park, CA, 738
CareMore Health Plan Cerritos, CA, 71
CareOregon Health Plan Portland, OR, 639
CarePlus Health Plans Miami, FL, 200
CareSource Indiana Dayton, OH, 290
CareSource Kentucky Louisville, KY, 339
CareSource Ohio Dayton, OH, 605
CareSource West Virginia Dayton, OH, 818
CDPHP Medicare Plan Albany, NY, 548
Central Health Medicare Plan Diamond Bar, CA, 74
Cigna-HealthSpring Nashville, TN, 722
Cigna-HealthSpring Medicare Bloomfield, CT, 172

Elderplan Brooklyn, NY, 554
Essence Healthcare Maryland Heights, MO, 467

First Health Part D Bethasda, MD, 375
Freedom Health Tampa, FL, 208

GEMCare Health Plan Bakersfield, CA, 91
GHI Medicare Plan New York, NY, 560

HAP-Health Alliance Plan: Senior Medicare Plan Detroit, MI, 414
Health Alliance Medicare Champaign, IL, 271
Health Alliance Medicare Detroit, MI, 415
Health First Health Plans Rockledge, FL, 209

Multiple

Magnolia Health Jackson, MS, 454

Martin's Point HealthCare Portland, ME, 362

MDwise Indianapolis, IN, 298

Medical Card System (MCS) San Juan, PR, 689

Mercy Care Plan/Mercy Care Advantage Phoenix, AZ, 32

Meritain Health Amherst, NY, 571

MHNet Behavioral Health Austin, TX, 756

Mid America Health Greenwood, IN, 299

Mid-Atlantic Behavioral Health Newark, DE, 183

MMM Holdings San Juan, PR, 690

Moda Health Alaska Anchorage, AK, 14

Moda Health Oregon Portland, OR, 646

MVP Health Care Schenectady, NY, 574

Nova Healthcare Administrators Williamsville, NY, 575

Ohio State University Health Plan Inc. Columbus, OH, 614

Optum Complex Medical Conditions Eden Prairie, MN, 446

Pacific Foundation for Medical Care Santa Rosa, CA, 120

PacificSource Health Plans Springfield, OR, 647

Piedmont Community Health Plan Lynchburg, VA, 800

Preferred Care Partners Miami, FL, 221

Preferred Mental Health Management Wichita, KS, 330

Primary Health Medical Group Garden City, ID, 256

Providence Health Plan Portland, OR, 649

QualCare Piscataway, NJ, 527

Regence BlueCross BlueShield of Oregon Portland, OR, 650

Regence BlueCross BlueShield of Utah Portland, OR, 781

Regence BlueShield of Idaho Lewiston, ID, 257

Samaritan Health Plan Operations Corvallis, OR, 651

Scott & White Health Plan Temple, TX, 760

Security Health Plan of Wisconsin Marshfield, WI, 848

Spectera Eyecare Networks Columbia, MD, 379

Sun Life Financial Kansas City, MO, 474

Taylor Benefits San Jose, CA, 133

TexanPlus Medicare Advantage HMO Austin, TX, 764

The Dental Care Plus Group Cincinnati, OH, 622

Trillium Community Health Plan Eugene, OR, 652

Tufts Health Plan Watertown, MA, 398

Tufts Health Plan: Rhode Island Providence, RI, 699

UCare Minneapolis, MN, 448

UniCare West Virginia Charleston, WV, 824

Unity Health Insurance Sauk City, WI, 851

UPMC Health Plan Pittsburgh, PA, 680

Valley Preferred Allentown, PA, 683

Wellmark Blue Cross & Blue Shield of South Dakota Sioux Falls, SD, 717

Wisconsin Physician's Service Madison, WI, 852

PPO

Aetna Health of Alabama Hartford, CT, 1

Aetna Health of Alaska Hartford, CT, 12

Aetna Health of California San Diego, CA, 54

Aetna Health of Colorado Hartford, CT, 144

Aetna Health of Connecticut Hartford, CT, 165

Aetna Health of District of Columbia Hartford, CT, 186

Aetna Health of Florida Sunrise, CT, 192

Aetna Health of Georgia Hartford, CT, 227

Aetna Health of Idaho Hartford, CT, 251

Aetna Health of Illinois Chicago, IL, 260

Aetna Health of Indiana Hartford, CT, 284

Aetna Health of Kansas Hartford, CT, 319

Aetna Health of Kansas Kansas City, KS, 320

Aetna Health of Kentucky Louisville, KY, 336

Aetna Health of Louisiana Kenner, LA, 346

Aetna Health of Maine Hartford, CT, 357

Aetna Health of Maryland Linthicum, MD, 366

Aetna Health of Massachusetts Hartford, CT, 383

Aetna Health of Michigan Detroit, MI, 401

Aetna Health of Minnesota Hartford, CT, 434

Aetna Health of Nevada Hartford, CT, 494

Aetna Health of New Jersey Princeton, NJ, 515

Aetna Health of New York Hartford, CT, 542

Aetna Health of North Carolina Hartford, CT, 583

Aetna Health of North Dakota Hartford, CT, 595

Aetna Health of Ohio New Albany, OH, 602

Aetna Health of Oklahoma Hartford, CT, 626

Aetna Health of Oregon Hartford, CT, 636

Aetna Health of Pennsylvania Philadelphia, PA, 656

Aetna Health of Rhode Island Hartford, CT, 693

Aetna Health of South Carolina Hartford, CT, 701

Aetna Health of Tennessee Hartford, CT, 718

Aetna Health of Texas Dallas, TX, 729

Aetna Health of Virginia Richmond, CT, 790

Aetna Health of Washington Hartford, CT, 803

Aetna Health of West Virginia Charleston, WV, 817

Aetna Health of Wisconsin Hartford, CT, 826

Aetna Health of Wyoming Hartford, CT, 853

Aetna Student Health Hartford, CT, 168

Alliance Regional Health Network Amarillo, TX, 730

Alliant Health Plans Dalton, GA, 228

American Health Care Alliance Kansas City, MO, 457

American Health Network Indianapolis, IN, 285

American National Insurance Company Galveston, TX, 731

American Postal Workers Union (APWU) Health Plan Glen Burnie, MD, 367

American PPO Irving, TX, 732

Americas PPO Bloomington, MN, 435

AmeriHealth New Jersey Cranbury, NJ, 516

AmeriHealth Pennsylvania Philadelphia, PA, 658

Anthem Blue Cross & Blue Shield of Colorado Denver, CO, 146

Anthem Blue Cross & Blue Shield of Connecticut Wallingford, CT, 169

Anthem Blue Cross & Blue Shield of Georgia Atlanta, GA, 230

Anthem Blue Cross & Blue Shield of Indiana Lafayette, IN, 287

Anthem Blue Cross & Blue Shield of Kentucky Lexington, KY, 337

Anthem Blue Cross & Blue Shield of Maine South Portland, ME, 358

Anthem Blue Cross & Blue Shield of Missouri St Louis, MO, 458

Anthem Blue Cross & Blue Shield of Nevada Las Vegas, NV, 495

Anthem Blue Cross & Blue Shield of New Hampshire Manchester, NH, 508

Health Care Service Corporation Chicago, IL, 272

Health Choice LLC Memphis, TN, 725

Health Choice of Alabama Birmingham, AL, 6

Health Link PPO Tupelo, MS, 452

Health New England Springfield, MA, 390

Health Partners of Kansas Wichita, KS, 326

Health Plans, Inc. Westborough, MA, 391

Healthchoice Orlando, FL, 211

HealthEZ Bloomington, MN, 440

HealthSmart Irving, TX, 751

Highmark BCBS Delaware Wilmington, DE, 181

Highmark BCBS West Virginia Triadelphia, WV, 820

Highmark Blue Cross Blue Shield Pittsburgh, PA, 667

Highmark Blue Shield Camp Hill, PA, 668

Horizon Blue Cross Blue Shield of New Jersey Newark, NJ, 522

Horizon Health Corporation Lewisville, TX, 752

Horizon NJ Health West Trenton, NJ, 523

Humana Health Insurance of Alabama Madison, AL, 7

Humana Health Insurance of Alaska Vancouver, WA, 13

Humana Health Insurance of Arizona Phoenix, AZ, 29

Humana Health Insurance of Arkansas Rogers, AR, 49

Humana Health Insurance of California Irvine, CA, 100

Humana Health Insurance of Colorado Colorado Springs, CO, 158

Humana Health Insurance of Connecticut Albany, NY, 176

Humana Health Insurance of Delaware Glen Allen, VA, 182

Humana Health Insurance of Florida Jacksonville, FL, 214

Humana Health Insurance of Georgia Atlanta, GA, 236

Humana Health Insurance of Hawaii Honolulu, HI, 248

Humana Health Insurance of Idaho Meridian, ID, 254

Humana Health Insurance of Illinois Oak Brook, IL, 273

Humana Health Insurance of Indiana Indianapolis, IN, 297

Humana Health Insurance of Iowa Bettendorf, IA, 311

Humana Health Insurance of Kansas Overland Park, KS, 327

Humana Health Insurance of Louisiana Baton Rouge, LA, 350

Humana Health Insurance of Massachusetts Albany, NY, 392

Humana Health Insurance of Michigan Detroit, MI, 417

Humana Health Insurance of Minnesota Minnetonka, MN, 443

Humana Health Insurance of Mississippi Ridgeland, MS, 453

Humana Health Insurance of Missouri Springfield, MO, 470

Humana Health Insurance of Montana Minnetonka, MN, 479

Humana Health Insurance of Nebraska Bettendorf, IA, 487

Humana Health Insurance of Nevada Las Vegas, NV, 501

Humana Health Insurance of New Hampshire Portsmouth, NH, 511

Humana Health Insurance of New Jersey Uniondale, NY, 524

Humana Health Insurance of New Mexico Albuquerque, NM, 535

Humana Health Insurance of New York Albany, NY, 564

Humana Health Insurance of North Carolina Charlotte, NC, 591

Humana Health Insurance of North Dakota Minnetonka, MN, 598

Humana Health Insurance of Ohio Cincinnati, OH, 608

Humana Health Insurance of Oklahoma Tulsa, OK, 633

Humana Health Insurance of Oregon Vancouver, WA, 642

Humana Health Insurance of Pennsylvania Mechanicsburg, PA, 669

Humana Health Insurance of Puerto Rico San Juan, PR, 687

Humana Health Insurance of Rhode Island Albany, NY, 697

Humana Health Insurance of South Carolina Columbia, SC, 706

Humana Health Insurance of South Dakota Bettendorf, IA, 715

Humana Health Insurance of Tennessee Memphis, TN, 726

Humana Health Insurance of Texas San Antonio, TX, 753

Humana Health Insurance of Utah Sandy, UT, 775

Humana Health Insurance of Virginia Glen Allen, VA, 797

Humana Health Insurance of Washington Vancouver, WA, 811

Humana Health Insurance of West Virginia , WV, 821

Humana Health Insurance of Wisconsin Waukesha, WI, 841

Humana Health Insurance of Wyoming Minnetonka, MN, 856

Humana Inc. Louisville, KY, 341

Independence Blue Cross Philadelphia, PA, 670

Independent Health Buffalo, NY, 565

Initial Group Nashville, TN, 727

InterGroup Services Pittsburgh, PA, 671

Island Group Administration, Inc. East Hampton, NY, 567

Kaiser Permanente Oakland, CA, 102

Kaiser Permanente Northern California Oakland, CA, 103

Kaiser Permanente Southern Colorado Colorado Springs, CO, 160

Landmark Healthplan of California Sacramento, CA, 109

LifeWise Mountlake Terrace, WA, 812

MagnaCare New York, NY, 570

Managed HealthCare Northwest Portland, OR, 645

MedCost Winston Salem, NC, 592

MedCost Virginia Richmond, VA, 798

Medical Mutual Services Copley, OH, 610

Midlands Choice Omaha, NE, 490

Mutual of Omaha Health Plans Omaha, NE, 492

National Imaging Associates St Paul, MN, 445

Nevada Preferred Healthcare Providers Reno, NV, 503

Noridian Insurance Services Inc. Fargo, ND, 600

North Alabama Managed Care Inc Huntsville, AL, 8

Northeast Georgia Health Partners Gainesville, GA, 238

NovaSys Health Little Rock, AR, 51

Ohio Health Choice Akron, OH, 613

OhioHealth Group Columbus, OH, 615

Optima Health Plan Virginia Beach, VA, 799

Oscar Health New York, NY, 576

Oxford Health Plans Trumbull, CT, 177

Pacific Health Alliance Burlingame, CA, 121

PacificSource Health Plans Springfield, OR, 648

Paramount Care of Michigan Dundee, MI, 421

Paramount Health Care Maumee, OH, 617

Parkview Total Health , IN, 300

PCC Preferred Chiropractic Care Wichita, KS, 329

Penn Highlands Healthcare DuBois, PA, 672

Physicians Health Plan of Mid-Michigan Lansing, MI, 422

Physicians Plus Insurance Corporation Madison, WI, 846

Preferred Health Care Lancaster, PA, 673

Preferred Healthcare System Duncansville, PA, 674

Preferred Network Access Darien, IL, 279

Preferred Therapy Providers Phoenix, AZ, 37

Premera Blue Cross Blue Shield of Alaska Anchorage, AK, 15

Premier Access Insurance/Access Dental Sacramento, CA, 38, 123, 504, 779

Prevea Health Network Green Bay, WI, 847
Prominence Health Plan Reno, NV, 505
ProviDRs Care Network Wichita, KS, 332
PTPN Calabasas, CA, 125
Public Employees Health Program Salt Lake City, UT, 780
Pueblo Health Care Pueblo, CO, 161

Quality Plan Administrators Washington, DC, 189

Rocky Mountain Health Plans Grand Junction, CO, 162
Rural Carrier Benefit Plan London, KY, 344

Sagamore Health Network Carmel, IN, 303
Sant, Community Physicians Fresno, CA, 128
Script Care, Ltd. Beaumont, TX, 761
Secure Health PPO Newtork Macon, GA, 239
South Central Preferred Health Network York, PA, 675
Stanislaus Foundation for Medical Care Modesto, CA, 131

The Health Plan of the Ohio Valley/Mountaineer Region , OH, 623
Trilogy Health Insurance Brookfield, WI, 849
Trustmark Companies Lake Forest, IL, 281

UniCare Illinois Chicago, IL, 282
UniCare Kansas Topeka, KS, 333
UniCare Massachusetts Andover, MA, 399
UniCare Texas Plano, TX, 766
UnitedHealthcare Community Plan Capital Area Hot Springs, AR, 190
UnitedHealthcare of Alabama Birmingham, AL, 10
UnitedHealthcare of Alaska Cypress, CA, 16
UnitedHealthcare of Arizona Phoenix, AZ, 42
UnitedHealthcare of Arkansas Little Rock, AR, 52
UnitedHealthcare of Colorado Centennial, CO, 164
UnitedHealthcare of Connecticut Hartford, CT, 179
UnitedHealthcare of Florida Maitland, FL, 224
UnitedHealthcare of Georgia Norcross, GA, 242
UnitedHealthcare of Hawaii Minneapolis, MN, 250
UnitedHealthcare of Idaho Meridian, ID, 259
UnitedHealthcare of Illinois Chicago, IL, 283
UnitedHealthcare of Indiana Indianapolis, IN, 306
UnitedHealthcare of Iowa West Des Moines, IA, 316
UnitedHealthcare of Kansas Overland Park, KS, 334
UnitedHealthcare of Kentucky Louisville, KY, 345
UnitedHealthcare of Louisiana Metairie, LA, 354
UnitedHealthcare of Maine Warwick, RI, 365
UnitedHealthcare of Maryland Columbia, MD, 382
UnitedHealthcare of Massachusetts Warwick, RI, 400
UnitedHealthcare of Michigan Kalamazoo, MI, 432
UnitedHealthcare of Minnesota Minnetonka, MN, 450
UnitedHealthcare of Mississippi Hattiesburg, MS, 456
UnitedHealthcare of Missouri Maryland Heights, MO, 475
UnitedHealthcare of Montana Spokane, WA, 482
UnitedHealthcare of Nebraska Omaha, NE, 493
UnitedHealthcare of Nevada Las Vegas, NV, 506

UnitedHealthcare of New Hampshire Warwick, RI, 513
UnitedHealthcare of New Jersey Iselin, NJ, 529
UnitedHealthcare of New Mexico Albuquerque, NM, 541
UnitedHealthcare of New York New York, NY, 580
UnitedHealthcare of North Carolina Raleigh, NC, 594
UnitedHealthcare of North Dakota Minnetonka, MN, 601
UnitedHealthcare of Northern California Concord, CA, 136
UnitedHealthcare of Ohio Columbus, OH, 625
UnitedHealthcare of Oklahoma Plano, TX, 635
UnitedHealthcare of Oregon Lake Oswego, OR, 654
UnitedHealthcare of Pennsylvania Pittsburgh, PA, 679
UnitedHealthcare of Puerto Rico Minnetonka, MN, 692
UnitedHealthcare of Rhode Island Warwick, RI, 700
UnitedHealthcare of South Carolina Columbia, SC, 710
UnitedHealthcare of South Dakota Minnetonka, MN, 716
UnitedHealthcare of South Florida Miramar, FL, 225
UnitedHealthcare of Southern California Anaheim, CA, 137
UnitedHealthcare of Tennessee Brentwood, TN, 728
UnitedHealthcare of Texas West Lake Hills, TX, 768
UnitedHealthcare of the District of Columbia Washington, DC, 191
UnitedHealthcare of Utah Salt Lake City, UT, 784
UnitedHealthcare of Vermont Warwick, VT, 789
UnitedHealthcare of Virginia Richmond, VA, 802
UnitedHealthcare of Washington Spokane, WA, 816
UnitedHealthcare of West Virginia Richmond, VA, 825
UnitedHealthcare of Wisconsin Green Bay, WI, 850
UnitedHealthcare of Wyoming Centennial, CO, 857
University Health Plans Murray, UT, 785
University HealthCare Alliance Newark, CA, 138
UPMC Susquehanna Williamsport, PA, 681
USA Managed Care Organization Austin, TX, 769

Vale-U-Health Belle Vernon, PA, 682
Value Behavioral Health of Pennsylvania Cranberry Township, PA, 684

Zelis Healthcare Bedminster, NJ, 530

Vision

Envolve Vision Rocky Mount, NC, 589
EyeMed Vision Care Mason, OH, 607

March Vision Care Los Angeles, CA, 112

Opticare of Utah Salt Lake City, UT, 778
Outlook Benefit Solutions Mesa, AZ, 34

Preferred Vision Care Overland Park, KS, 331

Superior Vision Rancho Cordova, CA, 132
SVS Vision Mount Clemens, MI, 425

Vision Plan of America Los Angeles, CA, 140
VSP Vision Care Rancho Cordova, CA, 141

Personnel Index

A

Abdi, Abdirahman Hennepin Health, 442

Abelman, David Dentaquest, 387

Abernathy, Jo Blue Cross Blue Shield of North Carolina, 584

Abrahamson, April Colorado Access, 152

Adams, Derek HAP-Health Alliance Plan: Flint, 413

Adams, Derick, Esq. Health Alliance Plan, 416

Adams, Gregory A. Kaiser Permanente Mid-Atlantic, 377

Adams, Joann Florida Health Care Plans, 207

Adams, Lavdena, MD AmeriHealth Caritas District of Columbia, 187

Adler, Jeremy Blue Cross & Blue Shield of Arizona, 21

Adler, Peter Molina Healthcare of Idaho, 255

Adorno, Niurka, Esq. Molina Healthcare of South Carolina, 708

Aga, Dr. Donald KelseyCare Advantage, 754

Agpaoa, Ronda Taylor Benefits, 133

Aguilar, Daniel Liberty Dental Plan of California, 110

Albert, Stephanie Delta Dental of Minnesota, 439

Aldrich, Mary Ann, RN Northeast Delta Dental, 512

Aliabadi, Karen Delta Dental of Washington, 808

All, Matt Blue Cross and Blue Shield of Kansas, 322

Allen, Ashley Health New England, 390

Allen, Calvin HealthPartners, 441

Allen, Greg Cigna HealthCare of Tennessee, 629

Allen, Klrk Ascension At Home, 2, 289, 321, 402, 627, 734, 829

Allen, Robert W. Intermountain Healthcare, 776

Allford, Allan Delta Dental of Arizona, 26

Allred, Steven Preferred Therapy Providers, 37

Almquist, Stacia Sun Life Financial, 474

Altman, Maya Health Plan of San Mateo, 98

Altmann, Lynn Medica, 444

Altmann, Lynn Medica with CHI Health, 488

Altmann, Lynn Medica: Nebraska, 489

Alvarado, Chuck MediGold, 611

Alvarez, Diana Health Choice Arizona, 28

Ambrose, David CenCal Health, 72

Amidei, Christopher Aetna Health of District of Columbia, 186

Amstutz, Karen Magellan Health, 30

Amstutz, Karen Magellan Complete Care of Florida, 217

Ancona, Vincent Amerigroup Maryland, 368

Anderl, Richard Mutual of Omaha Dental Insurance, 491

Anderl, Richard Mutual of Omaha Health Plans, 492

Anderson, David Delta Dental of Minnesota, 439

Anderson, David W. BlueCross BlueShield of Western New York, 545

Anderson, David W. BlueShield of Northeastern New York, 546

Anderson, Jann Aetna Health of Virginia, 790

Anderson, Joel Essence Healthcare, 467

Anderson, John Concentra, 743

Anderson, Kraig Moda Health Alaska, 14

Anderson, Mark Delta Dental of Arizona, 26

Anderson, William Assurant Employee Benefits Wisconsin, 830

Andrews, Colleen Coventry Health Care of the Carolinas, 586

Aponte Amador, Jos, Medical Card System (MCS), 689

Arakelian, Ronald, MD Stanislaus Foundation for Medical Care, 131

Armstrong, Cathleen HealthSCOPE Benefits, 48

Arnold, Greg Aetna Health of Georgia, 227

Arnold-Miller, Erica Colorado Health Partnerships, 153

Arrington Jr, Robyn James, MD Total Health Care, 426

Arrowood, Brian MDwise, 298

Arthur, Bill Blue Cross & Blue Shield of Arizona, 21

Arthur, Myron Amerigroup Maryland, 368

Asher, Drew WellCare Health Plans, 226

Atkins, Meera CoreSource, 267

Atwood, Michael, MD Blue Cross and Blue Shield of Kansas, 322

Auburn, Steve Trustmark Companies, 281

Aug, Matt Cox Healthplans, 464

Austen, Karla A. MVP Health Care, 574

Avery, Alan Kern Family Health Care, 105

Ayers, Kay AvMed, 194

B

Ba, Lisa Central California Alliance for Health, 73

Baackes, John L.A. Care Health Plan, 106, 107

Baasch, David A., DDS Northeast Delta Dental Vermont, 788

Bachmann, Anita UnitedHealthcare of North Carolina, 594

Bacon, Cindy Island Group Administration, Inc., 567

Bacus, Lisa Cigna Corporation, 171

Bagby, Rhonada Humana Health Insurance of Mississippi, 453

Bagby, Rhonda Humana Health Insurance of Louisiana, 350

Bahsin, Aman Alameda Medi-Cal Plan, 56

Bailey, Todd Health Plans, Inc., 391

Baird, Mark Medica, 444

Baird, Mark Medica with CHI Health, 488

Baird, Mark Medica: Nebraska, 489

Baker, William Coventry Health Care of Texas, 745

Balladeres, Victoria Contra Costa Health Services, 81

Ballard, Jeff Delta Dental of Tennessee, 724

Ballard, Tamara, LPC Colorado Health Partnerships, 153

Bank, Julie MagnaCare, 570

Barasch, Richard A Universal American Medicare Plans, 582

Barasch, Richard A. TexanPlus Medicare Advantage HMO, 764

Barbero, Monice MVP Health Care, 574

Barker, Dave SIHO Insurance Services, 304

Barlow, Jeff D., JD Molina Healthcare, 115

Barlow, Jeff D., JD Molina Medicaid Solutions, 117

Barnard, Mark L. Horizon Blue Cross Blue Shield of New Jersey, 522

Barnett, Curtis Arkansas Blue Cross Blue Shield, 45

Barnette, Donnell Amerigroup Washington, 804

Barney, Erin Blue Cross & Blue Shield of Texas, 736

Barrett, Matt MediGold, 611

Barrett, Tim Jai Medical Systems, 376

Barrueta, Anthony A. Kaiser Permanente, 102

Barth, Anthony S. Delta Dental of California, 83

Barth, Tony Delta Dental of Delaware, 180

Barth, Tony Delta Dental of the District of Columbia, 188

Borland, **Rob** Denver Health Medical Plan, 156

Born, **Rick** Aetna Health of Louisiana, 346

Boss, **Jessica** Opticare of Utah, 778

Bottrill, **Lorry** Mercy Care Plan/Mercy Care Advantage, 32

Boucher, **Francis** Northeast Delta Dental Maine, 364

Boucher, **Francis** Northeast Delta Dental, 512

Boudreaux, **Gail K.** Anthem, Inc., 288

Bowers, **Devon** Jai Medical Systems, 376

Boxer, **Mark** Cigna Corporation, 171

Boyd, **Branda** Care Plus Dental Plans, 831

Boyle, **Kathy** Denver Health Medical Plan, 156

Brach, **Karen** Meridian Health Plan of Illinois, 275

Bradshaw, **Lyndsay** Delta Dental of Illinois, 268

Brand, **Joe** Health Partners Plans, 665

Branson, **Kimberly** Medica, 444

Braswell, **Judi** Behavioral Health Systems, 3

Brawley, **Daniel** Cigna Healthcare Missouri, 462

Bray, **Greg** MedCost, 592

Breard, **Mike** Vantage Health Plan, 355

Breard, **Mike** Vantage Medicare Advantage, 356

Breckenridge, **Jim** Avera Health Plans, 711

Brehm, **Sara M.** Northeast Delta Dental, 512

Brennan, **Joseph** MagnaCare, 570

Brennan, **Maria Lariccia** Trinity Health of New Jersey, 528

Brennan, **Troyen A., MD** CVS CareMark, 696

Brennan Sapon, **Anne** New Mexico Health Connections, 537

Breskin, **William A.** BlueCross BlueShield Association, 263

Brewster, **William** Harvard Pilgrim Health Care New Hampshire, 510

Brice, **Kaitlin** Prevea Health Network, 847

Bridges, **David** Arkansas Blue Cross Blue Shield, 45

Briesacher, **Mark** Intermountain Healthcare, 776

Bright, **Yvette** Independence Blue Cross, 670

Briscione, **R.J.** Aetna Health of Georgia, 227

Britt, **Lisa** Well Sense Health Plan, 514

Britton, **Lynn** Mercy Clinic Missouri, 473

Brodrick, **Dr. Peter** Colorado Health Partnerships, 153

Brooks, **Dee Dee** Dominion Dental Services, 794

Brooks, **Lyn** Delta Dental of Virginia, 793

Broomfield, **Rob** UnitedHealthcare of Kansas, 334

Brosnan, **Patrick** Coventry Health Care of Missouri, 463

Broussard, **Bruce** Humana Health Insurance of Rhode Island, 697

Broussard, **Bruce D.** CompBenefits Corporation, 233

Broussard, **Bruce D.** Humana Inc., 341

Broussard, **Bruce Dale** CarePlus Health Plans, 200

Brown, **David** Wellmark Blue Cross Blue Shield, 317

Brown, **David** Wellmark Blue Cross & Blue Shield of South Dakota, 717

Brown, **Dewey** Coventry Health Care of the Carolinas, 586

Brown, **Diane** Trinity Health of Alabama, 9

Brown, **Jeff** Dentaquest, 387

Brown, **Jim** Script Care, Ltd., 761

Brown, **Keith, MD** Community Health Plan of Washington, 806

Brown, **Nathan** Humana Health Insurance of Utah, 775

Brown, **Roger** AHCCS/Medicaid, 18

Brown, **Roger** UnitedHealthcare of Arizona, 42

Brown, **Susan E.** Minuteman Health, 394

Brown, Jr., **John E.** Blue Cross and Blue Shield of Louisiana, 347

Browne, **Julie** Government Employees Health Association (GEHA), 468

Brumbaugh, **Brian** Preferred Healthcare System, 674

Bruno, **Michael B.** Blue Cross and Blue Shield of Louisiana, 347

Brusuelas, **Mary, RN** Central California Alliance for Health, 73

Bryan, **Tab** Script Care, Ltd., 761

Bryd, **Michael** Sharp Health Plan, 130

Buchert, **Greg, MD** Care1st Health Plan Blue Shield of California Promise, 69

Buck, **Eric E.** Preferred Health Care, 673

Budden, **Joan** Priority Health, 423

Budden, **Joan** PriorityHealth Medicare Plans, 424

Buggle, **Janet** QualCare, 527

Bunker, **Jonathan W** Health Plan of Nevada, 499

Buran, **Gregory, MD** Network Health Plan of Wisconsin, 845

Burdick, **Kenneth A.** WellCare Health Plans, 226

Burgin, **Meryl** CareFirst BlueCross BlueShield, 370

Burke, **Jonathan, MD** Valley Preferred, 683

Burke, **Richard P.** Fallon Health, 388

Burman, **Bill** Denver Health Medical Plan, 156

Burnett, **Brian** Presbyterian Medicare Advantage Plans, 539

Burnett, **David** Neighborhood Health Plan of Rhode Island, 698

Burnett, **Peg** Denver Health Medical Plan, 156

Burthay, **Darcy** Ascension At Home, 2, 289, 321, 402, 627, 734, 829

Busch, **David** BlueCross BlueShield of Western New York, 545

Busch, **David** BlueShield of Northeastern New York, 546

Bush, **Stephen** Scott & White Health Plan, 760

Butler, **James, III** Physicians Health Plan of Mid-Michigan, 422

Butler, **Martha** Essence Healthcare, 467

Butts, **Susan** Cox Healthplans, 464

Byndas, **Cynthia** United Concordia of Florida, 223

C

Cabanis, **Clara** Behavioral Healthcare, 147

Cabrera, **Jose L., Jr.** Humana Health Insurance of Delaware, 182

Cabrera, **Jose L., Jr.** Humana Health Insurance of Virginia, 797

Cade, **Lisa** Blue Cross Blue Shield of North Carolina, 584

Caldwell, **Joe, RN** Alliant Health Plans, 228

Callahan, **Chris, PharmD** MDwise, 298

Callender, **David L.** UTMB HealthCare Systems, 770

Camerlinck, **Bryan** Blue Cross and Blue Shield of Louisiana, 347

Cameron, **Dave** Santa Clara Family Health Foundations Inc, 127

Campanella, **Gary** On Lok Lifeways, 118

Campbell, **Craig** Wisconsin Physician's Service, 852

Campbell, **Donna L.** Trinity Health of Delaware, 184

Campbell, **Gemma** Trinity Health of Alabama, 9

Campbell, **Joe** Emi Health, 774

Campos, **Alina, MD** Leon Medical Centers Health Plan, 215

Canales, **Joe** Seton Healthcare Family, 762

Cantor, **Dr. Michael** CareCentrix, 170

Capezza, **Joseph C.** Health Net, Inc., 96

Capezza, **Joseph C.** Neighborhood Health Plan, 395

Capuano, **Pilar** Coventry Health Care of New Jersey, 520

Carlson, **Danita** Central California Alliance for Health, 73

Carmack, **Susan** Molina Healthcare of Texas, 757

Carpenter, **Theodore** TexanPlus Medicare Advantage HMO, 764

Carpenter Jr., **Theodore M.** Universal American Medicare Plans, 582

Carter, **Benjamin R.** Trinity Health, 427

Doumba, Laurend Delta Dental of Illinois, 268

Dow, Chuck Humana Health Insurance of South Dakota, 715

Dowdie, Andre Humana Health Insurance of New York, 564

Dowling, Angela Regence BlueCross BlueShield of Oregon, 650

Dowling, Angela Regence BlueCross BlueShield of Utah, 781

Downey, Mary Aetna Health of Texas, 729

Downey, Tom Coventry Health Care of New York, 550

Downing, Rebecca Western Health Advantage, 143

Downs, Barbara A. CDPHP: Capital District Physicians' Health Plan, 549

Drawdy, Donyale United Concordia of Georgia, 241

Drew, Julie InStil Health, 707

Drexler, Helen Delta Dental of Colorado, 155

Dreyfus, Andrew Blue Cross & Blue Shield of Massachusetts, 386

Driscoll, John CareCentrix, 170

Drohan, Mariann E. EmblemHealth, 555

Drohan, Mariann E. EmblemHealth Enhanced Care Plus (HARP), 556

Drohan, Mariann E. GHI Medicare Plan, 560

Drummond, Courntey Parkview Total Health, 300

Dudley, Debbie Cigna Healthcare Missouri, 462

Dunaway, Suzie Children's Mercy Pediatric Care Network, 461

Duncan, Erika Trinity Health of New York, 578

Duncan, Jodi The Dental Care Plus Group, 622

Duncan, Pat Rocky Mountain Health Plans, 162

Dunn, Lucille, RN Island Group Administration, Inc., 567

Dunn, Zon Superior Vision, 132

Dunnavant, Cindy Emi Health, 774

Dwyer, Jim Delta Dental of Washington, 808

Dwyer, Steve Humana Health Insurance of Wyoming, 856

E

Eadie, Dr. Reginald J. Trinity Health of Connecticut, 178

Eadie, Dr. Reginald J. Trinity Health of Massachusetts, 396

Eagan, Thomas AllCare Health, 637

Eames, Wendy Molina Medicaid Solutions, 363

Eapen, Zubin CareMore Health Plan, 71

Early, Karen Montana Health Co-Op, 480

Early, Karen Mountain Health Co-Op, 481

Ebeling, Brian, MD HealthEZ, 440

Ebenkamp, Bob Delta Dental of Kansas, 325

Eberle, Josiah Molina Healthcare of Michigan, 420

Ebert, Thomas H., MD Fallon Health, 388

Eckrich, Nancy CoreSource, 267

Eckstein, Michael Health Tradition, 840

Eddy, Paul Wellmark Blue Cross Blue Shield, 317

Eddy, Paul Wellmark Blue Cross & Blue Shield of South Dakota, 717

Edelen, Connie Aetna Health of Kentucky, 336

Edelman, Ann Colorado Access, 152

Edmonds, Daryl Amerigroup Washington, 804

Edwards, Brett HealthSCOPE Benefits, 48

Edwards, Joe HealthSCOPE Benefits, zzz
48

Eftekhari, Amir Araz Group, 384

Eftekhari, Amir Americas PPO, 435

Eftekhari, Amir HealthEZ, 440

Eftekhari, Nazie Araz Group, 384

Eftekhari, Nazie Americas PPO, 435

Eftekhari, Nazie HealthEZ, 440

Egerton, W. Eugene, MD Trinity Health of California, 134

Eichten, Mike Advance Insurance Company of Kansas, 318

Eig, Blair M. Trinity Health of Maryland, 380

Eller, Kim Peoples Health, 352

Ellertson, Chris Trillium Community Health Plan, 652

Elliott, David Baptist Health Services Group, 720

Ellis, Michael Delta Dental of Kansas, 325

Ellison, Edward M., MD Kaiser Permanente Northern California, 103

Engelman, Rebecca Select Health of South Carolina, 709

Enslinger, Lisa American Health Care Alliance, 457

Epstein, David Aetna Health of Georgia, 227

Epstein, Mark, MD New Mexico Health Connections, 537

ErkenBrack, Steven Rocky Mountain Health Plans, 162

Ertel, Albert Secure Health PPO Newtork, 239

Escobedo, Rene Community First Health Plans, 742

Escue, Dick Hawaii Medical Service Association, 247

Espeland, Kelly Amerigroup Iowa, 307

Esser, Debra Blue Cross & Blue Shield of Nebraska, 484

Esslinger, Laura AlohaCare, 243

Evanko, Brian Cigna Corporation, 171

Evans, Dave Moda Health Alaska, 14

Eve, Kathleen, MD Stanislaus Foundation for Medical Care, 131

Ewanchyna, Kevin, MD Samaritan Health Plan Operations, 651

Eze, E. Chris, MD Molina Healthcare of Illinois, 276

F

Faigin, Tracy Friday Health Plans, 157

Fair Taylor, Erin CareOregon Health Plan, 639

Fairley, Mimi Aetna of Illinois, 261

Fandrich, William M. Blue Care Network of Michigan, 403

Fann-Tucker, Jennifer Cigna HealthCare of Georgia, 232

Farnitano, Chris Contra Costa Health Services, 81

Farrell, Robert G., Jr. SVS Vision, 425

Farrell, Stephen UnitedHealthcare of Connecticut, 179

Farrell, Stephen UnitedHealthcare of Maine, 365

Farrell, Stephen UnitedHealthcare of Massachusetts, 400

Farrell, Stephen UnitedHealthcare of New Hampshire, 513

Farrell, Stephen UnitedHealthcare of Rhode Island, 700

Farrow, Peter Group Health Cooperative of Eau Claire, 837

Fasola, Barbara Careington Solutions, 739

Feagin, Cardwell VIVA Health, 11

Feinberg, David T., MD Geisinger Health Plan, 664

Feind, Julie Lakeside Community Healthcare Network, 108

Feldman, Karen Golden West Dental & Vision, 92

Feldstein, Eric Health Care Service Corporation, 272

Feliciano, Kristin Trinity Health of Maryland, 380

Felix, Carl Passport Health Plan, 343

Felix, John Henry Hawaii Medical Assurance Association, 246

Felkner, Joe Health First Health Plans, 209

Felkner, Joe Health First Medicare Plans, 210

Fennell, Charles J. Trinity Health of New York, 578

Ferguson, Margaret, MD Kaiser Permanente Northern Colorado, 159

Ferguson, Margaret, MD Kaiser Permanente Southern Colorado, 160

Ferguson, Mike Care1st Health Plan Arizona, 22

Ferik, Michael Guardian Life Insurance Company of America, 561

Fernandez, Luis Leon Medical Centers Health Plan, 215

Field, Catherine Humana Health Insurance of Alaska, 13

Field, Catherine Humana Health Insurance of Idaho, 254

Field, Catherine Humana Health Insurance of Oregon, 642

Field, Catherine Humana Health Insurance of Washington, 811

Fields, David Dean Health Plan, 834

Fields, Jordan Aetna Health of Oregon, 636

Figenshu, Bill Western Health Advantage, 143

Finerty, Kathryn Network Health Plan of Wisconsin, 845

Finerty, Jr., John Managed Health Services, 842

Finn, Mary Trinity Health of Delaware, 184

Finuf, Bob Children's Mercy Pediatric Care Network, 461

Fischer, John The Health Plan of the Ohio Valley/Mountaineer Region, 623

Fischer, Neal C., MD Humana Health Insurance of Illinois, 273

Fischer, Robyn Managed HealthCare Northwest, 645

Fish, Karyn CenCal Health, 72

Fish, Kathleen MVP Health Care, 574

Fishbein, Dan Sun Life Financial, 474

Fishbein, Dan Assurant Employee Benefits Wisconsin, 830

Fitzgerald, Kevin R, MD Rocky Mountain Health Plans, 162

Fitzsimmons, Andy CareFirst BlueCross BlueShield, 370

Flanagan, Shannon Behavioral Health Systems, 3

Flanders, Scott N. eHealthInsurance Services, Inc., 88

Flareau, Dr. Bruce Trinity Health of Florida, 222

Flaum, Amanda Care1st Health Plan Blue Shield of California Promise, 69

Fleming, William, PharmD Humana Inc., 341

Fletcher, Nathan AmeriHealth Caritas District of Columbia, 187

Flood, David L. Intermountain Healthcare, 776

Flott, Daniel Liberty Dental Plan of Illinois, 274

Flynn, Jordan Evolent Health, 796

Flynn, Susan Vale-U-Health, 682

Foels, Thomas J., MD, MMM Independent Health, 565

Foels, Thomas J., MD Independent Health Medicare Plan, 566

Fong, Jenny Health Partners Plans, 665

Fontaine, Steven M. Penn Highlands Healthcare, 672

Ford, Lawrence Avesis: Massachusetts, 385

Forrest, Bailey Amerigroup Iowa, 307

Forshee, James D., MD Priority Health, 423

Forsyth, John D. Wellmark Blue Cross Blue Shield, 317

Forsyth, John D. Wellmark Blue Cross & Blue Shield of South Dakota, 717

Fortner, Scott Central California Alliance for Health, 73

Foulkes, Helena B CVS CareMark, 696

Fowler, Patrina Aetna Health of Texas, 729

Fowler, Rosemary HCSC Insurance Services Company, 478

Fox, Annette Group Health Cooperative of South Central Wisconsin, 838

Fraiz, Juan MediGold, 611

Francis, Dave eHealthInsurance Services, Inc., 88

Frawley, Patrick Fidelis Care, 559

Freeman, Bob CenCal Health, 72

Frey, Robert Jai Medical Systems, 376

Friar, Wendy Trinity Health of Maryland, 380

Friedman, Jon, MD Optum Complex Medical Conditions, 446

Fritz, James S Baptist Health Plan, 338

Fronczek, Jodi The Dental Care Plus Group, 622

Frucella, Maureen Preferred Healthcare System, 674

Fusile, Jeff Anthem Blue Cross & Blue Shield of Georgia, 230

Fusile, Jeff Blue Cross Blue Shield of Georgia, 231

G

Gaffney, Tom CareCentrix, 170

Galatas, Bridget Molina Healthcare of Mississippi, 455

Gallagher, Michael P. AvMed, 194

Gallina, John E. Anthem, Inc., 288

Galt, Frederick B. CDPHP: Capital District Physicians' Health Plan, 549

Galvin, Eric ConnectiCare, 173

Garen, Kirsten Delta Dental of California, zzz

83

Garikes Schneider, Carol L. Trinity Health of Illinois, 280

Garnett, Robert Amerigroup Tennessee, 719

Garrigues, Brad Providence Health Plan, 649

Garzelli, Lisa Foundation f. Medical Care f. Kern & Santa Barbara Counties, 90

Gascey, Osjetta Texas HealthSpring, 765

Gaskill, Jeremy Humana Health Insurance of Arkansas, 49

Gaskill, Jeremy L. Humana Health Insurance of Kansas, 327

Gaudio, Joe AHCCS/Medicaid, 18

Gaudio, Joe UnitedHealthcare of Arizona, 42

Gauger, Tim Arkansas Blue Cross Blue Shield, 45

Geary, Emmet Peoples Health, 352

Geesaman, Brian AmeriHealth Caritas District of Columbia, 187

Gellert, Jay Health Net, Inc., 96

Genord, Michael, MD HAP-Health Alliance Plan: Flint, 413

Genord, Michael, MD Health Alliance Plan, 416

Gentile, James Fallon Health, 388

Gentile, Salvatore Friday Health Plans, 157

George, Don Blue Cross & Blue Shield of Vermont, 786

George, William S. Health Partners Plans, 665

Geraghty, Patrick Florida Blue, 206

Gerald, Pierre Aetna Health of Kentucky, 336

Gerbus, Dave, JD Delta Dental of Colorado, 155

Gessel, Barbara Mercy Health Network, 313

Gessells, Tom Ohio State University Health Plan Inc., 614

Ghaly, Christina, M.D. Health Services Los Angeles County, 99

Ghanayem, Darren WellCare Health Plans, 226

Gianturco, Laurie, MD Health New England, 390

Giasi, Steve Affinity Health Plan, 543

Gibb, Ron First Health, 89

Gibb, Ron Cofinity, 406

Gibboney, Liz Partnership HealthPlan of California, 122

Gibbs, Leslie Western Dental Services, 142

Giblin, John Blue Cross & Blue Shield of Tennessee, 721

Giese, Alexis, MD Colorado Access, 152

Gieseman, Greg Community First Health Plans, 742

Giesler, Scott eHealthInsurance Services, Inc., 88

Gilfillan, Richard J. Trinity Health of Idaho, 258

Gilfillan, Richard J. Trinity Health, 427

Gill, Laura Avesis: Arizona, 20

Gille, Larry Prevea Health Network, 847

Gilleland, Janna HealthNetwork, 212

Gilligan, Alison CareCentrix, 170

Gilligan, Patrick Blue Cross & Blue Shield of Massachusetts, 386

Gilliland, Robert Florida Health Care Plans, 207

Gillis, Anne Trinity Health of Maryland, 380

H

Hanlon, **Karen** Highmark Blue Cross Blue Shield, 667

Hannan, **Tim** eHealthInsurance Services, Inc., 88

Hanrahan, **Jennifer R.** Delta Dental of Wyoming, 855

Hansen, **David** UnitedHealthcare of Alaska, 16

Hansen, **David** UnitedHealthcare of Montana, 482

Hansen, **David** UnitedHealthcare of Washington, 816

Hard, **Chris** UnitedHealthcare of Utah, 784

Hardwick, **Debi** California Foundation for Medical Care, 66

Hardy, **Melvin** Arkansas Blue Cross Blue Shield, 45

Hargrave, **Vanessa** MagnaCare, 570

Hargreaves, **Diane** Trinity Health of Illinois, 280

Harlin, **Timothy J.** Denver Health Medical Plan, 156

Harrington, **Carly** Upper Peninsula Health Plan, 433

Harris, **Christopher** Amerigroup Texas, 733

Harris, **Cory R.** Wellmark Blue Cross Blue Shield, 317

Harris, **Cory R.** Wellmark Blue Cross & Blue Shield of South Dakota, 717

Harris, **Joe** Aetna Health of North Dakota, 595

Harris, **Pete** Dominion Dental Services, 794

Harris, **Ryan** MetroPlus Health Plan, 572

Harris, **Shelley** Trinity Health of Idaho, 258

Harrison, **A. Marc, MD** Intermountain Healthcare, 776

Harrison, **Samantha** CareSource Kentucky, 339

Harshman, **Eita** Delta Dental of Illinois, zzz
268

Hart, **Brian** Delta Dental of Kentucky, 340

Hart, **Erin** American HealthCare Group, 657

Harvey, **Christi** United Concordia of Texas, 767

Harvey, **Jonathan, MD** Martin's Point HealthCare, 362

Haslam, **Christine** Aetna Health of Maine, 357

Hauck, **Lisa** Central California Alliance for Health, 73

Havens, **Jim** LifeWise, 812

Hawkes, **Christie** Emi Health, 774

Hawks, **Ener** Coventry Health Care of North Dakota, 596

Haydel, **Augustavia** L.A. Care Health Plan, 106

Haydel, **Augustavia J.** L.A. Care Health Plan, 107

Hayden-Cook, **Melissa** Sharp Health Plan, 130

Hayes, **Bruce, CPA** MDwise, 298

Hayes, **Cain A.** Blue Cross & Blue Shield of Minnesota, 437

Haygood, **Rhonda** Vantage Health Plan, 355

Haygood, **Rhonda** Vantage Medicare Advantage, 356

Haynes, **Neil** Sun Life Financial, 474

Haynes, **Tadd** UniCare West Virginia, 824

Haynes, **Ted** Blue Cross & Blue Shield of Oklahoma, 628

Hayward, **Doug** Kern Family Health Care, 105

Haywood, **Trent** BlueCross BlueShield Association, 263

Hebenstreit, **Patricia, JD** MDwise, 298

Hebert, **Paul** Dental Benefit Providers, 374

Heckenlaible, **Mick** Delta Dental of South Dakota, 713

Hefley, **Debbie** Amerigroup Texas, 733

Heinze, **Dee** Humana Health Insurance of Montana, 479

Helmer, **Richard, MD** CalOptima, 67

Hemann, **Jenn** Consumers Direct Insurance Services (CDIS), 744

Hemsley, **Stephen** UnitedHealth Group, 449

Henderson, **Bill** Liberty Dental Plan of Texas, 755

Henderson, **Melissa** Molina Healthcare of Wisconsin, 844

Henderson, **William F.** NIA Magellan, 33

Henderson, **William F.** National Imaging Associates, 445

Hendrickson, **Brandon** Molina Healthcare of Idaho, 255

Hendrickson, **Brandon** Molina Healthcare of Utah, 777

Henningsen, **Rod** Beta Health Association, Inc., 148

Henriksen, **Majorie** Prominence Health Plan, 505

Herbert, **Michael** Delta Dental of Kansas, 325

Herman, **Ted** MVP Health Care, 574

Hermreck, **Irene** Aetna Health of Kansas, 320

Hernandez, **Al** Humana Health Insurance of Florida, 214

Hernandez, **Al** Humana Health Insurance of South Carolina, 706

Hernandez, **Henry** Leon Medical Centers Health Plan, 215

Herndon, **Matt** Medical Center Healthnet Plan, 393

Hern ndez, **In,s, MD** Medical Card System (MCS), 689

Heron, **Rick** Western Health Advantage, 143

Herren, **Todd** Delta Dental of Iowa, 309

Herrmann, **Katie** Behavioral Healthcare, 147

Hetu, **Maureen** Trinity Health of New Jersey, 528

Hickey, **JD** Blue Cross & Blue Shield of Tennessee, 721

Hickey, **Martin** New Mexico Health Connections, 537

Hickman, **Dave** Trinity Health of Iowa, 315

Hicks, **Dory** Central California Alliance for Health, 73

Higdon, **Kevin** Trinity Health of Indiana, 305

Hilbert, **Andy** Optima Health Plan, 799

Hilferty, **Daniel J.** Independence Blue Cross, 670

Hill, **Stephen** Valley Baptist Health Plan, 771

Hilliard, **Richard** New Mexico Health Connections, 537

Hillman, **Robert** Community Health Options, 359

Hinckley, **Robert R.** CDPHP: Capital District Physicians' Health Plan, 549

Hingst, **Jeanne** ProviDRs Care Network, 332

Hinton, **Dustin** UnitedHealthcare of Michigan, 432

Hinton, **Dustin** UnitedHealthcare of Wisconsin, 850

Hirasaki, **Ron** Christus Health Plan, 740

Hirsch, **Laura** Nova Healthcare Administrators, 575

Hiveley, **Jim** Unity Health Insurance, 851

Ho, **Sam** Oxford Health Plans, 177

Ho, **Sam** UnitedHealthcare Community Plan Delaware, 185

Ho, **Sam** Neighborhood Health Partnership, 219

Ho, **Sam** UnitedHealthcare of Illinois, 283

Ho, **Sam** UnitedHealthcare Great Lakes Health Plan, 431

Hodge, **Edmund F.** Trinity Health, 427

Hodges, **David** National Imaging Associates, 445

Hodges, **Deborah** Health Plans, Inc., 391

Hodgkins, **Robert C., Jr.** The Dental Care Plus Group, 622

Hogan, **John** Capital Health Plan, 198

Hoi, **Herman** Humana Health Insurance of Hawaii, 248

Holder, **Diane** UPMC Health Plan, 680

Hollingsworth, **Nancy, RN** Trinity Health of California, 134

Holmberg, **David L.** Highmark BCBS West Virginia, 820

Holmes, **Barbara** Community First Health Plans, 742

Holmes, **Dana** Blue Cross & Blue Shield of Illinois, 262

Holmquist, **Melissa** Upper Peninsula Health Plan, 433

Hopsicker, **Jim** MVP Health Care, 574

Horn, **Kim** Kaiser Permanente Mid-Atlantic, 377

Horowitz, **Steve** CareCentrix, 170

Horstmann, **Nancy** Christus Health Plan, 740

Horvath, **Steve** CoreSource, 267

Houghland, Stephen J., MD Passport Health Plan, 343
Houston, Daniel J. Employers Dental Services, 27
Howes, David, MD Martin's Point HealthCare, 362
Hoylman, Karen Molina Medicaid Solutions, zzz
822
Hoyt, Ann Group Health Cooperative of South Central Wisconsin, 838
Hrabchak, Richard Mutual of Omaha Health Plans, 492
Huber, Dave R. Horizon Blue Cross Blue Shield of New Jersey, 522
Hudson, Mike Independent Health, 565
Huffman, Sara Molina Healthcare of Ohio, 612
Hufford, Don Western Health Advantage, 143
Hulin, Colin Peoples Health, 352
Hummel, Jill Anthem Blue Cross & Blue Shield of Connecticut, 169
Humphrey, Craig FirstCarolinaCare, 590
Humphrey, Richard Parkland Community Health Plan, 759
Hunnicutt, JoAnne Amerigroup Tennessee, 719
Hunter, Eric C. CareOregon Health Plan, 639
Hunter, Robert L. First Choice Health, 477
Huotari, Mike Rocky Mountain Health Plans, 162
Hurst, David Health Plan of San Joaquin, 97
Husa, Sherry Managed Health Services, 842
Huss, Eric Health Partners Plans, 665
Hutchinson, Cheryl ConnectiCare, 173
Huth, Mark, MD Group Health Cooperative of South Central Wisconsin, 838
Hutton, Esq., Thomas A. Independence Blue Cross, 670
Huval, Tim CompBenefits Corporation, 233
Huval, Tim Humana Health Insurance of Rhode Island, 697

I

Iannelli, Lee Ann CHN PPO, 518
Ignagni, Karen M. EmblemHealth, 555
Ignagni, Karen M. EmblemHealth Enhanced Care Plus (HARP), 556
Ignagni, Karen M. GHI Medicare Plan, 560
Inge, Ronald E., DDS Delta Dental of Missouri, 465
Inge, Ronald E. Delta Dental of South Carolina, 705
Ingram, Carolyn Molina Healthcare of New Mexico, 536
Ingrum, Jeff Scott & White Health Plan, 760
Inzina, Tommy Trinity Health of Florida, 222
Ironside, Paula Coventry Health Care of Iowa, 308
Isaacs, Richard Kaiser Permanente Mid-Atlantic, 377
Iturriria, Louis Kern Family Health Care, 105
Ivanov, Joieta Coventry Health Care of Nevada, 498

J

Jackson, Amy Avesis: Arizona, 20
Jackson, Laura Wellmark Blue Cross & Blue Shield of South Dakota, 717
Jacobetti, Lorrie Prevea Health Network, 847
Jacobs, David Aetna Health of Colorado, 144
Jacobs, Kim UPMC Health Plan, 680
Jacobs, Seth, Esq Blue Shield of California, 62
Jacobson, Jim Medica, 444
Jacobson, Jim Medica with CHI Health, 488
Jacobson, Jim Medica: Nebraska, 489
Jacoby, Kathy Delta Dental of Colorado, 155
Jaconette, Paul CenCal Health, 72
Jain, Rashmi Careington Solutions, 739

Jain, Sachin H. CareMore Health Plan, 71
James, Jesse, MD Evolent Health, 796
James, Marcus Arkansas Blue Cross Blue Shield, 45
James, Valerie Cigna HealthSpring Maryland, 371
Januska, Jeff CenCal Health, 72
Jardine, Edie NIA Magellan, zzz
33
Jardine, Edie National Imaging Associates, 445
Jaroh, Jack Capital BlueCross, 660
Jasmer, Greg DakotaCare, 712
Javier Artau Feliciano, Francisco First Medical Health Plan, 686
Jelinek, Rick M. Aetna Inc., 166
Jenkins, Mary Beth UPMC Health Plan, 680
Jenkins, Nancy McLaren Health Plan, 418
Jennings, Jonathan R. Delta Dental of Missouri, 465
Jennings, Jonathan R. Delta Dental of South Carolina, 705
Jensen, Barbara Delta Dental of Nebraska, 486
Jeppesen, David Blue Cross of Idaho Health Service, Inc., 252
Jhawar, Sharon K. SCAN Health Plan, 129
Johansson, Ian Health Plan of San Mateo, 98
Johns, Nathan New Mexico Health Connections, 537
Johnson, Baretta Amerigroup Tennessee, 719
Johnson, Bruce, MD Pueblo Health Care, 161
Johnson, Eric H. UnitedHealthcare of Arkansas, 52
Johnson, Jennifer Trinity Health of Idaho, 258
Johnson, Mark Independent Health Medicare Plan, 566
Johnson, Pamela MK Children's Mercy Pediatric Care Network, 461
Johnson, Steven P. Health First Health Plans, 209
Johnson, Steven P. Health First Medicare Plans, 210
Johnson, Steven P., Jr UPMC Susquehanna, 681
Johnson, Thad Oxford Health Plans, 177
Johnson, Thad UnitedHealthcare Community Plan Delaware, 185
Johnson, Thad Neighborhood Health Partnership, 219
Johnson, Thad UnitedHealthcare of Illinois, 283
Johnson, Thad UnitedHealthcare Great Lakes Health Plan, 431
Johnson, William Moda Health Alaska, 14
Johnson, William, MD Moda Health Oregon, 646
Johnson-Mills, Rita UnitedHealthcare of Tennessee, 728
Johnston, Katherine AllCare Health, 637
Johnston, Lori Paramount Elite Medicare Plan, 616
Johnston, Lori Paramount Health Care, 617
Jones, Cathy Aetna Better Health of Kentucky, 335
Jones, David Delta Dental of Oklahoma, 631
Jones, Mary Anne Priority Health, 423
Jones, Mary Anne PriorityHealth Medicare Plans, 424
Jones, Melissa Avesis: Texas, 735
Jones, Michael UnitedHealthcare of Alabama, 10
Jones, Mike Molina Healthcare of Florida, 218
Jones, Nicole Cigna Corporation, 171
Jones, Patty Community Health Plan of Washington, 806
Jones, Rich DakotaCare, 712
Jones, Richard UnitedHealthcare of Idaho, 259
Jones, Richard Essence Healthcare, 467
Jones, Scott Delta Dental of South Dakota, 713
Jordan, Jennifer Aetna Health of Indiana, 284
Joseph Bell, Jill Passport Health Plan, 343

Joyce, Christopher InnovaCare Health, 688
Joyner, J David CVS CareMark, 696
Judy, Steve Primary Health Medical Group, 256
Julian, Marcus Dean Health Plan, 834
Junot, Deborah Coventry Health Care of Louisiana, 348
Jurevic, Jon Delta Dental of Idaho, 253
Jurkovic, Goran Delta Dental of Michigan, 409

K

Kaiser, Kelley C. Samaritan Health Plan Operations, 651
Kalin, Ian eHealthInsurance Services, Inc., 88
Kandalaft, Kevin UnitedHealthcare of Northern California, 136
Kandalaft, Kevin UnitedHealthcare of Southern California, 137
Kane, Brian CompBenefits Corporation, 233
Kane, Brian Humana Health Insurance of Rhode Island, 697
Kane, Brian A. Humana Inc., 341
Kane, Brian Andrew CarePlus Health Plans, 200
Kane, Edward J. Harvard Pilgrim Health Care Maine, 361
Kane, Sean Healthfirst, 562
Kao, John Alignment Health Plan, 57
Kapic, Maja Liberty Dental Plan of New York, 568
Kaplan, Alan Island Group Administration, Inc., 567
Kaplan, Lynn Island Group Administration, Inc., 567
Kapp, Keith Blue Cross and Blue Shield of Kansas, 322
Karl, Nick Peoples Health, 352
Karsten, Wendy Care N' Care, 737
Kasdagly, Dino L.A. Care Health Plan, 106, 107
Kashuba, Sheryl UPMC Health Plan, 680
Kastman, Chris, MD Group Health Cooperative of South Central Wisconsin, 838
Kastner, Rick Blue Cross Blue Shield of Kansas City, 459
Kasuba, Paul, MD Tufts Health Plan, 398
Kasuba, Pual, MD Tufts Health Medicare Plan, 397
Kates, Peter B Univera Healthcare, 581
Katich, Wanda Northeast Georgia Health Partners, 238
Katz, Mitchell, M.D. Health Services Los Angeles County, 99
Kaufman, Philip UnitedHealthcare of Minnesota, 450
Kaufman, Philip UnitedHealthcare of North Dakota, 601
Kaufman, Philip UnitedHealthcare of Puerto Rico, 692
Kaufman, Philip UnitedHealthcare of South Dakota, 716
Kavouras, Michael, Esq. Aetna of Illinois, 261
Kawano, Kie UnitedHealthcare of Hawaii, 250
Kaye, Michel PTPN, 125
Kayne, Jeremy HealthNetwork, 212
Keck, Kim A. Blue Cross & Blue Shield of Rhode Island, 694
Keeley, Larry Envolve Vision, 589
Keeling, Zach Medical Associates, 312
Keen, Marge DentalPlans.com Inc., 204
Kehaly, Pam Blue Cross & Blue Shield of Arizona, 21
Keller, Dixon Humana Health Insurance of Nevada, 501
Kelley, Sharon Gateway Health, 663
Kelly, Mary Jean Healthplex, 563
Kelly, Sarah American HealthCare Group, 657
Kemp, Kirt Partnership HealthPlan of California, 122
Kendall, Dani Concentra, 743
Kenney, Dave CoreSource, 267
Kenny, Becky Blue Cross & Blue Shield of New Mexico, 531

Kessel, Stacy Community Health Plan of Washington, 806
Ketner, Jennifer Cigna Healthcare North Carolina, 585
Khachatourian, Gaguik University HealthCare Alliance, 138
Khamseh, Ladan CalOptima, 67
Kilbreth, Will Community Health Options, 359
Kile, Gregory G. Valley Preferred, 683
Kinder, Deborah Liberty Dental Plan of Texas, 755
Kintu, Emmanuel AlohaCare Advantage Plus, 244
Kirby, Jennifer M. Trinity Health of Delaware, 184
Kirkpatrick, Mercy Leon Medical Centers Health Plan, 215
Kish, John Medical Mutual, 609
Klammer, Thomas P. Landmark Healthplan of California, 109
Kline, Teresa HAP-Health Alliance Plan: Flint, 413
Kline, Teresa Health Alliance Medicare, 415
Kline, Teresa Health Alliance Plan, 416
Kline, Teresa Presbyterian Health Plan, 538
Knight, Jeffrey M. The Health Plan of the Ohio Valley/Mountaineer Region, 623
Knight, Terry VIVA Health, 11
Knox, Mike Aetna Health of Oklahoma, 626
Knutson, Mark UnitedHealthcare of Northern California, 136
Knutson, Mark UnitedHealthcare of Southern California, 137
Kobylowski, Ken AmeriHealth New Jersey, 516
Koch, Tom The Dental Care Plus Group, 622
Koenig, Tere Medical Mutual, 609
Kokkinides, Penelope InnovaCare Health, 688
Kolli, Rama Blue Cross & Blue Shield of Nebraska, 484
Kolodgy, Robert BlueCross BlueShield Association, 263
Kornblatt, Janet SCAN Health Plan, 129
Kornwasser, Laizer CareCentrix, 170
Korth, Susan First Health, 89
Korth, Susan Cofinity, 406
Kotelon, Alexandra Delta Dental of Illinois, 268
Koushik, Srini Magellan Health, 30
Koushik, Srini Magellan Complete Care of Florida, 217
Kovaleski, Kerry Arizona Foundation for Medical Care, 19
Kowal, Nancy Total Health Care, 426
Koziara, Michael PriorityHealth Medicare Plans, 424
Kozik, Sue Blue Cross and Blue Shield of Louisiana, 347
Krajnovich, Dan UnitedHealthcare of Indiana, 306
Krawat, Tony Mercy Clinic Missouri, 473
Krawchuk, Shelley Aetna Health of Louisiana, 346
Krna, Catherine University HealthCare Alliance, 138
Krupinski, Steven J. Capital BlueCross, 660
Krzeminski, Kevin Assurant Employee Benefits Wisconsin, 830
Kudgis, Len Horizon NJ Health, 523
Kujawa, Kevin American Specialty Health, 286
Kunz, Eileen, MPH On Lok Lifeways, 118
Kurpad, Umesh Tufts Health Medicare Plan, 397
Kurpad, Umesh Tufts Health Plan, 398
Kushner, Joshua Oscar Health, 576
Kuss, Vincent J. Trinity Health of New York, 578
Kwan, Dennis Y.C. Hawaii Medical Assurance Association, 246
Kynalis, Paula Empire BlueCross BlueShield, 557

L

Lackner, Maria Care1st Cal MediConnect Plan, 68

M

S

Sade, Nikki ProviDRs Care Network, 332

Saelens, Holly Molina Healthcare of Ohio, 612

Salazar, Arnold Colorado Health Partnerships, 153

Salazar, Deanna Blue Cross & Blue Shield of Arizona, 21

Salmon, Kimberly Fallon Health, 388

Salzwedel, Jack American Family Insurance, 827

Samitt, Craig E. Blue Cross & Blue Shield of Minnesota, 437

Samuels, Michele A. Blue Cross Blue Shield of Michigan, 405

Sanborn, Pam Molina Healthcare of Illinois, 276

Sanchez, Ester M. California Foundation for Medical Care, 66

Sanchez Sierra, Manuel MMM Holdings, 690

Sanders, Henry Group Health Cooperative of South Central Wisconsin, 838

Santangelo, Andreana Blue Cross & Blue Shield of Massachusetts, 386

Saperstein, Arnold MetroPlus Health Plan, 572

Sarkari, Cherag Access Dental Services, 53

Sarma, Satya Care1st Health Plan Arizona, 22

Sarrel, Lloyd CoreSource, 267

Scaturro, Eileen Healthplex, 563

Schaefer, Dr. Joann Blue Cross & Blue Shield of Nebraska, 484

Schafer, Pepper HealthSCOPE Benefits, 48

Schandel, David Florida Health Care Plans, 207

Schechtman, Jay, MD Healthfirst, 562

Schenk, Thomas E., MD BlueCross BlueShield of Western New York, zzz 545

Schenk, Thomas E., MD BlueShield of Northeastern New York, 546

Schindelman, Simeon MagnaCare, 570

Schlosser, Mario Oscar Health, 576

Schmaltz, April Delta Dental of Iowa, 309

Schmidt, Brad Bright Now! Dental, 64

Schmidt, Christopher Healthplex, 563

Schmidt, Colleen Molina Healthcare of New York, 573

Schmidt, Loretta Trinity Health of Indiana, 305

Schmitz, James Care Plus Dental Plans, 831

Schneider-Stucky, Erin Blue Cross Blue Shield of Kansas City, 459

Schoen, Susan Humana Health Insurance of Ohio, 608

Scholl, Gloria J. Amerigroup Iowa, 307

Scholtz, Stacy Mutual of Omaha Health Plans, 492

Schrader, Michael CalOptima, 67

Schramm, Steve Soundpath Health, 814

Schrecengost, Jeff Amerigroup Florida, 193

Schrimsher, Megan VIVA Health, 11

Schrupp, Alison Providence Health Plan, 649

Schubach, Aaron Opticare of Utah, 778

Schubach, Stephen Opticare of Utah, 778

Schultz, Jason Trinity Health of Indiana, 305

Schultz, Rick Aetna Better Health of Kentucky, 335

Schultz, Rick Aetna Health of Kentucky, 336

Schum, Rick Blue Cross & Blue Shield of Wyoming, 854

Schumacher, Dan Oxford Health Plans, 177

Schumacher, Dan UnitedHealthcare Community Plan Delaware, 185

Schumacher, Dan Neighborhood Health Partnership, 219

Schumacher, Dan UnitedHealthcare of Illinois, 283

Schumacher, Dan UnitedHealthcare Great Lakes Health Plan, 431

Schutzen, Ron HealthSun, 213

Schwab, Jeff Dominion Dental Services, 794

Schwaninger, Tom L.A. Care Health Plan, 106, 107

Scono, Thomas E. EPIC Pharmacy Network, 795

Scott, Cory Coventry Health Care of Georgia, 234

Scott, Diana L. Guardian Life Insurance Company of America, 561

Scott, Kirby Delta Dental of South Dakota, 713

Sedgwick, Norman Coventry Health Care of California, 82

Sedita-Igneri, Jessica Care1st Health Plan Arizona, 22

Sedmak, Pamela Molina Healthcare, 115

Sedmak, Pamela Molina Medicaid Solutions, 117

Seereiter, Susan AllCare Health, 637

Segal, David Neighborhood Health Plan, 395

Segars, John Molina Healthcare of South Carolina, 708

Sehring, Bob OSF Healthcare, 278

Seidman, Richard L.A. Care Health Plan, 106, 107

Seifter, Esq., Lowell A. Trinity Health of New York, 578

Serota, Scott P. BlueCross BlueShield Association, 263

Serra, Steve Aetna Health of Tennessee, 718

Servais, Ann Cigna Healthcare New Jersey, 519

Shadle, Bridget Galaxy Health Network, 749

Shafer, Cheryl R., MD Molina Healthcare of South Carolina, 708

Shaffer, Ian, MD Managed Health Network, Inc., 111

Shah, Amit, MD CareOregon Health Plan, 639

Shah, Maria A., MD HealthEZ, 440

Shah, Rupesh Freedom Health, 208

Shah, Sanjiv, MD Fidelis Care, 559

Shames, Cary Sharp Health Plan, 130

Shanahan, Carolyn Delta Dental of Illinois, 268

Shane, Jr, P.J. Galaxy Health Network, 749

Shanley, Will UnitedHealthcare of Colorado, 164

Shannon, Allen Coventry Health & Life Ins. Co. of Tennessee, 723

Shannon, Lee Blue Cross & Blue Shield of Wyoming, 854

Sharbatz, Kim DenteMax, 411

Sharff, Samantha Able Insurance Agency, 507

Sharma, Vibhu Mutual of Omaha Dental Insurance, 491

Sharma, Vibhu Mutual of Omaha Health Plans, 492

Sheehan, Steve Golden West Dental & Vision, 92

Sheehy, Bob Bright Health Alabama, 5

Sheehy, Bob Bright Health Colorado, 150

Shepard, Kim Cigna HealthCare of Arizona, 24

Sheppard, Joel Public Employees Health Program, 780

Shiba, David, MD Stanislaus Foundation for Medical Care, 131

Shin, Amy Health Plan of San Joaquin, 97

Shinto, Richard InnovaCare Health, 688

Shinto, Richard MMM Holdings, 690

Shinto, Richard, MD PMC Medicare Choice, 691

Shipley, Kurt Blue Cross & Blue Shield of New Mexico, 531

Short, Marianna D. UnitedHealth Group, 449

Showalter, Kathryn MedCost, 592

Shumaker, L. Don Superior Dental Care, 621

Sideris, Wendy Careington Solutions, 739

Sigal, Steven J., CPA Health New England, 390

Sigel, Deena Care1st Health Plan Arizona, 22

Signor, Vicki Wellmark Blue Cross & Blue Shield of South Dakota, 717

Silverberg, Brian Superior Vision, 132

Silverman, Wayne, DDS Dominion Dental Services, 794

Simmer, Thomas, MD Blue Care Network of Michigan, 404

Simmer, Thomas L., MD Blue Care Network of Michigan, 403

W

Wachtelhaussen, Bert ConnectiCare, 173

Wada, Takashi Michael, MD CenCal Health, 72

Wagner, John J. Aetna Health of Alaska, 12

Wagner, Melissa DenteMax, 411

Waldron, Neil Rocky Mountain Health Plans, 162

Walker, Jennifer A. Hawaii Medical Service Association, 247

Walsh, Andrea HealthPartners, 441

Walsh, Tim Neighborhood Health Plan, 395

Walter, Dawn Essence Healthcare, 467

Walters, Laurel Rocky Mountain Health Plans, 162

Walton, Carolynn Blue Cross Blue Shield of Michigan, 405

Wang, Pat Healthfirst, 562

Ward, Karen Blue Cross & Blue Shield of Tennessee, 721

Wardena, Tonya Molina Healthcare of Michigan, 420

Warner, Syd Aetna Health of Kansas, 319

Warner, Syd Aetna Health of Wisconsin, 826

Warner, Venus Galaxy Health Network, 749

Waters, Glenn Trinity Health of Florida, 222

Wathen, Cheryl Deaconess Health Plans, 293

Watson, Chris One Call Care Management, 220

Watt, David Anthem Blue Cross & Blue Shield of Indiana, 287

Watts, Brian California Dental Network, 65

Wayne Barker, Robert Cigna Healthcare North Carolina, 585

Weaver, Jois J. Vale-U-Health, 682

Weber, Alissa UnitedHealthcare of Iowa, 316

Wecker, Allan Health Services Los Angeles County, 99

Wedin, Jeff UnitedHealthcare of Mississippi, 456

Weeks, John Delta Dental of Kentucky, 340

Wegleitner, James Avesis: Minnesota, 436

Wegner, Mike Trinity Health of Iowa, 315

Wehr, Ann O., MD, FACP AvMed, 194

Weickardt, Christina Molina Healthcare of Wisconsin, 844

Weidenkopf, Thomas W. Aetna Inc., 166

Weider, Drigan, MD Boulder Valley Individual Practice Association, 149

Weil, Stephanie Crescent Health Solutions, 587

Weinberg, Jonathan Evolent Health, 796

Weinper, Michael PTPN, 125

Weinraub, Helene UPMC Health Plan, 680

Weis, Brian Alliance Regional Health Network, 730

Weiss, Richard Aetna Health of Florida, 192

Welch, Jonathan, MD Medical Center Healthnet Plan, 393

Welch, Jonathan, MD Well Sense Health Plan, 514

Welch, Peter Cigna HealthCare of California, 77

Wells, Greg Blue Cross & Blue Shield of Arizona, 21

Wendling, Mark, MD Valley Preferred, 683

Wendorff, Daniel Trinity Health of Ohio, 624

Wenk, Philip A. Delta Dental of Tennessee, 724

Werksman, Diane Value Behavioral Health of Pennsylvania, 684

Wernicke, Mark Humana Health Insurance of Wisconsin, 841

West, Emily Fallon Health, 388

Westermeier, Stephanie Trinity Health of Idaho, 258

Whaley, Don American Dental Group, 145

Whaley, Kathy American Dental Group, 145

Wheatley, Alan Humana Medicare, 342

Wheeler, Brian Community First Health Plans, 742

Wheeler, Philip Mercy Clinic Missouri, 473

White, Kim Blue Cross Blue Shield of Kansas City, 459

White, Michael Providence Health Plan, 649

White, Robert American Specialty Health, 286

White, Todd Aetna Health of Virginia, 790

White, Todd Aetna Health of West Virginia, 817

White, William C. Humana Health Insurance of Texas, 753

Whitley, Kim R. Samaritan Health Plan Operations, 651

Whitmore, William Anthem Blue Cross & Blue Shield of Maine, 358

Whittle, Brenda Neighborhood Health Plan of Rhode Island, 698

Wichmann, David Neighborhood Health Partnership, 219

Wichmann, David UnitedHealthcare of Illinois, 283

Wichmann, David UnitedHealthcare Great Lakes Health Plan, 431

Wichmann, David S. Oxford Health Plans, 177

Wichmann, David S. UnitedHealth Group, 449

Wilkinson, Jeff Total Dental Administrators, 40

Wilkinson, Scott LifeMap, 644

Wilkosz, Diane Cigna Healthcare Florida, 201

Willett, Linda A. Horizon Blue Cross Blue Shield of New Jersey, 522

Willhoft, David UnitedHealthcare of New York, 580

Williams, Amy Trillium Community Health Plan, 652

Williams, Camille Opticare of Utah, 778

Williams, Clarence Aetna Health of Washington, 803

Williams, David Devon Health Services, 662

Williams, Frank Evolent Health, 796

Williams, Laurie, JD Molina Healthcare of Mississippi, 455

Williams, Lynne Delta Dental of Illinois, 268

Williams, Nessa Jai Medical Systems, 376

Williams-Brinkley, Ruth Kaiser Permanente Northwest, 643

Willis, Andrea D. Blue Cross & Blue Shield of Tennessee, 721

Willoughby, Brenda North Alabama Managed Care Inc, 8

Wilson, Andrew L. Crescent Health Solutions, 587

Wilson, Charlton Mercy Care Plan/Mercy Care Advantage, 32

Wilson, Danette Blue Cross Blue Shield of Kansas City, 459

Wilson, Dennis G. Delta Dental of New Jersey, 521

Wilson, Dora Molina Healthcare of South Carolina, 708

Wilson, Gary Humana Health Insurance of West Virginia, 821

Wilson, Greg Ohio State University Health Plan Inc., 614

Windfeldt, Ty Hometown Health Plan, 500

Wing, Christopher SCAN Health Plan, 129

Wingerter, Arthur G. Univera Healthcare, 581

Winn, Sharon Anthem Blue Cross & Blue Shield of Georgia, 230

Winn, Sharon Blue Cross Blue Shield of Georgia, 231

Winn, MD, Daniel CareFirst BlueCross BlueShield, 370

Winograd, Katharine Presbyterian Medicare Advantage Plans, 539

Winslow, Amy Magellan Rx Management, 31

Winton, Dakasha Blue Cross & Blue Shield of Tennessee, 721

Wise, Greg, MD MediGold, 611

Wissing, Deborah Dentcare Delivery Systems, 553

Wittenstein, Robin D. Denver Health Medical Plan, 156

Woelfert, Charles Humana Health Insurance of Indiana, 297

Wolf, Dale One Call Care Management, 220

Wolgemuth, Sherry Preferred Health Care, 673

Wolk, Anthony L. Universal American Medicare Plans, 582

Wolk, Anthony L. TexanPlus Medicare Advantage HMO, 764

Wong, Van San Francisco Health Plan, 126

Y

Z

Membership Enrollment Index

1,800,000	Wellmark Blue Cross & Blue Shield of South Dakota, 717
1,700,000	Dental Health Alliance, 466
1,700,000	Medica, 444
1,600,000	Medica: North Dakota, 599
1,500,000	Blue Cross & Blue Shield of Arizona, 21
1,500,000	Excellus BlueCross BlueShield, 558
1,500,000	OSF Healthcare, 278
1,500,000	Univera Healthcare, 581
1,326,000	MagnaCare, 570
1,300,000	Blue Cross and Blue Shield of Louisiana, 347
1,100,000	CoreSource, 267
1,018,589	Tufts Health Plan: Rhode Island, 699
1,000,000	CareSource Indiana, 290
1,000,000	CareSource Kentucky, 339
1,000,000	CareSource Ohio, 605
1,000,000	CareSource West Virginia, 818
1,000,000	Delta Dental of Oklahoma, 631
1,000,000	HealthSmart, 751
975,000	CHN PPO, 518
950,000	Blue Cross & Blue Shield of South Carolina, 702
942,000	American Health Care Alliance, 457
900,000	Anthem Blue Cross & Blue Shield of Indiana, 287
857,252	L.A. Care Health Plan, 107
807,000	Blue Care Network of Michigan, 403
800,000	Moda Health Alaska, 14
750,000	Intermountain Healthcare, 776
750,000	Meridian Health Plan, 419
750,000	Meridian Health Plan of Illinois, 275
750,000	QualCare, 527
737,411	Tufts Health Plan, 398
727,000	Horizon NJ Health, 523
717,000	Blue Cross & Blue Shield of Nebraska, 484
700,000	MVP Health Care, 574
670,000	MedCost, 592
650,000	HAP-Health Alliance Plan: Flint, 413
650,000	Health Alliance Plan, 416
625,000	Fidelis Care, 559
615,000	Midlands Choice, 490
614,350	Kaiser Permanente Mid-Atlantic, 377
600,000	Blue Cross & Blue Shield of Oklahoma, 628
600,000	Blue Cross & Blue Shield of Rhode Island, 694
596,220	Priority Health, 423
563,000	Blue Cross of Idaho Health Service, Inc., 252
560,000	Partnership HealthPlan of California, 122
555,405	BlueCross BlueShield of Western New York, 545
540,000	Geisinger Health Plan, 664
518,000	Health Choice LLC, 725
502,000	Behavioral Health Systems, 3
500,000	Aultcare Corporation, 604
500,000	CommunityCare, 630
500,000	HealthSCOPE Benefits, 48
475,000	Trustmark Companies, 281
430,000	Neighborhood Health Plan, 395
430,000	Optima Health Plan, 799
423,244	Baptist Health Services Group, 720
418,000	Health Plan of Nevada, 499

413,795	CalOptima, 67
400,000	CDPHP Medicare Plan, 548
400,000	Preferred Mental Health Management, 330
400,000	Presbyterian Health Plan, 538
390,000	Dental Alternatives Insurance Services, 84
390,000	SVS Vision, 425
383,000	Health Alliance Medicare, 415
380,000	The Health Plan of the Ohio Valley/Mountaineer Region, 623
370,000	Ohio Health Choice, 613
367,000	Blue Cross & Blue Shield of New Mexico, 531
365,000	Independent Health, 565
350,000	CDPHP: Capital District Physicians' Health Plan, 549
345,000	Cigna-HealthSpring, 722
340,000	AvMed, 194
340,000	AvMed Ft. Lauderdale, 195
340,000	AvMed Gainesville, 196
340,000	AvMed Orlando, 197
338,000	Pacific Health Alliance, 121
332,128	MetroPlus Health Plan, 572
330,000	Select Health of South Carolina, 709
326,000	Colorado Health Partnerships, 153
325,000	Mercy Care Plan/Mercy Care Advantage, 32
320,000	Care1st Health Plan Blue Shield of California Promise, 69
316,000	Preferred Network Access, 279
315,440	Western Dental Services, 142
300,000	Community Health Plan of Washington, 806
300,000	Medical Card System (MCS), 689
300,000	The Dental Care Plus Group, 622
275,000	PacificSource Health Plans, 647, 648
265,000	AmeriHealth New Jersey, 516
265,000	AmeriHealth Pennsylvania, 658
263,200	Health Partners Plans, 665
255,494	Health Alliance Medicare, 271
250,000	Araz Group, 384
250,000	Blue Cross & Blue Shield of Montana, 476
250,000	CareOregon Health Plan, 639
250,000	Lakeside Community Healthcare Network, 108
250,000	Santa Clara Family Health Foundations Inc, 127
247,881	Dean Health Plan, 834
240,890	Medical Center Healthnet Plan, 393
236,962	Rocky Mountain Health Plans, 162
210,000	Central California Alliance for Health, 73
210,000	Nova Healthcare Administrators, 575
205,677	Guardian Life Insurance Company of America, 561
205,000	American Postal Workers Union (APWU) Health Plan, 367
205,000	BlueChoice Health Plan of South Carolina, 703
200,000	Care Plus Dental Plans, 831
200,000	Health New England, 390
200,000	Initial Group, 727
200,000	Scott & White Health Plan, 760
193,498	BlueShield of Northeastern New York, 546
190,000	Neighborhood Health Plan of Rhode Island, 698
187,000	Paramount Care of Michigan, 421
187,000	Paramount Elite Medicare Plan, 616
187,000	Paramount Health Care, 617
187,000	Security Health Plan of Wisconsin, 848

185,000	Priority Partners Health Plans, 378	90,000	Quality Plan Administrators, 189
180,000	Blue Cross & Blue Shield of Vermont, 786	90,000	Total Health Care, 426
180,000	First Medical Health Plan, 686	90,000	Unity Health Insurance, 851
177,854	Public Employees Health Program, 780	90,000	VIVA Health, 11
175,000	Arizona Foundation for Medical Care, 19	88,366	MedCost Virginia, 798
175,000	CenCal Health, 72	87,740	Health Plan of San Mateo, 98
175,000	Wisconsin Physician's Service, 852	87,000	First Choice of the Midwest, 714
174,309	Valley Preferred, 683	86,000	University Health Plans, 785
170,000	Passport Health Plan, 343	80,000	Alliance Regional Health Network, 730
155,070	Health Link PPO, 452	80,000	First Choice Health, 477
154,162	Aetna Health of New York, 542	80,000	Group Health Cooperative of South Central Wisconsin, 838
152,000	ProviDRs Care Network, 332	80,000	UniCare West Virginia, 824
150,000	Atlanticare Health Plans, 517	75,000	Group Health Cooperative of Eau Claire, 837
150,000	ChiroCare of Wisconsin, 832	71,000	Asuris Northwest Health, 805
150,000	Landmark Healthplan of California, 109	70,000	AlohaCare, 243
150,000	Nevada Preferred Healthcare Providers, 503	70,000	Martin's Point HealthCare, 362
150,000	Opticare of Utah, 778	68,942	Physicians Health Plan of Mid-Michigan, 422
148,000	Altius Health Plans, 772	68,000	Secure Health PPO Newtork, 239
147,000	UCare, 448	66,000	North Alabama Managed Care Inc, 8
146,000	Community Health Group, 79	63,000	Avera Health Plans, 711
144,000	Medical Mutual Services, 610	60,000	Boulder Valley Individual Practice Association, 149
140,000	Alameda Alliance for Health, 55	60,000	Essence Healthcare, 467
140,000	Contra Costa Health Services, 81	55,000	MediGold, 611
136,472	Baptist Health Plan, 338	55,000	San Francisco Health Plan, 126
134,837	Affinity Health Plan, 543	54,418	Mutual of Omaha Health Plans, 492
134,000	Advance Insurance Company of Kansas, 318	54,000	AllCare Health, 637
130,000	Employers Dental Services, 27	53,000	GHI Medicare Plan, 560
130,000	Golden Dental Plans, 412	53,000	PMC Medicare Choice, 691
130,000	Managed Health Services, 842	52,000	Island Group Administration, Inc., 567
128,272	SCAN Health Plan, 129	52,000	Ohio State University Health Plan Inc., 614
126,000	MMM Holdings, 690	50,000	Care1st Health Plan Arizona, 22
125,000	Capital Health Plan, 198	50,000	Peoples Health, 352
125,000	Managed HealthCare Northwest, 645	50,000	Sanford Health Plan, 314
125,000	Premier Access Insurance/Access Dental, 123	50,000	Vantage Health Plan, 355
123,880	Access Dental Services, 53	49,976	Children's Mercy Pediatric Care Network, 461
120,000	Horizon Health Corporation, 752	49,000	Sharp Health Plan, 130
120,000	Sant, Community Physicians, 128	47,000	Upper Peninsula Health Plan, 433
119,712	Prevea Health Network, 847	45,000	Health Choice of Alabama, 6
118,600	DakotaCare, 712	45,000	Medical Associates, 312
118,000	Network Health Plan of Wisconsin, 845	45,000	Preferred Care Partners, 221
115,000	Health Choice Arizona, 28	44,000	Sterling Insurance, 763
112,000	Physicians Plus Insurance Corporation, 846	42,000	TexanPlus Medicare Advantage HMO, 764
111,000	CarePlus Health Plans, 200	40,000	Crescent Health Solutions, 587
110,000	Community First Health Plans, 742	34,000	Health Tradition, 840
109,000	Health Plan of San Joaquin, 97	33,000	South Central Preferred Health Network, 675
108,000	Neighborhood Health Partnership, 219	32,000	Hometown Health Plan, 500
101,000	UPMC Health Plan, 680	30,000	InStil Health, 707
100,000	Blue Cross & Blue Shield of Wyoming, 854	30,000	Piedmont Community Health Plan, 800
100,000	OhioHealth Group, 615	27,000	Leon Medical Centers Health Plan, 215
97,000	Kern Family Health Care, 105	26,000	SummaCare Medicare Advantage Plan, 620
95,000	Health Partners of Kansas, 326	22,000	Valley Baptist Health Plan, 771
92,000	Western Health Advantage, 143	20,000	Prime Time Health Medicare Plan, 618
90,000	BEST Life and Health Insurance Co., 61	19,000	Quality Health Plans of New York, 577
90,000	Dental Health Services of California, 86	17,000	ConnectCare, 407
90,000	Dental Health Services of Washington, 809	17,000	Primecare Dental Plan, 124
90,000	Gundersen Lutheran Health Plan, 839	17,000	Soundpath Health, 814

16,000 Elderplan, 554	**10,500** Hennepin Health, 442
15,000 Alliant Health Plans, 228	**10,000** Denta-Chek of Maryland, 373
15,000 Denver Health Medical Plan, 156	**6,000** Emi Health, 774
15,000 Seton Healthcare Family, 762	**5,000** Cox Healthplans, 464
14,600 Inter Valley Health Plan, 101	**5,000** Friday Health Plans, 157
14,000 HAP-Health Alliance Plan: Senior Medicare Plan, 414	**5,000** Trilogy Health Insurance, 849
14,000 Vantage Medicare Advantage, 356	**2,375** Vale-U-Health, 682
13,582 Chinese Community Health Plan, 75	**1,000** Heart of America Health Plan, 597
13,000 FirstCarolinaCare, 590	**1,000** On Lok Lifeways, 118
12,000 Medica HealthCare Plans, Inc, 114	**1,000** UTMB HealthCare Systems, 770

Primary Care Physician Index

4,500	CareFirst Blue Cross & Blue Shield of Virginia, 792
4,483	Nevada Preferred Healthcare Providers, 503
4,300	Cigna-HealthSpring, 722
4,300	Health New England, 390
4,200	Universal American Medicare Plans, 582
4,000	Alameda Alliance for Health, 55
4,000	Alameda Medi-Cal Plan, 56
4,000	Baptist Health Services Group, 720
4,000	NovaSys Health, 51
4,000	Prominence Health Plan, 505
4,000	The Health Plan of the Ohio Valley/Mountaineer Region, 623
3,800	Altius Health Plans, 772
3,800	Blue Cross & Blue Shield of Texas, 736
3,780	Phoenix Health Plan, 35
3,700	Trilogy Health Insurance, 849
3,600	Trinity Health, 427
3,555	L.A. Care Health Plan, 107
3,532	Anthem Blue Cross & Blue Shield of Indiana, 287
3,500	AlohaCare, 243
3,500	Aultcare Corporation, 604
3,500	CalOptima, 67
3,500	Emi Health, 774
3,500	Geisinger Health Plan, 664
3,500	PCC Preferred Chiropractic Care, 329
3,500	PTPN, 125
3,500	UniCare West Virginia, 824
3,434	Blue Cross & Blue Shield of South Carolina, 702
3,322	Blue Cross & Blue Shield of New Mexico, 531
3,300	Premera Blue Cross Blue Shield of Alaska, 15
3,250	Ohio State University Health Plan Inc., 614
3,200	Delta Dental of Colorado, 155
3,200	Golden Dental Plans, 412
3,100	Physicians Health Plan of Mid-Michigan, 422
3,000	Health Alliance Medicare, 271
3,000	Medical Center Healthnet Plan, 393
3,000	Parkland Community Health Plan, 759
2,855	Healthplex, 563
2,800	Neighborhood Health Plan, 395
2,691	Aetna Health of New York, 542
2,630	Rocky Mountain Health Plans, 162
2,500	Community Health Plan of Washington, 806
2,490	Blue Cross & Blue Shield of Tennessee, 721
2,300	San Francisco Health Plan, 126
2,000	Access Dental Services, 53
1,923	First Health, 89
1,900	Blue Cross & Blue Shield of Montana, 476
1,900	Crescent Health Solutions, 587
1,900	Paramount Care of Michigan, 421
1,900	Paramount Elite Medicare Plan, 616
1,900	Paramount Health Care, 617
1,900	Preferred Health Care, 673
1,750	University Health Plans, 785
1,700	Chinese Community Health Plan, 75
1,700	Western Dental Services, 142
1,631	Blue Cross of Idaho Health Service, Inc., 252
1,611	Blue Cross & Blue Shield of Arizona, 21

1,602	Prevea Health Network, 847
1,600	Intermountain Healthcare, 776
1,590	Central California Alliance for Health, 73
1,551	Blue Cross & Blue Shield of Oklahoma, 628
1,500	AllCare Health, 637
1,500	Bright Health Alabama, 5
1,500	Dean Health Plan, 834
1,500	Delta Dental of Oklahoma, 631
1,500	Health Link PPO, 452
1,500	Preferred Care Partners, 221
1,400	Affinity Health Plan, 543
1,400	EPIC Pharmacy Network, 795
1,400	Health Choice LLC, 725
1,400	Highmark BCBS West Virginia, 820
1,400	Medica with CHI Health, 488
1,400	Trinity Health of Idaho, 258
1,340	Employers Dental Services, 27
1,282	Neighborhood Health Partnership, 219
1,228	Managed HealthCare Northwest, 645
1,200	Elderplan, 554
1,200	Leon Medical Centers Health Plan, 215
1,200	Sant, Community Physicians, 128
1,161	Inter Valley Health Plan, 101
1,125	Independent Health, 565
1,121	Kaiser Permanente Northern Colorado, 159
1,121	Kaiser Permanente Southern Colorado, 160
1,100	Kaiser Permanente Mid-Atlantic, 377
1,090	UPMC Susquehanna, 681
1,050	MediGold, 611
1,000	Cox Healthplans, 464
1,000	Dental Health Services of California, 86
1,000	Dental Health Services of Washington, 809
1,000	Health Partners of Kansas, 326
1,000	Premier Access Insurance/Access Dental, 38, 123, 504, 779
1,000	Scott & White Health Plan, 760
983	Santa Clara Family Health Foundations Inc, 127
980	First Choice Health, 477, 641, 810
979	Delta Dental of New Mexico, 533
962	Blue Cross and Blue Shield of Louisiana, 347
950	CareOregon Health Plan, 639
950	Secure Health PPO Newtork, 239
908	Unity Health Insurance, 851
900	HAP-Health Alliance Plan: Flint, 413
900	HAP-Health Alliance Plan: Senior Medicare Plan, 414
900	Neighborhood Health Plan of Rhode Island, 698
900	Trinity Health of Connecticut, 178
880	Kaiser Permanente Northwest, 643
850	Gundersen Lutheran Health Plan, 839
825	DakotaCare, 712
800	Allied Pacific IPA, 58
800	Health Tradition, 840
778	Valley Preferred, 683
764	Baptist Health Plan, 338
750	Dentaquest, 387
750	Northeast Georgia Health Partners, 238
700	Mercy Clinic Arkansas, 50

Referral/Specialty Physician Index

2018 Title List

Visit www.GreyHouse.com for Product Information, Table of Contents, and Sample Pages

General Reference

America's College Museums
American Environmental Leaders: From Colonial Times to the Present
Encyclopedia of African-American Writing
Encyclopedia of Constitutional Amendments
Encyclopedia of Human Rights and the United States
Encyclopedia of Invasions & Conquests
Encyclopedia of Prisoners of War & Internment
Encyclopedia of Religion & Law in America
Encyclopedia of Rural America
Encyclopedia of the Continental Congress
Encyclopedia of the United States Cabinet, 1789-2010
Encyclopedia of War Journalism
Encyclopedia of Warrior Peoples & Fighting Groups
The Environmental Debate: A Documentary History
The Evolution Wars: A Guide to the Debates
From Suffrage to the Senate: America's Political Women
Gun Debate: An Encyclopedia of Gun Rights & Gun Control in the U.S.
Opinions throughout History: National Security vs. Civil and Privacy Rights
Opinions throughout History: Immigration
Opinions throughout History: Drug Abuse & Drug Epidemics
Political Corruption in America
Privacy Rights in the Digital Era
The Religious Right: A Reference Handbook
Speakers of the House of Representatives, 1789-2009
This is Who We Were: 1880-1900
This is Who We Were: A Companion to the 1940 Census
This is Who We Were: In the 1900s
This is Who We Were: In the 1910s
This is Who We Were: In the 1920s
This is Who We Were: In the 1940s
This is Who We Were: In the 1950s
This is Who We Were: In the 1960s
This is Who We Were: In the 1970s
This is Who We Were: In the 1980s
This is Who We Were: In the 1990s
This is Who We Were: In the 2000s
U.S. Land & Natural Resource Policy
The Value of a Dollar 1600-1865: Colonial Era to the Civil War
The Value of a Dollar: 1860-2014
Working Americans 1770-1869 Vol. IX: Revolutionary War to the Civil War
Working Americans 1880-1999 Vol. I: The Working Class
Working Americans 1880-1999 Vol. II: The Middle Class
Working Americans 1880-1999 Vol. III: The Upper Class
Working Americans 1880-1999 Vol. IV: Their Children
Working Americans 1880-2015 Vol. V: Americans At War
Working Americans 1880-2005 Vol. VI: Women at Work
Working Americans 1880-2006 Vol. VII: Social Movements
Working Americans 1880-2007 Vol. VIII: Immigrants
Working Americans 1880-2009 Vol. X: Sports & Recreation
Working Americans 1880-2010 Vol. XI: Inventors & Entrepreneurs
Working Americans 1880-2011 Vol. XII: Our History through Music
Working Americans 1880-2012 Vol. XIII: Education & Educators
Working Americans 1880-2016 Vol. XIV: Industry Through the Ages
Working Americans 1880-2017 Vol. XV: Politics & Politicians
World Cultural Leaders of the 20th & 21st Centuries

Education Information

Charter School Movement
Comparative Guide to American Elementary & Secondary Schools
Complete Learning Disabilities Directory
Educators Resource Handbook
Special Education: Policy and Curriculum Development

Health Information

Comparative Guide to American Hospitals
Complete Directory for Pediatric Disorders
Complete Directory for People with Chronic Illness
Complete Directory for People with Disabilities
Complete Mental Health Directory
Diabetes in America: Analysis of an Epidemic
Guide to Health Care Group Purchasing Organizations
Guide to U.S. HMO's & PPO's
Medical Device Market Place
Older Americans Information Directory

Business Information

Complete Television, Radio & Cable Industry Directory
Directory of Business Information Resources
Directory of Mail Order Catalogs
Directory of Venture Capital & Private Equity Firms
Environmental Resource Handbook
Financial Literacy Starter Kit
Food & Beverage Market Place
Grey House Homeland Security Directory
Grey House Performing Arts Directory
Grey House Safety & Security Directory
Hudson's Washington News Media Contacts Directory
New York State Directory
Sports Market Place Directory

Statistics & Demographics

American Tally
America's Top-Rated Cities
America's Top-Rated Smaller Cities
Ancestry & Ethnicity in America
The Asian Databook
Comparative Guide to American Suburbs
The Hispanic Databook
Profiles of America
"Profiles of" Series – State Handbooks
Weather America

Financial Ratings Series

Financial Literacy Basics
TheStreet Ratings' Guide to Bond & Money Market Mutual Funds
TheStreet Ratings' Guide to Common Stocks
TheStreet Ratings' Guide to Exchange-Traded Funds
TheStreet Ratings' Guide to Stock Mutual Funds
TheStreet Ratings' Ultimate Guided Tour of Stock Investing
Weiss Ratings' Consumer Guides
Weiss Ratings' Financial Literary Basic Guides
Weiss Ratings' Guide to Banks
Weiss Ratings' Guide to Credit Unions
Weiss Ratings' Guide to Health Insurers
Weiss Ratings' Guide to Life & Annuity Insurers
Weiss Ratings' Guide to Property & Casualty Insurers

Bowker's Books In Print® Titles

American Book Publishing Record® Annual
American Book Publishing Record® Monthly
Books In Print®
Books In Print® Supplement
Books Out Loud™
Bowker's Complete Video Directory™
Children's Books In Print®
El-Hi Textbooks & Serials In Print®
Forthcoming Books®
Law Books & Serials In Print™
Medical & Health Care Books In Print™
Publishers, Distributors & Wholesalers of the US™
Subject Guide to Books In Print®
Subject Guide to Children's Books In Print®

Canadian General Reference

Associations Canada
Canadian Almanac & Directory
Canadian Environmental Resource Guide
Canadian Parliamentary Guide
Canadian Venture Capital & Private Equity Firms
Canadian Who's Who
Financial Post Directory of Directors
Financial Services Canada
Governments Canada
Health Guide Canada
The History of Canada
Libraries Canada
Major Canadian Cities

Grey House Publishing | Salem Press | H.W. Wilson | 4919 Route, 22 PO Box 56, Amenia NY 12501-0056

2018 Title List

Visit www.SalemPress.com for Product Information, Table of Contents, and Sample Pages

Science, Careers & Mathematics

Ancient Creatures
Applied Science
Applied Science: Engineering & Mathematics
Applied Science: Science & Medicine
Applied Science: Technology
Biomes and Ecosystems
Careers in the Arts: Fine, Performing & Visual
Careers in Building Construction
Careers in Business
Careers in Chemistry
Careers in Communications & Media
Careers in Environment & Conservation
Careers in Financial Services
Careers in Green Energy
Careers in Healthcare
Careers in Hospitality & Tourism
Careers in Human Services
Careers in Law, Criminal Justice & Emergency Services
Careers in Manufacturing
Careers in Outdoor Jobs
Careers in Overseas Jobs
Careers in Physics
Careers in Sales, Insurance & Real Estate
Careers in Science & Engineering
Careers in Sports & Fitness
Careers in Social Media
Careers in Sports Medicine & Training
Careers in Technology Services & Repair
Computer Technology Innovators
Contemporary Biographies in Business
Contemporary Biographies in Chemistry
Contemporary Biographies in Communications & Media
Contemporary Biographies in Environment & Conservation
Contemporary Biographies in Healthcare
Contemporary Biographies in Hospitality & Tourism
Contemporary Biographies in Law & Criminal Justice
Contemporary Biographies in Physics
Earth Science
Earth Science: Earth Materials & Resources
Earth Science: Earth's Surface and History
Earth Science: Physics & Chemistry of the Earth
Earth Science: Weather, Water & Atmosphere
Encyclopedia of Energy
Encyclopedia of Environmental Issues
Encyclopedia of Environmental Issues: Atmosphere and Air Pollution
Encyclopedia of Environmental Issues: Ecology and Ecosystems
Encyclopedia of Environmental Issues: Energy and Energy Use
Encyclopedia of Environmental Issues: Policy and Activism
Encyclopedia of Environmental Issues: Preservation/Wilderness Issues
Encyclopedia of Environmental Issues: Water and Water Pollution
Encyclopedia of Global Resources
Encyclopedia of Global Warming
Encyclopedia of Mathematics & Society
Encyclopedia of Mathematics & Society: Engineering, Tech, Medicine
Encyclopedia of Mathematics & Society: Great Mathematicians
Encyclopedia of Mathematics & Society: Math & Social Sciences
Encyclopedia of Mathematics & Society: Math Development/Concepts
Encyclopedia of Mathematics & Society: Math in Culture & Society
Encyclopedia of Mathematics & Society: Space, Science, Environment
Encyclopedia of the Ancient World
Forensic Science
Geography Basics
Internet Innovators
Inventions and Inventors
Magill's Encyclopedia of Science: Animal Life
Magill's Encyclopedia of Science: Plant life
Notable Natural Disasters
Principles of Artificial Intelligence & Robotics
Principles of Astronomy
Principles of Biology
Principles of Biotechnology
Principles of Chemistry
Principles of Climatology
Principles of Physical Science
Principles of Physics
Principles of Programming & Coding
Principles of Research Methods
Principles of Sustainability
Science and Scientists
Solar System
Solar System: Great Astronomers
Solar System: Study of the Universe
Solar System: The Inner Planets
Solar System: The Moon and Other Small Bodies
Solar System: The Outer Planets
Solar System: The Sun and Other Stars
World Geography

Literature

American Ethnic Writers
Classics of Science Fiction & Fantasy Literature
Critical Approaches: Feminist
Critical Approaches: Multicultural
Critical Approaches: Moral
Critical Approaches: Psychological
Critical Insights: Authors
Critical Insights: Film
Critical Insights: Literary Collection Bundles
Critical Insights: Themes
Critical Insights: Works
Critical Survey of American Literature
Critical Survey of Drama
Critical Survey of Graphic Novels: Heroes & Super Heroes
Critical Survey of Graphic Novels: History, Theme & Technique
Critical Survey of Graphic Novels: Independents/Underground Classics
Critical Survey of Graphic Novels: Manga
Critical Survey of Long Fiction
Critical Survey of Mystery & Detective Fiction
Critical Survey of Mythology and Folklore: Heroes and Heroines
Critical Survey of Mythology and Folklore: Love, Sexuality & Desire
Critical Survey of Mythology and Folklore: World Mythology
Critical Survey of Novels into Film
Critical Survey of Poetry
Critical Survey of Poetry: American Poets
Critical Survey of Poetry: British, Irish & Commonwealth Poets
Critical Survey of Poetry: Cumulative Index
Critical Survey of Poetry: European Poets
Critical Survey of Poetry: Topical Essays
Critical Survey of Poetry: World Poets
Critical Survey of Science Fiction & Fantasy
Critical Survey of Shakespeare's Plays
Critical Survey of Shakespeare's Sonnets
Critical Survey of Short Fiction
Critical Survey of Short Fiction: American Writers
Critical Survey of Short Fiction: British, Irish, Commonwealth Writers
Critical Survey of Short Fiction: Cumulative Index
Critical Survey of Short Fiction: European Writers
Critical Survey of Short Fiction: Topical Essays
Critical Survey of Short Fiction: World Writers
Critical Survey of World Literature
Critical Survey of Young Adult Literature
Cyclopedia of Literary Characters
Cyclopedia of Literary Places
Holocaust Literature
Introduction to Literary Context: American Poetry of the 20th Century
Introduction to Literary Context: American Post-Modernist Novels
Introduction to Literary Context: American Short Fiction
Introduction to Literary Context: English Literature
Introduction to Literary Context: Plays
Introduction to Literary Context: World Literature
Magill's Literary Annual 2018
Masterplots
Masterplots II: African American Literature
Masterplots II: American Fiction Series
Masterplots II: British & Commonwealth Fiction Series
Masterplots II: Christian Literature
Masterplots II: Drama Series
Masterplots II: Juvenile & Young Adult Literature, Supplement
Masterplots II: Nonfiction Series
Masterplots II: Poetry Series
Masterplots II: Short Story Series
Masterplots II: Women's Literature Series
Notable African American Writers
Notable American Novelists
Notable Playwrights
Notable Poets
Recommended Reading: 600 Classics Reviewed
Short Story Writers

Grey House Publishing | Salem Press | H.W. Wilson | 4919 Route, 22 PO Box 56, Amenia NY 12501-0056

History and Social Science

The 2000s in America
50 States
African American History
Agriculture in History
American First Ladies
American Heroes
American Indian Culture
American Indian History
American Indian Tribes
American Presidents
American Villains
America's Historic Sites
Ancient Greece
The Bill of Rights
The Civil Rights Movement
The Cold War
Countries, Peoples & Cultures
Countries, Peoples & Cultures: Central & South America
Countries, Peoples & Cultures: Central, South & Southeast Asia
Countries, Peoples & Cultures: East & South Africa
Countries, Peoples & Cultures: East Asia & the Pacific
Countries, Peoples & Cultures: Eastern Europe
Countries, Peoples & Cultures: Middle East & North Africa
Countries, Peoples & Cultures: North America & the Caribbean
Countries, Peoples & Cultures: West & Central Africa
Countries, Peoples & Cultures: Western Europe
Defining Documents: American Revolution
Defining Documents: American West
Defining Documents: Ancient World
Defining Documents: Asia
Defining Documents: Civil Rights
Defining Documents: Civil War
Defining Documents: Court Cases
Defining Documents: Dissent & Protest
Defining Documents: Emergence of Modern America
Defining Documents: Exploration & Colonial America
Defining Documents: Immigration & Immigrant Communities
Defining Documents: LGBTQ
Defining Documents: Manifest Destiny
Defining Documents: Middle Ages
Defining Documents: Middle East
Defining Documents: Nationalism & Populism
Defining Documents: Native Americans
Defining Documents: Political Campaigns, Candidates & Discourse
Defining Documents: Postwar 1940s
Defining Documents: Reconstruction
Defining Documents: Renaissance & Early Modern Era
Defining Documents: Secrets, Leaks & Scandals
Defining Documents: 1920s
Defining Documents: 1930s
Defining Documents: 1950s
Defining Documents: 1960s
Defining Documents: 1970s
Defining Documents: The 17th Century
Defining Documents: The 18th Century
Defining Documents: The 19th Century
Defining Documents: The 20th Century: 1900-1950
Defining Documents: Vietnam War
Defining Documents: Women
Defining Documents: World War I
Defining Documents: World War II
Education Today
The Eighties in America
Encyclopedia of American Immigration
Encyclopedia of Flight
Encyclopedia of the Ancient World
Fashion Innovators
The Fifties in America
The Forties in America
Great Athletes
Great Athletes: Baseball
Great Athletes: Basketball
Great Athletes: Boxing & Soccer
Great Athletes: Cumulative Index
Great Athletes: Football
Great Athletes: Golf & Tennis
Great Athletes: Olympics

Great Athletes: Racing & Individual Sports
Great Contemporary Athletes
Great Events from History: 17th Century
Great Events from History: 18th Century
Great Events from History: 19th Century
Great Events from History: 20th Century (1901-1940)
Great Events from History: 20th Century (1941-1970)
Great Events from History: 20th Century (1971-2000)
Great Events from History: 21st Century (2000-2016)
Great Events from History: African American History
Great Events from History: Cumulative Indexes
Great Events from History: LGBTG
Great Events from History: Middle Ages
Great Events from History: Secrets, Leaks & Scandals
Great Events from History: Renaissance & Early Modern Era
Great Lives from History: 17th Century
Great Lives from History: 18th Century
Great Lives from History: 19th Century
Great Lives from History: 20th Century
Great Lives from History: 21st Century (2000-2017)
Great Lives from History: American Women
Great Lives from History: Ancient World
Great Lives from History: Asian & Pacific Islander Americans
Great Lives from History: Cumulative Indexes
Great Lives from History: Incredibly Wealthy
Great Lives from History: Inventors & Inventions
Great Lives from History: Jewish Americans
Great Lives from History: Latinos
Great Lives from History: Notorious Lives
Great Lives from History: Renaissance & Early Modern Era
Great Lives from History: Scientists & Science
Historical Encyclopedia of American Business
Issues in U.S. Immigration
Magill's Guide to Military History
Milestone Documents in African American History
Milestone Documents in American History
Milestone Documents in World History
Milestone Documents of American Leaders
Milestone Documents of World Religions
Music Innovators
Musicians & Composers 20th Century
The Nineties in America
The Seventies in America
The Sixties in America
Sociology Today
Survey of American Industry and Careers
The Thirties in America
The Twenties in America
United States at War
U.S. Court Cases
U.S. Government Leaders
U.S. Laws, Acts, and Treaties
U.S. Legal System
U.S. Supreme Court
Weapons and Warfare
World Conflicts: Asia and the Middle East

Health

Addictions & Substance Abuse
Adolescent Health & Wellness
Cancer
Complementary & Alternative Medicine
Community & Family Health
Genetics & Inherited Conditions
Health Issues
Infectious Diseases & Conditions
Magill's Medical Guide
Nutrition
Nursing
Psychology & Behavioral Health
Psychology Basics

Grey House Publishing | **Salem Press** | **H.W. Wilson** | 4919 Route, 22 PO Box 56, Amenia NY 12501-0056

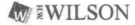
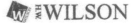

2018 Title List

Visit www.HWWilsonInPrint.com for Product Information, Table of Contents and Sample Pages

Current Biography
Current Biography Cumulative Index 1946-2013
Current Biography Monthly Magazine
Current Biography Yearbook: 2003
Current Biography Yearbook: 2004
Current Biography Yearbook: 2005
Current Biography Yearbook: 2006
Current Biography Yearbook: 2007
Current Biography Yearbook: 2008
Current Biography Yearbook: 2009
Current Biography Yearbook: 2010
Current Biography Yearbook: 2011
Current Biography Yearbook: 2012
Current Biography Yearbook: 2013
Current Biography Yearbook: 2014
Current Biography Yearbook: 2015
Current Biography Yearbook: 2016
Current Biography Yearbook: 2017

Core Collections
Children's Core Collection
Fiction Core Collection
Graphic Novels Core Collection
Middle & Junior High School Core
Public Library Core Collection: Nonfiction
Senior High Core Collection
Young Adult Fiction Core Collection

The Reference Shelf
Aging in America
Alternative Facts: Post Truth & the Information War
The American Dream
American Military Presence Overseas
The Arab Spring
Artificial Intelligence
The Brain
The Business of Food
Campaign Trends & Election Law
Conspiracy Theories
The Digital Age
Dinosaurs
Embracing New Paradigms in Education
Faith & Science
Families: Traditional and New Structures
The Future of U.S. Economic Relations: Mexico, Cuba, and Venezuela
Global Climate Change
Graphic Novels and Comic Books
Guns in America
Immigration
Immigration in the U.S.
Internet Abuses & Privacy Rights
Internet Safety
LGBTQ in the 21st Century
Marijuana Reform
The News and its Future
The Paranormal
Politics of the Ocean
Prescription Drug Abuse
Racial Tension in a "Postracial" Age
Reality Television
Representative American Speeches: 2008-2009
Representative American Speeches: 2009-2010
Representative American Speeches: 2010-2011
Representative American Speeches: 2011-2012
Representative American Speeches: 2012-2013
Representative American Speeches: 2013-2014
Representative American Speeches: 2014-2015
Representative American Speeches: 2015-2016
Representative American Speeches: 2016-2017
Representative American Speeches: 2017-2018
Rethinking Work
Revisiting Gender
Robotics
Russia
Social Networking
Social Services for the Poor
South China Seas Conflict
Space Exploration & Development
Sports in America

The Supreme Court
The Transformation of American Cities
U.S. Infrastructure
U.S. National Debate Topic: Educational Reform
U.S. National Debate Topic: Surveillance
U.S. National Debate Topic: The Ocean
U.S. National Debate Topic: Transportation Infrastructure
Whistleblowers

Readers' Guide
Abridged Readers' Guide to Periodical Literature
Readers' Guide to Periodical Literature

Indexes
Index to Legal Periodicals & Books
Short Story Index
Book Review Digest

Sears List
Sears List of Subject Headings
Sears: Lista de Encabezamientos de Materia

Facts About Series
Facts About American Immigration
Facts About China
Facts About the 20th Century
Facts About the Presidents
Facts About the World's Languages

Nobel Prize Winners
Nobel Prize Winners: 1901-1986
Nobel Prize Winners: 1987-1991
Nobel Prize Winners: 1992-1996
Nobel Prize Winners: 1997-2001

World Authors
World Authors: 1995-2000
World Authors: 2000-2005

Famous First Facts
Famous First Facts
Famous First Facts About American Politics
Famous First Facts About Sports
Famous First Facts About the Environment
Famous First Facts: International Edition

American Book of Days
The American Book of Days
The International Book of Days

Monographs
American Reformers
The Barnhart Dictionary of Etymology
Celebrate the World
Guide to the Ancient World
Indexing from A to Z
Nobel Prize Winners
The Poetry Break
Radical Change: Books for Youth in a Digital Age
Speeches of American Presidents

Wilson Chronology
Wilson Chronology of Asia and the Pacific
Wilson Chronology of Human Rights
Wilson Chronology of Ideas
Wilson Chronology of the Arts
Wilson Chronology of the World's Religions
Wilson Chronology of Women's Achievements

Grey House Publishing | Salem Press | H.W. Wilson | 4919 Route, 22 PO Box 56, Amenia NY 12501-0056